Prof.Dr.med.J.Flammer

D1700170

Prof.Dr.med.J.Flammer

Retinal Diseases

Retinal Diseases
Biomedical Foundations and Clinical Management

Edited by
Mark O. M. Tso, M.D.

Professor of Ophthalmology
Director, Macula Clinic
Director, Georgiana Theobald Eye Pathology Laboratory
Eye and Ear Infirmary
University of Illinois
College of Medicine at Chicago,
Chicago, Illinois

With 31 Contributors

J. B. Lippincott Company   *Philadelphia*
London   Mexico City   New York
St. Louis   São Paulo   Sydney

Sponsoring Editor: Delois Patterson
Indexer: Tony Greenberg
Design Coordinator: Caren Erlichman
Production Manager: Carol A. Florence
Production Coordinator: Kathryn Rule
Compositor: Progressive Typographers
Printer/Binder: Halliday Lithograph

6 5 4 3 2 1

Library of Congress Cataloging in Publication Data

Retinal diseases.

Based on the International Symposium on the Retina: Clinical and Basic Aspects, held in conjunction with the congress and
Scientific Meeting of the Chinese Medical Association in 1983
in Taipei, Taiwan, Republic of China; cosponsored by the Uni-
versity of Illinois at Chicago and others.
Both the 1981 and the 1983 meetings of the Chinese Medical
Association are called the 12th.
Includes bibliographies and index.
1. Retina—Diseases—Congresses. I. Tso, Mark
O. M. II. International Symposium on the Retina: Clinical
and Basic Aspects (1983: Taipei, Taiwan) III. Chung-hua i
hsüeh hui (China: Republic), Hui yüan ta hui (1983: Taipei,
Taiwan) IV. University of Illinois at Chicago. [DNLM: 1.
Retina—physiopathology—congresses. 2. Retinal Diseases—
diagnosis—congresses. 3. Retinal Diseases—therapy—
congresses.
WW 270 R438 1983]
RE551.R48 1988   617.7′3   87-31207
ISBN 0-397-50661-9

The authors and publisher have exerted every effort to ensure
that drug selection and dosage set forth in this text are in accord
with current recommendations and practice at the time of publication. However, in view of ongoing research, changes in government regulations, and the constant flow of information relating to drug therapy and drug reactions, the reader is urged to
check the package insert for each drug for any change in indications and dosage and for added warnings and precautions. This
is particularly important when the recommended agent is a new
or infrequently employed drug.

Contributors

Richard L. Abbott, M.D.
Consultant, Corneal and External Diseases
Department of Ophthalmology
Pacific Presbyterian Medical Center
San Francisco, California

Richard A. Alvarez, B.S.
Research Instructor
Baylor College of Medicine
Houston, Texas

Gustavo D. Aguirre, V.M.D.
Professor of Ophthalmology
School of Veterinary Medicine
University of Pennsylvania;
Scheie Eye Institute;
Director, Inherited Eye Disease Studies Unit
Veterinary Hospital
University of Pennsylvania
Philadelphia, Pennsylvania

Paul A. Blacharski, M.D.
Director, Vitreoretinal Service
Department of Ophthalmology
Naval Hospital
San Diego, California

Mark S. Blumenkranz, M.D.
Associate Professor of Ophthalmology
Chief, Vitreoretinal Surgery
Kresge Eye Institute
Wayne State University

School of Medicine;
Adjunct Associate Professor
Eye Research Institute of Oakland University
Detroit, Michigan

Dean Bok, Ph.D.
Professor of Anatomy
Dolly Green Professor of Ophthalmology
University of California
School of Medicine
Los Angeles, California

C. David Bridges, Ph.D., D.Sc.
Professor of Ophthalmology and Biochemistry
Baylor College of Medicine
Houston, Texas

Gerald J. Chader, Ph.D.
Chief, Laboratory of Retinal Cell and
  Molecular Biology
National Eye Institute
National Institutes of Health
Bethesda, Maryland

Stanley Chang, M.D.
Associate Professor of Clinical Ophthalmology
Cornell University Medical College;
Associate Attending Physician of
  Ophthalmology
New York Hospital
New York, New York

D. Jackson Coleman, M.D.
Chairman, Department of Ophthalmology
John Milton McLean Professor of
Ophthalmology
Cornell University Medical College
New York, New York

J. Terry Ernest, M.D., Ph.D.
Professor and Chairman
Department of Ophthalmology and Visual
Science
Michael Reese/University of Chicago School
of Medicine
Chicago, Illinois

Shao-Ling Fong, Ph.D.
Research Assistant Professor of Ophthalmology
Baylor College of Medicine
Houston, Texas

Robert N. Frank, M.D.
Professor of Ophthalmology
Wayne State University School of Medicine
Detroit, Michigan

Wayne E. Fung, M.D.
Consultant, Vitreoretinal Diseases
Pacific Presbyterian Medical Center
San Francisco, California

Federico Gonzalez-Fernandez, M.D.,
Ph.D.
Department of Pathology
University of Virginia School of Medicine
Charlottesville, Virginia

Michael K. Hartzer, Ph.D.
Visiting Assistant Professor of Ophthalmology
Eye Research Institute of Oakland University
Detroit, Michigan

Lee M. Jampol, M.D.
Professor and Chairman
Department of Ophthalmology
Northwestern University;
Chief of Ophthalmology
Northwestern Memorial Hospital
Chicago, Illinois

Henry J. Kaplan, M.D.
Professor of Ophthalmology
Director of Research
Emory University Medical School
Atlanta, Georgia

Dominic Man-Kit Lam, Ph.D.
Professor of Ophthalmology
Director, The Center for Biotechnology
Baylor College of Medicine
Houston, Texas

Charles Chia-Lee Lin, M.D.
Associate Professor of Ophthalmology
National Yang-Ming Medical College;
Section Chief of General Ophthalmology
Veterans General Hospital
Taipei, Taiwan
Republic of China

Gregory I. Liou, Ph.D.
Research Assistant Professor of Ophthalmology
Baylor College of Medicine
Houston, Texas

Jorn-Hon Liu, M.D.
Associate Professor of Ophthalmology
National Yang-Ming Medical College;
Chairman, Department of Ophthalmology
Veterans General Hospital
Taipei, Taiwan
Republic of China

Frederic L. Lizzi, Sc.D.
Research Director for Biomedical Engineering
Riverside Research Institute
New York, New York

David A. Newsome, M.D.
Professor of Ophthalmology
Louisiana State University School of Medicine;
Director, Clinical Research in Retinal
Dystrophies and Degenerations
Louisiana State University Eye Center
New Orleans, Louisiana

Somes Sanyal, Ph.D.
Assistant Professor of Anatomy
Erasmus University
Rotterdam, The Netherlands

Koichi Shimizu, M.D., Ph.D.
Professor and Chairman of Ophthalmology
Gunma University School of Medicine
Maebashi, Japan

Roy H. Steinberg, M.D., Ph.D.
Professor of Physiology and Ophthalmology
University of California School of Medicine
San Francisco, California

Wu-fu Tsai, M.D.
Professor of Ophthalmology
National Cheng Kong University;
Chief, Department of Ophthalmology
National Cheng Kong University Hospital
Taipei, Taiwan
Republic of China

Mark O. M. Tso, M.D.
Professor of Ophthalmology
Director, Macula Clinic

Director, Georgiana Theobald Eye Pathology
 Laboratory
Eye and Ear Infirmary
University of Illinois College of Medicine at
 Chicago
Chicago, Illinois

Liang-yen Wen, M.D.
Associate Professor and Chairman
Department of Ophthalmology
National Defense Medical Center;
Chief, Department of Ophthalmology
Tri-Service General Hospital
Taipei, Taiwan
Republic of China

Samuel M. Wu, Ph.D.
Assistant Professor of Ophthalmology
Baylor College of Medicine
Houston, Texas

Foreword

Like any good educational endeavor, this diverse and interesting book has its eye on the future. Awareness of its content will assist the reader in staying current with evolving ideas. Of course, knowledge of the past is essential if a clinician or scientist is to avoid intellectual or even pragmatic pitfalls. But an informed physician or investigator looks astern primarily to plan progress at the forefront. Modern ophthalmic curricula and other educational techniques should not only teach the resident-in-training and the practitioner those aspects of past and current knowledge that are valuable, but, more importantly, should also inculcate the techniques of self-education. Hopefully, re-education will occur continuously as ideas and techniques inexorably change. Indeed, they change over remarkably short periods of time. Especially in the fields of retinal and vitreous research, diagnosis, and therapy, it has not been unusual to see major tides of favored theories and techniques ebb and flow over intervals as short as 5 to 10 years.

How, then, does the retinal specialist (physiologist, surgeon, biochemist, or laser therapist, to name but a few of the specialists addressed in this book) not only stay abreast of knowledge but also prepare for the future? Active participation in retinal research or therapy, attendance at avant garde symposia, and assiduous study of the current literature are all essential. Another technique is to read compilations provided by highly specialized experts, depending upon their and their editor's sets of priorities and perspectives for inclusion and exclusion of specific bodies of knowledge. Dr. Tso's approach is that of an enthusiastic and erudite proselytizer. He and his distinguished colleagues are committed to their work, have contributed enormously to our current state of awareness, and generously want to share their knowledge and enjoyment of their specialized fields. Moreover, there is the implied wish to recruit acolytes and other experts into related efforts.

Dr. Tso places responsibilities where they belong; namely, on the reader. If you are sufficiently excited by some of these chapters, engage yourself in this work, either to confirm or refute an older idea or to develop an innovative one. If you are bemused by some of this material, think, discuss, and read some more, both in this book and elsewhere. If your horizons are expanded by one or another of these chapters, as surely most of ours will be, look to the future, standing securely on a massive base of information (some of which, to be sure, will shift a little over time), but be prepared to add to this solid intellectual edifice by personal contributions to the processes of creating and learning.

Morton F. Goldberg, M.D.
Eye and Ear Infirmary
University of Illinois
College of Medicine at Chicago

Preface

The retina is a portion of the central nervous system that is highly modified in structure, physiology, and biochemistry for the specialized function of visual perception. In the past 20 years, there has been an explosion of new information on the morphologic, physiologic, biochemical, immunologic, and pathologic processes of the retina at the cellular level associated with an increasing understanding of clinical diagnosis and therapy of retinal diseases. *Retinal Diseases: Biomedical Foundations and Clinical Management* attempts to summarize this body of new information so as to lay a firm foundation for its readers to seek new avenues for diagnosis and treatment of retinal diseases.

In this age of high technology, specialization has isolated experts of different disciplines in their own fields. The morphologist, physiologist, biochemist, pathologist, cell biologist, medical retina specialist, and retina surgeon do not have a common forum to discuss their work and to develop cross-fertilization of their expertise. The symposium that led to the publication of this book was developed to bring basic scientists and clinicians together for mutual education and exchange of information. Each of the clinicians and scientists who participated in the symposium and has authored a chapter in this book has attempted to outline new information in his field in relatively simple language that may be understood by those outside the subspecialty. Each chapter is written by specialists who have developed a passion for their subjects, and many have initiated the original investigations in their fields. In the world of medical literature, some copy, some compile, some edit, and others create. Each of these chapters has been created, and each shines with the style and originality of its authors.

This book was written for ophthalmologists who are interested in the basic biomedical information that led to clinical progress and for basic scientists who are interested in the various experiments that nature has performed in the human eye in the manifestation of disease processes. It is my hope that both basic scientists and clinicians may be stimulated by the new information in this book to plunge into a search for new answers in pathogenetic mechanisms, diagnosis, and therapy of retinal diseases in the 1980s and beyond.

Mark O. M. Tso

Acknowledgments

The International Symposium on the Retina: Clinical and Basic Aspects was held in conjunction with the Congress and Scientific Meeting of the Chinese Medical Association in the summer of 1983 in Taipei, Taiwan, Republic of China. It was cosponsored by the University of Illinois; the Chinese Medical Association; the Ophthalmological Society of the Republic of China; the Veterans' General Hospital, Taipei; the National Taiwan University; the Coordination Council for North American Affairs; and the Department of Health, Executive Yuan, of the Republic of China. I am deeply grateful for the leadership provided by Stanley O. Ikenberry, Ph.D., President, University of Illinois; Chi-Shuen Tsou, M.D., President of the Chinese Medical Association; Ho-Ming Lin, M.D., Professor of Ophthalmology, National Yang-Ming Medical College, Taiwan; Jorn-Hon Liu, M.D., Chief, Department of Ophthalmology, Veterans General Hospital, Taipei; and Chen-Wu Chen, M.D., President, Ophthalmological Society, Republic of China, for the meeting arrangements. Morton F. Goldberg, M.D., Eye and Ear Infirmary, Professor and Head of the Department of Ophthalmology, University of Illinois College of Medicine at Chicago provided me with an academic environment in which to pursue the project. Roberta O'Benar assisted me with the editing of these chapters. Delois Patterson of J.B. Lippincott Company patiently provided assistance with the publication details. I also would like to thank my wife, Petrina, and my children, Michael and Veleda, for their warm support at home during the time I spent in the organization of the symposium and the publication of this book.

Contents

1

Retinal Pigment Epithelium – Photoreceptor Complex

1

Structure and Function of the Retinal Pigment Epithelium–Photoreceptor Complex

Dean Bok

The retinal photoreceptors and pigment epithelium are highly specialized, polarized cells that lie adjacent to one another and interact in unique fashion. The photoreceptors are represented by two general cell types, rods and cones. They are capable of transducing light into electrochemical signals by virtue of their photopigments, which are present in high concentration (up to 10^9/cell in the rods of some lower vertebrates such as the leopard frog, *Rana pipiens*). Rods are more sensitive than cones and show measurable responses to relatively low light conditions; cones are less sensitive and therefore require higher levels of illumination.[83] Transduction of light by rods and cones into electrochemical signals is accomplished through a complex series of interactions among photons, the visual pigments that form a structural part of photoreceptor membranes, other phototransduction enzymes, cyclic nucleotides, and ions.[25,26,96,97,107,128,129,139,166,167,232,262] The photoreceptors exist in a state of relative depolarization in the dark,[243] where their neurotransmitters are released at a higher rate than in the light.[217,225,226] Light hyperpolarizes the cells and causes a decrease in transmitter release. The outer segments of the rods and cones, which contain the light-sensitive membranes and in which light trapping and transduction occur, are continually renewed and thereby kept young through incessant production of new photopigments, enzymes, and other structural components.[263,268,272] This synthesis takes place within the inner segment,[109,199,201,263,273] the part of the cell that lies adjacent to the outer segment and is connected to it by a modified cilium.[230] Components produced within the inner segment are then transported to the outer segment, where they are assembled into the plasma membrane, discs, and cytoplasmic components of that highly ordered organelle.[171,263,273]

The retinal pigment epithelium (RPE) is a monolayer of cells strategically situated between the choroidal blood supply and the photoreceptors. The RPE serves as a barrier between the choroidal circulation and the photoreceptors and, by virtue of this, regulates the transport of metabolites to and from the photorecep-

This research is supported by USPHS grants EY00444 and EY00331. The author was the Research to Prevent Blindness, Inc., William and Mary Greve International Research Scholar during 1982 and is currently Dolly Green Professor of Ophthalmology and Anatomy at the University of California at Los Angeles. The technical assistance of Marcia Lloyd, Caryl Lightfoot, and Orna Yaron is gratefully acknowledged, as is the photographic work by Alice Van Dyke. The author wishes to thank Ethel Mason for typing the manuscript.

tors.[65,68,206] It also plays a role in the generation of forces that cause the neural retina to adhere to the eye wall.[73,171,180,274] Owing to its melanin granules, the RPE protects the photoreceptors from light scatter and damaging levels of radiation. Finally, on a regular basis, the RPE phagocytizes and digests rod and cone outer-segment discs that are shed into the subretinal space as part of the photoreceptor renewal process.[134,272] Much of the information on photoreceptor structure and function has been gathered during the past two decades. It is the purpose of this chapter to give an overview of significant discoveries during this important period and to describe some very recent findings with respect to photoreceptor RPE interactions, namely the transport and utilization of retinol (vitamin A) and some of its derivatives (retinoids) by proteins that are found both inside and outside these two cell types.

PHOTORECEPTOR STRUCTURE AND FUNCTION

As was mentioned above, photoreceptors are highly polarized cells. Their component parts can be divided into several compartments,[62] each of which is highly specialized for the performance of its function (Fig. 1-1). They include the light-sensitive outer segment, the connecting cilium, the inner segment, the cell nucleus, and the synaptic terminal. With the exception of the nucleus, about which there is less to say, each of these cell compartments will be discussed in some detail.

Outer Segment

The light-sensitive outer segment is so specialized for the absorption of photons and phototransduction that all cell organelles whose functions are indirectly related to this process are excluded from this part of the cell. The outer segments of both rods and cones consist primarily of flattened saccules or discs that are derived by evagination of the outer segment plasma membrane.[233] The concept that the discs are, in fact, evaginations rather than invaginations[187] of the plasma membrane is a relatively new one

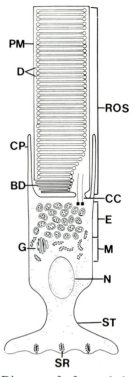

Figure 1-1. Diagram of a frog rod photoreceptor. The light-sensitive rod outer segment (ROS) is filled with photopigment-rich discs (D) which develop as evaginations of the plasma membrane near the ROS base. The basal discs (BD) thus formed are initially open to the extracellular space. The ROS is attached to the inner segment by a connecting cilium (CC). Calyceal processes (CP) extend distally from the inner segment. The inner segment is divided into an ellipsoid region (E), which is rich in mitochondria, and a myoid region (M), which contains a well-developed rough endoplasmic reticulum and Golgi apparatus (G). The cell nucleus (N) is located between the inner segment and synaptic terminal. The synaptic terminal in this species contains multiple synaptic ribbons (SR), which, characteristically, are surrounded by synaptic vesicles. (Modified from Basinger S et al: J Cell Biol 69:29–42, 1976)

introduced by Steinberg et al.[233] In addition to the fact that membrane evagination is more easily reconciled with what is currently known about mechanisms of outer segment disc assembly, the concept as outlined by these authors also posits a separate mechanism for assembly of the disc rim, a structure that is chemically distinct from the rest of the disc membrane. More will be said about this interesting feature of outer segment morphology and its implications later in this section. Rods and cones differ rather dramatically in terms of the physical relationship between their discs and plasma membranes in fully differentiated regions of their respective outer segments (Fig. 1-2). The continuity that exists between the plasma membrane and disc membrane as a consequence of the evagination process persists for all of the discs in the cone outer segment, as evidenced by transmission electron microscopy and tracer studies which have shown quite convincingly that electron-opaque substances and fluorescent dyes can diffuse readily from the extracellular space into the spaces between cone outer-segment discs.[66,158,159] The situation is quite different in the rods (Fig. 1-2*A*). Recently developed discs remain continuous with the plasma membrane at the rod outer-segment base, a situation analogous to that in cones. However, as the discs mature, the extent of attachment to the plasma membrane reduces gradually until, ultimately, the discs detach completely and become physically isolated from the membrane. Thus, the more mature discs of the rod outer segment are, by virtue of this detachment, no longer open to the extracellular space.

The utility of this separate organization for rod and cone outer segments remains in question in the minds of retinal cell biologists and electrophysiologists. Yet one cannot help but feel that these rather different morphologies for rods and cones may someday help to explain why some of the electrophysiological features of rods and cones are so different. Rods, for example, show a high level of sensitivity with relatively long dark-adaptation characteristics, whereas cones exhibit relatively low sensitivity and rapid dark adaptation.[83] The molecular and ionic mechanisms for these properties remain to be described completely, but part of the answer may lie in the distinct morphological differences between the two cell types.

Since the initial discovery that the photosensitivity of visual cells is mediated by visual pigments whose photon-catching chromophore is the 11-*cis* aldehyde (11-*cis* retinal) derivative of vitamin A (retinol),[246] biochemists with an interest in photoreceptors have directed most of their attention to these visual pigments, particularly the rod pigment rhodopsin, which is the

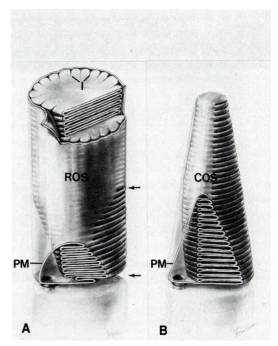

Figure 1-2. Diagrams of frog rod and cone photoreceptors. *(A)* The basal discs region between arrows of the rod outer segment (ROS) exhibit a gradient in the extent of their continuity with the plasma membrane (PM) from which they are derived. The newest, most basal discs, show extensive continuity with the plasma membrane. As these discs are displaced distally, they gradually lose their attachment to the plasma membrane and ultimately pinch off completely, thereby obliterating their continuity with the extracellular space. Frog rods are very rich in disc incisures (I), the function of which remains unknown. *(B)* Unlike the disks of the ROS, discs of the cone outer segment (COS) remain attached to the plasma membrane (PM) irrespective of their position within the outer segment, thereby remaining open to the extracellular space. (Young, RW: Sci Am 223:80–91, 1970)

most plentiful. Rhodopsin molecules are densely packed within the disc membranes (about $30,000/\mu m^2$) where they reside as intrinsic, transmembrane proteins.[141] The term *intrinsic* is applied to proteins that can be partitioned away from the membrane lipid bilayer with aqueous solutions only by the use of detergents. The term *transmembrane* refers to the fact that the rhodopsin molecule spans the membrane lipid bilayer with portions of it exposed on both surfaces of that bilayer (Fig.

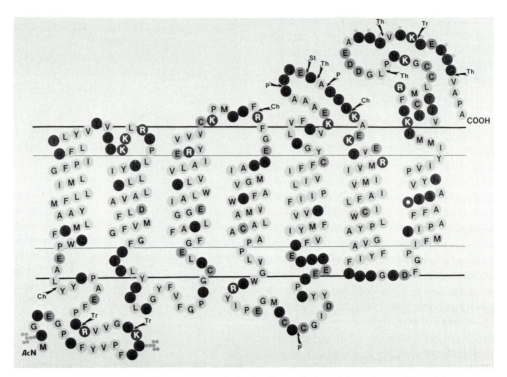

Figure 1-3. The transmembrane nature of rhodopsin as deduced from its amino acid sequence. The rhodopsin polypeptide is thought to thread its way back and forth across the disc's lipid bilayer. The carboxyl terminus (COOH) and phosphorylation sites *(small dots)* on the protein protrude from the extradiscal side of the disc lipid bilayer; the acetylated amino terminus (AcN) is found on the intradiscal side as are the glycosylated regions. (Oligosaccharide chains are indicated by branched arrays of small dots.) The seven portions of the polypeptide that span the most hydrophobic portion of the lipid bilayer are thought to be alpha helical. The lysine residue to which 11-*cis* retinal is attached is indicated with an open circle on the alpha helix at the extreme right. The positions along the extradiscal and intradiscal surface of the polypeptide that are labeled with small arrows and letters indicate proteolytic cleavage sites that are not germane to the topic of this discussion. (Baldwin, PA: Rhodopsin–lipid interactions: I. The effects of lipid environment on the light-induced conformational changes of rhodopsin. II. The motion of the lipid at the rhodopsin interface. Doctoral dissertation, University of California, Berkeley, 1983)

1-3).[95] Rhodopsin is a conjugated glycoprotein with a molecular weight of 41,800, based on the recently acquired amino acid sequence[112,198] plus the carbohydrate and retinaldehyde content. The carboxy terminus of the protein protrudes from the lipid bilayer on the cytoplasmic surface (interdiscal space) of the disc membrane; the amino terminus projects from the surface of the membrane that faces the disc interior (intradiscal space).[95] Carbohydrate chains are linked to amino acids 2 and 15 near the amino terminus and thereby reside within the intradiscal space.[94,110] The precise location of the 11-*cis* retinal moiety remains a matter of

conjecture, but it clearly is attached to a hydrophobic portion of the rhodopsin molecule that is buried in the lipid bilayer. Because the length and diameter of rod outer segments vary so dramatically among species, the actual amount of rhodopsin per rod can vary by orders of magnitude. Because much has been written about the photochemistry of rhodopsin the subject will not be covered in this short review. The reader is referred to other resources for information on this subject.[71]

There is, as far as we know, only one other intrinsic membrane glycoprotein in the outer segment disc membrane. This is the so-called edge or rim protein discovered by Papermaster and coworkers (mol. wt. 290,000 in frogs, 240,000 in cattle) and shown by immunocyto-chemical methods to be present at disc edges and incisures.[200-202] The discs of all vertebrate species are complicated by the fact that, rather than forming precise circular cross-sectional images, their margins are indented by incisures (see Figs. 1-2, 1-6), which vary from one to many, depending on the species. The purpose of these structures remains to be determined. Their function may someday be deduced when a role is discovered for the rim protein.

The interest in photopigment biochemistry took on a new dimension following Young's classic study on outer-segment renewal.[263] Injection of ³H-amino acids into a variety of species followed by light- and electron-microscopic radioautography revealed quite dramatically the dynamic nature of photorecep-tors.[263,268,272,273] Amino acids were rapidly incor-porated into protein synthesized in the rough endoplasmic reticulum (RER) of the myoid. The radioactive product was transported from there to the Golgi apparatus and subsequently distributed throughout the cell (Fig. 1-4), the majority of it destined for the outer segment.[273] In the case of rods, there was a striking accumu-lation of radioactivity at the outer-segment base manifested in radioautograms in the form of a band of silver grains arranged at right angles to the long axis of the outer segment.[263,272,273] Su-perimposed upon this was a pattern of radioac-tivity randomly distributed along the length of the outer segment.[37] Over time, the band of silver grains persisted in intensity, migrated dis-tally, and ultimately disappeared at the outer segment – RPE interface.[263] The randomly dis-tributed radioactivity faded rapidly; its half-life about 24 hours.[37] Subsequent higher-resolution autoradiographic studies showed that the radio-active bands that disappeared at the RPE – photoreceptor interface were included in bits of distal outer segment that were shed by the pho-toreceptor and phagocytized by the RPE. These structures, once within the RPE, were termed *phagosomes* by Young and Bok.[38,272] In Young's original work the phenomenon of ra-dioactive band displacement in rods was cor-rectly interpreted by him as a process of mem-

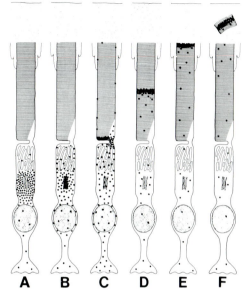

Figure 1-4. Summary of the ROS renewal process as revealed by tissue radioautography. *(A)* Protein synthesis begins in the RER of the myoid region. In the case of opsin, this includes the initial stages of glycosylation. *(B)* Some of the proteins, including opsin, are then routed through the Golgi apparatus, where post-translational modifications such as additional glycosylation occurs. *(C)* Proteins are then distributed throughout the cell, but many of them are transported through the inner segment, across the connecting cilium, and into the outer segment. *(D, E)* Over the course of days in mammals (weeks in cold-blooded animals), radio-active discs are displaced to the distal end of the outer segment. *(F)* Ultimately, they are shed into the extracellular space along with their enveloping plasma membrane and phagocytized by the retinal pigment epithelium. (Young, RW: Invest Ophthal-mol Vis Sci 15:700 – 725, 1976)

brane renewal in which new discs are continually assembled at the outer-segment base and subsequently displaced by newer discs assembled thereafter.[263] Continual assembly at one end of the cell is balanced by intermittent shedding of outer-segment tips so that the net length of the outer segment remains relatively constant.[272]

Young and coworkers observed radioauto-graphic labeling patterns to be random in cone outer segments (Fig. 1-5).[37,264,272,273] This radio-activity disappeared rather rapidly (half-life about 24 hours).[37] In addition, cones showed no evidence whatsoever for a migrating band of ra-

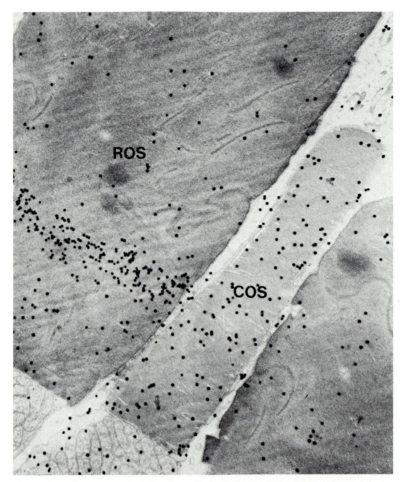

Figure 1-5. Electron microscopic radioautograph of protein renewal in an axolotl *(Ambystoma mexicanum)* rod and cone outer segment. Rod outer-segment (ROS) renewal is characteristically observed as a band of silver grains extending from edge to edge of the outer segment. Radioactive opsin, once synthesized from ^{3}H-amino acids and assembled into the rod disc membrane, can diffuse in the plane of the membrane but cannot leave the disc owing to the isolation of the latter from the plasma membrane. Radioactive proteins, represented by silver grains distal to the band are cytoplasmic proteins that are not similarly confined. Cone outer segments (COS) show random labeling. All proteins, including photopigments, have the freedom to move from disc to disc in the cone. Intrinsic membrane proteins like opsin can diffuse from one end of the outer segment to the other in the plane of the lipid bilayer because each disc is part of a continuous sheet of folded membrane (see Fig. 1-2). Extrinsic membrane proteins and others that may not be membrane bound can diffuse in the plane of the disc surface or in the small volume of cytoplasm that exists between the discs ($\times$6825; courtesy of N. Custer).

dioactivity that would have implied *de novo* membrane assembly and disc displacement, even in differentiating cone outer segments where membrane assembly was clearly taking place. Young's original conclusion with regard to this observation was that cones did not assemble new discs or shed them *in toto,* but rather that cones carried out their renewal process by random molecular replacement of proteins.[267] The current interpretation of observed rod and cone outer segment labeling patterns is based on the important observation (not available to Young at the time of his original observations) that photopigments are highly mobile within the plane of the lipid bilayer which, because of its unique fatty acid composition,[4-6] has a low viscosity (~ 1 poise).[165,209] Consequently, because of the continuity of cone disc membranes, the photopigments are free to diffuse in the plane of the cone disc membrane from one disc to the next, thereby explaining the randomization of labeled photopigments over time.

The rapid diminution of cone outer segment label can be explained on the basis of current knowledge as well. Like rods, cones are now known to shed their discs.[3,122,195,269,270] Thus a "pulse" of radioactive photopigments and soluble proteins arriving at and randomizing within the cone outer-segment disc membranes and cytosol is rather quickly diminished in concentration by a combination of the inherently shorter half-life of the soluble components and the shedding of disc membranes. The shedding of rod and cone disc membranes follows a diurnal rhythm, the majority of rods shedding their membranes in the morning[13,160,161] and the majority of cones shedding their membranes at night,[195,269,270] although variations on this theme have been reported.[87]

The fascinating and extensive subject of outer segment disc shedding and factors that control it was recently reviewed by Besharse[19] and therefore will not be discussed here. One new and intriguing development bears mention however: the hormone melatonin may play a role in the control of disc shedding.[21] *Xenopus* eyecups placed *in vitro* in the dark were primed to undergo light-evoked rod outer-segment shedding when melatonin was added to the medium.[21] Additionally, Bubenik and coworkers have demonstrated melatonin-like immunoreactivity in photoreceptors and have provided evidence that melatonin levels vary during the diurnal cycle and that the highest levels occur at night.[45] Finally, Wiechmann and associates have now shown with immunocytochemistry that the terminal enzyme for the synthesis of melatonin, hydroxyindole-0-methyltransferase (HIOMT, E.C. 2.1.1.4), is present in the photoreceptors (except in the outer segment) in multi-

ple vertebrate species.[248] The molecular mechanism for melatonin function in disc shedding must still be determined, but the evidence is building for a significant role for this hormone in retinal function.

It was apparent from the outer segment renewal studies of Young and associates that rhodopsin must be continually renewed along with the rest of the outer segment. This was quickly verified by radiobiochemical methods,[109] and the multistep process involving the biosynthesis of rhodopsin and its assembly into disc membranes was elucidated thereafter.[33,192] During the course of this renewed focus on rhodopsin biochemistry, it became apparent that additional proteins must share in the process of phototransduction, and interest began to focus on the chemistry and function of proteins other than rhodopsin. Consequently our understanding of the chemistry of rod outer segment membranes has expanded significantly in recent years. A seminal contribution in this regard was the discovery that light initiates a reduction in the cyclic nucleotide content of rod outer segments.[25,26,178] It was shown that this reduction is produced by a light-activated cGMP phosphodiesterase (PDE) that is unique to photoreceptors.[178] Thus began the study of outer segment enzymes that are now thought to play some role in the phototransduction process itself. Biochemical evidence strongly indicates that light-activated PDE belongs to a class of membrane components commonly referred to as peripheral or extrinsic proteins, an operational description that simply denotes that they can be washed from the disc membranes with aqueous buffers of the appropriate ionic composition and strength. From a physiological, and therefore more significant, perspective, they can associate with and dissociate from other membrane proteins and thereby perform a role in important biological processes. Two additional proteins of this class have now been isolated from rod outer segments and partially characterized. One is guanosine triphosphate (GTP)-binding protein[103] (G-binding protein or transducin[96,97]), which is bound by rhodopsin in the dark and, when released during light exposure, activates the PDE by some unresolved mechanism. The other is rhodopsin kinase,[179] an enzyme that catalyzes the phosphorylation of rhodopsin. Other extrinsic proteins of unknown function have been detected in the outer segment; more will undoubtedly be discovered as methods of detection improve.

PDE and G-binding protein participate in the enzyme cascade that controls cyclic nucleotide metabolism, and they are thought to be involved somehow in phototransduction.[26,118,166,167,232] Rhodopsin kinase, as stated above, is involved in the phosphorylation of rhodopsin.[55,93,143–146] It is not yet understood why the phosphorylation of this photopigment occurs. It takes place over minutes and, so, is far too slow to be implicated in the transduction process. The subjects of phototransduction and phosphorylation are extensive and complicated and certainly beyond the purview of this chapter. Nonetheless, it should be mentioned that cell biologists have developed an interest in the peripheral proteins that are thought to contribute to these processes and have begun to localize them within the outer segment by a variety of sophisticated methods. Recently, with the aid of deep-etch, rotary shadowing techniques for the production of high-resolution carbon-platinum replicas, it has been suggested that G-binding protein is randomly distributed on the rod disc surface at a density of about $300/\mu$.[2,219,220] This is consistent with biochemical evidence that suggests that G-binding protein is present in the outer segment at a concentration one tenth that of rhodopsin. Similar methods were unsuccessful in localizing light-activated PDE, perhaps because of its low concentration (the PDE : rhodopsin estimates range from 1 : 40 to 1 : 170 in the rod) or other geometric factors that prevented its identification.[219,220]

Additional outer segment disc components assumed to be proteins have been discovered by morphological methods. Ultrathin sections of rapidly frozen, freeze-substituted outer segments (Fig. 1-6) or carbon-platinum replicas of deep-etched and rotary shadowed specimens exhibit filamentous structures that run from margin to margin of adjacent rod discs, including those edges that follow the disc incisures.[219,220,245] The filaments are evenly spaced at approximately 140-nm intervals and are displaced from the disc margin in the direction of the disc

center by approximately 1500 nm. Additional filaments oriented at right angles to those just described attach the disc margins to the outer segment plasma membrane. Although nothing is currently known about the chemical nature of these structures, their discovery aids significantly in explaining why the disc incisures remain in register for relatively long distances along the outer segment. Their attachment to the plasma membrane explains why disc edges tend to adhere to the plasma membrane in osmotically swollen or partially disrupted outer segments.[67]

Cytoskeletal elements, not previously thought to be in the outer segment, have recently been demonstrated by electron microscopic immunocytochemistry in amphibian and mammalian species by Chaitin and co-workers.[56,59] A heavy concentration of actin was localized at the junction between the outer segment and connecting cilium in frog, rat, cow, rhesus monkey, and human retina.[56,59] This is the site where the connecting cilium plasma membrane evaginates to form new outer-segment discs (Fig. 1-7). This suggests that actin, as part of a contractile mechanism, mediates outer segment disc morphogenesis. Chaitin and Bok, also using electron microscopic immunocytochemical methods, have shown that myosin is found in this region as well, but the scope of its distribution differs from that of actin.[56] Whereas actin was found only at the site of disc evagination, myosin extended from the ciliary axoneme distally along the length of the outer segment. Myosin was found only on the ciliary side of the cell. No other region of the outer segment was labeled with antimyosin antibodies. The significance of this observation can only be suggested at this point. Nonetheless, it is noteworthy that photoreceptors possess the ability to align their outer segments toward the entrance pupil of the eye.[79,155,156,158] Myosin is located in the outer segment in a strategic position for mediation of this process. Contraction or relaxation of contractile elements asymmetrically disposed within the outer segment cylinder could cause movement of that structure in opposing directions. Recently, Chaitin and Bok have observed the localization of calmodulin antibodies in portions of the outer segment as

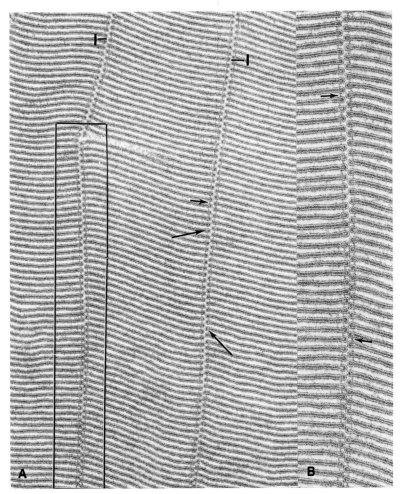

Figure 1-6. Frog ROS and interdisc filaments. The outer segment was rapidly frozen against a polished copper block cooled to about 4 °Kelvin and then freeze-substituted at −80 °C in acetone containing 2% osmium tetroxide. *(A)* Disc incisures (I) in register along most of the outer segment's length have been sectioned longitudinally, exposing the hairpin-like loops *(long arrows)* characteristic of disc edges. This process of fixation reveals delicate filaments *(small arrows)* that extend from neck to neck of the stacked membrane loops (magnification ×53,800). *(B)* The disc incisures outlined in this figure are shown at higher magnification (×82,800), which shows the delicate filaments *(arrows)* connecting disc edges more clearly. (Courtesy of J. Usukura)

well, specifically, those regions that contain myosin.[56] Calmodulin, as its name implies, is a calcium-binding regulatory protein for many cellular processes. Its localization in the outer segment is consistent with our knowledge that, through its binding of calcium, it regulates myosin light-chain kinase.[70] Calmodulin antibodies were not associated with outer segment discs. Those with a knowledge of PDE function in other systems might be surprised by this observation since some PDE types are activated by calcium. However the light-activated PDE that is unique to photoreceptors does not require calcium for its function.[39] Thus the role of calmodulin in the cilium and outer segment appears to be related to contractile mechanisms rather than to cyclic nucleotide metabolism. In this context, it is worth noting that actin and myosin

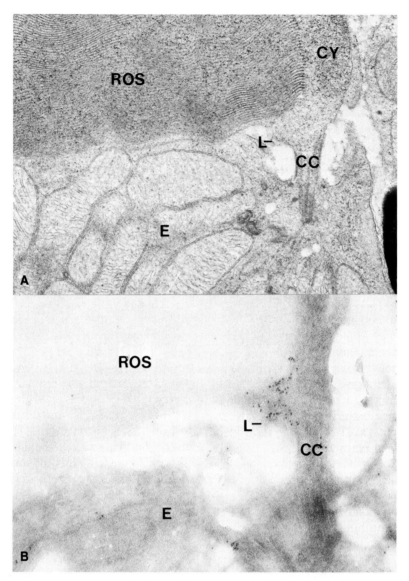

Figure 1-7. Electron micrographs of thin sectioned frog rods fixed in aldehydes and embedded and sectioned in epoxy resin by conventional methods, *A*, and from tissue fixed in adehydes and embedded and sectioned in glutaraldehyde cross-linked albumin, *B*. The section in *B* was stained successively with affinity-purified rabbit antiactin immunoglobulin G (IgG), sheep antirabbit biotinyl-IgG and avidin-conjugated ferritin. *(A)* This figure is shown for purposes of orientation to *B*. The rod outer segment (ROS) and mitochondria-rich ellipsoid (E) are joined by the connecting cilium (CC). Distal to the cilium, a zone of cytoplasm (CY) free of discs is evident. Immediately distal to the cilium, this cytoplasmic zone expands to form a lip-shaped structure (L). The region just distal to the lip is the area of membrane evagination. (Original magnification ×49,000) *(B)* Bovine serum albumin-embedded tissue lacks the contrast of conventionally prepared material. Nonetheless, the rod outer segment (ROS), ellipsoidal mitochondria (E), and connecting cilium (CC) are visible. The liplike expansion distal to the connecting cilium and the zone of membrane evagination are stained with the ferritin-antibody complex. These findings suggest that actin may be involved in the generation of motive forces involved in disc formation. (×34,300; courtesy of M. Chaitin)

have recently been demonstrated in the motile cilia of quail oviduct.[224]

Before ending this discussion of the outer segment, a few comments should be added about the plasma membrane that surrounds this organelle. To the extent that it contains rhodopsin,[14,75,135,190] the chemistry of the plasma membrane resembles that of the disc membrane, although the purpose of a photopigment in the plasma membrane is not clear. When bound to rhodopsin in the disc, 11-*cis* retinal is oriented with its long axis at approximately right angles to the incoming photons, thereby maximizing its quantum-catching efficiency.[163] Rhodopsin molecules in the plasma membrane (as well as their chromophores) are oriented at right angles to their counterparts in the disc membrane. Therefore, one would assume that the light-trapping efficiency would be less for 11-*cis* retinal in the plasma membrane.

Clearly, although the plasma membrane resembles the outer segment disc with respect to its rhodopsin content, it must be quite different from the disc membrane in other respects. Classic electrophysiological studies have shown that the outer segment plasma membrane contains light-sensitive channels that control the influx of sodium under dark and light conditions.[107,203,262] Dark-adapted photoreceptors exist in a state of relative depolarization, owing to the relatively high permeability of sodium ions in the dark.[243] When the photoreceptor is illuminated, this sodium permeability is dramatically decreased, perhaps owing to blockage by calcium ions or alteration in some manner by cyclic nucleotides (herein lies the controversy alluded to earlier with respect to the mechanism for phototransduction).[25,26,96,97,129,139,166,167,232,262]

One of the frustrations of biochemists and cell biologists has been their inability to isolate quantities of photoreceptor plasma membrane sufficient for the study of its biochemistry. Technological advances in this area will aid significantly in attempts to characterize the proteins of the outer-segment plasma membrane. Andrews and Cohen recently used the sterol-specific antibiotic filipin and freeze-fracture technology to demonstrate the differential distribution of cholesterol in the plasma membrane of the outer and inner segment and disc

membranes.[8,9] Quantitative biochemical methods are needed to supplement these elegant morphological techniques.

Inner Segment

We will postpone a description of the connecting cilium until the next section, in the interest of clarity, because a discussion of this structure will have considerably more meaning if we first describe the cytology and function of the inner segment.

The inner segment of the cell can rightfully be considered the biosynthetic center since it is filled with all of the organelles essential for that process (see Fig. 1-1). The inner segment is usually divided into an ellipsoid and a myoid region. The ellipsoid is the region closest to the outer segment and is joined to it by the connecting cilium. In addition, plasma membrane extensions called *calyceal processes* project distally from the inner segment circumference and caress the lateral surface of the outer segment. The major distinguishing feature of the inner segment ellipsoid, however, is its high density of mitochondria, and, in the cones of some lower vertebrates such as birds and turtles, oil droplets of various colors. The myoid lies between the ellipsoid and the nucleus. It is rich in endoplasmic reticulum and Golgi apparatus. One purpose for its wealth of biosynthetic organelles became apparent with the discovery of outer segment renewal, namely the biosynthesis and transport of molecules for the maintenance of outer segment structure and function. The biosynthesis of one of those components, rhodopsin, has been studied in detail.

It was discovered in the early 1970s that rhodopsin is a glycoprotein.[114,117] As described earlier, the protein was subsequently found to contain two oligosaccharide chains linked through asparagine residues at the 2nd and 15th amino acid positions from the amino terminus.[94,110] Owing to its tripartite composition of polypeptide, oligosaccharide, and 11-*cis* retinal, the multistep synthesis of rhodopsin and the cellular organelles involved in that process became a subject of interest. It was demonstrated by a combination of biochemical, radioautographic, and immunocytochemical methods that rho-

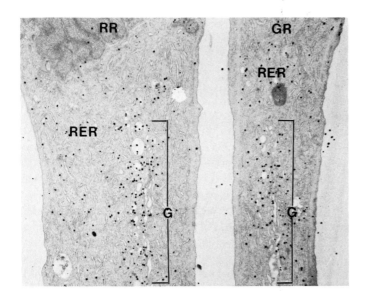

Figure 1-8. Frog red (RR) and green (GR) rod inner segments labeled with ^{3}H-glucosamine. Isolated neural retina incubated in ^{3}H-glucosamine, a precursor for asparagine-linked glycosylation, shows simultaneous labeling of the rough endoplasmic reticulum (RER) and the Golgi apparatus (G) after 10 minutes of incubation. This, along with biochemical and immunocytochemical evidence, indicates dual intracellular glycosylation sites for rhodopsin. ($\times$7800)

dopsin, like other glycoproteins of the asparagine-linked type, begins its glycosylation on the RER; further additions take place in the Golgi apparatus (Fig. 1-8).[29,33,192] The rhodopsin oligosaccharides consist exclusively of N-acetylglucosamine and mannose.[111,117] Recent investigations have shown that a lipid carrier (dolichol phosphate) transfers presynthesized oligosaccharide units consisting of glucosamine, mannose, and N-acetylglucosamine $[(Glc)_3 (Man)_9 (Glc NAc)_2]$ to asparagine 2 and 15 of the growing polypeptide chain while it is still in the RER.[140] These oligosaccharides are then processed or "edited" in the RER and Golgi apparatus by the successive removal of the terminal glucosamines and some of the terminal mannoses. Additions of terminal N-acetylglucosamine and mannose follow this process to yield oligosaccharides consisting exclusively of N-acetylglucosamine and mannose ranging in size from six to eight residues per oligosaccharide $[(Man)_5 (Glc NAc)_3, (Man)_4 (Glc NAc)_3,$ or $(Man)_3 (Glc NAc)_3]$.[94,110,111] Rhodopsin, like many glycoproteins, shows microheterogeneity in its oligosaccharide structure.

Unlike amino acids and sugars, the 11-*cis* retinal moiety of rhodopsin is not added to the growing molecule in the rod inner segment (Fig. 1-9).[33,72] This event awaits the arrival of the fully glycosylated opsin molecule at the base of the outer segment. This subject will be discussed in

greater detail near the end of this chapter when we discuss new discoveries and concepts regarding the transport and utilization of the retinoids (vitamin A and its derivatives) by the retina.

The contributions of Papermaster, Schneider, and coworkers have been invaluable to our understanding of mechanisms whereby opsin is transported from the inner to outer segment and how membrane assembly occurs.[200,201,204] The indispensable technique in their studies has been electron microscopic immunocytochemistry. These authors have shown quite convincingly that, in amphibians at least, opsin-rich membranous vesicles pinch off from Golgi lamellae and are transported to the apical (distal) region of the inner segment plasma membrane. En route, the vesicles make their way between ellipsoid mitochondria and fuse with the apical plasma membrane of the inner segment. In this region of the amphibian rod, there exists a well-developed complex array of plasma membrane-lined ridges and grooves called the *periciliary ridge complex.*[204] The complex has ninefold symmetry, apparently reflecting the nine-plus-zero microtubule organization of the connecting cilium. Crowning the ridges are double rows of intramembrane particles, somewhat reminiscent of the structures observed at the neuromuscular junction. Andrews has suggested that these structures, like their counterparts in the neuromuscular junction, may serve as fusion points

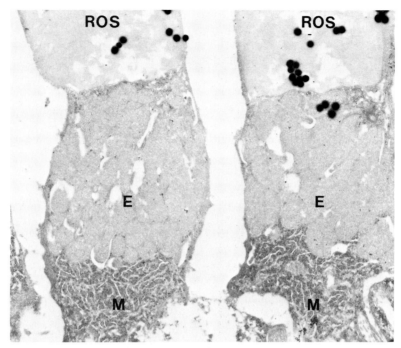

Figure 1-9. Frog red rods labeled with ^{3}H-retinol bound to its natural carrier protein, plasma retinol-binding protein, and injected into dark-adapted animals. After allowing time for incorporation into rhodopsin, as evidenced by parallel biochemical analysis, the retinas were fixed in the dark in formaldehyde. Thereafter, the retinal–opsin Schiff–base double–bond linkage was reduced *in situ* to a single bond to irreversibly bind the retinal to opsin. The tissue was then extracted with chloroform and methanol to remove free retinoids and lipids. (The latter step plus the lack of osmium fixation accounts for the poor morphology.) Only the rod outer segments show incorporation of ^{3}H-retinol. It is therefore concluded that the binding of 11-*cis* retinal during rhodopsin synthesis does not occur until the glycosylated opsin reaches the outer segment. ($\times$9800)

for opsin-rich transport vesicles that carry the components for outer segment disc assembly.[7] It is not currently known whether these periciliary complexes are widespread among vertebrate species, but Andrews has demonstrated rows of intramembranous particles in the vicinity of the connecting cilium in toads and goldfish as well.[7] The ridges and grooves that are so prominent in the frog are not as apparent in these animals however.

In the adult retina, opsin is highly restricted in terms of its distribution in the inner segment plasma membrane. Apparently, by an undefined process, the opsin, following its assembly into the apical inner segment plasma membrane, diffuses in the plane of the membrane in the direction of the outer segment. To reach the outer segment, it presumably must traverse the plasma membrane of the connecting cilium. Paradoxically, immunocytochemical studies show heavy labeling of opsin in the distal plasma membrane of the connecting cilium but very little in the proximal region.[201,204] More about this phenomenon will be said and illustrated when the cilium is discussed in the next section.

Conceptually, it is rather easy to correlate growing, evaginating discs at the outer segment base with the continual arrival of new membrane components in the region, aided, perhaps, by a cytoskeletal motor in the form of actin and myosin and their regulatory proteins.[56,59] The process of opsin synthesis and assembly into disc membrane is unceasing, although, as recently demonstrated by Matsumoto and Bok using immunochemical methods, the rate of synthesis and assembly follows diurnal fluctuations, the highest rates for each occurring shortly after light onset in *Rana pipiens*.[173] Hollyfield and associates, on the other hand, in their studies of *Xenopus* retina, found little difference in the biosynthetic rates of opsin in light and dark.[124] There is indirect evidence to suggest that opsin builds up within the inner segment during the night, in preparation for a rapid assembly of disc membranes following light onset.[173] Again, it is tempting to draw an analogy between the neuromuscular junction and specialized components in the apical inner-segment plasma membrane. As we are reminded by Andrews, neurotransmitter vesicles are released as a function of a change in local membrane potential.[7] Could it be that changes in inner segment membrane potential elicited by light onset foster an enhanced rate of fusion between the periciliary ridge complex and opsin transport vesicles that have accumulated during the night? Indeed, in *Xenopus* rods there is a dramatic increase in the number of open basal discs following light onset, an index of the accelerated rate of membrane assembly.[22] This correlates, in turn, with an accelerated rate of radioactive band displacement following the injection of ^{3}H-amino acids at light onset.

Mechanisms whereby the photoreceptor maintains its remarkable state of membrane polarization remain a mystery at this point. We have already mentioned that, following fusion of opsin transport vesicles with the apical inner segment plasma membrane, the protein is immediately directed to the outer segment and not allowed to randomize within the inner segment plasma membrane. There is evidence to suggest that this state of polarization exists even when the rod first begins to differentiate its outer segment, although there is disagreement on this point. Forestner and Besharse have shown that opsin antibodies localize to the distal connecting cilium from the time that it begins its differentiation of an outer segment.[92] Nir and coworkers, on the other hand, claim that opsin is initially distributed throughout the inner segment plasma membrane, and only subsequently polarized to the distal connecting cilium after several hundred discs have formed.[188]

The difference in their results is difficult to resolve at this point. Nonetheless, a state of strict polarization is ultimately achieved. Unlike opsin, Na-K ATPase, the intrinsic plasma membrane enzyme responsible for the Na$^+$ dark current in photoreceptors, is segregated to the photoreceptor inner segment plasma membrane (Fig. 1-10).[30,238] How cells achieve and maintain this state of polarization and how they direct these membrane components to their respective membrane domains remains one of the major unresolved problems in cell biology. The photoreceptor (because of its polarity) serves as an excellent cellular model for the study of this important process.

The subject of cytoskeletal proteins should be included at this point because it is relevant to the subject of inner segment elongation and contraction in some of the lower vertebrates. Indeed, the term *myoid* is derived from the observation that this portion of the cell is contractile in some species. Although this contractile system is not prevalent in man and lower mammals, it reaches its zenith in teleost fish, where cone myoid length can vary from 5 to 85 μm, depending on the state of light adaptation.[48] The cones shorten in response to light, presumably in an effort to place themselves in a favorable position for photic stimulation. By shortening, they evade the screening effects of melanin granules that occupy the microvilli of the RPE. The rods, on the other hand, elongate in the light, presumably to reduce their exposure to photons. In the teleost cone, actin filaments are present throughout the length of the cell with the exception of most of the outer segment.[48,54] They are present in the calyceal processes as well.[48,59] In the midregion of the cell, there is a switch in the polarity of the actin filaments as judged by their decoration with myosin subfragment-1. The cytochemical procedure for myosin subfragment decoration produces "arrowhead" arrays along the actin filament that indicate the direction of movement that that region of the cell would take if it were free to move during contraction.[48] In fact, only the inner segment and its attached outer segment are free to move since the remainder of the cell is anchored at the outer limiting membrane by intercellular junctions. In the dark-adapted

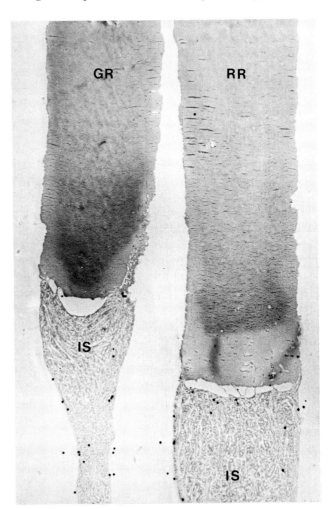

Figure 1-10. Green (GR) and red (RR) frog rods labeled with ^{3}H-ouabain, a specific ligand for Na$^+$-K$^+$ ATPase. The neural retina was incubated in ^{3}H-ouabain, rinsed free of unbound ouabain and rapidly frozen in liquid Freon 22. The tissue was then freeze dried, further fixed in osmium tetroxide vapors, embedded in epoxy resin, and analyzed by electron microscopic autoradiography. The special fixation protocol was necessary because ouabain is not bound covalently and conventional fixation and dehydration protocols would have removed or translocated the radioactive ligand. Silver grains are localized exclusively to the inner segment (IS) plasma membrane. No binding of ouabain is observed on the ROS plasma membrane. ($\times$ 5400)

state, the distal half of the cone, which includes the myoid, displays actin filaments whose direction of pull is proximal, whereas the proximal portion of the cell (roughly from the axon terminal to the nucleus) exhibits filaments of the opposite polarity. When the cone contracts, the myoid shortens, and these two groups of actin filaments of opposing polarity overlap.[54] Whether or not myosin plays a role in this process remains a matter of conjecture. Another class of thicker filaments has been identified in the teleost cone, but its chemical identity has not yet been determined.[48] Because cone contraction is linear, slow ($1 - 3$ μm/min), and repetitive, Burnside and coworkers used this system to great advantage in the study of the contractile properties of nonmuscle cells. Warren and Burnside suggested that cone elongation is me-

diated by closely associated microtubules located in the inner segment.[247] This prediction rests primarily on the observation that colchicine inhibits elongation. In addition, they have provided morphological evidence for lateral interaction between overlapping microtubules and have suggested a sliding mechanism reminiscent of the axoneme in sperm flagella. Elongation and contraction in teleost rods have been studied by Burnside and coworkers as well.[54, 193,194] Again, the change in inner segment length is formidable in these cells and easy to quantify. (Changes greater than threefold are common.) Whereas contraction in rods is similar to that in cones in that it appears to involve an actomyosin system, elongation appears to be controlled by actin as well. In the latter case the process appears to involve actin assembly rather than microtubule interaction. Finally, photoreceptor elongation and contraction, like so many cellular processes, follow a circadian rhythm modulated by light and cyclic nucleotides.[20,49,51,162,194]

Connecting Cilium

Since the discovery of the connecting cilium during early electron microscopic studies of photoreceptors,[230] this portion of the cell has been a subject of interest, but its true importance has only recently become apparent. The connecting cilium serves as the only normal link between inner and outer segment and therefore must serve as the bridge for the passage of electrical information that originates in the outer segment. Furthermore, with the advent of the concept of photoreceptor renewal,[263] it is recognized that this structure must also play a major role in the transport of membrane and cytoplasmic constituents and metabolites to the outer segment.[23,201,204] Aside from early observations that the connecting cilium resembles nonmotile cilia with respect to its nine-plus-zero microtubular arrangement, surprisingly little was learned about this important structure for the first two decades following its discovery. However, several significant observations have been made recently regarding its structure.

The connecting cilium is asymmetrically positioned between the outer and inner segment so that the curvature of the cilium representing its eccentric surface lies nearly parallel with the contiguous lateral surfaces of the inner and outer segment. In cross section, the cilium displays nine microtubule doublets arranged in a circular pattern.[64] As mentioned earlier, the central pair of microtubules commonly present in motile cilia is classically described as absent in the photoreceptor connecting cilium, although Matsusaka[175] has reported "paired helical microtubules" in the center of the cilium. In cross section, the central cytoplasmic core of the cilium appears somewhat empty with the vacancy outlined by a ring of material that connects the microtubule doublets along their center-facing curvatures. Proceeding distally, the nine doublets make a sharp transition into nine singlets, whereas, proximally, the doublets change into triplets as the centriole is reached.[64]

Matsusaka and Rohlich made independent and important new observations regarding the plasma membrane of the connecting cilium based on freeze-fracture studies.[174,176,218] In order to appreciate their observations, a few general comments must first be made concerning the structure of motile cilia. Motile cilia, of course, have a central pair of microtubules in their axonemes, the so-called nine-plus-two arrangement. In addition, as pointed out initially by Flowers and in greater detail by Gilula and Satir, motile cilia display a striking arrangement of intramembranous particles (IMPS) within the portion of the plasma membrane surrounding the transition zone that joins the cilium to the cell body.[91,102] These IMPS are arranged circumferentially around the cilium in rows and have therefore been named the *ciliary necklace.*[102] The number of strands comprising the necklace varies with the species. Extending radially between the intramembranous particles and the ciliary doublets are structures resembling champagne glasses, with the stems attached to the doublets and the cups attached to the necklace region of the plasma membrane. Matsusaka and Rohlich have shown that the majority of the plasma membrane of the connecting cilium in the rat retina resembles the ciliary necklace or transition zone of motile cilia.[174,176,218] Because the rat cilium is very long ($> 1 \mu$m), 30 to 40 strands of ciliary necklace can be observed in this structure (Fig. 1-11*A*). Only in the most distal region of the cilium does the necklace arrangement finally give way to a random arrangement of particles. Unlike motile cilia, the IMPS of the photoreceptor ciliary necklace partition with the E (extracellular) face (rather than the P [protoplasmic] face) of the lipid bilayer during freeze fracture. The significance of this difference in partitioning (and, for that matter, the significance of the ciliary necklace itself) is not known. The chemical identity of the ciliary necklace IMPS remains a mystery. The particles are probably not opsin molecules since only the most distal cilium plasma membrane labels heavily with antiopsin antibodies, namely the portion of the cilium lacking a necklace.[201,204]

The IMPS that form the ciliary necklace appear to be anchored in place by linkers (Fig.

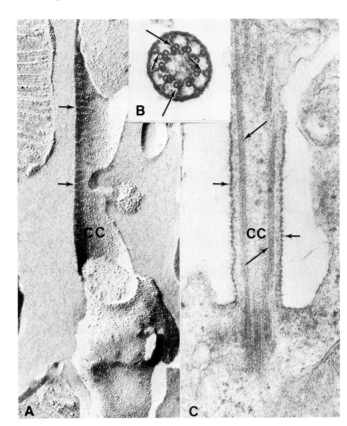

Figure 1-11. Freeze-fracture replica and thin-section electron micrographs of rat connecting cilia. *(A)* Freeze-fracture replica. The ciliary necklace is represented by rows of intramembranous particles *(arrows)* that partition with the E-face of the connecting cilium (CC) plasma membrane. (×46,200) *(B)* Cross section of the rat connecting cilium showing nine microtubule doublets *(long arrows)* and the linkers *(small arrows)* that connect the doublets with intramembranous particles in the plasma membrane. (×59,700) *(C)* Section of rat connecting cilium shown for comparison with the freeze-fracture replica in *A*. Longitudinally sectioned microtubules *(long arrows)* are evident as are "fuzzy" globular structures *(short arrows)* with a repeat periodicity similar to that for the rows of intramembranous particles shown in *A*. (×47,400) (Modified from Besharse JC et al.: J Neurosci 5:1035–1048, 1985)

1-11*B*) that extend between them and the microtubule doublets.[102,176,218] The rows of 10-nm particles have a periodicity of about 32 nm with 25-nm center-to-center spacing between particles in individual rows. Therefore, even though they are fixed in position by the radial linkers, the particles presumably allow sufficient space between them for translational diffusion within the lipid bilayer of opsin and the large rim protein of the disc.

Recent cytochemical studies show a significant glycocalyx on the surface of the connecting cilium.[92,189] In transmission electron micrographs this can be observed as a layer of "fuzz" on the surface of the cilium (Fig. 1-11*C*). In addition, colloidal gold-labeled lectins bind at high density to the entire surface of the plasma membrane, in sharp contrast to the labeling patterns observed for opsin antibody (Fig. 1-12) labeling.[92] As stated earlier, the paucity of opsin in the region of the proximal cilium remains an enigma to cell biologists in view of the fact that opsin is moving in the plane of the cilium

against an opsin concentration gradient. Perhaps there is some motive element in the axoneme of this region of the cilium that rapidly propels the diffusing opsin molecules along. In this context, it is noteworthy that myosin and calmodulin have now been localized to the axoneme and to points distal as well.[56-58] Actin, on the other hand, is observed only in the distal cilium, at the point of disc evagination[59] (see Fig. 1-7*B*).

It was mentioned earlier that the subject of cyclic nucleotide metabolism has become important from the standpoint of visual transduction. The cyclic nucleotide that has been implicated most heavily in both issues has been cGMP.[129,166,167,232] The site of synthesis of this important molecule therefore becomes a matter of considerable importance. A significant factor in this regard is the localization of the synthesizing enzyme for cGMP, guanylate cyclase. Surprisingly, about half of the guanylate cyclase activity of bovine photoreceptors copurifies with connecting cilium axonemes.[89,90,212] A signifi-

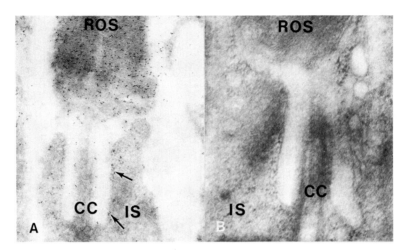

Figure 1-12. Electron-microscopic immunocytochemical localization of opsin in the cow rod. Tissues were fixed in aldehydes and, without further fixation in osmium tetroxide, embedded and sectioned in Lowicryl K4M (Polysciences), a hydrophilic embedding resin that allows retention of considerable tissue antigenic activity. The sections were stained successively with affinity-purified rabbit antibovine opsin IgG and F(ab)₂-ferretin. *(A)* Rod outer-segment (ROS) discs are heavily stained with ferritin-antibody, but the plasma membrane of the connecting cilium (CC) is only lightly stained. Presumed membrane assembly sites for opsin on the inner segment (IS) apical plasma membrane *(arrows)* are also lightly labeled. (×25,500) *(B)* Control section for *A*, in which immune antibovine opsin IgG was substituted with nonimmune IgG. Rod outer segment (ROS), cilium (CC), and inner segment (IS) are unstained. (×38,500)

cant portion of outer segment cGMP must therefore be synthesized within the connecting cilium. Whether this nucleotide is utilized locally within the cilium remains to be seen.

Finally, to end this discussion of the connecting cilium, it should be added that photoreceptor cilia are associated with prominent ciliary rootlets (Fig. 1-13), a structural feature present with other types of cilia as well.

Nuclear Region

The nuclear region of the photoreceptor varies significantly among species in terms of its morphology and the manner in which this region is linked to the rest of the cell. In human and rat rods, an axonlike fiber attaches the nuclear zone to the inner segment distally and to the synaptic terminal proximally. In other species, such as the frog red rod, the distal fiber does not exist.[265] Instead, the nuclear and myoid regions of the inner segment are in continuity. In the human and rat retina and in other species that have

many layers of nuclei in their outer nuclear layer, the lengths of the proximal and distal fibers are determined by the position of the nucleus within that layer. Photoreceptors with nuclei near the outer plexiform layer have short proximal fibers and long distal fibers. Those with nuclei near the outer limiting membrane display the opposite arrangement. Some species such as the axolotl *(Ambystoma mexicanum)* have their cone nuclei positioned so close to the outer plexiform layer that there is no proximal fiber.[69] Proximal and distal fibers, when present, are filled with cytoskeletal elements, including actin, microtubules, and neurofilaments.[121] The presumed roles for these structures include cell structural support and transport of materials destined for the synaptic terminal.

The nucleus is perhaps the least studied of all photoreceptor cell organelles. Its morphology varies considerably from species to species, in terms of its euchromatin and heterochromatin patterns. In some species (the rat, for example) most of the rod nucleoprotein is compacted into large heterochromatin clumps, regions of the genome that are presumably not undergoing expression. In other photoreceptors, such as those of the human, the heterochromatin regions are much smaller but more numerous. The significance of these different patterns is not currently understood since one would expect the number of genes active in the human and rat rod to be about equal and the number of proteins expressed by each, about the same.

From the early radioautographic studies of Sidman, it is known that the nuclei of presumptive photoreceptor cells cease their synthesis of DNA prior to differentiation and, so, thereafter do not synthesize DNA *de novo*.[229] Like other cells, however, the photoreceptor is able to repair its DNA following damage by ultraviolet radiation.[271] The photoreceptor nucleus also synthesizes the RNA that is required for the support of protein synthesis in the myoid.[27] Radioautographic studies demonstrate that this RNA migrates from the nucleus to the myoid region over a period of hours. The rate of RNA synthesis is higher in the light than it is in the dark.[27] Like other eukaryotic cells, other constituents of the photoreceptor nucleus include nonhistone chromosomal proteins (NHCPs) and histones.[271] The former include a heterogeneous population of proteins, including enzymes, that mediate the DNA repair process. The histones are a highly conserved group of proteins that are electrostatically bound to DNA and, by virtue of their binding to and dissociation from that molecule through reversible acylation, contribute to the control of DNA transcription. Whereas NHCPs are dynamic components that undergo rapid renewal, the histones are synthesized only during the DNA synthetic phase of the cell cycle. Histones are synthesized in the cytoplasm and transported to the nucleus. Thereafter, they appear to be the only class of molecule in nucleated cells, including photoreceptors, that does not turn over through repair or renewal.[271]

Synaptic Terminal

Classically, the synaptic terminals of rods are described as spherules because of their somewhat spherical shape (Fig. 1-14*A*); the terminals

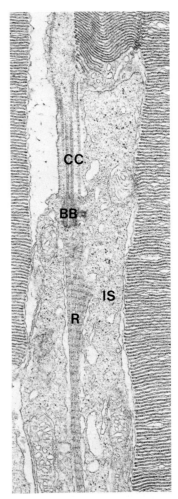

Figure 1-13. Rat rod photoreceptor. The ciliary rootlet (R) is a striated structure that extends from the basal body (BB) of the connecting cilium (CC) into the cytoplasm of the inner segment (IS). (×19,500)

of cones are described as pedicles (Fig. 1-14*B*) because of their broad pyramidal shape, the base of the pyramid facing the neurites of the outer plexiform layer.[62,182] There are many exceptions to this scheme however. The rod and cone synaptic terminals of the domestic pigeon (*Columba livia domestica*), for example, are all of the pedicle type.[63] Hence, as is frequently the case with other regions of photoreceptor cells, one cannot generalize about the respective morphologies of rod and cone synaptic terminals. In recent years, cell biologists and electrophysiologists have turned their attention to the intramembrane specializations, synaptic circuitry,

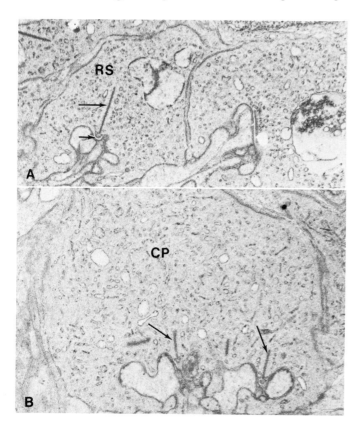

Figure 1-14. Goldfish rod and cone synaptic terminals. *(A)* Rod spherule (RS) containing a single synaptic ribbon *(long arrow)* with an arciform density *(short arrow)* intervening between the edge of the ribbon and the plasma membrane of the synaptic terminal. The spherule is rich in synaptic vesicles and membranous cisterns that are involved in neurotransmitter release and the recycling of synaptic plasma membrane. *(B)* Cone pedicle (CP) containing multiple synaptic ribbons *(arrows)*. Aside from its shape and size, it exhibits features in common with the rod spherule. (×15,600)

and functions of these terminals rather than to their shape. A discussion of circuitry is beyond the scope of this review, but a brief discussion is in order with respect to photoreceptor synaptic terminal dynamics and their presynaptic specializations.

One observation that has been crucial to our understanding of synapse function in photoreceptors is the discovery in the late 1960s that photoreceptors *hyperpolarize* in response to light stimulation.[243] Conventionally, it is understood that neurons release their neurotransmitters in response to cell *depolarization*. The question then arose: what happens to the release of neurotransmitter when light falls upon a visual cell? It was established in other systems that active synapses could be labeled with horseradish peroxidase (HRP) and other macromolecular tracers.[120] This is by virtue of the fact that the synaptic vesicle membrane, which fuses with the plasma membrane during the exocytic process, is ultimately retrieved by the cell through endocytic mechanisms. This process is neces-

sary to prevent the constant growth of the synaptic terminal plasma membrane owing to the addition of new membrane to its surface. Schacher and associates incubated isolated frog retinas in HRP and showed that the uptake of HRP into vesicles of rod and cone terminals was much higher in the dark than in the light.[225,226] In keeping with the observation that cones are less sensitive than rods, it was also observed that more light was required to suppress HRP uptake by cones than was required for rods.[217,226] These observations, along with additional experiments involving the control of synaptic activity by manipulation of the ion content of the bathing media, were consistent with the interpretation that photoreceptors release less neurotransmitter when they are illuminated.[125,217] There is now also ample and elegant evidence to indicate that retrieval of the synaptic-vesicle membrane is mediated by an endocytic mechanism.[227] Interestingly, this retrieval mechanism is inoperative in cold-blooded animals maintained at 4 °C, but the fusion process attendant upon synaptic-vesicle release continues with a concomitant swelling of the terminal. Schaeffer and Raviola have used this effect to advantage in the study of membrane retrieval of the synaptic surface.[227] Turtle eyecups were incubated at 4 °C in the presence of HRP, a condition conducive to synaptic vesicle fusion but not retrieval. When these eyecups were warmed to 22 °C, there was a transient increase in HRP-labeled cisterns, coated vesicles, and vacuoles concomitant with a reduction in synaptic-terminal volume, thereby providing strong evidence that membrane retrieval is achieved by an endocytic process.

Where do vesicle release and retrieval occur? These processes have been observed only along the synaptic ridges that take part in the interaction between rod and cone terminals and invaginating processes of horizontal and bipolar cells.[214] There are three fundamental types of contact between photoreceptors and the dendrites of second-order neurons: synapses made with invaginating processes, such as those of horizontal and bipolar cells; basal contacts, such as those observed between the basal surfaces of cone pedicles and flat or diffuse bipolar dendrites; and gap junctions[216] (which occur between rods and cones and between cones). Gap junctions subserve electrical coupling between cells, and therefore no synaptic vesicles are involved. More will be said about the structure and function of gap junctions when they are discussed again in the section on the RPE. Synaptic vesicles have not been observed in relation to basal contacts, so the mode of intercellular signalling is not known for this type of junction, although Nelson and Kolb recently showed that cat bipolars communicate with cones at these junctions.[186] At the invaginating synapse, on the other hand, the case for chemical synaptic transmission is quite clear. Here rods and cones make contact with horizontal and bipolar cell dendrites through a synaptic ridge bisected by an unusual ribbonlike structure (Fig. 1-14*A* and *B*).[152,214] Intervening between one edge of the ribbon and the plasma membrane of the synaptic ridge is a trough-shaped structure called the *arciform density*.[152] Synaptic vesicles are bound to the synaptic ribbon in an orderly hexagonal array, which has prompted some to suggest that

the ribbon holds the vesicles in this strategic location and guides them to their point of fusion thought to be on the plasma membrane slope that extends from either side of the arciform density to the base of the synaptic ridge.[46,214] Vesicle fusion sites can be observed on this slope in specimens studied by freeze fracture. These fusion sites are similar to those observed in the neuromuscular junction.[120] Membrane retrieval is thought to take place at points remote from the slope of the synaptic ridge, near the mouth of the synaptic invagination and at points along the basal surface of the synaptic terminal.

Although it was at one time widely believed that retinal photoreceptors are isolated units, electrically independent of one another, this is no longer thought to be true.[81] Gap junctions are now known to electrically couple cones to cones and cones to rods.[69,82,104,214] In monkey retina, these intercellular junctions are present in regions where the respective cell types come together in close apposition with no intervening glial processes.[214] It is known from electrophysiological studies in lower vertebrates that the signals generated in dark-adapted toad rods result from the bleaching of an average of less than one rhodopsin molecule.[81] This is taken as evidence of the electrical coupling among photoreceptors. In the case of amphibians, however, this current spread may well occur through gap junctions between radial cytoplasmic fins that extend between adjacent inner segments in some species.[69,82] Nonetheless, since photoreceptors are believed to be isopotential throughout their cytoplasm,[10] gap junctions positioned anywhere along the cell, be it at the inner segment or at the synapse, should cause the spread of current to adjacent partners.

Finally, a brief comment should be made concerning putative photoreceptor neurotransmitters. Although this subject has been under active investigation for a number of years, information on the subject is extremely limited. Reports have been published concerning the synthesis of acetylcholine by turtle photoreceptors,[154] and alpha-bungarotoxin, a specific probe for acetylcholine at the neuromuscular junction, has been observed to bind to elements postsynaptic to both rods and cones in turtle and goldfish retina.[228,260] Nonetheless, the most recent evidence to date is derived from the observation of L-glutamate effects on goldfish cone horizontal cells.[133,257] L-aspartate and L-glutamate both depolarize cone horizontal cells. Although these amino acids exert their effects about equally when applied independently and at relatively high concentration (in the millimolar range), the effect of L-glutamate is enhanced about 15-fold by D-aspartate, which is known to act as a competitive inhibitor on the high-affinity uptake system for L-glutamate, thus raising the effective concentration of L-glutamate at the cone–horizontal cell synapse.[132,133] Enhancement of L-aspartate action was not observed under similar circumstances, even though D-aspartate is known to compete with the high-affinity uptake system for L-aspartate as well. The conclusion is that cone horizontal cells are much more sensitive to L-glutamate than they are to L-aspartate and that the former is a good neurotransmitter candidate for goldfish cones, at least for the type that synapses with H-1 horizontal cells.[132,133] Another laboratory has presented evidence that favors L-aspartate as a photoreceptor neurotransmitter.[257] Obviously this issue awaits resolution.

RETINAL PIGMENT EPITHELIUM — STRUCTURE AND FUNCTION

The retinal pigment epithelium (RPE) intervenes between the wide-bore, fenestrated capillaries of the choroidal layer and the photoreceptors of the neurosensory retina (Fig. 1-15). By virtue of this strategic location and by means of its plasma membrane permeability properties and intercellular junctions, the RPE controls the flow of nutrients and metabolites into and out of the neurosensory retina. For example, with the aid of specialized retinoid-binding proteins (*retinoid* is a generic term that includes retinol and its derivatives), the RPE receives retinol from the blood and transports it to the subretinal space or internalizes it from that space during the visual cycle.[15,34,43,47,115,116,169,250,255] If the retinoids are not needed immediately, they are esterified and stored in the RPE.[40,41,43] By enveloping the photoreceptor outer segments

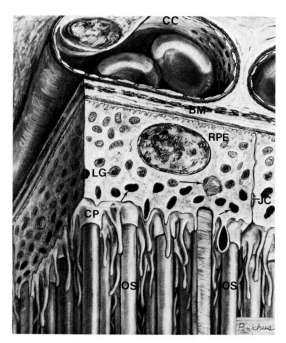

Figure 1-15. Rendition of the retinal photoreceptor–pigment epithelial complex and its adjacent blood supply. The light-sensitive outer segments (OS) of photoreceptors are in very close association with cellular processes (CP) of the retinal pigment epithelium (RPE). The RPE rests on Bruch's membrane (BM), a fibroelastic layer that separates the photoreceptor–RPE unit from its blood supply, the latter represented here by a layer of choroidal capillaries (CC). Melanin granules *(small arrows)* within the cytoplasm of the RPE prevent the scattering of excess light by absorbing it. Lipofuscin granules (LG), incompletely digested portions of phagosomes and various intracellular components, are visible, as is a phagosome *(large arrow)* itself. Phagosomes are recently ingested tips of photoreceptor outer segments. The RPE cells are joined together at their lateral surfaces by junctional complexes (JC). Included in these complexes are tight junctions which, in concert with similar junctions between endothelial cells of retinal vessels, serve as the extracellular site of the blood–retinal barrier. (Adapted from Young RW, Sears ML (eds): New Directions in Ophthalmic Research. New Haven, Yale University Press, 1981)

with its apical processes, secreting complex proteoglycans and glycosaminoglycans,[16,18] and moving water from the subretinal space,[171,180,274] the RPE creates the forces necessary to hold itself against the neurosensory retina with an intimacy sufficient to its nutritional role. This melanin-rich epithelial layer absorbs pho-

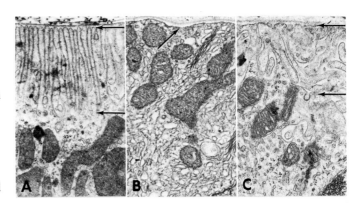

Figure 1-16. Basal RPE infoldings in chicken, frog, and rat. *(A)* The basal infoldings of the chicken RPE are among the deepest *(distance between upper and lower arrows)* encountered in common laboratory animals. *(B)* Frog RPE has virtually no basal infoldings; the basal surface *(arrow)* shows only mild undulations. *(C)* Rat RPE basal infoldings are intermediate in depth *(distance between upper and lower arrows)* when compared to chicken and frog. (×12,000)

tons that are not caught by the photoreceptors during transduction, thereby reducing their scatter and reflection. Finally, as mentioned earlier, the RPE plays a crucial role in photoreceptor renewal.[263] Daily, it phagocytizes the shed fragments of outer segments of rods and cones.[3,13,122,160,161,195,269,270,272]

Like the visual cells, the RPE cells are highly polarized in terms of their plasma membrane and cytoplasmic content.[28] Each cell is organized into a basal portion that rests upon a basement membrane, which in turn is attached to Bruch's membrane, the fibroelastic layer that is interposed between the RPE and the choroidal capillaries. The apical portion of the cell interacts with the photoreceptors. Laterally, the cell interacts with its neighbors through junctional complexes that form part of the blood–retina barrier.[65,68,130,206] Within the cell, organelles and inclusions are somewhat less polarized than the photoreceptor organelles. Nonetheless, melanin granules and mitochondria, for example, occupy fairly distinct regions of the cell. We will outline the organization of various domains of the RPE plasma membrane and elements of the cytoplasm independently and describe their function.

Basal Plasma Membrane

The basal plasma membrane of the RPE cell is thrown into numerous folds, the magnitude of which varies among species.[148] The most dramatic basal infoldings encountered by this author are seen in the RPE of the chicken (Fig. 1-16*A*), and the least pronounced are those ob-

served in the frog (*Rana pipiens;* Fig. 1-16*B*), where the surface shows only moderate undulations. Human and rodent RPE basal infoldings (Fig. 1-16*C*) are intermediate between these two extremes. The purpose of the basal infoldings is unproved, but the prevailing hypothesis is that they increase the surface area in the region of the cell. Although this would be a useful feature for transporting epithelia such as the RPE, one wonders why the magnitude of the infoldings varies so much among species. Korte has recently reported a new feature of the basal plasma membrane in rats, namely, tubular structures that are continuous with the extracellular spaces.[142] Again, the function of these structures is not known.

In 1976, Bok and Heller[34,116] showed with radioautographic methods (Fig. 1-17) that both the basal and lateral plasma membranes of the RPE are rich in receptors for the retinol-binding protein that circulates in the blood, the so-called plasma or serum retinol-binding protein (SRBP). This protein is secreted by liver hepatocytes as a tight complex with all-*trans* retinol (*t*-retinol);[106,136,205] in fact, *t*-retinol is required for its secretion.[185] The 1:1 retinol–SRBP complex is, in turn, bound in a 1:1 ratio to prealbumin. The purpose of this protein–protein association is thought to involve the conservation of circulating holo-SRBP, which has a molecular weight of 21,000, well within the limit for glomerular filtration.[106] The larger prealbumin (mol. wt. 55,000) gives the complex an effective molecular weight of about 75,000, which is well above the glomerular limit of approximately 45,000. Prealbumin has recently

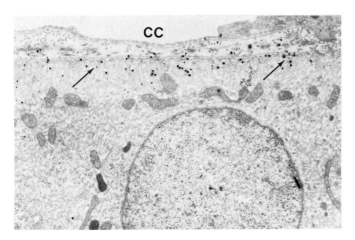

Figure 1-17. Rat RPE basal surface labeled with ^{125}I-retinol-binding protein (^{125}I-RBP). The radioactive protein was injected into the animal to allow binding to its membrane receptor. Unbound ^{125}I-RBP and blood were then flushed from the animal and the ^{125}I-RBP was fixed to its membrane receptor with glutaraldehyde. Silver grains *(arrows)* indicate the sites of association of RBP with basal infoldings. The radioactive carrier protein does not appear to enter the cell. The flushed choriocapillaris (CC) is free of radioactivity. (×7800)

been renamed transthyretin (TTR) because, in addition to binding retinol indirectly through SRBP, it binds one molecule of thyroxin (T_4) as well. For an excellent account of TTR and the retinoid-binding proteins, the reader is referred to recent reviews on the subject.[43,106]

Current evidence would indicate that SRBP, having bound to its membrane receptor on the basolateral surface of the RPE cell, releases the *t*-retinol into the cell but does not itself enter the cytoplasm. This interpretation is based on displacement studies with [125]I – labeled and nonradioactive SRBP and on the observation from electron-microscopic radioautograms that radioactive SRBP is not found in the cytoplasm following its binding to the cell surface.[34,115] This process deserves further study, however, in light of our current knowledge from other systems that involve ligand – receptor interactions. Asialoglycoprotein, after it binds to its membrane receptor on hepatocytes, enters the cell for a short distance through receptor-mediated endocytosis and is quickly cycled back to the plasma membrane.[61,101] The short intracellular distances traveled in this case would not be resolved by radioautographic methods. High-resolution electron-microscopic immunocytochemical studies are needed to resolve this question for the RPE. The subject of other intra- and extracellular retinoid-binding proteins, in terms of their localization and proposed function in the retina, will be presented later in this chapter.

Lateral Plasma Membrane

The lateral plasma membrane is quite different in appearance from its basal counterpart. The membrane surface is ordinarily quite straight with little evidence of infoldings. Electron-microscope radioautographic studies suggest that SRBP receptors are present on the lateral plasma membrane,[34] but beyond that we have no direct information regarding the comparative biochemistry of basal and lateral membranes. Their morphologies would indicate different chemical compositions, but transport physiologists generally refer to the basal and lateral membranes as a single functional unit, hence the term *basolateral.*

As one approaches the boundary between the basal and apical surface of the cell, striking alterations are observed in membrane ultrastructure, for it is at this point that the interepithelial junctional complexes express themselves. Hudspeth and Yee have shown that the complexes are similar in composition among vertebrate classes ranging from primates to teleost fish, although, unlike other epithelia, the domains of the respective junctional components overlap.[130] These junctional components include gap junctions, which lie near the apical surface, a *zonula adherens* (adhering junction) situated in a more basal direction, and a *zonula occludens* (tight junction) which overlaps the others. Thus, in freeze-fracture images of the protoplasmic face (P-face) of the lateral RPE plasma

Figure 1-18. Freeze-fracture electron micrographs of mouse RPE. *(A)* The lateral plasma membrane (upper region of figure) of the RPE cell is involved in the formation of junctional complexes near the apical portion of the cell body. Tight junctions consist of interconnecting elevated ridges *(long arrows)* on the P-face and complementary grooves *(short arrows)* on the E-face of the cleaved plasma membranes. Interspersed among the tight junction components are clusters of intramembranous particles *(arrowheads)* that represent gap junctions. Each particle within the cluster is thought to represent a hexameric transmembrane channel called a *connexon,* which allows the controlled transfer of ions and small molecules from one cell to its neighbor. These structures thereby subserve the phenomenon of electrical coupling and metabolic cooperation among cells. (×33,000). *(B)* Higher magnification of area outlined in *A.* The interconnecting ridges *(arrows)* of the tight junction and gap junctions *(arrowheads)* with their connexons are more easily seen. (×79,200; courtesy of M. Matthes)

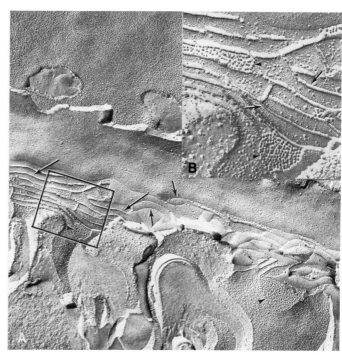

membrane, dislike patches of intramembranous particles characteristic of gap junctions are mingled with the anastomosing ridges typical of zonulae occludentes (Fig. 1-18). Both the zonula adherens and zonula occludens form unbroken belts around each epithelial cell. Since the ridges of the zonula occludens represent points of membrane fusion, the result is focal obliteration of the extracellular space and formation of a barrier to the diffusion of molecules and even ions in this region of the complex.[234] Thus the zonula occludens represents the anatomical substrate for the high resistance that is measured across the RPE (350–600 ohms/cm^2)[65,235] and a point at which blood constituents are prevented from entering the neural retina. (The other component of the blood-retinal barrier is found at the level of zonulae occludentes between endothelial cells of retinal blood vessels).[68] The gap junctions contribute very little to the barrier function of the com-

plex.[216] Instead, they represent low electrical resistance pathways and sites for metabolic cooperation between adjacent epithelial cells.[74,98,137,170] Each component in the array of intramembranous particles (connexon) is thought to represent a transmembrane channel that lies in series with an identical channel in the adjacent cell.[105] As a result, the cells are connected by tiny intercellular tubes with an inner diameter of about 1 nm through which ions and small molecules are allowed to pass under permissive conditions. It is believed that calcium ions or protons control the patency of these channels.[170,221,244] Like the gap junctions, the zonulae adherentes provide little in the way of a barrier. These junctions leave no imprint on freeze-fracture replicas on the plasma membrane, hence no intramembranous particles are discernible. By transmission electron microscopy, however, the junctions exhibit a rather uniform extracellular space of about 10 nm as

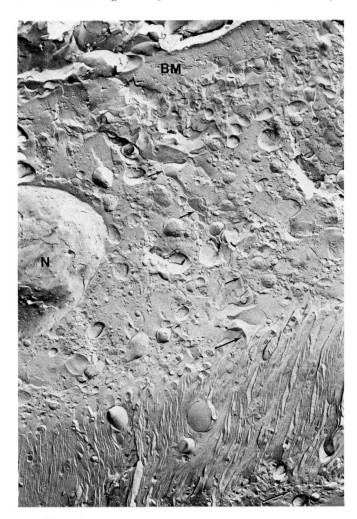

Figure 1-19. Freeze-fracture electron micrograph of the RPE layer detached from the neural retina. Bruch's membrane (BM), the nucleus (N) of an RPE cell, and the step-fractured interface between two adjacent cells *(short arrows)* are observed. The long and numerous apical microvilli *(region between two long arrows)* are also seen. (×8400; courtesy of M. Matthes)

well as complex interaction with cytoskeletal elements.[130] Some structural role is therefore implied for them.

Apical Plasma Membrane

The apical plasma membrane of the RPE is clearly the most complex in terms of topography. This region of the cell is thrown into complex arrays of microvilli (Fig. 1-19) and sheaths (see Fig. 1-15) that increase its surface area greatly. Steinberg and Miller have compared the apical and basal surface areas in the bullfrog *(Rana catesbeiana)* RPE.[235] The apical processes increase the cell surface by about 30-fold, whereas the basal infoldings increase that surface by a factor of only three. The values will

undoubtedly vary among species, but the point is well made by these figures.

The cell processes that mediate the increase in surface area differ among species. Some are slender projections that truly resemble microvilli; others are sheetlike and therefore lamellar in form.[11,231,236,237] The lamellar form ensheathes the distal outer segments of rods and cones and, particularly in the case of the latter, forms elaborate leaflets much like the calyces (husks) that surround an ear of corn.[88,207] The lamellar processes participate in the phagocytosis of shed distal rod and cone outer segment packets (presumptive phagosomes) during the renewal process.[237]

The precise role played by the apical RPE during the phagocytosis of distal outer segment fragments remains a matter of conjecture. It is generally assumed that the apical plasma membrane contains specific receptors for ligands on the outer segment plasma membrane.[191] These ligands are believed to be either added or unmasked at some point prior to the phagocytic event. This hypothesis, although unproved, is a reasonable one since uptake of presumptive phagosomes does not take place at a regular pace throughout the day, a consequence, no doubt, of the fact that a given photoreceptor does not shed discs on a daily basis. Under normal circumstances, a given rod photoreceptor will shed a portion of its outer segment every fourth day. Thus there are quiet periods when that complement of discs and its investing plasma membrane are not recognized as foreign (using an analogy from immunology). These periods are interrupted by active episodes that probably involve some form of receptor – ligand interaction between the plasma membranes of the RPE and the outer segment.[13,160,161,195,269,270] Indeed, Hall has shown that cultured rat RPE cells preferentially phagocytize light-exposed outer segment fragments over dark-adapted ones.[108]

The sequence of events that takes place during the shedding and ingestion process has been beautifully demonstrated by transmission electron microscopy of rods in rhesus monkey and nonfoveal cones in the human retina.[237,266] The reader is referred to these studies for details. It would appear that the shedding process is initiated in the outer segment by a curling of distal discs and invagination of the outer segment plasma membrane at the point of scission. Secondarily, the plasma membrane of enveloping RPE processes surrounds the presumptive phagosome and draws it into the RPE soma. Cytoskeletal elements are intimately involved in this process.[58] Their role will be discussed later.

The apical RPE membrane is rich in sodium – potassium ATPase (Na$^+$-K$^+$ ATPase).[28,30,181,197,234] Evidence for this was initially established by the work of Steinberg and Miller, in which the effects of ouabain, a cardiac glycoside, on Na$^+$-K$^+$ ATPase were measured on the apical and basolateral plasma membranes of isolated, perfused bullfrog *(Rana catesbeiana)* RPE – choroid preparations.[181,234] Biochemical

and morphological evidence was subsequently provided from microdissected RPE and from tissue radioautograms of RPE – choroid preparations exposed to ^{3}H-ouabain.[28,30,197] Polarization of Na$^+$-K$^+$ ATPase on the apical plasma membrane is rather unusual for epithelial cells, and in addition to the RPE has been observed only in choroid plexus epithelium,[211] a cell monolayer that has a close developmental kinship with the RPE. In other epithelia such as kidney proximal tubules, Na$^+$-K$^+$ ATPase predominates on the basolateral plasma membrane.[150,151] In the RPE, this intrinsic membrane enzyme, which is, in fact, the Na$^+$-K$^+$ exchange pump common to all eukaryotic cells, is thought to provide the motive force for maintaining adhesion of the RPE to the neural retina.[171,180,274] Other factors, such as the extracellular matrix and interdigitations between photoreceptor outer segments and RPE apical processes apparently play a role in this important function as well.[171,274]

Cytoplasmic Organelles and Inclusions

This discussion of RPE organelles and inclusions is not intended to be exhaustive because the subject has been well covered in earlier reviews. The reader is directed to two contributions that deal with the subject in great detail, particularly with respect to human RPE and species differences.[121,148] Several features that are somewhat unusual for epithelia, however, deserve mention.

The RPE contains, in addition to the standard organelles and inclusions, two types of pigment granules, one containing melanin[85,100] and the other lipofuscin.[86,240] Within the RPE cell soma, melanin and lipofuscin granules tend to be intermixed within the apical two thirds of the cell (see Fig. 1-15). In addition, melanin granules occupy apical microvilli which vary in length among species. In mammals, melanin granules that occupy microvilli are not capable of movement during dark adaptation.[52,148] The melanin of reptiles is able to migrate only slightly. In teleost fish, amphibians, and some birds, however, dramatic melanin movement is observed.[53] RPE melanin in the leopard frog *(Rana pipiens),* for example, is crowded into the apical two thirds of the soma in the dark-adapted state, but during light adaptation it extends along with the long apical microvilli nearly as far as the outer limiting membrane, which is comprised of junctional complexes between Müller and photoreceptor cells.

Melanin is, of course, a biosynthetic product.[121] Lipofuscin, on the other hand, is residual material derived from phagocytic and autophagic activity and can therefore be derived from the incomplete digestion of intracellular organelles or outer segment discs. The lipofuscin content of the RPE increases with age and can, in extreme cases, fill the cell and impair its function.[86,113] A dietary deficiency in vitamin E, an antioxidant[242] present in photoreceptors, has been shown to result in elevated levels of lipofuscin in the RPE.[84,113] The dearth of antioxidant allows the formation of free radicals which, in turn, participate in the formation of peroxides.[138,249] Unsaturated fatty and side chains in outer segment disc phospholipids are cross-linked by these peroxides and are thereby rendered somewhat refractory to the action of lysosomal hydrolytic enzymes. The rapid exchange of old fatty acids for new ones in the outer segment[24] probably protects against this process as does the presence of vitamin E and other antioxidants.[24]

Because of its vigorous and lifelong phagocytic and autophagic[215] activity, the RPE is rich in hydrolytic lysosomal enzymes.[17,80] The effectiveness of this system is appreciated when one considers that a single rat RPE cell is in contact with 250–300 rods.[38] About one fourth of these rods shed approximately 100 discs each day (one tenth of the total outer segment length) soon after light onset. Yet by the end of the day, there is very little evidence of this episode within the cytoplasm of the RPE cell. The phagolysosomal system has considerable reserve. Following laser treatment or other types of light injury to the photoreceptor layer, the phagosomes derived from the resulting photoreceptor debris can occupy over 70 percent of the RPE cell's volume.[149,172] This material is quickly digested by the lysosomal system.

The subject of myeloid bodies should be discussed briefly in light of their superficial resemblance to phagosomes. Myeloid bodies (Fig. 1-20) are components of the smooth endoplasmic reticulum and are particularly pronounced in the RPE of some of the lower vertebrates (fish, amphibians, reptiles, and birds). Although they have been reported recently in a mammalian retina as well, they are small and normally go undetected.[241] The function of myeloid bodies has never been determined. Porter and Yamada suggested a photoreceptive function which might serve to trigger photomechanical movements.[210] Until recently, it was held that all animals that exhibit this phenomenon do, in fact, have myeloid bodies in their RPE cells. The recent observation of small myeloid bodies in the squirrel retina,[241] however, challenges this otherwise neat correlation since mammalian retinas do not exhibit photomechanical movement.[53] Furthermore, Liebman and coworkers have provided rather convincing evidence that RPE photomechanical movements are triggered by the photoreceptors.[164] Some amphibians show remarkable diurnal variations in myeloid body morphology suggestive of a significant role in or response to changes in RPE metabolic activity.[177,261]

Finally, the RPE of some species contains prominent lipid droplets that are rich in retinyl esters, the storage form of retinol.[44] Injection of ^{3}H-labeled retinoids into the circulation causes the RPE oil droplets to rapidly accumulate ^{3}H-retinyl esters. The lipid droplets also receive esterified retinol that migrates to the RPE following photoreceptor illumination.

Cytoskeleton

The RPE cytoskeleton is a subject that has received only modest attention during the past decade, but some excellent reports have appeared nonetheless, particularly with regard to its role in melanin granule movement and phagocytosis. For an informative and engaging review of the RPE cytoskeleton the reader is directed to a contribution by Burnside and Laties.[53]

Actin is the only RPE cytoplasmic filament (diameter 4–7 nm) that has been studied in detail. Myosin (diameter 12–20 nm) and intermediate filaments (diameter 10 nm) are present, but little is currently known about their

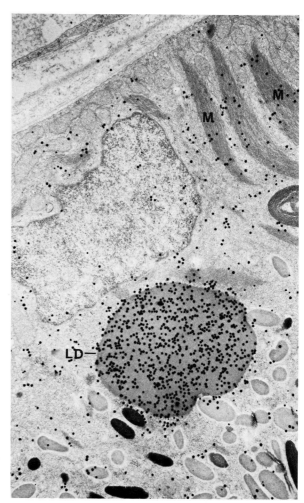

Figure 1-20. Autoradiogram of frog RPE following intravascular injection of ³H-retinol. The RPE of some vertebrates contains lipid droplets (LD) that serve as storage sites for retinyl esters. These depots of retinyl ester, which are used in the regeneration of photopigments during the visual cycle, are in a dynamic state and therefore are readily labeled with exogenous ³H-retinol as evidenced by the heavy concentration of silver grains over the LD. Myeloid bodies (M) are also prominent organelles in some lower vertebrates. (×9600)

function and distribution in the RPE.[208] Likewise, microtubules have been studied to a limited extent.[50,131]

The role of actin and microtubules in pigmentary migration has been re-examined in the context of an old controversy—namely, do melanin granules move independently within the apical microvilli or do they migrate as a result of microvillar contraction? Burnside and coworkers recently confirmed the original observation by Kuhne that the melanin granules move within fixed apical process.[50,147] Pigment migration is an energy-requiring event that is currently thought to involve actin filaments alone rather than in combination with microtubules, although both types of filament are present.[50] The current evidence for the involvement of actin is pharmacological, namely that cytochalasins B and D abolish pigmentary movement within the microvilli but colchicine does not. Interestingly, cytochalasins inhibit only pigment dispersion and not retraction into the cell body.[50] The mechanisms for maintenance of pigmentary dispersion within the apical microvilli and contraction of same are currently hypothetical. Even the issue of microtubule involvement in melanin granule migration within the microvilli remains open. Initially, Murray and Dubin reported that microtubules were not present in the apical microvilli and concluded that they do not play a role in migration.[184] However, with appropriate fixation methods, microtubules can be observed, at least in certain teleost fish.[50,52,53] Unlike the microtubules in the cell soma, they demonstrate a high stability to colchicine, so their effects on pigmentary migration cannot be tested by pharmacological experiments.[50]

Evidence for the role of microtubules in melanin movement within the RPE soma is quite convincing, on the other hand.[50] When colchicine is injected intraocularly into light-adapted fish and the animals are subsequently dark adapted, melanin granules migrate from the most distal regions of apical microvilli but do not continue their migration into the soma. Ultrastructural analysis following colchicine treatment indicates that somal microtubules are depolymerized by the drug. Thus, the evidence strongly suggests that somal microtubules are involved in the movement of pigment granules within the soma and that the stability and perhaps the function of these microtubules is quite different from that of those in the apical processes. Colchicine binds to depolymerized tubulin monomers. Hence when the equilibrium between the depolymerized and polymerized state shifts in the direction of the former, microtubules are more readily dispersed by colchicine and its related alkaloids.

Contributions by cytoskeletal elements to RPE phagocytosis have been studied with respect to actin only, and in this context certain analogies have been drawn between the RPE and wandering macrophages. In macrophages, it has been shown that actin is involved in engulfment of particles, whereas microtubules somehow mediate the delivery of new phagosomes to primary lysosomes for digestion.[239] Chaitin and Hall recently studied the distribution of actin filaments in cultured rat RPE cells in the nonphagocytic state and after feeding them rod outer segment fragments.[58] The results were consistent with those observed by others for the macrophage. Immunofluorescence of spreading cells showed parallel and crossed arrays of actin bundles traversing the length of the cell at multiple focal planes. Confluent cells exhibited actin along intercellular margins in addition to the patterns described for isolated spreading cells. Upon challenge with rod outer segment fragments, the filament bundle arrangements persisted and, in addition, "feltworks" of actin filaments similar to those observed in macrophages were indicated by intense foci of fluorescence assembled under the domains of the plasma membrane to which the outer segment fragments were attached. Scanning electron microscopy revealed that, following attachment, the rod outer segment fragments were surrounded by an "attachment saucer." Numerous microvilli emanated from the cell surface and from the edge of the saucer as well. These microvilli fused during the engulfment step. The actin feltwork persisted for a while around the phagosome and then dissipated. The precise relationship between this process *in vitro* and that which takes place *in vivo* remains to be examined. *In vivo,* distal rod and cone outer segments are in close contact with apical RPE processes at all times, but it is only following the shedding event that recognition, attachment, and engulfment take place.

It has been known for some time that the dystrophic rat RPE has a phagocytic defect, and it has been assumed that the problem was a failure in recognition of shed distal outer segments.[31,32,119,183] Interestingly, Chaitin and Hall[57] have shown that cultured dystrophic rat RPE cells are capable of what appears to be normal recognition and attachment of rod outer segment fragments although, as predicted from a variety of earlier studies, internalization of the particles occurs only rarely.[31,32,119,183] They have interpreted this as a defect in the transmembrane signalling that is thought to precede the engulfment process. In the rare cases when engulfment did occur in their cell cultures, normal actin feltwork patterns were observed in association with the phagosome. Therefore, it was concluded that the contractile apparatus necessary for ingestion is normal in the dystrophic retina.

RETINOID TRANSPORT: THE ROLE OF BINDING PROTEINS IN THIS PROCESS

Historical Aspects

The final segment of this chapter reviews recent evidence that has accumulated regarding retinoid-binding proteins and their presumed role in the delivery of retinol and its derivatives from the blood to the retina. This (currently) very active field has been reviewed in other chapters of this book in terms of its biochemical aspects. We will deal primarily with immunocytochemical localization of these proteins, a subject that is very new. However it will be useful to first provide some background to these studies by briefly reviewing the biochemical experiments that led to their detection in the retina and to define the group of binding proteins that are now known to reside there.

The laboratories of Chader and Wiggert, Saari, and Futterman, were the first to explore the subject of cellular retinoid-binding proteins in the retina.[99,222,223,250-255] Chader, Wiggert, and coworkers used classical sucrose-density techniques for the initial detection of retinoid-binding proteins in the RPE and neural retina. The technique involved the addition of ^{3}H-labeled retinoids to supernatants from homogenized RPE choroid and neural retina. The supernatants were then centrifuged in a continuous sucrose gradient until equilibrium was achieved. Radioactive samples from the gradient were correlated with sedimentation coefficients for proteins of known molecular weight. The specificity of binding for various retinoids was also tested by competition with nonradioactive retinoids. Using this approach, Wiggert, Bergsma, Chader, and coworkers were able to demonstrate two binding proteins in the neural retina, one with a sedimentation coefficient of 2S and another, larger 7 — 8S species.[15,254] The 2S protein was specific in its binding of retinol, that is to say, ^{3}H-retinol was displaced from its binding site by excess nonradioactive retinol but not by other retinoids. The 7 — 8S protein bound retinol but was less specific. Within the RPE choroid, only the retinol-specific, 2S species was found. The 2S-binding protein resembled an intracellular retinol-binding protein first reported by Bashor and associates in nonocular rat tissues, including testis and liver.[12] It is now known that this 2S protein, named *cellular retinol binding protein* (CRBP), is present in all tissues except blood.[60] Its molecular weight is approximately 16,600, and it is distinct from RBP (mol. wt. 21,000) which was discovered by Goodman and colleagues.[106,136] Futterman, Saari, and colleagues, meanwhile, were detecting and characterizing still other retinoid-binding proteins in the RPE and neural

retina. Cellular retinoic acid – binding protein (CRABP), initially described by Ong and Chytil[196] in rat nonocular tissues, was detected in the bovine neural retina by gel filtration techniques.[223] In addition, these authors confirmed the presence of CRBP in the bovine neural retina and purified both CRBP and CRABP from that source.[223] The molecular weights for the two proteins were similar (16,600 and 16,300, respectively), and it was determined that CRBP was present in both neural retina and RPE choroid, whereas CRABP was found only in the neural retina. Subsequently, this group identified and purified yet another binding protein from the bovine neural retina which is specific for 11-*cis* isomers of retinol and retinal.[99] This unique binding protein has a molecular weight of 33,000 which is far removed from that of CRBP and CRABP. Initially, it was believed that the binding protein was specific for 11-*cis* retinal only and it was therefore given the name *cellular 11-*cis *retinal-binding protein* (CRALBP). Later these investigators found that CRALBP in the neural retina carries 11-*cis* retinol as well, whereas its only endogenous retinoid in the RPE is retinal. Nonetheless, the original nomenclature has been retained for convenience.

Finally, in providing a current list of retinoid-binding proteins that have been isolated from the retina, we must return to the 7 — 8S-binding protein described by Wiggert and associates.[15,251] Adler and coworkers[1,2] recently purified a large glycoprotein (subunit mol. wt. ≈ 140,000)[169] from the neural retina that carries relatively small amounts of *t*-retinol, 11-*cis* retinol[169] and 11-*cis* retinal* although with no great specificity. Chader and associates named this protein interphotoreceptor retinol-binding protein; Liou and colleagues called it interstitial retinol-binding protein (IRBP).[153,169] This protein is probably the 7 — 8S-binding protein first described by Wiggert and colleagues, although at the time these authors were uncertain of its extracellular location since they were working with retinal homogenates.[15,251] As described below, its extracellular location has recently

* J. Saari, Personal communication

been unequivocally demonstrated by immuno-cytochemical methods.

Immunocytochemical Studies of Retinoid-Binding Proteins in the Retina

Bunt-Milam and Saari were the first to localize retinoid-binding proteins in the retina by immunocytochemical means.[47] Peroxidase – anti-peroxidase (PAP) localization was performed using both light- and electron microscopy. IRBP, as predicted by its extraction properties from intact retina, was shown to be extracellular. Its localization within the neural retina was sharply limited to the region between the apical RPE surface and the outer limiting membrane. Thus, both its retinoid-binding properties and its localization within the interphotoreceptor matrix are consistent with a role for the intercellular transport of retinol, the directionality of which remains an open question. The localization of CRALBP was also reported by Bunt-Milam and Saari.[47] This binding protein was present in RPE as predicted from the earlier biochemical studies of Saari and coworkers in which it was shown that CRALBP could be extracted from the RPE choroid as well as from the neural retina.[223] However, its distribution in the neural retina was surprising.[47] CRALBP was found in Müller cells only. This finding is remarkable for two reasons. One would have expected an 11-*cis* retinal-binding protein to be present in the one cell type of the neural retina that requires the 11-*cis* isomer for its function, namely the photoreceptor. Furthermore, the Müller cell, heretofore unrecognized as a factor in the visual cycle, now has to be viewed from a new perspective.

Bok and coworkers have also recently studied the localization of retinoid-binding proteins by immunocytochemistry.[35,36] Like CRALBP, CRBP proved to be highly localized in the retina.[36] Light microscopic examination of the rat retina with the aid of rabbit – anti-rat antibodies and the PAP method indicated that CRBP is expressed in the RPE as predicted from earlier biochemical data. In the peripheral retina, however, there was a dramatic reduction in the amount of CRBP as the transition was made from the RPE to the epithelium covering the

pars plicata and pars plana of the ciliary body. Within the neural retina, the localization of CRBP, like that of CRALBP, was a surprise. The only cell type of the neural retina positive for antibody staining was the Müller cell. Within the rat neural retina, CRBP was most prominently displayed in Müller cell end-feet that abut the vitreal surface. PAP-positive staining also was observed as a bilaminar pattern within the inner plexiform layer. The cellular source of this stain could not be resolved by light microscopic methods, therefore ferritin-conjugated antibody analysis of ultrathin sections was performed. Ferritin labeling in the inner plexiform layer was limited to processes of Müller cells that ramify in that region. It should be added at this point that CRBP in the rat neural retina may not be limited to Müller cell end-feet and processes in the inner plexiform layer but may simply not be sufficiently concentrated in other regions of the cell to allow detection by our methods. Indeed, recent unpublished studies on human retina (Bok and Ong) have shown that rabbit antibodies directed against human CRBP stain the entire Müller cell. Bok and associates have further investigated the ultrastructural localization of CRBP in the rat RPE by ferritin-labeled antibody methods.[36] CRBP was uniformly distributed throughout the cytosol of the RPE (Fig. 1-21) including basal infoldings and apical microvilli. In addition, a significant amount of CRBP was found within the nucleus, in keeping with the current theory from Ong and Chytils's laboratories that retinol may somehow be involved in the control of gene expression.[60] Thus a dual role is suggested for CRBP in the RPE, namely intracellular transport of retinol and maintenance of the appropriate differentiated state of the cell through gene interaction.

Bok and associates have studied the localization of IRBP in the cow (Fig. 1-22) and monkey (Fig. 1-23) retina as well.[35] Their light-microscopic PAP results confirm the observations of Bunt-Milam and Saari with respect to the extracellular location of IRBP.[47] Their electron microscopic localizations differ from those of Bunt-Milam and Saari, however, with respect to cones. The latter authors, based on their PAP ultrastructural studies, reported that IRBP was

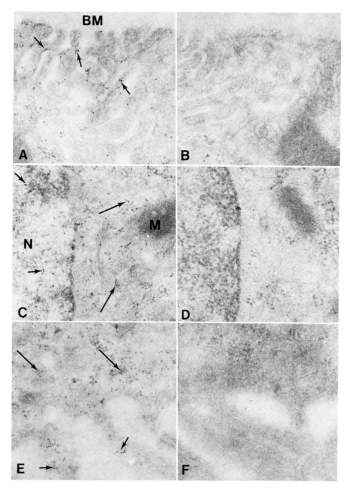

Figure 1-21. Electron microscopic immunocytochemistry of cellular retinol-binding protein in the rat RPE. The tissue was fixed, embedded, and sectioned as described in Figure 1-12. The sections shown in *A, C,* and *E* were reacted successively with affinity-purified rabbit antirat CRBP IgG, biotinyl goat antirabbit IgG, and avidin-conjugated ferritin. The sections shown in *B, D,* and *F* are controls that were treated the same way except that nonimmune rabbit IgG was substituted for immune rabbit anti-CRBP IgG. *(A)* Bruch's membrane (BM) and basal infoldings of the RPE. Bruch's membrane is not stained, but the cytoplasm of the basal infoldings is stained with ferritin-antibody complexes *(arrows).* *(B)* Nonimmune control for *A. (C)* An area from the middle portion of an RPE cell. The nucleus (N) is stained *(short arrows)* as well as the cytoplasm *(long arrows).* Mitochondria (M) are negative. *(D)* Nonimmune control for *C. (E)* The cytoplasm of the apical cell body binds ferritin antibody complexes *(long arrows)* as does the cytoplasm of the apical microvilli *(short arrows). (F)* Nonimmune control for *E.* (×33,000)

present between cone outer segment discs, perhaps owing to its ability to diffuse into that region from the interphotoreceptor space. The immunoferritin localizations of Bok and colleagues did not confirm this, since no ferritin labeling was observed over cone outer segment discs of either cow or monkey. In light of the relatively great molecular weight of IRBP, it is doubtful that this glycoprotein could gain entry to the cone intradiscal space. Bok and colleagues were unable to determine the cellular source of the IRBP with immunoferritin staining, but reports from several laboratories indicate that it is secreted by cells in the neural retina and not the RPE. Hollyfield and coworkers recently provided indirect radioautographic and biochemical data from *Xenopus* retina that implicate the rod photoreceptors in the secretion of IRBP.[123] Bunt-Milam and Saari have localized IRBP in

bovine rod and cone inner segments.* The protein is present in vesicles positioned near the junctional complexes of the outer limiting membrane.

Purification of specific retinoid-binding proteins resident within the retina, analysis of their endogenous retinoids, and localization of the binding proteins to specific cell types have helped significantly in our understanding of the visual cycle and, like any new endeavor, have raised new questions as well. The embryonic scheme that is emerging with respect to the various binding proteins and their role in the visual cycle is described below and summarized in Figure 1-24.

Holo-RBP interacts with specific membrane receptors on the basolateral surface of the RPE

* Personal communication

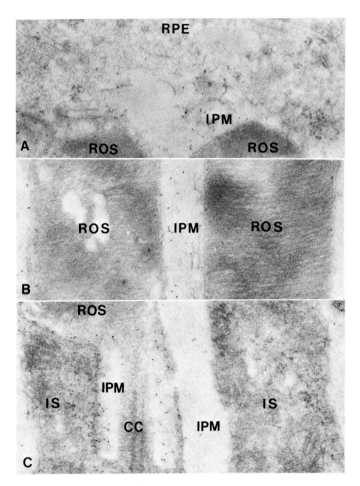

Figure 1-22. Electron-microscopic immunocytochemistry of interphotoreceptor retinol-binding protein in the cow retina. Tissues and sections were processed as in Figure 1-12, except that affinity-purified rabbit antibovine-IRBP IgG was used in place of antiopsin IgG. *(A)* Interface between retinal pigment epithelium (RPE) and rod outer segment (ROS) distal ends. IRBP is present in the extracellular space as evidenced by the presence of ferritin over the interphotoreceptor matrix (IPM). *(B)* Interphotoreceptor matrix (IPM) and rod outer segments (ROS) about half the distance between distal ends and bases of the outer segments. IRBP staining is uniform. *(C)* Rod outer segment (ROS), inner segments (IS), and connecting cilium (CC) of adjacent rods. The interphotoreceptor matrix (IPM) surrounding the CC and between apical IS and ROS is labeled. ($\times$ 33,000)

and, by a mechanism that remains to be elucidated, delivers *t*-retinol into the cell.[34,115,116] Current evidence suggests that the RBP remains outside the cell.[34] The most likely binding protein to receive *t*-retinol following its entry into the RPE cell is CRBP, because its endogenous retinoid is also *t*-retinol.[60] CRALBP carries only 11-*cis* retinal in the RPE (recall that this protein in the neural retina carries both 11-*cis* retinal and 11-*cis* retinol).[222] The source of 11-*cis* retinal in the RPE remains unresolved, but one likely origin is from unbleached rhodopsin carried into the RPE by phagocytized outer segment disc packets.[47] Theoretically, this 11-*cis* retinal could be salvaged from digested phagosomes, although it is not known whether it would survive the acid conditions in the phagolysosome. In addition, the 11-*cis* retinal could arise through the combined action of an alcohol dehydrogenase[168,222,275,276] that has been re-

ported in the RPE and a *t*-retinal isomerase.[168,222,275,276] CRALBP serves as an effective substrate carrier for the action of RPE alcohol dehydrogenase,[222] but there is no current evidence that the RPE is capable of isomerizing *t*-retinol.

By virtue of its distribution within the cell, CRBP is in a position to transport *t*-retinol into the nucleus for gene interaction and to move it across the epithelium into the apical projections for delivery into the subretinal space.[36] The mode and form of retinoid delivery across the apical plasma membrane have not yet been determined, but CRBP itself does not appear to be secreted since there is no immunocytochemical evidence for its presence in the interphotoreceptor space.[36] Within the interphotoreceptor space, the only current candidate for acceptance of retinoids from the RPE during dark adaptation or for the delivery of *t*-retinol to the RPE

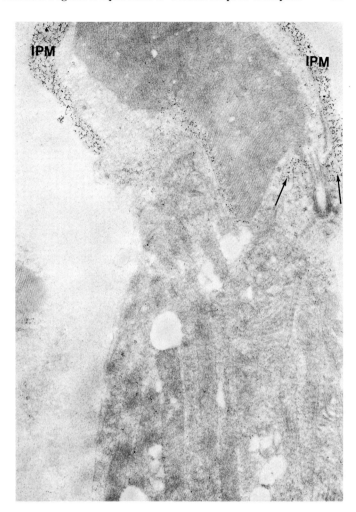

Figure 1-23. Electron-microscopic immunocytochemistry of IRBP localization in the vicinity of a monkey cone. The tissue was fixed and processed as in Figure 1-22. The interphotoreceptor matrix (IPM) stains heavily with ferritin-antibody complexes including the matrix that surrounds the connecting cilium *(arrows)*. The cone outer segment, however, is not labeled. The uneven distribution of IPM was observed both in Lowicryl K4M and Araldite-embedded tissue from this retina. This could be due to shrinkage or partial extraction of the IPM during tissue processing. ($\times$ 16,500)

following its release from photoreceptors during the bleaching of photopigments is IRBP.[47,153,169] IRBP could serve as a multidirectional shuttle protein with the ability to interact with the plasma membranes of RPE, Müller cell, and photoreceptor alike. As stated earlier, IRBP contains, in addition to *t*-retinol, small amounts of 11-*cis* retinol[169] and 11-*cis* retinal* the source of which has not been determined. In part, 11-*cis* retinol could originate from the photoreceptor outer segment during dark exchange of this retinoid.[72]

Where, then, do the 11-*cis* isomerization of *t*-retinol and the oxidation of retinol take place? This remains one of the great unresolved mysteries of the visual cycle.[76,127] An early report

* J. Saari, Personal communication

implicated the RPE in this process,[126] but this was never substantiated. In light of current evidence for an abundance of retinoid-binding proteins in the Müller cell and evidence for endogenous 11-*cis* retinal and retinol bound to CRALBP in the neural retina, the Müller cell must be given serious consideration along with the RPE as an isomerization site.[36,47] It is conceivable that the Müller cell is the source of the small amount of 11-*cis* retinol bound to IRBP in the interphotoreceptor space. Following its production in the Müller cell, 11-*cis* retinol could be delivered to photoreceptors that could, in turn, perform the final oxidation step to 11-*cis* retinal. Bridges showed that outer segments of the frog retina contain significant amounts of 11-*cis* retinol.[42] Furthermore, the frog photoreceptors, unlike those of mammals, can synthe-

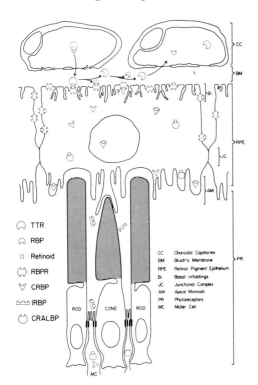

TTR
RBP
Retinoid
RBPR
CRBP
IRBP
CRALBP

ROD   CONE   ROD

CC	Choroidal Capillaries
BM	Bruch's Membrane
RPE	Retinal Pigment Epithelium
Bi	Basal Infoldings
JC	Junctional Complex
AM	Apical Microvilli
PR	Photoreceptors
MC	Müller Cell

Figure 1-24. Retinoid-binding proteins and their putative roles in the transport of retinoids into and within the retina. The retinol-binding protein (RBP) present in blood is secreted by the liver as a complex with all-*trans* retinol. This holo-RBP circulates as a complex with transthyretin (TTR), formerly called prealbumin. The binding of TTR and RBP is strongest when retinol is present on RBP. In the eye, the holo-RBP–TTR complex passes through fenestrations in the choroidal capillaries and the holo-RBP binds to its specific membrane receptor (RBPR) on the basolateral surface of the retinal pigment epithelium (RPE), thereby delivering retinol into that cell layer. Apo-RBP and TTR dissociate and return to the choroidal capillaries. The RBP (mol. wt. 21,000), with its reduced affinity for TTR is now unprotected from kidney filtration. Following its entry into the RPE, *trans*-retinol is probably bound initially to cellular retinol-binding protein (CRBP) since the endogenous retinoid for CRBP is the same as that of RBP, whereas the endogenous retinoid for cellular retinaldehyde-binding protein (CRALBP) in the RPE is 11-*cis* retinal. The binding of retinol to CRALBP requires oxidation to retinal as well as 11-*cis* isomerization. Although it is known that the RPE can oxidize retinol to retinal, the cellular site and mechanism for 11-*cis* isomerization are currently unknown. CRBP apparently delivers *trans*-retinol to the nucleus where it may play a role in gene expression. Neither the mode of delivery of retinoid(s) to the

size 11-*cis* retinal from 11-*cis* retinol.[43] In the frog, IRBP could in fact have a high affinity for photoreceptor plasma membranes when its bound retinoids are in the 11-*cis* configuration and a high affinity for apical RPE plasma membrane when its bound retinoid is *t*-retinol. This speculation is testable by radioautographic techniques of the type performed by Bok and Heller with [125]IRBP on the basolateral membrane of the RPE.[34,116] The situation in mammals is different from that in frogs. Mammalian photoreceptors lack an 11-*cis* oxidoreductase system.[168,276] Therefore in the mammalian retina, the above scheme would have to be altered to include an additional pathway for 11-*cis* retinol that would take it from the Müller cell to the RPE for oxidation prior to being delivered to the photoreceptors.

Although the story remains far from complete, the study of retinoid-binding proteins has significantly enhanced our understanding of the intraretinal transport of vitamin A and its derivatives. Still lacking in the scheme is a well-characterized retinyl ester–binding protein for the RPE, although Wiggert and associates have recently reported a 6S binding species that shows some specificity for esters.[252] A major surprise to investigators in the field has been the lack of soluble retinoid-binding proteins in photoreceptors, the ultimate target cells in the visual cycle. To date, the only apparent binding pro-

interphotoreceptor space nor the form of retinoid delivered there by the RPE is known. Interphotoreceptor retinol-binding protein (IRBP) carries not only *trans*-retinol and 11-*cis* retinol but 11-*cis* retinal as well.* The source of the *trans*-retinol bound to IRBP in the interphotoreceptor space is probably the illuminated photoreceptor since *trans*-retinol is the ultimate photoproduct of that cell. The source of 11-*cis* retinol and 11-*cis* retinal that are bound to IRBP remains a matter of conjecture, but both the RPE and Müller cell would have to be considered potential contributors since each contains CRALBP. The form of retinoid(s) delivered to the photoreceptor during photopigment biosynthesis and regeneration and its cellular source are not currently known, but further studies of retinoid-binding proteins and their endogenous retinoids should aid significantly in the resolution of this question.

* J. Saari, Personal communication

teins in visual cell outer segments are the membrane-bound photopigments. Because of the presence of visual pigments in high concentration within the outer segment (10^7–10^9 copies per cell, depending on the species), soluble binding proteins may not be necessary for the protection and solubilization of the hydrophobic, unstable retinoids during their short transit from the plasma membrane to the discs. In addition, soluble binding proteins are apparently not required in the photoreceptor inner segment. Bok and colleagues have reported that the chromophore for visual pigments is not added during their biosynthesis until nascent opsin molecules reach the outer segment.[33] Defoe and Bok have shown, however, that once within the outer segment, the chromophores exchange among opsin molecules, even in the fully dark-adapted state.[72] The exchange rate has been calculated to be approximately 2000/min/rod in the mouse. Since this exchange rate is much more rapid than the dark noise or "quantum bumps" that have been measured in individual frog outer segments,[258,259] and since the exchange therefore is not mediated by thermal isomerizations, it is assumed that it is the 11-*cis* isomer that exchanges among opsin molecules in the dark.[72] The process clearly involves the breaking of covalent bonds between the chromophore and opsin. Such a process, it seems, would require the action of an exchange protein, perhaps of the type that mediates the exchange of phospholipids in the retina and other membrane systems.[78,256] Thus, although there may not be soluble retinoid-binding proteins *per se* in the outer segment, other soluble or membrane proteins may yet be found that mediate chromophore exchange.

The subject of RPE and photoreceptor cell biology is a broad one. One can expect with considerable confidence that the next two decades will be even more fruitful and exciting than the last.

REFERENCES

1. Adler AJ, Klucznik KM: Proteins and glycoproteins of the bovine interphotoreceptor matrix: Composition and fractionation. Exp Eye Res 34:423–434,1982

2. Adler AJ, Severin KM: Proteins of the bovine interphotoreceptor matrix: Tissues of origin. Exp Eye Res 32:755–769, 1981
3. Anderson DH, Fisher SK: The photoreceptors of diurnal squirrels: Outer segment disc shedding and protein renewal. J Ultrastruct Res 55:119–141, 1976
4. Anderson RE, Maude MB: Phospholipids of bovine rod outer segments. Biochemistry 9:3624–3628, 1970
5. Anderson RE, Maude MB: Lipids of ocular tissues. VIII. The effects of essential fatty acid deficiency on the phospholipids of the photoreceptor membranes of rat retina. Arch Biochem Biophys 151:270–276, 1972
6. Anderson RE, Sperling L: Lipids of ocular tissues. VII. Positional distribution of the fatty acids in the phospholipids of bovine retinal rod outer segments. Arch Biochem Biophys 144:673–677, 1971
7. Andrews LD: Freeze-fracture studies of vertebrate photoreceptor membranes. In Hollyfield JG (ed): The Structure of the Eye, pp 11–23. New York, Elsevier North-Holland, 1982
8. Andrews LD, Cohen AI: Freeze-fracture evidence for the presence of cholesterol in particle-free patches on basal disks and the plasma membrane of retinal rod outer segments of mice and frogs. J Cell Biol 81:215–288, 1979
9. Andrews LD, Cohen AI: Freeze-fracture studies of photoreceptor membranes: new observations bearing upon the distribution of cholesterol. J Cell Biol 97:749–755, 1983
10. Bader CR, MacLeish PR, Schwartz EA: Responses to light of solitary rod photoreceptors isolated from tiger salamander retina. Proc Natl Acad Sci 75:3507–3511, 1978
11. Bairati A, Orzalesi N: The ultrastructure of the pigment epithelium and of the photoreceptor-pigment epithelium junction in the human retina. J Ultrastruct Res 9: 484–496, 1963
12. Bashor MM, Toft DO, Chytil F: In vitro binding of retinol to rat-tissue components. Proc Natl Acad Sci 70:3483–3487, 1973
13. Basinger S, Hoffman R, Matthes M: Photoreceptor shedding is initiated by light in the frog retina. Science 194:1074–1076, 1976
14. Basinger SF, Bok D, Hall MO: Rhodopsin in the rod outer segment plasma membrane. J Cell Biol 69:29–42, 1976
15. Bergsma DR, Wiggert BN, Funahashi M, et al: Vitamin A receptors in normal and dystrophic human retina. Nature 265:66–67, 1977
16. Berman ER: The biosynthesis of mucopolysaccharides and glycoproteins in pigment epithelial cells of bovine retina. Biochem Biophys Acta 83:371–373, 1964
17. Berman ER: Acid hydrolyases of the retinal pigment epithelium. Invest Ophthalmol 10:64–68, 1971

18. Berman ER, Bach G: The acid mucopolysaccharides of cattle retina. Biochem J 108:75–88, 1968
19. Besharse JC: The daily light-dark cycle and rhythmic metabolism in the photoreceptor-pigment epithelial complex. In Osborne NN, Chader GJ (eds): Progress in Retinal Research, pp 81–124. New York, Pergamon Press, 1982
20. Besharse JC, Dunis DA, Burnside B: Effects of cyclic adenosine 3',5'-monophosphate on photoreceptor disc shedding and retinomotor movement. J Gen Physiol 79:775–790, 1982
21. Besharse JC, Dunis DA: Methoxyindoles and photoreceptor metabolism: Activation of rod shedding. Science 219:1341–1343, 1983
22. Besharse JC, Hollyfield JG, Rayborn ME: Turnover of rod photoreceptor outer segments. II. Membrane addition and loss in relationship to light. J Cell Biol 75:507–527, 1977
23. Besharse JC, Pfenninger KH: Membrane assembly in retinal photoreceptors. I. Freeze-fracture analysis of cytoplasmic vesicles in relationship to disc assembly. J Cell Biol 87:451–463, 1980
24. Bibb C, Young RW: Renewal of fatty acids in the membranes of visual cell outer segments. J Cell Biol 61:327–343, 1974
25. Bitensky MW, Gorman RE, Miller WH: Adenyl cyclase as a link between photon capture and changes in membrane permeability of frog photoreceptors. Proc Natl Acad Sci 68:561–562, 1971
26. Bitensky MW, Miki N, Keirns JJ, et al: Activation of photoreceptor disk membrane phosphodiesterase by light and ATP. Adv Cyclic Nucleotide Res 5:213–240, 1975
27. Bok D: The distribution and renewal of RNA in retinal rods. Invest Ophthalmol 9:516–523, 1970
28. Bok D: Autoradiographic studies on the polarity of plasma membrane receptors in retinal pigment epithelial cells. In Hollyfield JG (ed): The Structure of the Eye, pp 245–256. New York, Elsevier North-Holland, 1982
29. Bok D, Basinger SF, Hall MO: Autoradiographic and radiobiochemical studies on the incorporation of [63H] glucosamine into frog rhodopsin. Exp Eye Res 18:225–240, 1974
30. Bok D, Filerman B: Localization of Na⁺,K⁺ ATPase in retinal photoreceptors and RPE with 3H ouabain (abstr). Invest Ophthalmol Vis Sci 18:224, 1979
31. Bok D, Hall MO: The etiology of retinal dystrophy in RCS rats (abstr). Invest Ophthalmol 8:648, 1969
32. Bok D, Hall MO: The role of the pigment epithelium in the etiology of inherited retinal dystrophy in the rat. J Cell Biol 49:664–682, 1971
33. Bok D, Hall MO, O'Brien PJ: The biosynthesis of rhodopsin as studied by membrane renewal in rod outer segments. In Brinkley BR, Porter KR (eds): International Cell Biology, pp 608–617. New York, Rockefeller University Press, 1976–1977
34. Bok D, Heller J: Transport of retinol from the blood to the retina: An autoradiographic study of the pigment epithelial cell surface receptor for plasma retinol-binding protein. Exp Eye Res 22:395–402, 1976
35. Bok D, Horwitz J, Ong DE, Chytil F: Immunocytochemical localization of retinol binding proteins in the retina (abstr). Invest Ophthalmol Vis Sci 25:276, 1984
36. Bok D, Ong DE, Chytil F: Immunocytochemical localization of cellular retinol binding protein in the rat retina. Invest Ophthalmol Vis Sci 25:1–7, 1984
37. Bok D, Young RW: The renewal of diffusely distributed protein in the outer segments of rods and cones. Vision Res 12:161–168, 1972
38. Bok D, Young RW: Phagocytic properties of the retinal pigment epithelium. In Marmor MF, Zinn KM (eds): The Retinal Pigment Epithelium, pp 148–174. Cambridge, Harvard University Press, 1979
39. Bownds D, Dawes J, Miller J, et al: Phosphorylation of frog photoreceptor membranes induced by light. Nature 237:125–127, 1972
40. Bridges CDB: Effects of light and darkness on the visual pigments of amphibian tadpoles. Vision Res 14:779–793, 1974
41. Bridges CDB: Vitamin A and the role of the pigment epithelium during bleaching and regeneration of rhodopsin in the frog eye. Exp Eye Res 22:435–455, 1976
42. Bridges CDB: 11-*cis* Vitamin A in dark-adapted rod outer segments is a probable source of prosthetic groups for rhodopsin biosynthesis. Nature 259:247–248, 1976
43. Bridges CDB: Retinoids in photosensitive systems. In Sporn MB, Roberts AB, Goodman DS (eds): The Retinoids, pp 125–176. Orlando, Academic Press, 1984
44. Bridges CDB: Storage distribution and utilization of Vitamin A in the eyes of adult amphibians and their tadpoles. Vision Res 15:1311–1323, 1975
45. Bubenik GA, Purtill RA, Brown GM, et al: Melatonin in the retina and the harderian gland. Ontogeny, diurnal variations and melatonin treatment. Exp Eye Res 27:323–333, 1978
46. Bunt AH: Enzymatic digestion of synaptic ribbons in amphibian retinal photoreceptors. Brain Res 25:571–577, 1971
47. Bunt-Milam AH, Saari JC: Immunocytochemical localization of two retinoid-binding proteins in vertebrate retina. J Cell Biol 97:703–712, 1983
48. Burnside B: Thin (actin) and thick (myosinlike)

Structure and Function of the Retinal Pigment Epithelium – Photoreceptor Complex   41

filaments in cone contraction in the teleost retina. J Cell Biol 78:227–246, 1978

49. Burnside B, Ackland N: Circadian and cAMP effects on retinomotor movement. Invest Ophthalmol Vis Sci 25:539–545, 1984

50. Burnside B, Adler R, O'Connor P: Retinomotor pigment migration in the teleost retinal pigment epithelium. Invest Ophthalmol Vis Sci 24:1–15, 1983

51. Burnside B, Evans M, Fletcher RT, et al: Induction of dark-adaptive retinomotor movement (cell elongation) in teleost retinal cones by cyclic adenosine 3′,5′-monophosphate. J Gen Physiol 79:759–774, 1982

52. Burnside B, Laties AM: Actin filaments in apical projections of the primate pigmented epithelial cell. Invest Ophthalmol 15:570–575, 1976

53. Burnside B, Laties AM: Pigment movement and cellular contractility in the retinal pigment epithelium. In Marmor MF, Zinn KM (eds): The Retinal Pigment Epithelium, pp 175–191. Cambridge, Harvard University Press, 1979

54. Burnside B, Nagle B: Retinomotor movements of photoreceptors and retinal pigment epithelium: Mechanisms and regulation. In Osborne NN, Chader GJ (eds): Progress in Retinal Research, pp 67–109. Oxford, Pergamon Press, 1983

55. Chader GJ, Fletcher RT, Krishna G: Light-induced phosphorylation of rod outer segments by guanosine triphosphate. Biochem Biophys Res Comm 64:535–538, 1975

56. Chaitin M, Bok D: EM immunocytochemical localization of actin, myosin and calmodulin in mammalian photoreceptors (abstr). Invest Ophthalmol Vis Sci 25:63, 1984

57. Chaitin MH, Hall MO: Defective ingestion of rod outer segments by cultured rat pigment epithelial cells. Invest Ophthalmol Vis Sci 24:812–820, 1983

58. Chaitin MH, Hall MO: The distribution of actin in cultured normal and dystrophic rat pigment epithelial cells during the phagocytosis of rod outer segments. Invest Ophthalmol Vis Sci 24: 821–831, 1983

59. Chaitin MH, Schneider BG, Hall MO, et al: Actin in the photoreceptor connecting cilium: Immunocytochemical localization to the site of outer segment disk formation. J Cell Biol 99:239–247, 1984

60. Chytil F, Ong DE: Cellular retinoid-binding proteins. In Sporn MB, Roberts AB, Goodman DS (eds): The Retinoids, pp 89–123. Orlando, Academic Press, 1984

61. Ciechanover A, Schwartz AL, Lodish HF: The asialoglycoprotein receptor internalizes and recycles independently of the transferrin and insulin receptors. Cell 32:267–275, 1983

62. Cohen AI: Vertebrate retinal cells and their organization. Biol Rev 38:427–459, 1963

63. Cohen AI: The fine structure of the extrafoveal receptors of the pigeon. Exp Eye Res 2:88–97, 1963

64. Cohen AI: New details of the ultrastructure of the outer segments and ciliary connectives of the rods of human and macaque retinas. Anat Rec 152:63–80, 1965

65. Cohen AI: A possible cytological basis for the "R" membrane in the vertebrate eye. Nature 205:1222–1223, 1965

66. Cohen AI: New evidence supporting the linkage to extracellular space of outer segment saccules of frog cones but not rods. J Cell Biol 37:424–444, 1971

67. Cohen AI: Electron microscopic observations on form changes in photoreceptor outer segments and their saccules in response to osmotic stress. J Cell Biol 48:547–565, 1971

68. Cuhna-Vaz JG, Shakib M, Ashton N: Studies on the permeability of the blood retinal barrier. I. On the existence, development and site of the blood retinal barrier. Br J Ophthalmol 50:441–453, 1966

69. Custer NV: Structurally specialized contacts between the photoreceptors of the retina of the axolotl. J Comp Neurol 151:35–56, 1973

70. Dabrowska R, Hartshorne DJ: A Ca^{2+} and modulator-dependent myosin light chain kinase from non-muscle cells. Biochem Biophys Res Commun 85:1352–1359, 1978

71. Dartnall HJA: Handbook of Sensory Physiology: Photochemistry of Vision. Berlin, Springer-Verlag, 1972

72. Defoe DM, Bok D: Rhodopsin chromophore exchanges among opsin molecules in the dark. Invest Ophthalmol Vis Sci 24:1211–1226, 1983

73. De Guillebon H, Zauberman H: Experimental retinal detachment: Biophysical aspects of retinal peeling and stretching. Arch Ophthalmol 87:545–598, 1972

74. Dewey MM, Barr L: Intercellular connection between smooth muscle cells: The nexus. Science 137:670–672, 1962

75. Dewey MM, Davis PK, Blasie JK, et al: Localization of rhodopsin antibody in the retina of the frog. J Molec Biol 39:395–405, 1969

76. Dowling JE: Chemistry of visual adaptation in the rat. Nature 188:114–118, 1960

77. Droz B: Dynamic condition of proteins in the visual cells of rats and mice as shown by radioautography with labeled amino acids. Anat Rec 145:157–168, 1963

78. Dudley PA, Anderson RE: Phospholipid transfer protein from bovine retina with high activity towards retinal rod disc membranes. FEBS Lett 95:57–60, 1978

79. Enoch JM, Birch DG: Evidence for alteration in

photoreceptor orientation. Ophthalmology 87: 821–833, 1980

80. Essner E, Gorin M, Griewski R: Localization of lysosomal enzymes in retinal pigment epithelium of rats with inherited retinal dystrophy. Invest Ophthalmol Vis Sci 17:278–288, 1978

81. Fain GL: Quantum sensitivity of rods in the toad retina. Science 187:838–841, 1975

82. Fain GL, Gold GH, Dowling JE: Receptor coupling in the toad retina. Cold Spring Harbor Symposia on Quantitative Biology XL: 547–561, 1976

83. Fain GL, Lisman JE: Membrane conductances of photoreceptors. Prog Biophys Molec Biol 37:91–147, 1981

84. Farnsworth CC, Dratz EA: Oxidative damage of retinal rod outer segment membranes and the role of vitamin E. Biochem Biophys Acta 443:556–570, 1976

85. Feeney L, Grieshaber JA, Hogan M: Studies on human ocular pigment. In Rohen JW (ed): The Structure of the Eye, pp 535–548. Stuttgart, FK Schattauer-Verlag, 1965

86. Feeney-Burns L, Hildebrand ES, Eldridge S: Aging human RPE: Morphometric analysis of macular, equatorial, and peripheral cells. Invest Ophthalmol Vis Sci 25:195–200, 1984

87. Fisher SK, Pfeffer BA, Anderson DH: Both rod and cone disc shedding are related to light onset in the cat. Invest Ophthalmol Vis Sci 24:844–856, 1983

88. Fisher SK, Steinberg RH: Origin and organization of pigment epithelial apical projections to cones in cat retina. J Cell Biol 206:131–145, 1982

89. Fleischman D, Denisevich M: Guanylate cyclase of isolated bovine retinal rod axonemes. Amer Chem Soc 18:5060–5066, 1979

90. Fleischman D, Denisevich M, Raveed D, et al: Association of guanylate cyclase with the axoneme of retinal rods. Biochem Biophys Acta 630:176–186, 1980

91. Flowers NE: Particles within membranes: A freeze-etch view. J Cell Sci 9:435–441, 1971

92. Forestner DM, Besharse JC: Membrane assembly in photoreceptors: Spatially differentiated labeling of developing photoreceptor cilia with antiopsin and lectins (abstr). Invest Ophthalmol Vis Sci 24:287, 1983

93. Frank RN, Cavanaugh HD, Kenyon KR: Light-stimulated phosphorylation of bovine visual pigments by adenosine triphosphate. J Biol Chem 248:596–609, 1973

94. Fukuda MN, Papermaster DS, Hargrave PA: Rhodopsin carbohydrate. Structure of small oligosaccharides attached at two sites near the NH2 terminus. J Biol Chem 254:8201–8207, 1979

95. Fung BK-K, Hubbell WL: Organization of rhodopsin in photoreceptor membranes. 2. Trans-

membrane organization of bovine rhodopsin: evidence from proteolysis and lactoperoxidase-catalyzed iodination of native and reconstituted membranes. Biochemistry 17: 4403–4410, 1978

96. Fung BK-K, Hurley JB, Stryer L: Flow of information in the light-triggered cyclic nucleotide cascade of vision. Proc Natl Acad Sci 78:152–156, 1981

97. Fung BK-K, Stryer L: Photolyzed rhodopsin catalyzes the exchange of GTP for bound GDP retinal rod outer segments. Proc Natl Acad Sci 77:2500–2504, 1980

98. Furshpan EJ, Potter D: Transmission at the giant motor synapse of the crayfish. J Physiol 145:289–325, 1959

99. Futterman S, Saari JC, Blair S: Occurrence of a binding protein for 11-*cis*-retinal in retina. J Biol Chem 252:3267–3271, 1977

100. Garcia RI, Szabo G, Fitzpatrick TB: Molecular and cell biology of melanin. In Marmor MF, Zinn KM (eds): The Retinal Pigment Epithelium, pp 124–147. Cambridge, Harvard University Press, 1979

101. Geuze HJ, Slot JW, Strous GJAM, et al: Intracellular site of asialoglycoprotein receptor-ligand uncoupling: Double-label immunoelectron microscopy during receptor-mediated endocytosis. Cell 32:277–287, 1983

102. Gilula NB, Satir P: The ciliary necklace. A ciliary membrane specialization. J Cell Biol 53:494–509, 1972

103. Godchaux W III, Zimmerman WF: Membrane-dependent guanine nucleotide binding and GTPase activities of soluble protein from bovine rod cell outer segments. J Biol Chem 254:7874–7884, 1979

104. Gold GH: Photoreceptor coupling in retina of the toad *Bufo marinus.* J Neurophysiol 42:311–328, 1979

105. Goodenough DA: The structure of cell membranes involved in intercellular communication. Am J Clin Pathol 63:636–645, 1975

106. Goodman DS: Plasma retinol-binding protein. In Sporn MB, Roberts AB, Goodman DS (eds): The Retinoids, pp 41–88. Orlando, Academic Press, 1984

107. Hagins WA, Penn RD, Yoshikami S: Dark current and photocurrent in retinal rods. Biophys J 10:380–412, 1970

108. Hall MO: Phagocytosis of light- and dark-adapted rod outer segments by cultured pigment epithelium. Science 202:526–528, 1978

109. Hall MO, Bok D, Bacharach ADE: Biosynthesis and assembly of the rod outer segment membrane system. Formation and fate of visual pigment in the frog retina. J Mol Biol 45:397–406, 1969

110. Hargrave PA: The amino-terminal tryptic peptide of bovine rhodopsin. A glycopeptide con-

taining two sites of oligosaccharide attachment. Biochem Biophys Acta 492:83–94, 1977

111. Hargrave PA: Rhodopsin chemistry, structure and topography. In Osborne NN, Chader GJ (eds): Progress in Retinal Research, pp 1–52. Oxford, Pergamon Press Ltd, 1982

112. Hargrave PA, McDowell JH, Curtis DR, et al: The structure of bovine rhodopsin. Biophys Struct Mech 9:235–244, 1983

113. Hayes KC: Retinal degeneration in monkeys induced by deficiencies of Vitamin E or A. Invest Ophthalmol 13:499–510, 1974

114. Heller J: Structure of visual pigments. I. Purification, molecular weight and composition of bovine visual pigment 500. Biochemistry 7:2906–2913, 1968

115. Heller J: Interactions of plasma retinol-binding protein with its receptor. J Biol Chem 250:3613–3619, 1975

116. Heller J, Bok D: A specific receptor for retinol binding protein: binding of human and bovine retinol binding protein to pigment epithelial cells. Am J Ophthalmol 81:93–97, 1976

117. Heller J, Lawrence MA: Structure of the glycopeptide from bovine visual pigment 500. Biochemistry 9:864–869, 1970

118. Hermolin J, Karell MA, Hamm HE, Bownds MD: Calcium and cyclic GMP regulation of light-sensitive protein phosphorylation in frog photoreceptor membranes. J Gen Physiol 79:633–655, 1982

119. Herron WL, Riegel BW, Myers OE: Retinal dystrophy in the rat: A pigment epithelial disease. Invest Ophthalmol 8:595–604, 1969

120. Heuser JE, Reese TS: Evidence for recycling of synaptic vesicle membrane during transmitter release at the frog neuromuscular junction. J Cell Biol 57:315–344, 1973

121. Hogan MJ, Alvarado JA, Waddell JE: Histology of the Human Eye. Philadelphia, WB Saunders, 1971

122. Hogan MJ, Wood I, Steinberg RH: Phagocytosis by pigment epithelium of human retinal cones. Nature 252:305–307, 1974

123. Hollyfield JG, Fliesler SJ, Rayborn ME, et al: Synthesis and secretion of interstitial retinol-binding protein by the human retina. Invest Ophthalmol Vis Sci 26:58–67, 1985

124. Hollyfield JG, Rayborn ME, Verner GE, Maude MB: Membrane addition to rod photoreceptor outer segments: Light stimulates membrane assembly in the absence of increased membrane biosynthesis. Invest Ophthalmol Vis Sci 22:417–427, 1982

125. Holtzman E, Schacher S, Evans J, et al: Origin and fate of the membranes of secretion granules and synaptic vesicles: Membrane circulation in neurons, gland cells and retinal photoreceptors. In Poste G, Nicolson GL (eds): The Synthesis, Assembly and Turnover of Cell Surface Components, pp 167–246. Elsevier, North-Holland, 1977

126. Hubbard R: Retinene isomerase. J Gen Physiol 39:935–962, 1956

127. Hubbard R: Vitamin-A content of the frog eye during light and dark adaptation. Science 130:977–978, 1959

128. Hubbell W, Fung BK-K: Molecular anatomy and light-dependent processes in photoreceptor membranes. In Barlow HB, Fatt P (eds): Vertebrate Photoreception, pp 41–59. London, Academic Press, 1977

129. Hubbell WL, Bownds MD: Visual transduction in vertebrate photoreceptors. Ann Rev Neurosci 2:17–34, 1979

130. Hudspeth AJ, Yee AG: The intercellular junctional complexes of retinal pigment epithelia. Invest Ophthalmol 12:354–365, 1973

131. Irons M, Kalnins VI: Distribution of microtubules in cultured RPE cells from normal and dystrophic RCS rats. Invest Ophthalmol Vis Sci 25:434–439, 1984

132. Ishida AT: Selective potentiation of retinal horizontal cell responses to L-glutamate by D-aspartate. Comp Biochem Physiol 72C:241–247, 1982

133. Ishida AT, Fain GL: D-aspartate potentiates the effects of L-glutamate on horizontal cells in goldfish retina. Proc Natl Acad Sci 78:5890–5894, 1981

134. Ishikawa T, Yamada E: The degradation of the photoreceptor outer segment within the pigment epithelial cell of rat retina. J Electron Microsc 19:85–99, 1970

135. Jan LY, Revel J-P: Ultrastructural localization of rhodopsin in the vertebrate retina. J Cell Biol 2:257–273, 1974

136. Kanai M, Raz A, Goodman DS: Retinol-binding protein: The transport protein for vitamin A in human plasma. J Biol Chem 47:2025–2044, 1968

137. Karrer HE: The striated musculature of blood vessels, cell interconnections and cell surfaces. Cytology 8:135–150, 1960

138. Katz ML, Stone WL, Dratz EA: Fluorescent pigment accumulation in retinal pigment epithelium of antioxidant deficient rats. Invest Ophthalmol Vis Sci 17:1049–1058, 1978

139. Kaupp UB, Schnetkamp PPM: Calcium metabolism in vertebrate photoreceptors. Cell Calcium 3:83–112, 1982

140. Kean EL: Stimulation by GDP-mannose of the biosynthesis of N-acetylglucosaminylpyrophosphoryl polyprenols by the retina. J Biol Chem 255:1921–1927, 1980

141. Korenbrot JI: Signal mechanisms of phototransduction in retinal rods. Crit Rev Biochem 17:223–256, 1985

142. Korte GE: New ultrastructure of rat RPE cells:

basal intracytoplasmic tubules. Exp Eye Res 38:399–410, 1984

143. Kuhn H, Dreyer WJ: Light dependent phosphorylation of rhodopsin by ATP. FEBS Lett 20:1–6, 1972

144. Kuhn H: Phosphorylation of rhodopsin in bovine photoreceptor membranes. A dark reaction after illumination. Biochemistry 12:2495–2501, 1973

145. Kuhn H: Light-dependent phosphorylation of rhodopsin in living frogs. Nature 250:588–590, 1974

146. Kuhn H: Light-regulated binding of rhodopsin kinase and other proteins to cattle photoreceptor membranes. Biochemistry 17:4389–4395, 1978

147. Kuhne W: Fortgesetzte Untersuchungen über die Retina und die Pigmente des Auges. Untersuch Physiol Instit Univ Heidelberg 2:89, 1877

148. Kuwabara T: Species differences in the retinal pigment epithelium. In Marmor MF, Zinn KM (eds): The Retinal Pigment Epithelium, pp 58–82. Cambridge, Harvard University Press, 1979

149. Kuwabara T, Gorn RA: Retinal damage by visible light. Arch Ophthalmol 79:69–78, 1968

150. Kyte J: Immunoferritin determination of the distribution of (Na$^+$ + K$^+$) ATPase over the plasma membranes of renal convoluted tubules. I. Distal segment. J Cell Biol 68:287–303, 1976

151. Kyte J: Immunoferritin determination of the distribution of (Na$^+$ + K$^+$) ATPase over the plasma membranes of renal convoluted tubules. II. Proximal segment. J Cell Biol 68:304–318, 1976

152. Ladman AJ: The fine structure of the rod-bipolar cell synapse in the retina of the albino rat. J Biophys Biochem Cytol 4:459–466, 1958

153. Lai Y-L, Wiggert B, Liu Y-P, et al: Interphotoreceptor retinol-binding proteins: Possible transport vehicles between compartments of the retina. Nature 298:848–849, 1982

154. Lam DMK: Biosynthesis of acetylcholine in turtle photoreceptors. Proc Natl Acad Sci 69:1987–1991, 1972

155. Laties A, Liebman P, Campbell C: Photoreceptor orientation in the primate eye. Nature 218:172–173, 1969

156. Laties AM: Histochemical techniques for the study of photoreceptor orientation. Tissue Cell 1:63–81, 1969

157. Laties AM, Bok D, Liebman P: Procion yellow: A marker dye for outer segment disc patency and for rod renewal. Exp Eye Res 23:139–148, 1976

158. Laties AM, Enoch JM: An analysis of retinal receptor orientation: Angular relationship of neighboring photoreceptors. Invest Ophthalmol Vis Sci 10:69–77, 1971

159. Laties AM, Liebman PA: Cones of living amphibian eye: Selective staining. Science 168:1475–1477, 1970

160. LaVail MM: Rod outer segment disc shedding in relation to cyclic lighting. Exp Eye Res 23:277–280, 1976

161. LaVail MM: Rod outer segment disk shedding in rat retina: Relationship to cyclic lighting. Science 194:1071–1074, 1976

162. Levinson G, Burnside B: Circadian rhythms in teleost retinomotor movements. Invest Ophthalmol Vis Sci 20:294–303, 1981

163. Liebman PA: In situ microspectrophotometric studies on the pigments of single retinal rods. Biophys J 2:161–178, 1962

164. Liebman PA, Carroll S, Laties A: Spectral sensitivity of retinal screening pigment migration in the frog. Vision Res 9:377–384, 1969

165. Liebman PA, Entine G: Lateral diffusion of visual pigment in photoreceptor disk membranes. Science 185:457–459, 1974

166. Liebman PA, Pugh EN Jr: The control of phosphodiesterase in rod disk membranes: Kinetics, possible mechanisms and significance for vision. Vision Res 19:375–380, 1979

167. Liebman PA, Pugh EN Jr: Control of rod disk membrane phosphodiesterase and a model of visual transduction. Curr Top Membr Trans 15:157–170, 1981

168. Lion R, Rotmans JP, Daemen FJM, et al: Biochemical aspects of the visual process. XXVII. Stereospecificity of ocular retinal dehydrogenases and the visual cycle. Biochem Biophys Acta 384:282–292, 1975

169. Liou GI, Bridges CDB, Fong S-L: Vitamin A transport between retina and pigment epithelium — An interstitial protein carrying endogenous retinol (interstitial retinol binding protein). Vision Res 22:1457–1468, 1982

170. Lowenstein WR, Kanno Y: Studies on an epithelial gland cell junction; modifications of surface membrane permeability. J Cell Biol 22:565–586, 1964

171. Marmor MF, Abdul-Rahim AS, Cohen DS: The effect of metabolic inhibitors on retinal adhesion and subretinal fluid resorption. Invest Ophthalmol Vis Sci 19:893–903, 1980

172. Marshall J: Acid phosphatase activity in the retinal pigment epithelium. Vision Res 10:821–824, 1970

173. Matsumoto B, Bok D: Diurnal variations in the incorporation of tritiated amino acids into nascent inner segment opsin. Invest Ophthalmol Vis Sci 25:1–9, 1984

174. Matsusaka T: Membrane particles of the connecting cilium. J Ultrastruct Res 48:305–312, 1974

175. Matsusaka T: Cytoplasmic fibrils of the connecting cilium. J Ultrastruct Res 54:318–324, 1976

176. Matsusaka T: Fine structure of the connecting

cilium in the rat eye. In Yamada E, Mishima S (eds): The Structure of the Eye III, pp 261–271. Tokyo, Japanese J Ophthalmol, 1976

177. Matthes MT, Basinger SF: Myeloid body associations in the frog pigment epithelium. Invest Ophthalmol Vis Sci 19:298–302, 1980

178. Miki N, Baraban J, Keirns JJ, et al: Purification and properties of the light-activated cyclic nucleotide phosphodiesterase of rod outer segments. J Biol Chem 250:6320–6327, 1975

179. Miller JA, Paulsen R: Phosphorylation and dephosphorylation of frog rod outer segment membranes as part of the visual process. J Biol Chem 250:4427–4432, 1975

180. Miller SS, Hughes BA, Machen TE: Fluid transport across retinal pigment epithelium is inhibited by cyclic AMP. Proc Natl Acad Sci 79:2111–2115, 1982

181. Miller SS, Steinberg RH: Active transport of ions across frog retinal pigment epithelium. Exp Eye Res 25:235–248, 1977

182. Missoten L, Appelmans M, Michiels J: L'ultrastructure des synapses des cellules vissuelles de la retine humaine. Bull Soc Franc Ophthal 76:59–82, 1963

183. Mullen RJ, LaVail MM: Inherited retinal dystrophy: Primary defect in pigment epithelium determined with experimental rat chimeras. Science 192:799–801, 1976

184. Murray RL, Dubin MW: The occurrence of actin-like filaments in association with migrating pigment granules in frog retinal pigment epithelium. J Cell Biol 64:705–710, 1975

185. Muto Y, Smith JE, Milch PO, et al: Regulation of retinol-binding protein metabolism by vitamin A status in the rat. J Biol Chem 247:2542–2550, 1971

186. Nelson R, Kolb H: Synaptic patterns and response properties of bipolar and ganglion cells in the cat retina. Vision Res 23:1183–1195, 1983

187. Nilsson SEG: Receptor cell outer segment development and ultrastructure of the disc membranes in the retina of the tadpole *(Rana pipiens)*. J Ultrastruct Res 11:581–620, 1964

188. Nir I, Cohen D, Papermaster DS: Immunocytochemical localization of opsin in the cell membrane of developing rat retinal photoreceptors. J Cell Biol 98:1788–1795, 1984

189. Nir I, Cohen D, Rabinowitz H, et al: Lectin binding to the surface of the connecting cilium of photoreceptors (abstr). Invest Ophthalmol Vis Sci 24:287, 1983

190. Nir I, Papermaster DS: Differential distribution of opsin in the plasma membrane of frog photoreceptors: An immunocytochemical study. Invest Ophthalmol Vis Sci 24:868–878, 1983

191. O'Brien PJ: Rhodopsin as a glycoprotein: A possible role for the oligosaccharide in phagocytosis. Exp Eye Res 23:127–138, 1976

192. O'Brien PJ, Muellenberg CG: The biosynthesis of rhodopsin in vitro. Exp Eye Res 18:241–252, 1974

193. O'Connor P, Burnside B: Actin-dependent cell elongation in teleost retinal rods: Requirement for actin filament assembly. J Cell Biol 89:517–524, 1981

194. O'Connor P, Burnside B: Elevation of cyclic AMP activates an actin-dependent contraction in teleost retinal rods. J Cell Biol 95:445–452, 1982

195. O'Day WT, Young RW: Rhythmic daily shedding of outer-segment membranes by visual cells in the goldfish. J Cell Biol 76:593–604, 1978

196. Ong DE, Chytil F: Cellular retinoic acid-binding protein from rat testis (purification and characterization). J Biol Chem 253:4551–4554, 1978

197. Ostwald TJ, Steinberg RH: Localization of frog retinal pigment epithelium Na$^+$-K$^+$ ATPase. Exp Eye Res 31:351–369, 1980

198. Ovchinnikov YA, Abdulaev NG, Feigina MY, et al: The complete amino acid sequence of visual rhodopsin. Bioorg Khim 8:1011–1014, 1982

199. Papermaster DS, Converse CA, Siu J: Membrane biosynthesis in the frog retina: Opsin transport in the photoreceptor cell. Biochemistry 14:2438–2442, 1975

200. Papermaster DS, Reilly P, Schneider BG: Cone lamellae and red and green rod outer segment disks contain a large intrinsic membrane protein on their margins: An ultrastructural immunocytochemical study of frog retinas. Vision Res 22:1417–1428, 1982

201. Papermaster DS, Schneider BG: Biosynthesis and morphogenesis of outer segment membranes in vertebrate photoreceptor cells. In McDevitt DS (ed): Cell Biology of the Eye, pp 475–531. New York, Academic Press, 1982

202. Papermaster DS, Schneider BG, Zorn MA, et al: Immunocytochemical localization of a large intrinsic membrane protein to the incisures and margins of frog rod outer segment disks. J Cell Biol 78:415–425, 1978

203. Penn RD, Hagins WA: Kinetics of the photocurrent of retinal rods. Biophys J 12:1073–1094, 1972

204. Peters K-R, Palade GE, Schneider BG, et al: Fine structure of a periciliary ridge complex of frog retinal rod cells revealed by ultrahigh resolution scanning electron microscope. J Cell Biol 96:265–276, 1983

205. Peterson PA: Characteristics of a vitamin A-transporting protein complex occurring in human serum. J Biol Chem 246:34–43, 1971

206. Peyman GA, Bok D: Peroxidase diffusion in the normal and laser-coagulated primate retina. Invest Ophthalmol Vis Sci 11:35–45, 1972

207. Pfeffer BA, Fisher SK: Development of retinal pigment epithelial surface structures ensheathing cone outer segments in the cat. J Ultrastruct Res 76:158–172, 1981

208. Philp N, Nachmias VT: Identification and localization of cytoskeletal proteins in chick RPE cells (abstr). Invest Ophthalmol Vis Sci 25:287, 1984

209. Poo M-M, Cone RA: Lateral diffusion of rhodopsin in the photoreceptor membrane. Nature 247:438–441, 1974

210. Porter KR, Yamada E: Studies on the endoplasmic reticulum. V. Its form and differentiation in pigment epithelial cells of the frog retina. Biophys Biochem Cytol 8:181–205, 1960

211. Quinton PM, Wright EM, Tormey JMcd: Localization of sodium pumps in the choroid plexus epithelium. J Cell Biol 58:724–730, 1973

212. Raveed D, Fleischman D: The basal apparatus of bovine retinal rods (abstr). Proc Electron Microscopy Soc Am 33:478–479, 1975

213. Raviola E, Gilula NB: Gap junctions between photoreceptor cells in the vertebrate retina. Proc Natl Acad Sci 70:1677–1681, 1973

214. Raviola E, Gilula NB: Intramembrane organization of specialized contacts in the outer plexiform layer of the retina. J Cell Biol 65:192–222, 1975

215. Reme CE: Autophagy in visual cells and pigment epithelium. Invest Ophthalmol Vis Sci 16:807–814, 1977

216. Revel JP, Karnovsky KJ, Hexagonal array of subunits in intercellular junctions of the mouse heart and liver. J Cell Biol 33:C7–C12, 1967

217. Ripps H, Shakib M, MacDonald ED: Peroxidase uptake by photoreceptor terminals of the skate retina. J Cell Biol 70:86–96, 1976

218. Rohlich P: The sensory cilium of retinal rods is analogous to the transitional zone of motile cilia. Cell Tiss Res 161:421–430, 1975

219. Roof DJ, Heuser JE: Surfaces of rod photoreceptor disk membranes: Integral membrane components. J Cell Biol 95:487–500, 1982

220. Roof DJ, Korenbrot JI, Heuser JE: Surfaces of rod photoreceptor disk membranes: Light-activated enzymes. J Cell Biol 95:501–509, 1982

221. Rose B, Lowenstein WR: Permeability of cell junctions depends on local cytoplasmic activity. Nature 254:250–252, 1975

222. Saari JC, Bredberg L: Enzymatic reduction of 11-*cis* retinal bound to cellular retinal-binding protein. Biochem Biophys Acta 716:266–272, 1982

223. Saari JC, Futterman S, Bredberg L: Cellular retinol- and retinoic acid-binding proteins of bovine retina. J Biol Chem 253:6432–6436, 1978

224. Sandoz D, Gounon P, Karsenti E, et al: Immunocytochemical localization of tubulin, actin, and myosin in axonemes of ciliated cells from quail oviduct. Proc Natl Acad Sci 79:3198–3202, 1982

225. Schacher S, Holtzman E, Hood DC: Synaptic activity of frog retinal photoreceptors. A peroxidase uptake study. J Cell Biol 70:178–192, 1976

226. Schacher SM, Holtzman E, Hood DC: Uptake of horseradish peroxidase by frog photoreceptor synapses in the dark and the light. Nature 249:261–263, 1974

227. Schaeffer SF, Raviola E: Membrane recycling in the cone cell endings of the turtle retina. J Cell Biol 79:802–852, 1978

228. Schwartz IR, Bok D: Electron microscopic localization of [^{125}I] alpha-bungarotoxin binding sites in the outer plexiform layer of the goldfish retina. J Neurocytology 8:53–66, 1979

229. Sidman: Histogenesis of mouse retina studies with thymidine-^{3}H. In Smelser GK (ed): The Structure of the Eye, pp 487–505. New York, Academic Press, 1961

230. Sjostrand FS: The ultrastructure of the inner segments of the retinal rods of the guinea pig eye as revealed by electron microscopy. J Cell Comp Physiol 42:45–70, 1953

231. Spitznas M, Hogan MJ: Outer segments of photoreceptors and the retinal pigment epithelium. Arch Ophthalmol 84:810–819, 1970

232. Stein PJ, Rasenick MM, Bitensky MS: Biochemistry of the cyclic nucleotide-related enzymes in rod photoreceptors. In Osborne NN, Chader GJ (eds): Progress in Retinal Research, pp 227–243. Oxford, Pergamon Press, 1982

233. Steinberg RH, Fisher SK, Anderson DH: Disc morphogenesis in vertebrate photoreceptors. J Comp Neurol 190:501–518, 1980

234. Steinberg RH, Miller S: Aspects of electrolyte transport in frog pigment epithelium. Exp Eye Res 16:365–372, 1973

235. Steinberg RH, Miller SS: Transport and membrane properties of the retinal pigment epithelium. In Marmor MF, Zinn KM (eds): The Retinal Pigment Epithelium, pp 205–225. Cambridge, Harvard University Press, 1979

236. Steinberg RH, Wood I: Pigment epithelial ensheathment of cone outer segments in the retina of the domestic cat. Proc Roy Soc Lond (Biol) 187:461–478, 1974

237. Steinberg RH, Wood I: The relationship of the retinal pigment epithelium to photoreceptor outer segments in human retina. In Marmor MF, Zinn K (eds): The Retinal Pigment Epithelium, pp 32–44. Cambridge, Harvard University Press, 1979

238. Stirling CE, Lee A: [^{3}H] ouabain autoradiography of frog retina. J Cell Biol 85:313–324, 1980

239. Stossel TP: Phagocytosis. New Eng J Med 290:833–839, 1974

240. Streeten BW: The sudanophilic granules of the

human retinal pigment epithelium. Arch Ophthalmol 66:391–398, 1961

241. Tabor GA, Fisher SK: Myeloid bodies in the mammalian retinal pigment epithelium. Invest Ophthalmol Vis Sci 24:288–391, 1983

242. Tappel AL: Biological antioxidant protection against lipid peroxidation damage. Am J Clin Nutr 23:1137–1139, 1970

243. Tomita T: Electrical activity of vertebrate photoreceptors. Q Rev Biophys 3:179–222, 1970

244. Turin L, Warner A: Intracellular pH in early Xenopus embryos: its effect on current flow between blastomeres. J Physiol 300:489–504, 1980

245. Usukura J, Yamada E: Molecular organization of the rod outer segment. A deep-etching study with rapid freezing using unfixed frog retina. Biomedical Res 2:177–193, 1981

246. Wald G: Carotenoids and the visual cycle. J Gen Physiol 19:351–371, 1935

247. Warren RH, Burnside B: Microtubules in cone myoid elongation in the teleost retina. J Cell Biol 78:247–259, 1978

248. Wiechmann AF, Bok D, Horwitz J: Localization of hydroxyindole o-methyltransferase in the mammalian pineal gland and retina. Invest Ophthalmol Vis Sci 26:253–265, 1985

249. Wiegand RD, Giusto NM, Rapp LM, et al: Evidence for rod outer segment lipid peroxidation following constant illumination of the rat retina. Invest Ophthalmol Vis Sci 24:1433–1435, 1983

250. Wiggert B, Bergsma DR, Helmsen R: Retinoic acid binding in ocular tissues. Biochem J 169:87–94, 1978

251. Wiggert B, Bergsma DR, Lewis M, et al: Vitamin A receptors: Retinol binding in neural retina and pigment epithelium. J Neurochem 29:947–954, 1977

252. Wiggert B, Derr JE, Israel P, et al: Cytosol binding of retinyl palmitate and palmitic acid in pigment epithelium and retina. Exp Eye Res 32:187–196, 1981

253. Wiggert BO, Bergsma DR, Chader GJ: Retinol receptors of the retina and pigment epithelium: Further characterization and species variation. Exp Eye Res 22:411–418, 1976

254. Wiggert BO, Chader GJ: A receptor for retinol in the developing retina and pigment epithelium. Exp Eye Res 21:143–151, 1975

255. Wiggert EM, Israel P, Chader GJ: Differential retinoid binding in chick pigment epithelium and choroid. Invest Ophthalmol Vis Sci 18:306–310, 1979

256. Wirtz KWA: Transfer of phospholipids between membranes. Biochem Biophys Acta 344:95–117, 1974

257. Wu SM, Dowling JE: L-Aspartate: Evidence for a role in cone photoreceptor synaptic transmission in the carp retina. Proc Natl Acad Sci 75:5205–5209, 1978

258. Yau K-W, Lamb TD, Baylor DA: Light-induced fluctuations in membrane current of single toad rod outer segments. Nature 269:78–80, 1977

259. Yau K-W, Matthews G, Baylor DA: Thermal activation of the visual transduction mechanism in retinal rods. Nature 279:806–807, 1979

260. Yazulla S, Schmidt J: Radioautographic localization of ^{125}I-alpha-bungarotoxin binding sites in the retinas of goldfish and turtle. Vision Res 16:878–880, 1976

261. Yorke MA, Dickson DH: Diurnal variations in myeloid bodies of the newt retinal pigment epithelium. Cell Tissue Res 235:177–186, 1984

262. Yoshikami S, Hagins WA: Light, calcium and the photocurrent of rods and cones. Biophys J 11:47a, 1971

263. Young RW: The renewal of photoreceptor cell outer segments J Cell Biol 33:61–72, 1967

264. Young RW: A difference between rods and cones in the renewal of outer segment protein. Invest Ophthalmol 8:222–231, 1969

265. Young RW: The organization of vertebrate photoreceptor cells. In Straatsma BR, Hall MO, Allen RA, et al (eds): The Retina: Morphology, Function, and Clinical Characteristics, pp 177–210. Berkeley, University of California Press, 1969

266. Young RW: Shedding of discs from rod outer segments in the rhesus monkey. J Ultrastruct Res 34:190–203, 1971

267. Young RW: An hypothesis to account for a basic distinction between rods and cones. Vision Res 11:1–5, 1971

268. Young RW: Visual cells and the concept of renewal. Invest Ophthalmol 15:700–725, 1976

269. Young RW: The daily rhythm of shedding and degradation of cone outer segment membranes in the lizard retina. J Ultrastruct 61:172–185, 1977

270. Young RW: The daily rhythm of shedding and degradation of rod and cone outer segment membranes in the chick retina. Invest Ophthalmol 17:105–116, 1978

271. Young RW: The chemistry of the retina: Function, renewal, rhythms, and the nucleus. In Bazan NG, Lolley RN (eds): Neurochemistry of the Retina, pp 123–142. Oxford, Pergamon Press, 1980

272. Young RW, Bok D: Participation of the retinal pigment epithelium in the rod outer segment renewal process. J Cell Biol 42:392–402, 1969

273. Young RW, Droz B: The renewal of protein in retinal rods and cones. J Cell Biol 39:169–184, 1968

274. Zauberman H: Adhesive forces between the retinal pigment epithelium and sensory retina. In

Zinn KM, Marmor MF (eds): The Retinal Pigment Epithelium, pp 192–204. Cambridge, Harvard University Press, 1979

275. Zimmerman WF: Subcellular distribution of 11-*cis* retinol dehydrogenase activity in bovine pigment epithelium. Exp Eye Res 23:159–164, 1976

276. Zimmerman WF, Lion F, Daemen FJM, et al: Biochemical aspects of the visual process. XXX. Distribution of stereospecific retinol dehydrogenase activities in subcellular fractions of bovine retina and pigment epithelium. Exp Eye Res 21:325–332, 1975

2

Vitamin A: Utilization, Metabolism, and Role in Retinal Disease

C. David Bridges
Gregory I. Liou
Federico Gonzalez-Fernandez
Richard A. Alvarez
Shao-Ling Fong

All light-initiated events in the eye depend on the absorption of quanta of incident radiation by visual pigment molecules in the photoreceptor outer segments. Visual pigments are transmembrane glycoproteins that have retinaldehyde (vitamin A_1 aldehyde) or 3,4-didehydroretinaldehyde (vitamin A_2 aldehyde) as their prosthetic groups. In the rhodopsins the prosthetic group is 11-*cis* retinaldehyde, and in the porphyropsins, which are present in the eyes of amphibians and fishes, this is replaced by 11-*cis*-3,4-didehydroretinaldehyde.[11,44]

In bovine rhodopsin, 11-*cis* retinaldehyde is covalently attached to Lys-296 of the glycoprotein moiety (opsin) by an aldimine linkage.[68] Light isomerizes the 11-*cis* isomer to all-*trans* and sets in train a succession of intermediate products, many of which have only a transient existence at room temperature.[67] The structures of these intermediates are still not understood. They include hypsorhodopsin, bathorhodopsin, lumirhodopsin, metarhodopsins I and II, pararhodopsin, and *N*-retinylideneopsin.[4,71] The final intermediate, usually identified as *N*-retinylideneopsin, is unstable at physiological pH and temperature and hydrolyzes to opsin and all-*trans* retinaldehyde. In the isolated human retina at 36°C, free retinaldehyde has a half-life of 23 seconds and is reduced to all-*trans* retinol.[5] The oxidoreductase involved in this reaction differs from the zinc-dependent liver-alcohol dehydrogenase (which can also reduce retinaldehyde to retinol) in that it is membrane-bound, requires NADP rather than NAD as a cofactor, and is more specific in that it has preference for the all-*trans* isomer and cannot use ethanol as a substrate.[14,36,48]

Because it is the precursor of the retinaldehyde prosthetic group of rhodopsin, retinol is needed to maintain the visual process. Retinoids must therefore be supplied to the eye from the circulation, transported within its cells and between its layers, and stored in its tissues.

This investigation was supported by the Retina Research Foundation of Houston, National Institutes of Health (National Eye Institute), National Retinitis Pigmentosa Foundation, Baltimore, Maryland, and an unrestricted departmental grant from Research to Prevent Blindness. The authors thank Dr. D.M.K. Lam and Ms. Pat Glazebrook for carrying out the immunocytochemical localization of IRBP.

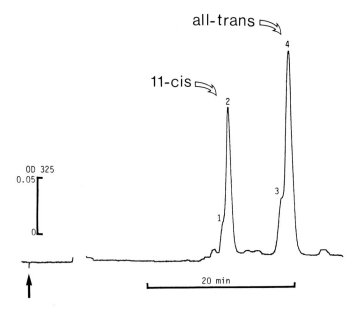

all-trans

11-cis

OD 325
0.05

0

20 min

Figure 2-1. Vitamin A esters in the human pigment epithelium, high-performance liquid chromatography on normal-phase columns: 11-*cis* retinyl palmitate, peak 2; all-*trans* retinyl palmitate, peak 4. The shoulders labeled 1 and 2 indicate the positions of the 11-*cis* and all-*trans* retinyl stearates, respectively. Columns, mobile phase, equipment, and other conditions are as described by Bridges and colleagues.[18]

STORAGE OF VITAMIN A IN THE HUMAN EYE

In the body, the highest concentrations of vitamin A are found in the liver and pigment epithelium (RPE). The RPE from a pair of human eyes contains 4.5 ± 2.6 μg of vitamin A. On a molar basis, this is equivalent to between two and three times the quantity of rhodopsin in the retina.[18]

Most of the vitamin A in the RPE consists of retinyl palmitate and stearate in the approximate ratio of 5:1. As much as 75% of these esters may be in the 11-*cis* configuration. A typical chromatogram obtained by high-performance liquid chromatography of the retinyl esters stored in human RPE is illustrated in Figure 2-1. Two major peaks are evident, representing 11-*cis* retinyl palmitate and all-*trans* retinyl palmitate. The shoulders are attributable to the corresponding stearates. These were not fully resolved in the present system, which was optimized for isomer separation.

In the dark-adapted eyes of most animals, the amount of vitamin A in the RPE represents between 1 and 6 molecular equivalents of the visual pigment in the retina. It is not known whether the magnitude of these stores depends on vitamin A nurture, but it is probable that they serve as a reserve that protects the visual system from depletion under conditions of dietary deficiency.

DELIVERY OF VITAMIN A TO THE RPE

Extracellular Retinoid-Binding Proteins

In the form of retinol, vitamin A enters the RPE cells through their apical surfaces from the interphotoreceptor space and through their basal surfaces from the choroidal blood vessels. Extracellular retinoid-binding proteins appear to be involved in both delivery routes (Fig. 2-2).

In the bloodstream, all-*trans* retinol is carried by a 21,000-dalton protein known as serum retinol-binding protein (RBP).[38] This protein circulates as a 1:1 complex with transthyretin (prealbumin). RBP solubilizes retinol, protects it from oxidative degradation, and provides the means for targeting its delivery to cells that have RBP receptors on their plasma membranes. Receptors for RBP have been found on the surfaces of intestinal mucosa, testicular and corneal epithelial cells, and on the basement membranes of RPE cells.[9,10,52,56,57]

The all-*trans* retinol that is generated when rhodopsin is bleached flows outward from the rod outer segments (ROS) and enters the RPE cells through their apical membranes. It accumulates in the RPE in the form of all-*trans* retinyl esters.[13,29] The transfer of retinol between the ROS and the RPE entails passage through the interphotoreceptor matrix, which has been shown to contain a glycoprotein that carries endogenous all-*trans* and 11-*cis* retinol.[2,50] It is a major component of the interphotoreceptor matrix, where it is present in concentrations of 30 to 100 μM.[35] This glycoprotein is known as interphotoreceptor matrix or interstitial retinol-binding protein (IRBP).[49,50] IRBP from human and bovine eyes has been purified and characterized.[34,35] Bovine IRBP has an apparent molecular weight of 144,000 daltons on sodium dodecyl sulfate polyacrylamide gels, binds about two molecules of retinol, and has four to five sialated, fucosylated oligosaccharide chains. It exhibits an anomalously high molecular weight of 250,000 daltons on gel-filtration columns because it is an elongated molecule with an axial ratio of about 10:1.*

Very recently, the structure of human IRBP has been elucidated from its cDNA.[50A] It appears to have evolved by a succession of gene duplication events that generated four homologous segments. These segments may fold and interact to generate two retinol-binding pockets. Isolation of cloned cDNA probes has permitted mapping of the IRBP structural gene to the centromere region of chromosome 10.[50A]

Figure 2-3 illustrates the first purification of human IRBP using single-step high-performance size-exclusion chromatography.[50] The peak at 205,000 daltons corresponds to IRBP and displays a single polypeptide band at 135,000 daltons when collected and examined by sodium dodecyl sulfate polyacrylamide gel electrophoresis. The fluorescence characteristics of the native protein show that it carries endogenous retinol, but its isomeric configuration could not be determined because sufficient quantities of the human protein were not available. Therefore, it was necessary to examine bovine IRBP instead.[21,35,50] The normal-phase high-performance liquid chromatogram shows that while the endogenous ligand of bovine

* A. Adler and J. C. Saari, personal communications

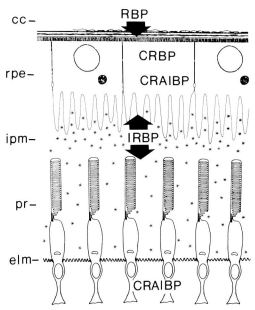

Figure 2-2. Binding proteins for the retinoids of the visual cycle (endogenous ligands shown below in parentheses): RBP, plasma retinol-binding protein (all-*trans* retinol); CRBP, cellular retinol-binding protein (all-*trans* retinol); IRBP, interstitial retinol-binding protein (all-*trans* and 11-*cis* retinol); CRALBP, cellular retinaldehyde-binding protein (11-*cis* retinol and 11-*cis* retinaldehyde); cc, choriocapillaris; rpe, retinal pigment epithelium; ipm, interphotoreceptor matrix; pr, photoreceptors; elm, external limiting membrane.

CRABP, cellular retinoic acid-binding protein, is not shown; retinoic acid is not convertible to retinol or retinaldehyde and hence cannot participate directly in the visual cycle.

IRBP consists mainly of all-*trans* retinol, 11-*cis* retinol is also present. The small amount of 13-*cis* retinol was probably an artifact of extraction. The proportion of 11-*cis* retinol was found to vary from preparation to preparation and may have depended on the degree of light adaptation.

Human IRBP is immunologically cross-reactive with bovine IRBP (Fig. 2-4) and has a similar amino acid composition and complement of oligosaccharide chains.[34] Its electrophoretic mobility is slightly greater than that of bovine IRBP. The molecular weight of IRBP obtained from the rhesus monkey appears to be identical with that from humans.

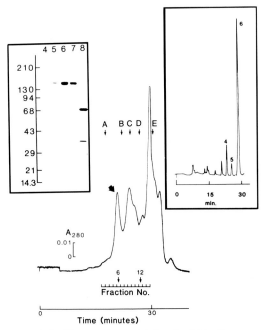

Figure 2-3. Human interstitial retinol-binding protein. The chromatogram obtained by high-performance size-exclusion liquid chromatography of human interphotoreceptor matrix shows a peak *(arrow)* due to IRBP at a molecular weight of 205,000 daltons. The protein in this peak was collected and found to display fluorescence due to endogenous retinol: the chromatogram obtained by normal-phase high-performance liquid chromatography of the endogenous retinol extracted from a similar sample of bovine IRBP is shown in the inset *(top right)*. Fractions were also collected and examined by sodium dodecyl sulfate polyacrylamide gel electrophoresis, as illustrated in the inset *(top left)*. Fraction 6, which corresponded to IRBP, displays a single polypeptide band of 135,000 daltons mol. wt. (Data from Fong S-L, Liou GI, Landers RA, et al: The characterization, localization and biosynthesis of an interstitial retinol-binding glycoprotein in the human eye. J Neurochem 42, 1667–1676, 1984)

Rat IRBP has also been purified and found to have a molecular weight (144,000 daltons) that is identical with that of bovine IRBP.[39] Its occurrence in rat IPM is demonstrable by immunohistochemistry with rabbit antibodies directed against the bovine protein (Fig. 2-5). Sections of adult Sprague-Dawley rat eyes were incubated with rabbit antibovine IRBP serum or with preimmune serum followed by an FITC-conjugated goat antirabbit secondary antibody. The sections were examined under fluorescent and

transmitted light. Immunospecific fluorescence was observed between the apical surface of the RPE and the external limiting membrane. The fluorescence was most intensely localized in a thin band adjacent to the RPE. The fluorescence was less intense over the ROS layer and was comparatively faint in the inner-segment region. No immunofluorescence was visible elsewhere in the retina or in the section treated with preimmune serum. In the region of the ora serrata the fluorescence terminated abruptly at the point where the photoreceptors disappear and the external limiting membrane merges with Verhoeff's membrane (Fig. 2-5).

Experiments where labeled sugar- and amino-acid precursors were incubated with rat, monkey, human, and bovine tissue showed that IRBP was synthesized and secreted into the extracellular space by the neural retina.[19,34,35,40] The cell of origin appeared to be the photoreceptor. Secretion was not prevented by tunicamycin, an antibiotic that inhibits the assembly of oligosaccharides linked N-glycosidically to proteins.

Prior to the demonstration that IRBP carried endogenous retinol, it was suggested that this protein might function in neural retina – RPE adhesion in a manner comparable to the role of fibronectin in other systems.[1,69] However, because the amount of retinol bound to IRBP increases when rhodopsin is bleached in the retina

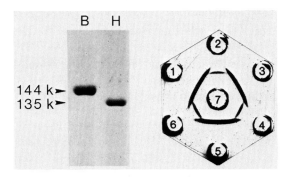

Figure 2-4. Human and bovine IRBP: comparison of electrophoretic mobility and immunological properties. *(Left)* Sodium dodecyl sulfate polyacrylamide gel electrophoresis of bovine (B) and human (H) IRBP. *Right:* Ouchterlony immunodiffusion plate showing partial cross-reactivity of human IRBP (wells 2, 4, 6) with rabbit antibovine IRBP serum (well 7); bovine IRBP was placed in wells 1, 3, 5. (Conditions as described by Fong[34,35])

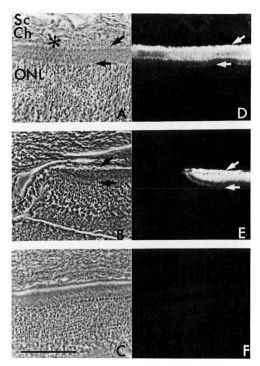

Figure 2-5. Immunocytochemical localization of IRBP in the retina of the rat. The antigen was visualized with rabbit antibovine IRBP serum and FITC-labeled goat antirabbit IgG. *(A, D)* Immune serum, area near posterior pole. *(B, E)* Immune serum, ora serrata. *(C, F)* Preimmune serum, area near posterior pole. Slanted arrows indicate the apical surface of the RPE cells; horizontal arrows indicate the position of the external limiting membrane. A line of more intense fluorescence is visible adjacent to the RPE. Sc, sclera; Ch, choroid; ONL, outer nuclear layer; ILM, internal limiting membrane; asterisk, RPE: scale bar, 100 μm.

it is now believed that the primary function of this protein, like that of RBP, is to transport retinol extracellularly.[2,49,50]

Intracellular Retinoid-Binding Proteins

When retinol passes from the plasma membrane to its intracellular sites of esterification and utilization, it is apparently bound to an intracellular protein, cellular retinol-binding protein (CRBP).[53] CRBP is distinct from RBP immunologically, spectroscopically, by its lower molecular weight (15,000 daltons), and by its failure to complex with transthyretin. CRBP occurs in many tissues, but most of the CRBP in

the eye is found in the RPE.[25] Very little, if any, is associated with the cells of the neural retina.[61] Its endogenous ligand is exclusively all-*trans* retinol.[62]

Binding proteins for other retinoids are also present in the retina and RPE. They include cellular retinoic acid binding protein (CRABP) and cellular retinal-binding protein (CRALBP).[61,64] CRABP also occurs in many other tissues but not in the RPE.[25] Its endogenous ligand consists of all-*trans* retinoic acid. CRALBP is restricted to the RPE and the Müller cells of the retina.[22] Its endogenous ligands consist of 11-*cis* retinaldehyde and 11-*cis* retinol.[62]

THE VISUAL CYCLE: REGENERATION OF RHODOPSIN

Nearly all studies on the visual cycle have been carried out on frogs and rats.[13,29,72] When dark-adapted, rats have very little vitamin A in the RPE, but frogs store about 2 moles of retinyl palmitate per mole of rhodopsin in the retina. After 24 hours of dark adaptation about half of this ester may be in the 11-*cis* conformation.[13] In both species it has been demonstrated that when a large fraction of rhodopsin is bleached by intense light adaptation, there is a corresponding accumulation of all-*trans* retinyl ester in the RPE. In frogs, it has also been shown that pre-existing supplies of 11-*cis* retinyl ester are consumed over several cycles of bleaching and regeneration.[13] Therefore, at the end of a period of strong light adaptation, rats and frogs are faced with the task of carrying out an overall conversion of all-*trans* retinyl ester to 11-*cis* retinaldehyde. In frogs and rats, the retinoid that is isomerized appears to be all-*trans* retinol, the isomerase being in the pigment epithelium.[7A,16A] Photo-isomerization of all-*trans* retinoid does not appear to play a role in the physiological process of dark adaptation in vertebrates.[15] Recent observations have suggested that the apparently straightforward exchange of retinoids between the ROS and RPE may be more complicated, perhaps involving the Müller cells.[21,22]

Any proposed description of the *vertebrate*

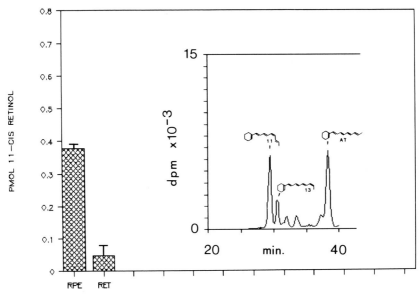

Figure 2-6. Isomerization of all-*trans* to 11-*cis* retinol by microsomal fractions from dark-adapted frog RPE and retina. The low level of activity in the retina (12.7 percent of the RPE) may be due to contamination by RPE. The ordinate represents pmol of 11-*cis* retinol formed over a 3-hour incubation. The inset shows the radioactivity profile of an hplc chromatogram obtained in a typical experiment. A microsomal fraction (approximately 600 μg protein $\times$ ml^{-1}) from dark-adapted RPE and retina was incubated with 8.5 pmol of (^{3}H) all-*trans* retinol (about 10^6 dpm). After 3 hours, the prominent radioactive peak corresponding to 11-*cis* retinol demonstrates that this isomer has been formed in the incubation mixture. The smaller peak due to 13-*cis* retinol is formed by nonenzymatic isomerization. (Data of Bridges and Alvarez[16A])

visual cycle must take account of the following observations. (1) CRALBP, which binds 11-*cis* retinoids, occurs only in the RPE and Müller cells.[22] (2) The major endogenous ligand of CRALBP is 11-*cis* retinaldehyde in the RPE but mainly 11-*cis* retinol in the retina.[21,50,62] Unidentified membrane fractions from the retina (but not the ROS and RPE) also contain 11-*cis* retinol.[21] (3) Eleven-*cis* retinol oxidoreductase, which is necessary to form 11-*cis* retinaldehyde from 11-*cis* retinol, is absent from the retina of mammals but present in the RPE.[48,73]

The RPE is generally acknowledged to have a role in visual pigment regeneration. Until recently however, no isomerase has been demonstrated in fresh or cultured RPE cells.[33] Therefore, it had been suggested that the site of isomerization must lie in the retina.[12,13,33] The difficulty with this idea is that, except for one unconfirmed observation in the rat, isolated retinas do not regenerate rhodopsin.[26] As noted

above, this question has now been resolved by the finding that retinol isomerase is concentrated in the pigment epithelium.[7A,16A]

The 11-*cis* retinol found in the *retina* may have been delivered to the Müller cells, perhaps after IRBP has transported 11-*cis* retinol from the RPE to their apical membranes. As noted above, 11-*cis* retinaldehyde cannot be formed from 11-*cis* retinol in the mammalian retina because this tissue lacks 11-*cis* retinol oxidoreductase.[48,54,70,73] The occurrence of this stereospecific enzyme in the RPE coupled with the predominance of 11-*cis* retinaldehyde bound to CRALBP in the RPE cytosol suggests that another important role of the RPE in the mammalian visual cycle is to convert 11-*cis* retinol to 11-*cis* retinaldehyde (Fig. 2-6).[48,73] Clearly, IRBP may be implicated in the transport of 11-*cis* retinoids as well as all-*trans* retinol.

In the scheme in Figure 2-7, any 11-*cis* retinol that is not immediately utilized by the pathway

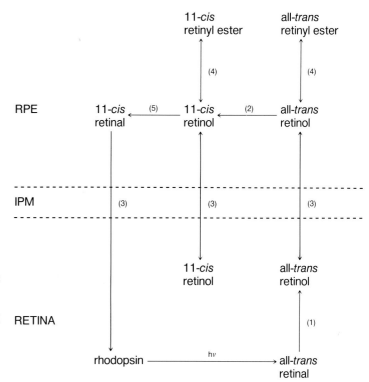

Figure 2-7. Proposed visual cycle in the vertebrate eye. 1, all-*trans* retinol oxidoreductase.[38,48,73] 2, isomerase.[7A,16A] 3, transport of retinoid through the IPM, possibly bound to IRBP. 4, ester synthase and hydrolase.[23,45] 5, 11-*cis* retinol oxidoreductase.[48,73]

leading to rhodopsin regeneration would be esterified and stored, thus accounting for the observed accumulation of 11-*cis* retinyl esters in dark-adapted eyes.[3,45] This pool may also exchange with opsin molecules in the dark.[17,28] Strong illumination would release large quantities of all-*trans* retinol that could bypass the isomerization reaction in the RPE by being esterified, as observed experimentally.[13,29]

In summary, in the vertebrate visual cycle 11-*cis* retinol is generated from all-*trans* retinol in the pigment epithelium, where (at least in mammals) it is converted to 11-*cis* retinol. IRBP appears to be implicated in delivering all-*trans* retinol to the RPE and in returning 11-*cis* retinoids to the retina (Müller cells, rod outer segments).

HUMAN RETINAL DISEASE

The association of night-blindness with vitamin A deficiency is well documented.[8] In its initial stages, nutritional night-blindness appears to be caused by loss of rhodopsin.[32] In rats, this is followed by degeneration of the ROS and loss of the photoreceptors.[30] Degeneration occurs even in animals that are maintained on a retinoic-acid-supplemented diet. Because of the resemblance between the histopathology of the retina in retinitis pigmentosa and in vitamin-A deficiency, there have been several attempts to find a link between the disease and some malfunction in the absorption, transport, delivery, or utilization of vitamin A. Thus retinal degeneration is observed in abetalipoproteinemia, where there is an inability to form chylomicrons.[23,41,63] Retinitis pigmentosa patients, however, have normal serum-retinol and RBP levels, and the RBP molecule itself is not abnormal.[37,51] These findings, as well as the failure to arrest or reverse the progression of the disease by vitamin-A therapy make it unlikely that retinitis pigmentosa arises from a defect in the absorption of vitamin A or in its delivery to the eye.[6] There is the possibility that retinitis pigmentosa is associated

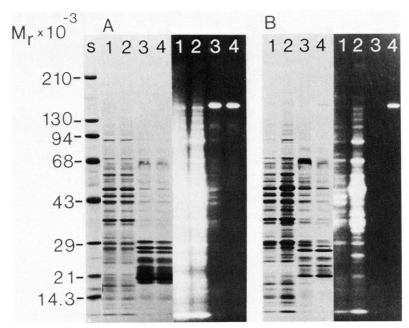

Figure 2-8. Evidence that the photoreceptors synthesize and secrete IRBP. Fluorograms show the synthesis *in vitro* of IRBP by the retinas of RCS rats and their congenic controls (RCS/rdy$^+$). Incubations were carried out with (^{3}H)-leucine as described by Gonzalez-Fernandez and colleagues.[40] Lanes 1, RCS retina cystosols; lanes 2, control retina cytosols; lanes 3, RCS retina media; lanes 4, control retina media. *(A)* P15 RCS, P18 controls; *(B)* P99 RCS, P100 controls.

with a defect in the transport of vitamin A within the ocular tissues or in an enzyme responsible for its isomerization or conversion to one of its derivatives. Work that has been carried out to investigate this question has included therapy with 11-*cis* vitamin A to remedy any possible deficiency in the isomerization system and studies in retinitis pigmentosa patients of the ERG and the relationship between rhodopsin and visual sensitivity.[8,24,42,55,60] The results have not been clear cut.[15] However, more recent studies on eyes donated by patients with hereditary chorioretinal degeneration have provided further insights into the possible role of vitamin A in these diseases.[16,19]

An early suggestion that was prompted by observations on the Royal College of Surgeons (RCS) rat model of retinal dystrophy was that there might be a defect in the ability of the RPE to esterify retinol.[7,59] This could lead to a damaging accumulation of free retinol in the RPE. The human disease does not seem to be associated with this problem, because Bridges and

colleagues were unable to identify any abnormality in the storage or formation of retinyl esters in RPE from a patient with retinitis pigmentosa.[19] This tissue also contained 11-*cis* retinyl esters in proportions that were close to normal. On the other hand, while the vitamin A stores in the RPE of another patient with a retinal degeneration resembling retinitis pigmentosa were essentially normal in amount, they were selectively depleted in the 11-*cis* isomer.[16,27,58] It was not determined whether this depletion was a primary cause of the degeneration or whether it was secondary to it.

Recent studies on the RCS rat have provided new information on the role of IRBP in retinal dystrophy.[39,40] During the first three weeks of postnatal life the amount of IRBP in RCS rats was found to increase with the elongation of the rod outer segments, but subsequently (as demonstrated by immunocytochemical and biochemical means) it declined rapidly. This proved to be an important finding because Bridges and coworkers had earlier reported that they were unable to detect IRBP in the eye of a patient with retinitis pigmentosa.[19] Thus although it appears that the hereditary defect in the RCS rat (viz., failure to phagocytize shed rod outer-segment tips) is not the defect in retinitis pigmentosa, there may be some common features to these conditions.[46,65,66]

In the dystrophic rats the retina ceased to synthesize and secrete IRBP when the photoreceptors had degenerated, suggesting that these cells were its source (Fig. 2-8). This suggestion has been confirmed by Hollyfield and coworkers.[43]

The possibility that loss of IRBP plays a role in photoreceptor cell death in the RCS rat was considered by Gonzalez-Fernandez and associates.[40] Although reduction in the amount of IRBP was not observed until after the appearance of pyknotic nuclei in the outer nuclear layer, they suggested that depletion of IRBP could permit a potentially damaging accumulation of retinol in the photoreceptor layers and that this might account for the observation that cell death is retarded in darkness.[29,47] IRBP is also capable of binding α-tocopherol: loss of IRBP could therefore accelerate the degradation of photoreceptor membranes by depriving them of an agent that may protect them from oxidative damage.[35]

In summary, the cause or causes of retinitis pigmentosa are yet to be found. At present, a possible role for vitamin A in this condition has not been established, but recent observations on IRBP in an animal model of retinal dystrophy and in the eye of a patient with retinitis pigmentosa are new and intriguing developments. Much more work is needed to provide further insights into the problem.

REFERENCES

1. Adler AJ, Klucznik KM: Proteins and glycoproteins of the bovine interphotoreceptor matrix: Composition and fractionation. Exp Eye Res 34:423–434, 1982
2. Adler AJ, Martin KJ: Retinol-binding proteins in bovine interphotoreceptor matrix. Biochem Biophys Res Comm 108:1601–1608, 1982
3. Alvarez RA, Bridges CDB, Fong S-L: High-pressure liquid chromatography of fatty acid esters of retinol isomers — Analysis of retinyl esters stored in the eye. Invest Ophthalmol Vis Sci 20:304–313, 1981
4. Applebury ML, Rentzepis PM: Picosecond spectroscopy of visual pigments. Methods Enzymol 81:354–368, 1982
5. Baumann C, Bender S: Kinetics of rhodopsin bleaching in the isolated retina. J Physiol 235:761–773, 1973
6. Bergsma DR, Wolf ML: A therapeutic trial of vitamin A in patients with pigmentary retinal degeneration: A negative study. In Landers, MA et al (eds): Retinitis Pigmentosa, pp 197–209. New York, Plenum Press, 1976
7. Berman ER, Segal N, Photiou S, et al: Inherited retinal dystrophy in RCS rats: A deficiency in vitamin A esterification in pigment epithelium. Nature 293:217–220, 1981
7A. Bernstein PS, Law WC, Rando RR: Isomerization of all-*trans* retinoids to 11-*cis* retinoids in vitro. Proc. Natl Acad Sci USA 84: 1849–1853, 1987
8. Berson EL: Nutrition and retinal degenerations: Vitamin A, taurine, ornithine, and phytanic acid. The Retina 2:236–255, 1982
9. Bhat MK, Cama HR: Gonadal cell surface receptor for plasma retinol binding protein: A method for its radioassay and studies on its level during spermatogenesis. Biochim Biophys Acta 587:273–281, 1979
10. Bok D, Heller J: Transport of retinol from the blood to the retina: An autoradiographic study of the pigment epithelial cell surface receptor for plasma retinol binding protein. Exp Eye Res 22:395–402, 1976
11. Bridges CDB: The rhodopsin–porphyropsin visual system. In Dartnall HJA (ed): Handbook of Sensory Physiology 7/1A, pp 418–480. Berlin, Springer-Verlag, 1972
12. Bridges CDB: 11-*cis* Vitamin A in dark-adapted rod outer segments is a probable source of prosthetic groups for rhodopsin biosynthesis. Nature 259:247–248, 1976
13. Bridges CDB: Vitamin A and the role of the pigment epithelium during bleaching and regeneration of rhodopsin in the frog eye. Exp Eye Res 22:435–455, 1976
14. Bridges CDB: Rhodopsin regeneration in rod outer segments: Utilization of 11-*cis* retinal and retinol. Exp Eye Res 24:571–580, 1977
15. Bridges CDB: Retinoids in Photosensitive Systems. In Sporn MB, Roberts AB, Goodman, DS (eds): The Retinoids, vol 2, pp 125–176. New York, Academic Press, 1984
16. Bridges CDB, Alvarez RA: Selective loss of 11-*cis* vitamin A in an eye with hereditary chorioretinal degeneration similar to sector retinitis pigmentosa. Retina 2:256–260, 1982
16A. Bridges CDB, Alvarez RA: The visual cycle operates through an isomerase acting on all-*trans* retinol in the pigment epithelium. Science (in press)
17. Bridges CDB, Yoshikami S: Uptake of tritiated

retinaldehyde by the visual pigment of dark-adapted rats. Nature 221:275–276, 1970

18. Bridges CDB, Alvarez RA, Fong S-L: Vitamin A in human eyes—Amount, distribution and composition. Invest Ophthalmol Vis Sci 22:706–714, 1982

19. Bridges CDB, O'Gorman S, Fong SL, et al: Vitamin A and interstitial retinol-binding protein in an eye with recessive retinitis pigmentosa. Invest Ophthalmol Vis Sci 26:684–691, 1985

20. Bridges CDB, Fong S-L, Liou GI, et al: A retinol-binding glycoprotein synthesized and secreted by mammalian neural retina. Society for Neuroscience. Abstract. 13th Annual Meeting

21. Bridges CDB, Alvarez RA, Fong S-L, et al: Visual cycle in the mammalian eye: Retinoid-binding proteins and the distribution of 11-*cis* retinoids. Vision Res 24,1581–1594, 1984

22. Bunt-Milam AH, Saari JC: Immunocytochemical localization of two retinoid-binding proteins in vertebrate retina. J Cell Biol 97:703–712, 1983

23. Carr RE: Abetalipoproteinemia and the eye. In Bergsma D, Bron AJ, Cotlier E (eds): The Eye and Inborn Errors of Metabolism. Birth Defects: Original Article Series XII.3, pp 385–399. New York, Alan Liss Inc., 1976

24. Chatzinoff A, Nelson E, Stahl N, et al: Eleven-*cis* vitamin A in the treatment of retinitis pigmentosa: A negative study. Arch Ophthalmol 80:417–419, 1968

25. Chytil F, Ong DE: Cellular Retinoid Binding Proteins. In Sporn MB, Roberts AB, Goodman DS: The Retinoids. New York, Academic Press, 1984

26. Cone RA, Brown PK: Spontaneous regeneration of rhodopsin in the isolated rat retina. Nature 221:818–820, 1969

27. Cope LA, Teeters VW, Borda RP, et al: Sector retinitis pigmentosa with chronic disc edema. Doc Ophthal Proc Ser Int Symp on Fluorescein Angiography, pp 431–437. The Hague, Dr. W. Junk b.v. Publishers, 1976

28. Defoe DM, Bok, D: Rhodopsin chromophore exchanges among opsin molecules in the dark. Invest Ophthalmol Vis Sci 24:1211–1226, 1983

29. Dowling JE: Chemistry of visual adaptation in the rat. Nature, 188:114–118, 1960

30. Dowling JE, Gibbons IR: The effect of vitamin A deficiency on the fine structure of the retina. In Smelser GK (ed): The Structure of the Eye, pp 85–99. New York, Academic Press, 1961

31. Dowling JE, Sidman RL: Inherited retinal dystrophy in the rat. J Cell Biol 14:73–109, 1962

32. Dowling JE, Wald G: Vitamin A deficiency and night blindness. Proc Natl Acad Sci Wash 44:648–661, 1958

33. Flood MT, Bridges CDB, Alvarez RA, et al: Vitamin A utilization in human retinal pigment epi-

thelial cells *in vitro.* Invest Ophthalmol Vis Sci 24:1227–1235, 1983

34. Fong S-L, Liou GI, Landers RA, et al: The characterization, localization and biosynthesis of an interstitial retinol-binding glycoprotein in the human eye. J Neurochem 42:1667–1676, 1984

35. Fong S-L, Liou GI, Alvarez RA, et al: Purification and characterization of a retinol-binding glycoprotein synthesized and secreted by bovine neural retina. J Biol Chem 259:6534–6542, 1984

36. Futterman S: Metabolism of the retina. III. Role of reduced triphosphopyridine nucleotide in the visual cycle. J Biol Chem 238:1145–1150, 1963

37. Futterman S, Swanson D, Kalina RE: Retinol in retinitis pigmentosa: Evidence that retinol is in normal concentration in serum and the retinol-binding protein complex displays unaltered fluorescence properties. Invest Ophthalmol Vis Sci 13:798–801, 1974

38. Goodman DS: Plasma retinol-binding protein. In Sporn MB, Roberts AB, Goodman DS (eds): The Retinoids. New York, Academic Press, 1984

39. Gonzalez-Fernandez F, Fong S-L, Liou GI, et al: A retinol-binding glycoprotein of the interphotoreceptor matrix: Localization, synthesis and secretion in normal and dystrophic rat retinas. J Cell Biol 97:454a, 1983

40. Gonzalez-Fernandez F, Landers RA, Glazebrook PA, et al: An extracellular retinol-binding glycoprotein in the eyes of mutant rats with retinal dystrophy—development, localization and biosynthesis. J Cell Biol 99:2092–2098, 1984

41. Gouras P, Carr RE, Gunkel RD: Retinitis pigmentosa in abetalipoproteinemia: Effects of vitamin A. Invest Ophthalmol Vis Sci 10:784–793, 1971

42. Highman VN, Weale RA: Rhodopsin density and visual threshold in retinitis pigmentosa. Am J Ophthalmol 75:822–832, 1973

43. Hollyfield JG, Fliesler SJ, Rayborn ME, et al: Synthesis and secretion of interstitial retinol-binding protein by the human retina. Invest Ophthalmol Vis Sci 26:58–67, 1985

44. Knowles A, Dartnall HJA: In Davson H (ed): The Eye, Vol 2B. The photobiology of vision. New York, Academic Press, 1977

45. Krinsky NI: The enzymatic esterification of vitamin A. J Biol Chem 232:881–894, 1958

46. LaVail MM: Analysis of neurological mutants with inherited retinal degeneration. Invest Ophthalmol Vis Sci 21:638–657, 1981

47. LaVail MM, Battelle B-A: Influence of eye pigmentation and light deprivation on inherited retinal dystrophy in the rat. Exp Eye Res 21:167–192, 1975

48. Lion F, Rotmans JP, Daemen FJM, et al: Stereospecificity of ocular retinol dehydrogenases and

the visual cycle. Biochim Biophys Acta 384:283–292, 1975

49. Liou GI, Bridges CDB, Fong S-L: Vitamin A transport between retina and pigment epithelium—An interphotoreceptor matrix protein carrying endogenous retinol (IRBP). Invest Ophthalmol Vis Sci 22 (Suppl):65, 1982

50. Liou, GI, Bridges CDB, Fong S-L: Vitamin A transport between retina and pigment epithelium—An interstitial protein carrying endogenous retinol (interstitial retinol-binding protein). Vision Res 22:1457–1468, 1982

50A. Liou GI, Fong SL, Gosden J, et al: Human interstitial retinol-binding protein (IRBP): cloning, partial sequence and chromosomal localization. Somatic Cell Mol Genet (in press)

51. Maraini G, Fadda G, Gozzoli F: Serum levels of retinol-binding protein in different genetic types of retinitis pigmentosa. Invest Ophthalmol Vis Sci 14:236–237, 1975

52. McGuire BW, Orgebin-Crist MC, Chytil F: Autoradiographic localization of serum retinol-binding protein in rat testis. Endocrinology 108:658–667, 1981

53. Ong DE, Chytil F: Cellular retinol-binding protein from rat liver: Purification and characterization. J Biol Chem 253:828–832, 1978

54. Pepperberg DR, Masland RH: Retinal-induced sensitization of light-adapted rabbit photoreceptors. Brain Res 151:194–200, 1978

55. Perlman I, Auerbach E: The relationship between visual sensitivity and rhodopsin density in retinitis pigmentosa. Invest Ophthalmol Vis Sci 20:758–765, 1981

56. Rask L, Peterson P: *In vitro* uptake of vitamin A from the retinol-binding plasma protein to mucosal epithelial cells from the monkey's small intestine. J Biol Chem 251:6360–6366, 1976

57. Rask L, Geijer C, Bill A, et al: Vitamin A supply of the cornea. Exp Eye Res 31:201–211, 1980

58. Rayborn ME, Moorhead LC, Hollyfield JG: A dominantly inherited chorioretinal degeneration resembling sectoral retinitis pigmentosa. Ophthalmology 89:1441–1454, 1982

59. Reading HW: Retinal and retinol metabolism in hereditary degeneration of the retina. Biochem J 100:34, 1966

60. Ripps H, Brin KP, Weale, RA: Rhodopsin and visual threshold in retinitis pigmentosa. Invest Ophthalmol Vis Sci 17:735–745, 1978

61. Saari JC, Futterman S, Bredberg L: Cellular retinol- and retinoic-acid binding proteins of bovine retina: Purification and properties. J Biol Chem 253:6432–6436, 1978

62. Saari JC, Bredberg L, Garwin GC: Identification of the endogenous retinoids associated with three cellular retinoid-binding proteins from bovine retina and retinal pigment epithelium. J Biol Chem 257:13329–13333, 1982

63. von Sallmann L, Gelderman AH, Laster L: Ocular histopathologic changes in a case of abetalipoproteinemia (Bassen–Kornzweig syndrome). Doc Ophthal 26:451–460, 1969

64. Stubbs GW, Saari JC, Futterman S: 11-*cis*-Retinal-binding protein from rat retina. Isolation and partial characterization. J Biol Chem 254:8529–8533, 1979

65. Szamier RB, Berson EL: Retinal ultrastructure in advanced retinitis pigmentosa. Invest Ophthalmol Vis Sci 16:947–962, 1977

66. Szamier RB, Berson EL, Klein R, et al: Sex-linked retinitis pigmentosa: Ultrastructure of the photoreceptors and pigment epithelium. Invest Ophthalmol Vis Sci 18:145–160, 1979

67. Wald G: The molecular basis of visual excitation. Nature 219:800–807, 1968

68. Wang JK, McDowell JH, Hargrave PA: Site of attachment of 11-*cis* retinal in bovine rhodopsin. Biochemistry 19:5111–5117, 1980

69. Yamada KM: Cell surface interactions with extracellular materials. Ann Rev Biochem 52:761–799, 1983

70. Yoshikami S, Noll GN: Isolated retinas synthesize visual pigments from retinol congeners delivered by liposomes. Science 200:1393–1395, 1978

71. Yoshizawa T, Shichida Y: Low-temperature spectrophotometry of intermediates of rhodopsin. Methods Enzymol 81:333–354, 1982

72. Zimmerman WF: The distribution and proportions of vitamin A compounds during the visual cycle in the rat. Vision Res 14:795–802, 1974

73. Zimmerman WF, Lion R, Daemen FJM, et al: Distribution of stereospecific retinol dehydrogenase activities in sub-cellular fractions of bovine retina and pigment epithelium. Exp Eye Res 21:325–332, 1975

3

Electrical Interactions Between the RPE and the Photoreceptors

Roy H. Steinberg

The retinal pigment epithelium (RPE) can be described as a simple epithelium that separates a cavity, the subretinal space (or paraventricular space), from the blood (choriocapillaris) (Fig. 3-1). In its principal functions the RPE interacts with the photoreceptor layer, which it faces across the subretinal space. In considering its remarkably diverse array of functions we can view the RPE as behaving as three cell types with respect to the photoreceptors—epithelium, macrophage, and glia (Fig. 3-2). These three modes of cell function are, of course, not totally separate, but they can help to organize the way we view the many functions of these cells.

As an epithelium the RPE bounds the subretinal space, separating it from the blood and acting as a barrier. Like other epithelia its apical and basal membranes face completely different environments and are anatomically and functionally very different. The villous nature of its apical surface suggests the epithelial functions of absorption and secretion. Both membranes function together to transport metabolites, water, and salt between the blood and the subretinal space.

RPE cells are also macrophages serving the photoreceptors by phagocytizing the shed tips of outer segments. Here it is a special macrophage

This research was supported by a grant from the National Institutes of Health EY 01429. The author is indebted to his colleagues, S.S. Miller, B. Oakley II, E.R. Griff, and R.A. Linsenmeier, for their contributions to this work.

en place. But in case of damage to the neural retina, RPE cells can detach from Bruch's membrane, multiply, and rove the neural retina cleaning up debris in the manner typical of macrophages elsewhere in the body.

As a cell providing support for neurones, the photoreceptors, RPE–photoreceptor interactions suggest the glia–neuron relationship. The qualities of all four classes of glia can be observed in this association. In location, forming the lining of a ventricular space, it is *ependymal.* In the structural specialization of the apical surface, ensheathing photoreceptor outer segments, it acts like *oligodendrocytes.* In function, it resembles *astrocytes,* providing metabolic support and determining the contents of the extracellular environment. Finally, like *microglia,* it is a "professional" macrophage.

RPE cells are especially similar to glial cells in the way they respond electrically to changes in the extracellular concentration of potassium ($[K^+]_o$) that result from photoreceptor activity.[13] There is also evidence from research on the light peak (see below) that the RPE probably also responds electrically to substances other than K^+.[36] These electrical responses, which are changes in the membrane potentials and membrane resistances of the RPE, are of interest for at least two reasons. First, we can imagine that they may be involved in the functional interactions between RPE cells and photoreceptors. By studying these electrical events, we hope to link them to cellular mechanisms, such as changes in

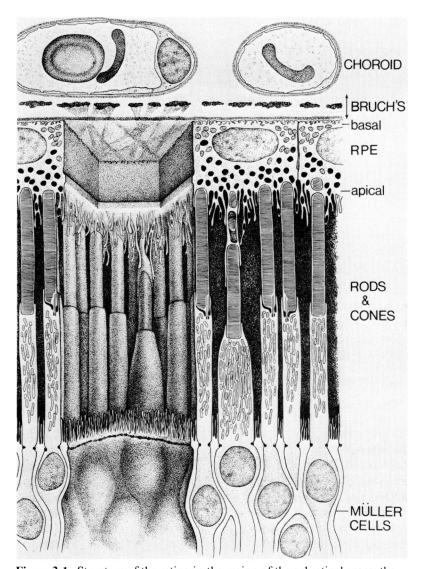

Figure 3-1. Structure of the retina in the region of the subretinal space: the subretinal space is the extracellular space surrounding the photoreceptors (rods and cones). Its proximal (vitreal) boundaries are the basal portions of photoreceptor inner segments and the Müller cells at the outer limiting membrane. Distally (sclerally) it is bounded by the apical membranes of RPE cells, a single layer of cells bounded proximally by the neural retina and distally by the choroid. Its basal surface rests on Bruch's membrane. Belts of tight junctions encircle the RPE cells dividing their membranes into basal (basolateral) and apical portions. The basal membranes and the tight junctions form the RPE portion of the barrier between the blood and the neural retina. The apical membrane extrudes profuse villous and sheetlike processes that are closely apposed to and ensheath portions of the outer segments of the rods and cones. This drawing generally follows retinal structure as observed in electron micrographs of human retina. (Steinberg RH, Linsenmeier L, Griff ER: Three light-evoked responses of the retinal pigment epithelium. Vis Res 11:1315, 1983)

Functions of RPE

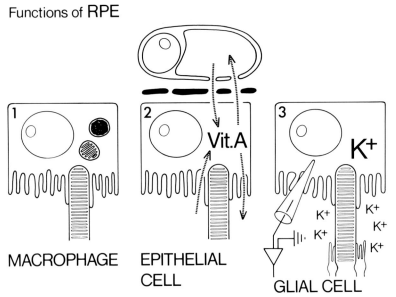

Figure 3-2. The RPE can be seen to function as three distinct cells. *(1)* As a macrophage it phagocytizes and degrades the shed tips of photoreceptor outer segments. *(2)* As an epithelial cell it transports molecules between the blood and the subretinal space. *(3)* As a glial cell, its apical membrane ensheaths portions of the photoreceptor outer segments and responds to changes in subretinal $[K^+]_0$. (Steinberg RH, Linsenmeier L, Griff ER: Three light-evoked responses of the retinal pigment epithelium. Vis Res 11:1315, 1983)

ion, metabolite, and water transport between the RPE and the blood or the RPE and the neural retina. Second, the electrical responses contribute to changes in the corneoretinal potential recorded in the human DC–electroretinogram (DC–ERG) and electro-oculogram (EOG). In a sense the photoreceptors and RPE cells carry on a conversation that can be monitored at the cornea. The clinician is provided with information about RPE–photoreceptor interactions whose value may depend on how well he understands the physiological mechanisms that cause these interactions. Let us look at these electrical responses as they are observed in the DC–ERG.

DC–ERG

Absorption of light by the photoreceptors produces three ERG components that have substantial RPE contributions: c-wave, fast oscillation, and light peak. In cat, these responses depend predominantly on the rods, but small cone contributions, particularly at photopic light levels, cannot be ruled out.[15,17,31] All three responses have time-courses considerably slower than the a- and b-waves.[27] Figure 3-3 shows a vitreal DC–ERG from the cat retina in response to 5 minutes of illumination. Following the b-wave, the potential rises to a positive peak at 2 to 4 seconds, the c-wave. Following the c-wave there is a return to baseline (or to below baseline at higher illumination) that peaks at 20 seconds, which we call the fast-oscillation trough. (The term *fast oscillation* is also used in a different sense, in EOG recordings.) After this trough, the potential rises to the light peak. The peak voltage is reached at 5 to 6 minutes and then diminishes, whether or not illumination is maintained. The end of illumination is accompanied by a relatively rapid decrease in potential, an "OFF c-wave."[3,27,37] This recording is very similar to DC recordings made from the human eye.[40]

The c-wave, fast oscillation, and light peak

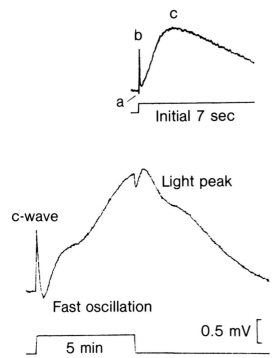

Figure 3-3. A DC–ERG (cat) in response to a 5-minute period of illumination at 9.3 log quanta/deg²/sec showing the c-wave, fast oscillation, and light peak. Inset shows initial 7 seconds at an expanded time scale. (Modified from Linsenmeier RA, Steinberg RH: Delayed basal hyperpolarization of cat retinal pigment epithelium and its relation to the fast oscillation of the DC electroretinogram. J Gen Physiol 83:213, 1984; by permission of Rockefeller University Press)

will be considered, in turn, in the ensuing paragraphs. Our attention will be given to the location and mechanism of each RPE generator and how the ERG wave forms are determined by events in the RPE and neural retina.

EXPERIMENTAL METHODS AND STRATEGIES

The majority of the experiments have been performed on experimental animals using two different types of preparations: intraocular recordings from the eye of the cat or *in-vitro* preparations of ocular tissues from cold-blooded vertebrates, either the bullfrog *(R. catesbeiana)* or a lizard, the gecko *(Gekko gekko).*[5,6,17,23,37]

To determine the cellular origin of any ERG

component, it is first necessary to determine whether it can be recorded across the neural retina, the RPE, or both. The experimental approach is to place extracellular electrodes that will record potentials originating either in the neural retina or in the RPE. The recording configuration for these experiments is diagrammed in Figure 3-4. The arrow on the left side of the figure represents a microelectrode that has been placed in the subretinal space (between the neural retina and the RPE). In the cat, microelectrodes used for intraretinal and intracellular recordings were advanced into the eye through a hypodermic needle. The DC–ERG was recorded between the vitreal electrode and the reference behind the eye. In an experiment the microelectrode penetrated the retina at its vitreal border, the internal limiting membrane, and passed through the entire thickness of the neural retina. It was then positioned accurately in the subretinal space by first penetrating an RPE cell and then withdrawing a few microns. By referring this electrode to the back of the eye, the potential across the RPE, the transepithelial potential (TEP), was recorded. By referring the electrode to the vitreous, the potential across the neural retina, the transretinal potential, was recorded.

In the gecko experiments a 3.0-mm square piece of tissue, consisting of the neural retina, RPE, and choroid, was excised from the eye and mounted in a Lucite chamber. The retinal and choroidal surfaces were each separately perfused by a modified Ringer's solution. The transtissue potential, equivalent to the vitreal recording in cat, was recorded between agar–Ringer bridges placed in the baths on each side of the tissue. The transepithelial and transretinal potentials were simultaneously recorded between a microelectrode in the subretinal space and references in each of the baths.

Transepithelial Potential

The transepithelial potential (TEP) is determined by the potentials of both membranes of the RPE, the apical membrane potential and the basal membrane potential. Since the electrical responses of the RPE are recorded as changes of the TEP, such changes could originate from

Recordings

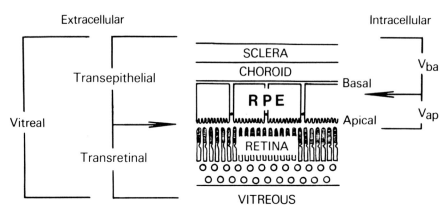

Figure 3-4. Recording configurations. As shown, for cat, vitreal recordings were made between an electrode in the vitreous and a reference behind the eye. The arrow *(left)* represents a microelectrode placed within the subretinal space that when referenced behind the eye recorded the transepithelial potential. The transretinal recording was obtained by subtraction (by computer) of the vitreal and transepithelial recordings. Intracellular recordings were obtained by placing the microelectrode in the cytoplasm of an RPE cell *(arrow, right)*. The basal membrane potential, V_{ba}, was recorded between this microelectrode and the reference behind the eye. The apical membrane potential, V_{ap}, was obtained from subtraction of a basal membrane response from a transepithelial response obtained subsequently. In gecko, the recording configurations were essentially the same. The transtissue potential was essentially equivalent to the vitreal recording in cat, while the transretinal and transepithelial potentials were recorded simultaneously as were the apical and basal RPE membrane potentials. (Steinberg RH, Griff ER, Linsenmeier RA: The cellular origin of the light peak. Doc Ophthal Proc Series 37:1, 1983)

changes in either or both membrane potentials. Let us consider how the TEP is generated (Fig. 3-5). The TEP is the difference between the apical and basal membrane potential that occurs because of differences in the passive and active ionic transport characteristics of the two cell membranes.[35] In the frog, for example, the apical membrane potential is more hyperpolarized (more "inside negative") than the basal membrane potential. The difference is a TEP of about 10 mV whose polarity is apical-side- (or vitreal-) positive.

An increase in TEP, as will be shown for the c-wave and light peak, can originate at the two cell membranes in one of two ways. If it originates at the apical membrane, then this membrane must *hyperpolarize* with respect to the basal membrane. If it originates at the basal membrane, this membrane must *depolarize* with respect to the apical. Conversely, a decrease in TEP, as will be shown for the fast-oscillation

trough, can originate in either an apical depolarization or a basal hyperpolarization. (One additional possibility is that the response originates as a diffusion potential across the paracellular shunt, a condition that has not yet been observed for any ERG potential.) The mechanisms in each case are clearly quite different, and finding out which one is responsible for the response is an important step toward understanding its mechanism.

If we are to interpret intracellular recordings from the RPE, we must also take into account the effects of passive voltage drops at the cell membranes produced by current flow across the *shunt* resistances. In the circuit diagram of Figure 3-5A it is clear that the apical and basal membranes are connected through R_s, primarily the resistance of the tight junctions between cells. This means that current must flow around the circuit that will modify the apical and basal membrane potentials. More importantly this

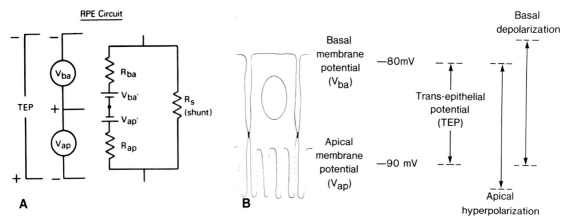

Figure 3-5. Schematic circuit of the retinal pigment epithelium and mechanisms for an increase in transepithelial potential. *(A)* Circuit components: R_{ap}, apical membrane resistance; R_{ba}, basal membrane resistance; R_s, shunt resistance; V'_{ap}, apical membrane battery; V'_{ba}, basal membrane battery; V_{ap}, measured apical membrane potential; V_{ba}, measured basal membrane potential. TEP, transepithelial potential. *(B)* A TEP increase may result either from a hyperpolarization of V_{ap} relative to V_{ba} or from a depolarization of V_{ba} relative to V_{ap}. (Steinberg RH, Griff ER, Linsenmeier RA: The cellular origin of the light peak. Doc Ophthal Proc Series 37:1, 1983)

current will change whenever a potential is initiated at either cell membrane. The size and relative importance of this effect varies depending on the relative size of all three resistances in this circuit (R_{ap}, R_{ba}, R_s). The practical effect of shunting is to reduce the magnitude of the voltage at the membrane generating it and to produce a smaller voltage of the same polarity at the opposite membrane.

COMPONENTS OF THE DC–ERG

C-Wave

The c-wave as recorded at the cornea or in the vitreous humor of animals is the sum of two components.[30] One component, generated by the RPE, is called here the *TEP c-wave;* the other component, generated in the neural retina, is usually called *slow PIII.*[3,38] When measured with a vitreal positive recording polarity, the components are as shown in the solid lines in Figure 3-6. The TEP c-wave in the cat has a maximum amplitude of about 6 mV, and slow PIII has a maximum of about 5 mV. The vitreal c-wave is the sum of these, about 1 mV.

The dual origin of the c-wave leads to some rather simple but important observations on how its amplitude is affected by changes in its components. The vitreal c-wave, as the sum, has an amplitude of 1 mV. Obviously, the vitreal c-wave will become larger when the TEP c-wave increases, when slow PIII decreases, or both occur, or if the TEP c-wave increases more than slow PIII. It is important to recognize that if only one component changes while the other remains constant the *percentage* change in the vitreal response will be much larger than in the component, although the absolute change is the same in both this component and in the vitreal c-wave. For instance, if the TEP c-wave increases from 6 to 7 mV, the vitreal c-wave will double. Thus, the vitreal c-wave can magnify changes that occur in one component. On the other hand, if both components change, it is possible for the vitreal c-wave to be unaffected. For instance, if the TEP c-wave were reduced from 6 to 3 mV, and slow PIII were reduced from 5 to 2 mV, the vitreal c-wave would still be 1 mV.

So far, enhancement of the c-wave has been observed in a number of conditions: during the light peak, in systemic hypoxia, and after sodium azide infusion.[14,15,20,24] In each case the increase in c-wave amplitude resulted solely from an increase in the TEP component.

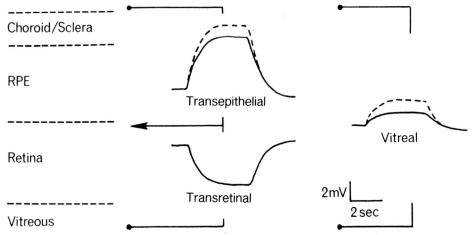

Figure 3-6. The vitreal c-wave (cat) and the effect of changes in the amplitude of its components. Both the transepithelial and transretinal (slow PIII) components are shown. The solid lines show the normal maximum amplitudes of the potentials; the dashed lines show that a small increase in the TEP c-wave causes a large change in the vitreal c-wave. The c-wave was evoked by 4-second flashes of diffuse white light. This figure is a tracing with approximately the time-course and amplitudes observed. (Linsenmeier RA, Steinberg RH: Variations of c-wave amplitude in the cat eye. Doc Ophthal Proc Series 37:21, 1983)

Both c-wave components are thought to be responses to a light-evoked decrease in $[K^+]_o$ in the subretinal space.[29,37] The TEP c-wave is known to be generated by the hyperpolarization

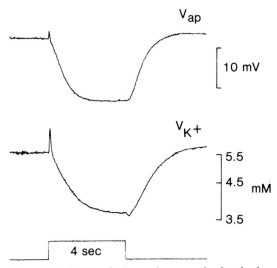

Figure 3-7. RPE apical membrane and subretinal $[K^+]_o$ in response to 4.0 seconds of illumination in cat. These responses were obtained in separate experiments at an illumination of 8.3 log quanta/deg²/sec. The apical membrane potential, V_{ap}, was derived by subtracting an intracellular recording of basal membrane potential from the transepithelial recording.

of the RPE apical membrane.[38] This hyperpolarization is the expected response of the cell to the change in the K^+ equilibrium potential across the apical membrane. The records in Figure 3-7 show that the initial light-evoked $[K^+]_o$ decrease is accompanied by a hyperpolarization of the apical membrane, while the return of $[K^+]_o$ at light-off is accompanied by repolarization. Details of the generation of slow PIII are less clear, but it is probably the extracellular sign of the hyperpolarization of Müller cells elicited by the same change in $[K^+]_o$.[3,7,43]

Recordings of the depth profile of the light-evoked $[K^+]_o$ decrease show that it is maximal outside the inner segments of the photoreceptors both in the eyecup preparation and in the isolated retina.[28,29] This targets the photoreceptors as the principal generator of the $[K^+]_o$ decrease. A model successfully predicts for brief flashes (<0.3 sec) that the $[K^+]_o$ decrease originates from a decrease in the passive efflux from the rods during the light-evoked hyperpolarization coupled to an unchanged inward-active K^+ pumping by the Na^+/K^+ pump of the inner segments.[4,22,28]

We can describe in detail how the RPE hyperpolarization gives rise to the TEP c-wave (Fig. 3-8). The apical membrane hyperpolarization

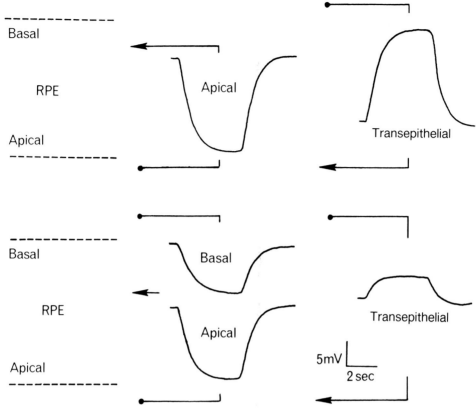

Figure 3-8. The origin of the TEP c-wave. *(Top)* An apical membrane hyperpolarization leads to a TEP increase. Shunting has been ignored. *(Bottom)* A smaller TEP c-wave is actually observed, because part of the apical hyperpolarization is shunted to the basal membrane. The c-wave was evoked by 4-second flashes of diffuse white light. This figure is a tracing with approximately the time-course and amplitudes observed. (Linsenmeier RA, Steinberg RH: Variations of c-wave amplitude in the cat eye. Doc Ophthal Proc Series 37:21, 1983)

leads to a change in current flow through the tight junctions between RPE cells and through the basal membrane, causing a basal hyperpolarization, also; in turn, the apical hyperpolarization is reduced by the current flowing out. Since the basal hyperpolarization effectively subtracts from the apical hyperpolarization, the TEP c-wave is reduced. (Compare upper and lower parts of Fig. 3-8.) Clearly, factors that influence shunting can change the TEP c-wave. A circuit analysis of the RPE shows that the electrical resistances of the apical and basal membranes and of the paracellular pathway are the important variables.[16,23] (Each resistance is the reciprocal of the sum of ionic conductances.) If, for example, the basal membrane resistance decreased, the shunted basal hyperpolarization would decrease but the TEP c-wave would *increase.*

It is now known that the increase in c-wave amplitude that occurs during the light peak and during systemic hypoxia experimentally produced in the cat originates from just this mechanism — a decrease in the resistance of the RPE's basal membrane.[16,18] While a full understanding of the mechanism is not yet available, in both cases the resistance change accompanies a depolarization of the basal membrane. Since the basal-membrane depolarization in systemic hypoxia and also in sodium azide infusion produces prominent c-wave increases by this mechanism it would not be surprising to find the same effect occurring in diseases that affect the epithelium.[18-20]

MECHANISM OF C-WAVE

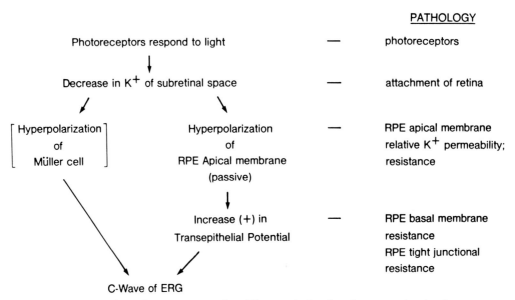

Figure 3-9. Mechanism of c-wave generation. The step in brackets has yet to be clearly demonstrated. Possible pathologies associated with each step are shown at the right. (Linsenmeier RA, Steinberg RH: Variations of c-wave amplitude in the cat eye. Doc Ophthal Proc Series 37:21, 1983)

Figure 3-9 summarizes the stages in c-wave generation and suggests how pathology could modify each stage. Similar figures are presented below for the fast oscillation and light peak. For a normal c-wave to occur, light absorbed by the photoreceptors must produce the usual decrease in subretinal $[K^+]_o$; this will depend upon the integrity of the photoreceptors and their attachment to the RPE. Of course, the RPE itself must be intact. Interestingly, as discussed above, changes in RPE resistance originating at the basal membrane that are functional in nature lead to prominent effects on c-wave amplitude. The sensitivity of c-wave amplitude to this effect again suggests that it could be an important mechanism for altering the c-wave in disease.

Fast Oscillation

Using the technique of electro-oculography in humans and animals, Kolder and Brecher and Kolder and North described a fast oscillation of the EOG potential that differed from the slow oscillation that had been described earlier, of which the light peak is the most prominent component.[1,9-12] The stimuli consisted of equal durations of light and darkness, and while the slow oscillation was largest when each phase was about 12.5 minutes (man), the fast oscillation was most prominent with repeated light and dark phases of 1.1 minutes each (man and rabbit). DC–ERG recordings in response to maintained illumination contain a trough in the potential following the c-wave, which also has been identified as the fast oscillation (see Fig. 3-3).[12,21,25,40] It is now known that the fast oscillation produced either in the EOG or DC–ERG has a unique origin in delayed basal membrane responses of the RPE. In either recording the particular appearance of the fast oscillation depends upon the duration of stimulation, which influences the relative magnitudes and temporal spacing of the ON and OFF phases of the fast oscillation. The specific appearance of the fast oscillation in the ERG (or EOG) will be determined in part by its algebraic addition with the transretinal potential, even though the latter does not appear to have a specific fast-oscillation component.

In order to understand the origin of the fast

oscillation and light peak it is first necessary to consider how subretinal $[K^+]_o$ changes during maintained illumination as well as the time-courses of the apical and basal membrane responses.

The lower two records of Figure 3-10 compare the response of the apical membrane with the light-evoked change in subretinal space $[K^+]_o$ during 5 minutes of illumination of the cat retina. There is first a decrease of $[K^+]_o$ to a minimum at 4.0 seconds followed by a reaccumulation to a new steady-state level in the light. With the cessation of illumination there is an overshoot of $[K^+]_o$ above the dark-adapted level and then a gradual return.

There is a remarkable correlation between these changes in $[K^+]_o$ and the apical membrane response, V_{ap}: the apical membrane potential first hyperpolarizes to a peak as $[K^+]_o$ decreases and then repolarizes as $[K^+]_o$ reaccumulates. Parallel V_{ap} and $[K^+]_o$ events also occur at the cessation of illumination. The apical membrane responses to K^+ are the origin of the RPE component of the ERG c-wave and off c-wave as just described.

Although the apical membrane follows subretinal $[K^+]_o$, the TEP, which is the sum of apical and basal responses, exhibits a more complex time-course. This additional complexity results from the presence of two distinct responses of the basal membrane that appear in the V_{ba} recording of Figure 3-10. The first basal response, called the *delayed basal hyperpolarization,* makes the initial hyperpolarization and subsequent repolarization of V_{ba} slower than the V_{ap} response. The second basal response, called the *light-peak depolarization,* produces a very slow depolarization of V_{ba} as illumination continues.

The fast-oscillation response that originated at the basal membrane appeared in Figure 3-10 combined with the change in V_{ba} that was due to shunting of the V_{ap} response. In order to describe responses that originate basally, therefore, it is helpful to isolate them from the passive voltage drop due to shunting of the apical response. (In cat, the relative resistances of the membranes are such that there is little or no shunting of basal-membrane responses to the apical membrane.) This is accomplished by esti-

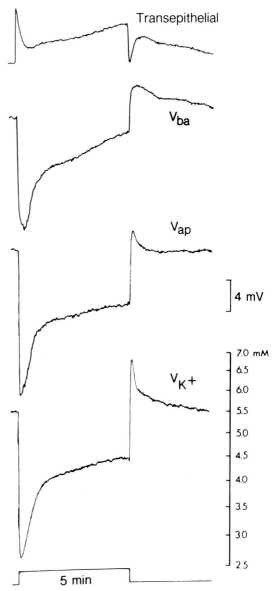

Figure 3-10. Light-evoked responses in cat to 5 minutes of illumination: transepithelial potential, basal membrane potential (V_{ba}), apical membrane potential (V_{ap}), and subretinal potassium concentration (V_{K+}). For the top three traces illumination was diffuse white light, 9.3 log quanta/deg²/sec. For the V_{K+} trace illumination was a large spot (75 deg²), 440 nm, 8.1 log quanta/deg²/sec. (Steinberg RH, Linsenmeier L, Griff ER: Three light-evoked responses of the retinal pigment epithelium. Vis Res 11:1315, 1983)

mating the basal response that is due to shunting alone, as a constant fraction of the apical response.[17] Figure 3-11 presents the initial 135

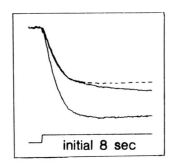

initial 8 sec

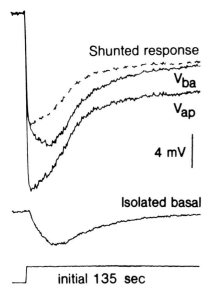

Shunted response

V_{ba}

V_{ap}

4 mV

Isolated basal

initial 135 sec

Figure 3-11. Isolation of the delayed basal hyperpolarization in cat. The initial 135 seconds of responses to 5 minutes of illumination are shown. Intracellular recordings of the apical (V_{ap}) and basal (V_{ba}) membrane potentials are superposed with an estimate of the shunted response at the basal membrane *(interrupted line)*. Subtraction of the shunted response from the basal response gave the isolated basal response *(bottom trace)*. The inset *(top)* shows the initial 8 seconds of the responses at one half gain, demonstrating that the shunted response accounts for V_{ba} over the initial 3 to 4 seconds of the response. Illumination at 9.3 log quanta/deg^2/sec. (Steinberg RH, Linsenmeier L, Griff ER: Three light-evoked responses of the retinal pigment epithelium. Vis Res 11:1315, 1983)

seconds of the response to a 5-minute stimulus, showing the shunted response superimposed on the actual apical and basal responses. The peak hyperpolarization of V_{ba} occurs later than that of V_{ap} and after the initial 3 to 4 seconds, V_{ba} departs significantly from the response expected

due to shunting. By subtracting the shunted response from V_{ba} we obtain an estimate of events originating at the basal membrane. This *delayed hyperpolarization* has a much slower time-course than the apical response to $[K^+]_o$, peaking about 20 seconds after the onset of illumination and then slowly repolarizing to the dark-adapted level. The delayed hyperpolarization is the origin of the fast-oscillation trough seen between the c-wave and light peak during maintained illumination.[17]

It was possible to study the mechanism of the basal hyperpolarization in an isolated RPE-choroid preparation (neural retina removed) of gecko.[6] RPE responses equivalent to the RPE c-wave and fast oscillation were produced simply by decreasing the $[K^+]_o$ in the RPE apical

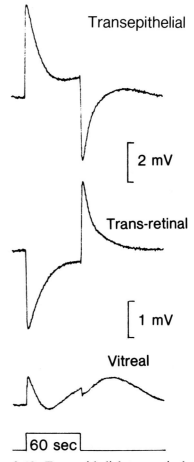

Transepithelial

2 mV

Trans-retinal

1 mV

Vitreal

60 sec

Figure 3-12. Transepithelial, transretinal, and vitreal recordings (cat) of the response to 60 seconds' illumination at 8.3 log quanta/deg^2/sec.

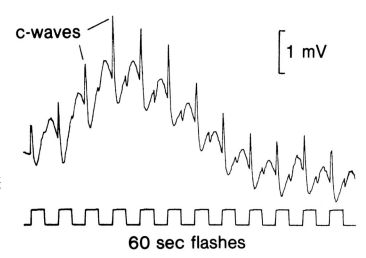

c-waves

1 mV

Figure 3-13. Vitreal DC–ERG to alternating 60-second periods of light and dark in cat. The positive peak of each fast oscillation appears prior to each c-wave. These flashes also have produced a light peak. The illumination was 8.8 log quanta/deg²/sec.

60 sec flashes

bathing solution by an amount equal to the light-evoked $[K^+]_o$ decrease that occurred in the intact retina. In the isolated RPE, this $[K^+]_o$ decrease first hyperpolarized the apical membrane so that the TEP increased (c-wave) and subsequently led to a basal hyperpolarization that produced a TEP decrease (fast oscillation). The apical hyperpolarization was the expected response to a change in the potassium equilibrium potential.[23] The basal hyperpolarization, recorded in isolation or evoked by light in the intact retina, is a *delayed* consequence of the decrease in apical (or subretinal) $[K^+]_o$.

In cat, the fast oscillation also can be recorded using 1-minute stimuli, approximating the technique used for recording it in humans (Fig. 3-12). With 1 minute of illumination a trough follows the c-wave that is, in turn, followed by a peak and then a decline of potential. The trough in the vitreal trace is formed from declines in both the TEP and transretinal potentials. The TEP declines more rapidly because of two mechanisms, the delayed basal hyperpolarization and the K^+-dependent apical membrane repolarization (see Fig. 3-10). If the delayed basal hyperpolarization did not bring the TEP down so rapidly, the vitreal trough would be much smaller or absent.[17]

The peak following stimulus OFF in Figure 3-12 corresponds to the peak in the fast oscillation in response to repetitive stimuli. Figure 3-13 shows this in cat for stimuli with repeated 60-second light and dark phases, fast-oscillation

peaks appearing just prior to each c-wave.[25] This peak is produced at stimulus offset mainly by a delayed basal-membrane *depolarization* triggered by the increase in subretinal $[K^+]_o$ at that time. Thus, a 60-second stimulus evokes the delayed basal hyperpolarization at light onset, producing the fast-oscillation trough, and the delayed basal depolarization at light cessation, producing the fast-oscillation peak. These appear at the vitreal level to be one rather simple, nearly smooth wave, rather than the separate responses they actually are. Both basal events, therefore, contribute to each cycle of the fast oscillation evoked with relatively brief stimuli.

Figure 3-14 summarizes the mechanism of fast oscillation and demonstrates how it might be affected by disease at each step; the major pathway is shown in the center column. Light absorbed by the photoreceptors leads to a decrease in subretinal $[K^+]_o$ that initiates potentials in the neural retina and RPE, in particular a delayed basal membrane hyperpolarization that decreases TEP. The decrease in extracellular $[K^+]$ leads to a decrease in RPE intracellular $[K^+]$ that may be necessary to produce the basal response.[6] The mechanism of the delayed basal hyperpolarization, however, and its relationship to intracellular $[K^+]$ are still unknown.

Light Peak

The light peak is the first of a series of slow oscillations in potential in response to illumina-

MECHANISM OF FAST OSCILLATION

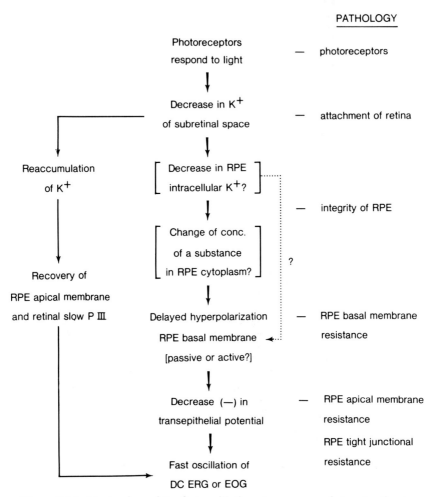

PATHOLOGY

Photoreceptors
respond to light — photoreceptors

Decrease in K^+
of subretinal space — attachment of retina

Reaccumulation
of K^+

Decrease in RPE
intracellular K^+? — integrity of RPE

Change of conc.
of a substance
in RPE cytoplasm? ?

Recovery of
RPE apical membrane
and retinal slow P III

Delayed hyperpolarization
RPE basal membrane — RPE basal membrane
[passive or active?] resistance

Decrease (—) in — RPE apical membrane
transepithelial potential resistance

RPE tight junctional
Fast oscillation of resistance
DC ERG or EOG

Figure 3-14. Mechanism of the fast oscillation. A sequence of steps leading to the fast oscillation of the DC–ERG or EOG is outlined. The mechanism for the fast-oscillation trough only is shown. An opposite set of events is thought to occur at light offset to produce the fast-oscillation peak. Steps in brackets have yet to be demonstrated; the dashed line indicates an alternate path. Possible pathologies associated with each step are shown at the right. (Griff ER, Linsenmeier RA, Steinberg RH: The cellular origin of the fast oscillation. Doc Ophthal Proc Series 37:13, 1983)

tion that are usually recorded in humans by electro-oculography but can also be studied by DC recording.[1,9,12,32,39,40] The "dark trough" is an off response to maintained illumination that is also considered to be one of the slow oscillations. It has a latency and time-course resembling the light peak but is opposite in polarity; the voltage going to a minimum well below the dark-adapted baseline of the standing potential.[8,21] In general, it is the light peak that can be

most readily studied experimentally because it is the first and the largest of the slow oscillations and the most reliable to appear in the DC–ERG.

Figure 3-15 shows the transepithelial and transretinal as well as the vitreal DC–ERG recordings in response to a 5-minute stimulus. In every case, there was a slow rise and fall of the TEP that followed the c-wave and had the time-course of the vitreal light peak. By contrast, the transretinal recordings never showed a response of this type. The light peak, therefore, originates in the RPE as a change in the transepithelial potential. This finding was obtained at about the same time in the cat and gecko and in the intact eye of rhesus monkey by Valeton and van Norren.[5,15,42]

The origination of the TEP light peak at the basal membrane of the RPE can be seen more clearly in Figure 3-16, which shows the initial 8.5 minutes of responses to 10 minutes of illumination. The dashed line shows a scaled version of V_{ap}, which is an estimate of the portion of the basal response that is due to shunting. Superimposition of the shunted response shows that the basal membrane undergoes a slow de-

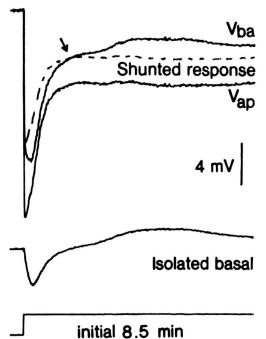

Figure 3-16. Isolation of the light-peak depolarization in cat. The initial 8.5 min. of responses to 10 minutes of illumination are shown; the format is as in Figure 3-11. The arrow at 2 minutes indicates the approximate time at which the basal membrane begins to depolarize relative to the apical. Subtraction of the shunted response from the basal response shows the delayed basal hyperpolarization followed by the light-peak depolarization. Illumination at 9.3 log quanta/deg²/sec. (Steinberg RH, Linsenmeier L, Griff ER: Three light-evoked responses of the retinal pigment epithelium. Vis Res 11:1315, 1983)

CAT

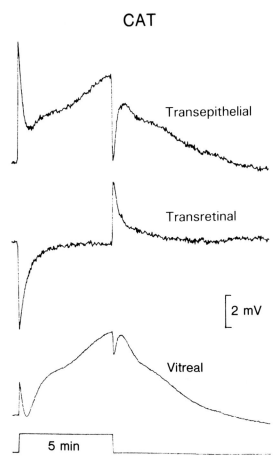

Figure 3-15. DC–ERG components in response to maintained illumination. The vitreal DC–ERG, transepithelial, and transretinal responses were recorded in response to a 5-minute period of illumination at 9.3 log quanta/deg²/sec (cat).

polarization that appears to begin at about 2 minutes and, in this example, peaks 5 minutes after the onset of illumination. The isolated basal response, obtained by subtracting the shunted response from V_{ba}, shows that the slower light-peak depolarization follows the previously described delayed basal hyperpolarization. Because the two responses overlap in time a precise latency of onset cannot be assigned to the light-peak depolarization. During the time that the light peak rises and falls the apical membrane potential is essentially flat. The TEP light peak quite faithfully reflects the basal membrane event. It does, therefore, originate at the RPE as a depolarization of the basal membrane.

MECHANISM OF LIGHT PEAK

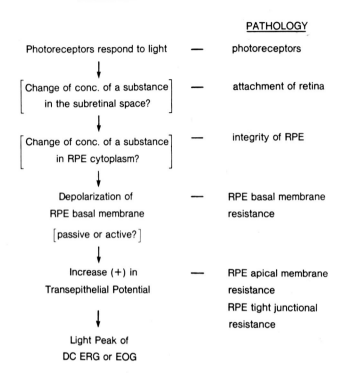

Figure 3-17. Mechanism of the light peak. A sequence of steps leading to the light peak of the DC–ERG or EOG is outlined. Steps in brackets have yet to be demonstrated. Possible pathologies associated with each step are shown at the right. (Steinberg RH, Griff ER, Linsenmeier RA: The cellular origin of the light peak. Doc Ophthal Proc Series 37:1, 1983)

Our understanding of the mechanism that generates the light peak is essentially limited to knowledge about the location of the voltage change (i.e., that the *light-peak depolarization* is generated at the basal membrane of the RPE). Of the mechanism at the basal membrane and from there on back into the RPE cell, across the apical membrane, and into the subretinal space and neural retina we know almost nothing. Figure 3-17 shows a hypothetical sequence of events. From its spectral properties and sensitivity we know that the initial event must be absorption of light by the photoreceptors.[2,15,41] We have speculated that a substance is produced (or consumed) by the neural retina and diffuses to (or away from) the *apical* membrane. This would resemble the $[K^+]_o$ change, which is initiated by the photoreceptors and which then hyperpolarizes the apical membrane during the c-wave.[28] Unfortunately, we do not yet know the nature of the "light-peak substance" or even where it originates. The time-course of $[K^+]_o$ changes in the cat retina suggested that it is probably not K^+.[36] Following its change in concentration in the subretinal space the *basal membrane* must somehow be affected. The route to the basal membrane could be direct (the substance reaching there after being transported into the cell) or one or more intracellular messengers might be responsible for the effect at the basal membrane. The depolarization of the basal membrane could result from a change in the concentration of a permeant ion, from a change in the membrane's permeability to one or more ions, or from a change in the rate of an electrogenic ion pump. Current pulses can be passed across the RPE of gecko during the light peak to determine whether there are changes in RPE resistances that might reveal a change in permeability at the basal membrane. Figure 3-18 shows that both the transepithelial resistance (R_t) and the ratio of apical- to basal-cell-membrane resistances (R_{ap}/R_{ba}) change with the time-course of the light peak. The direction of these changes is consistent with a decrease in basal membrane resistance (and an increase in permeability) during the light peak, but this might be a voltage-dependent effect and therefore a consequence of the basal membrane depolarization instead of its cause.

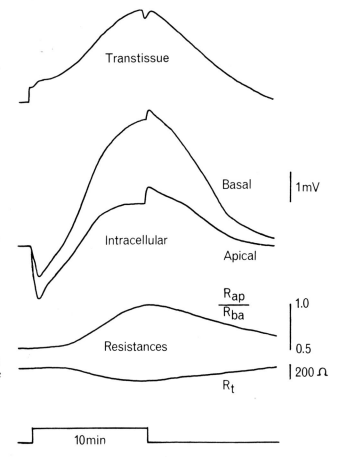

Figure 3-18. Resistance changes during the light peak and the RPE origin of the light peak in gecko. Intracellular RPE recordings *(middle)* show that the transtissue *(top)* light peak originates from the RPE cell as a basal membrane depolarization. Because of shunting the apical membrane also depolarizes with the same time course. Responses are to 10 minutes of illumination. To measure R_t, transepithelial resistance, and R_{ap}/R_{ba}, 1.0 μA, 1.0 second square current pulses were passed across the tissue and the iR drops of the cell membranes gives R_{ap}/R_{ba}. These measurements show that R_{ap}/R_{ba} increases and R_t decreases with the time-course of the light peak. This is most consistent with a decrease in the resistance of the basal membrane, R_{ba}, during the light peak. (Steinberg RH, Griff ER, Linsenmeier RA: The cellular origin of the light peak. Doc Ophthal Proc Series 37:1, 1983)

Does the light-peak mechanism, described here in animal models, also apply to the human response? As indicated above the cat and human light peaks are similar in form and in stimulus–response characteristics. The similarity extends, further, to the presence in cat of at least one additional slow oscillation following the light peak, which also has been shown to originate from a change in TEP.[15] In addition, the resistance changes just described for gecko have been found also in cat, where they are the basis for the changes in c-wave amplitude that occur during the light peak.[16] Most strikingly, identical effects on the c-wave occur in the human retina, where they actually had been described much earlier.[26,33] The c-wave effects indicate that similar changes in resistance occur also in the human RPE during the light peak. There is now very strong evidence that RPE participation in the light peak is very similar in lizard, cat, and human.

CONCLUSIONS

Three changes in membrane potential of the RPE contribute to the DC–ERG. As shown in Figure 3-19, the three responses peak at progressively longer latencies (4, 20, and 300 seconds [cat]) and exhibit progressively slower time constants. The first two events clearly depend upon photoreceptor-initiated changes in subretinal $[K^+]_o$, and the best available evidence indicates that the light-peak depolarization is also closely linked to photoreceptor activity.[15] The cessation of illumination initiates a repetition of the sequence but the responses have the opposite polarity from those at light onset.

It is assumed that each of the three responses participates in one of the RPE functions that serve the needs of the photoreceptors, but this has yet to be demonstrated for each response. We know that light and dark initiate changes in a number of RPE and photoreceptor cellular

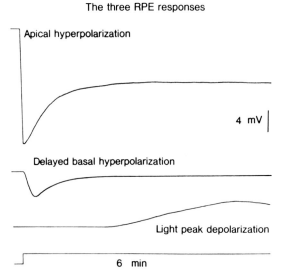

The three RPE responses

Apical hyperpolarization

4 mV

Delayed basal hyperpolarization

Light peak depolarization

6 min

Figure 3-19. Summary of the three light-evoked responses in cat showing their relative time-courses and amplitudes. The initial 6 minutes of the response to maintained illumination are shown. The first response *(top)* is a hyperpolarization of the apical membrane that reaches its maximum at 4 seconds. This is followed by two responses of the basal membrane: the delayed basal hyperpolarization, peaking at 20 seconds, and the light-peak depolarization reaching its peak at 300 seconds. The offset of illumination produces a similar sequence of response but of the opposite polarity (not shown). (Modified from Steinberg RH, Linsenmeier L, Griff ER: Three light-evoked responses of the retinal pigment epithelium. Vis Res 11:1315, 1983)

functions, and for the moment it seems best to view these responses in the broad context of light – dark differences. These responses could, for example, represent membrane events that can be observed electrically during metabolite, ion, or water transport, melanin migration, photoreceptor membrane turnover, or control of the extracellular milieu. It is hoped that precise knowledge of the mechanism of each response (e.g., whether it represents a change in an ionic conductance or transport) will eventually lead to knowledge of its functional significance.

We are fortunate that human DC – ERG and EOG recordings can inform us through the c-wave, fast oscillation, and light peak about these three RPE membrane events. Ultimately, of course, these responses depend upon the activity of the photoreceptors as well as the RPE. It is

significant that the nature of the contributions from the neural retina and the RPE differ for each response. It is also important to distinguish between the origin of the voltage contributions and the origin of the chemical mechanisms for each response (Fig. 3-20, 3-21).

For the c-wave, two voltages of very similar time-course originate in the neural retina and the RPE. The ERG c-wave, therefore, always reflects the relative magnitudes of its two components. The c-wave is initiated, however, by only one chemical mechanism, a photoreceptor-dependent decrease in subretinal $[K^+]_o$. The fast oscillation depends upon this same K^+ event, but in addition there must be one or more intracellular chemical step in the RPE. Although the voltage of the fast oscillation has a unique origin at the basal membrane, it sums in the ERG with the ongoing change in potential of the neural retina. Finally, we know little about the chemical mechanisms for the light peak except that a chemical event in the subretinal space and intracellular chemical steps in the RPE must be involved. The light-peak voltage is simplest in origin since it originates only at the RPE basal membrane, there being no neural retinal voltage.

That each of the three responses reflects events in and around the subretinal space in a special way should contribute to their clinical usefulness. Relatively little is known, however, about how they are altered by diseases that affect the RPE, the photoreceptors, and their interactions. Recent studies on experimental systemic hypoxia in cat are helpful in providing an initial understanding of hypoxic effects in the subretinal region.[14] In relatively mild hypoxia, PaO_2 60 – 80 in cat, c-wave and fast-oscillation amplitude are increased while the light peak becomes smaller. There is no change in the ERG a- and b-waves at these levels of hypoxia. We now know that K^+ homeostasis in the subretinal space is affected by mild hypoxia and that the c-wave and fast oscillation reflect these effects.[18,19] The origin of the sensitivity of the light peak to mild hypoxia is not yet understood. These responses respond differently to hypercapnia. The fast oscillation, for example, does not change, while the c-wave amplitude is increased and the light peak, depressed.[14] In this

MECHANISMS OF THREE RPE RESPONSES

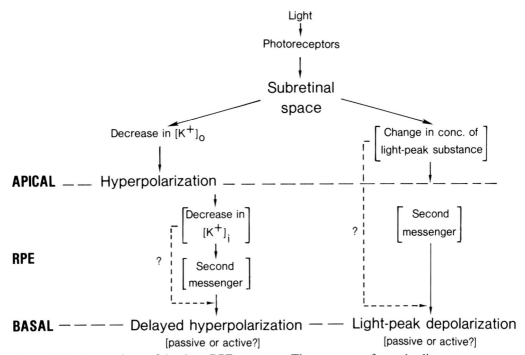

Figure 3-20. Mechanisms of the three RPE responses. The sequence of steps leading to each response is shown. Steps in brackets have yet to be demonstrated. Interrupted lines indicate alternative pathways. (Steinberg RH, Linsenmeier L, Griff ER: Three light-evoked responses of the retinal pigment epithelium. Vis Res 11:1315, 1983)

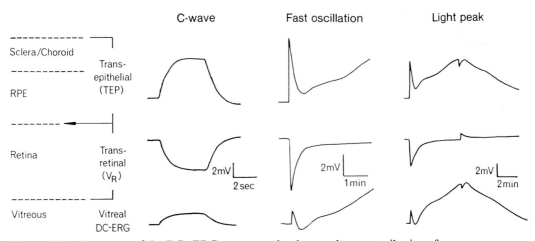

Figure 3-21. Summary of the DC–ERG responses that have voltage contributions from the retinal pigment epithelium. Transepithelial and transretinal recordings are shown. Flash durations: c-wave, 4 seconds; fast oscillation and light peak, 5 minutes. The responses are tracings with the approximate time-courses and amplitudes of the actual responses. (Modified from Steinberg RH, Griff ER, Linsenmeier RA: The cellular origin of the light peak. Doc Ophthal Proc Series 37:1, 1983; Linsenmeier RA, Steinberg RH: Variations of c-wave amplitude in the cat eye. Doc Ophthal Proc Series 37:21, 1983; Griff ER, Linsenmeier RA, Steinberg RH: The cellular origin of the fast oscillation. Doc Ophthal Proc Series 37:13, 1983)

case the pathophysiological mechanisms are not yet known, but an effect on K^+ homeostasis, as in hypoxia, does not seem to be involved.* We are hopeful that the clinical usefulness of these RPE-related DC–ERG and EOG responses will be increased by an understanding of the normal mechanisms of each response and how the physiology is altered by pathological conditions.

REFERENCES

1. Arden GB, Kelsey JH: Changes produced by light in the standing potential of the human eye. J Physiol 161:189, 1962
2. Arden GB, Kelsey JH: Some observations on the relationship between the standing potential of the human eye and the bleaching and regeneration of visual purple. J Physiol 161:205, 1962
3. Faber, DS: Analysis of the Slow Transretinal Potentials in Response to Light, Ph.D. dissertation, State University of New York, 1969
4. Fujimoto M, Tomita T: Reconstruction of the slow PIII from the rod potential. Invest Ophthalmol Vis Sci 18:1090, 1979
5. Griff ER, Steinberg RH: Origin of the light peak: *In vitro* study of *Gekko gekko.* J Physiol London 331:637, 1982
6. Griff ER, Steinberg RH: Changes in apical $[K^+]_o$ produce delayed basal membrane responses of the retinal pigment epithelium in the gecko. J Gen Physiol 83:193, 1984
7. Karwoski CJ, Proenza LM: Relationship between Müller cell responses, a local transretinal potential, and potassium flux. J Neurophysiol 40:244, 1977
8. Kikawada N: Variations in the corneo-retinal standing potential of the vertebrate eye during light and dark adaptations. Jpn J Physiol 18:687, 1968
9. Kolder H: Spontane und experimentale Änderungen des Bestandpotentials des menschlichen Auges. Pflügers Arch Ges Physiol 268:258, 1959
10. Kolder H, Brecher GA: Fast oscillations of the corneo-retinal potential in man. Arch Ophthalmol 75:232, 1966
11. Kolder H, North AW: Oscillations of the corneo-retinal potential in animals. Ophthalmologica, Basel 152:149, 1966
12. Kris CH: Corneo-fundal potential variations during light and dark adaptation. Nature 182:1027, 1958
13. Kuffler SW, Nicholls JG: The physiology of neuroglial cells. Ergebn Physiol 57:1, 1966
14. Linsenmeier RA, Mines AH, Steinberg RH: Effects of hypoxia and hypercapnia on the light peak and electroretinogram of the cat. Invest Ophthalmol Vis Sci 24:37, 1983
15. Linsenmeier RA, Steinberg RH: Origin and sensitivity of the light peak of the intact cat eye. J Physiol London 331:653, 1982
16. Linsenmeier RA, Steinberg RH: A light-evoked interaction of the apical and basal membranes of the retinal pigment epithelium: The c-wave and the light peak. J Neurophysiol 50:136, 1983
17. Linsenmeier RA, Steinberg RH: Delayed basal hyperpolarization of cat retinal pigment epithelium, and its relation to the fast oscillation of the DC ERG. J Gen Physiol 83:213, 1984
18. Linsenmeier RA, Steinberg RH: Effects of hypoxia on potassium homeostasis and pigment epithelial cells in the cat retina. J Gen Physiol 84:945, 1984
19. Linsenmeier RA, Steinberg RH: Mechanisms of hypoxic effects on the cat DC electroretinogram. Invest Ophthalmol Vis Sci 27:1385, 1986
20. Linsenmeier RA, Steinberg RH: Mechanisms of azide induced increases in the c-wave and standing potential of the intact cat eye. Vision Res 27:1, 1987
21. Marmor MF, Lurie M: Light-induced electrical responses of the retinal pigment epithelium. In Zinn KM, Marmor MF (eds): The Retinal Pigment Epithelium, p 226. Cambridge, Harvard University Press, 1979
22. Matsuura T, Miller WH, Tomita T: Cone-specific c-wave in the turtle retina. Vision Res 18:767, 1978
23. Miller SS, Steinberg RH: Passive ionic properties of frog retinal pigment epithelium. J Membr Biol 36:337, 1977
24. Niemeyer G, Nagahara K, Demant E: Effects of changes in arterial Po_2 and Pco_2 on the ERG in the cat. Invest Ophthalmol Vis Sci 23:678, 1982
25. Nikara T, Sato S, Mita T, et al: An analysis of oscillatory potentials elicited by slow repetitive light stimulation in cat eye. J Iwate Med Ass 26:414, 1974
26. Nilsson SEG, Skoog K-O: Covariation of the simultaneously recorded c-wave and standing potential of the human eye. Acta Ophthalmol 53:721, 1975
27. Noell WK: Studies on the Electrophysiology and Metabolism of the Retina. Randolph Field, TX, USAF School of Aviation Med Project No 21-1201-0004, 1953
28. Oakley B II, Flaming DG, Brown KT: Effects of the rod receptor potential upon extracellular potassium ion concentration. J Gen Physiol 74:713, 1979
29. Oakley B II, Green DG: Correlation of light-induced changes in retinal extracellular potassium concentration with the c-wave of the electroretinogram. J Neurophysiol 39:1117, 1976
30. Rodieck RW: Components of the electroretinogram—A reappraisal. Vision Res 12:773, 1972

* RA Linsenmeier, RH Steinberg: Personal communication

31. Schmidt R, Steinberg RH: Rod-dependent intracellular responses to light recorded from the pigment epithelium of the cat retina. J Physiology 217:71, 1971

32. Skoog KO: The directly recorded standing potential of the human eye. Acta Ophthalmol 53:120, 1975

33. Skoog K-O, Nilsson SEG: The c-wave of the human DC registered ERG. II. Cyclic variations of the c-wave amplitude. Acta Ophthalmol 52:904, 1974

34. Steinberg RH, Linsenmeier RA, Griff ER: Three light-evoked responses of the retinal pigment epithelium. Vision Res 23:1315, 1983

35. Steinberg RH, Miller SS: Transport and membrane properties of the retinal pigment epithelium. In Zinn KM, Marmor MF (eds): The Retinal Pigment Epithelium, p 205. Cambridge, Harvard University Press, 1979

36. Steinberg RH, Niemeyer G: Light peak of cat DC electroretinogram: Not generated by a change in $[K^+]_o$. Invest Ophthalmol 20:414, 1981

37. Steinberg RH, Oakley B II, Niemeyer G: Light-evoked changes in $[K^+]_o$ in retina of the intact cat eye. J Neurophysiol 44:897, 1980

38. Steinberg RH, Schmidt R, Brown KT: Intracellular responses to light from the cat retinal pigment epithelium: Origin of the electroretinogram c-wave. Nature 227:728, 1970

39. Taümer R: Electro-oculography—Its clinical importance. Taümer, R (ed): Bibl Ophthalmol 85:1–134, 1976

40. Taümer R, Hennig J, Wolff L: Further investigations concerning the fast oscillation of the retinal potential. Bibl Ophthalmol 85:57, 1976

41. Taümer R, Rohde N, Pernice D: The slow oscillation of the retinal potential. Bibl Ophthalmol 85:40, 1976

42. Valeton JM, van Norren D: Intraretinal recordings of slow electrical responses to steady illumination in monkey: Isolation of receptor responses and the origin of the light peak. Vision Res 22:393, 1982

43. Witkovsky P, Dudek FE, Ripps H: Slow PIII component of the carp electroretinogram. J Gen Physiol 65:119, 1975

4

Studies on Animal Models of Retinal Degeneration

Gerald J. Chader
Gustavo D. Aguirre
Somes Sanyal

RETINITIS PIGMENTOSA

Retinitis pigmentosa (RP) in man is a disease that results in progressive visual impairment and eventual blindness. The disease is not a single entity but rather a family of allied diseases that affect the retina and have a common end result, loss of vision. Genetically, morphologically, and electrophysiologically several distinct types of RP have now been identified.[13,54]

RP was first reported in the 1800s as a form of night blindness associated with pigmentary changes. Because it was initially thought to be a result of an inflammatory process the term *retinitis pigmentosa* was coined. Clinically, patients most often present with night blindness and loss of the mid-peripheral visual field. With progression of this disease, the visual field further constricts, producing the characteristic tunnel vision of RP. ERG studies in patients with ophthalmoscopically visible lesions demonstrated that the ERG is nonrecordable or "extinguished." However, electrophysiological studies early in the disease process indicate that rod ERG responses are affected before cone responses, although cone abnormalities are also observed.[13,42] Onset is usually in the second decade of life, occasionally earlier. The disease course is variable but progressive, gradually involving the central visual field and color vision. Funduscopically, bone spicule pigment clumps are observed along with attenuated blood vessels and a waxy pallor of the disc.[30] Pigment epithelial involvement is often an important early manifestation; cataracts often develop, perhaps as a secondary event.[1] In later stages pigment accumulates in the retina, and gliosis is observed.[26]

It is generally agreed that the disease has a strong hereditary component, although the genetic picture is not clear in many cases. In typical RP, three major modes of transmission have been identified: sex-linked, autosomal-recessive, and autosomal-dominant. In males affected with the X-linked form, the disease progresses rapidly with blindness often occurring by the beginning of the third decade. Even female carriers of the sex-linked form may demonstrate some signs of the disease including pigmentary changes, reduced ERG, and reduced rhodopsin content as assessed by fundus reflectometry.[14,15,48] In the autosomal-recessive form of RP, differences in the clinical manifestations of the disease and times of onset may indicate different modes of inheritance even within this subgrouping. The causes of typical RP have yet to be determined.

Owing to the scarcity of human RP ocular

tissues most work in this area has been done on animal models; it is this work that is the subject of the present review.

General Disease Characteristics

Table 4-1 lists several characteristics of RP that are useful in attempts to pinpoint the cause(s) of the disease. It is primarily a hereditary disease that is present, at least electrophysiologically, in very young patients.[13] Since nonocular gross abnormalities or malformations generally are not associated with the disease, one would suspect some type of a localized metabolic disorder in the retina. Second, the disease primarily affects the photoreceptor and pigment epithelium (PE) cell, both of which are highly specialized neuroepithelial cells involved in the visual process. Third, other extraocular somatic cell types generally appear to be unaffected. Thus, biochemically, it is reasonable to assume that one of the unique enzymes or enzyme systems of the retina–PE complex might be involved in the disease rather than a more ubiquitous enzyme found in all (or most) cells and tissues. The most obvious candidates, therefore, are the enzyme systems involved in the visual process in the photoreceptor cell. One of the most intensively studied of these is the phosphodiesterase enzyme system, which controls cyclic GMP metabolism and is mainly compartmentalized in the outer segment. It is this enzyme, in particular, on which the present review focuses.

ANIMAL MODELS OF RP

The diversity of the disease in the human is mirrored by the diversity of retinal degenerative diseases observed in animals. Rodent and canine species have been particularly well studied in this regard, the disease(s) generally being thought to be controlled by different autosomal-recessive genes. It is thought that the visual cells of the retina are the primary site of expression in these neurological mutants, although the pigment epithelium is known to be the primary tissue affected in some cases.

Severe limitations on the usefulness of these

Table 4-1. General Disease Characteristics of RP

Hereditary Nature

Dominant, recessive, sex-linked forms
Specific hereditary pattern not defined in all RP types

Primarily Affects Photoreceptor Cells

Outer segment generally affected first
Possible pigment epithelial origin in some RP types

Generally Selective to Retina

Other tissues usually not affected
Sometimes associated with nonocular diseases (e.g., deafness, mental retardation, others)

animal models is apparent. In many respects, they have been studied simply because they are readily available for laboratory experimentation rather than for their compelling similarity to human RP. Morphologically, the retinas of lower species differ from that of the human in important characteristics (e.g., rod–cone density and distribution and the absence of a well-defined macular–foveal area). The lack of substantial numbers of cones in the rodent models, in particular, limits their usefulness in studying cone pathology and rod–cone interactions. The dog retina is somewhat more like the human retina in its composition of photoreceptor types and organization, although it also lacks a discrete macular-foveal area. In spite of these limitations, there are cogent reasons for studying these models. The understanding of any genetic disease that affects the retina adds to our total knowledge of normal and abnormal retinal function. The complexity of the human RP diseases suggests a different genetic and biochemical basis for each one, making it likely that studies on at least one of the animal models will be directly relevant to the human condition. It is certainly true that the same biochemical and physiological processes underlie retinal function in all higher animals. From a purely practical point of view, the limited availability of human RP retinal tissue makes the tissues from

Table 4-2. Types of Pathology in Animal Models of RP and Allied Retinal Degenerations

Photoreceptor Degeneration

Normal development
Full maturation of retina
Slow degeneration, in adult animal

Photoreceptor Dysplasia

Abnormal development
Fully normal developed retina not achieved
Rapid disease course, usually in early postnatal period

PE – Choroid Diseases

Affect PE – choroid in primary manner
Visual cells affected secondarily

Unknown Etiology

Normal morphology often observed
Photoreceptor cells, other retinal cells may be involved
Extraocular components?

the animal models the only ones readily available for study.

General Pathology

The terms *retinal degeneration* and *retinal dystrophy* have been used indiscriminately to describe any or all of the various diseases involving the retinal photoreceptor layer. Somewhat more logical and correct terminology is given in Table 4-2. Most of the better-studied diseases are not of general retinal etiology but are, more precisely, of photoreceptor origin (Table 4-3). Depending on whether pathological changes are observed before or after morphological maturation, the term *dysplasia* or *degeneration* is applied. Dysplasia signifies that overt signs of pathology appear before morphological maturity. The photoreceptor dysplasias are specific models of abnormal visual-cell differentiation.

As mentioned above, human RP is usually quite specific in that it affects only the retina – PE complex. Several interesting animal mutants, however, demonstrate retinal degeneration as well as an array of other neurological manifestations. Two of the best studies of this class of mutants are the nervous *(nr)* and Purkinje cell degeneration *(pcd)* mice.[57] The *pcd* mutant, for example, exhibits a gradual photoreceptor loss over the first 12 months of life, and virtually all of the cerebellar Purkinje cells are lost by 5 weeks of age. These mutants are perhaps better models of human diseases that exhibit more generalized neurological involvement.

In the RCS rat and several other animal models it is known that the PE – choroid is the primary site of the genetic mutation, with the visual cells and, subsequently, inner retinal neurons affected as secondary events. In other animal models, the exact site of the lesion is unknown. In recessively inherited congenital stationary night blindness in the Appaloosa horse, for example, a defect in synaptic vesicle recycling or, alternatively, a faulty neurotransmitter is suspected of producing the severe functional deficits present.[65,77] Systemic factors certainly could play a role in the disease, either by precipitating the overt signs of a latent abnormality or by exacerbating a relatively mild condition.

THE VISUAL PROCESS AND CYCLIC GMP

The retinal photoreceptor outer segment contains a high concentration of a unique membrane protein, rhodopsin, that is able to interact with photic energy and (in a manner that is poorly understood) translate and amplify the photic signal into an electrophysiological response. The cascade of intermediates resulting from the initial interaction of light with rhodopsin is depicted in Figure 4-1. It is now known that a second photosensitive system is closely coupled with the rhodopsin cycle at the metarhodopsin II level, one that involves cyclic GMP metabolism.[11] Specifically, this results in the light activation of the enzyme phosphodiesterase, reducing the cyclic GMP concentration in the photoreceptor.[21,55]

Cyclic GMP phosphodiesterase activity is much higher in photoreceptor rod outer segments than in other retinal areas.[22] Likewise,

Table 4-3. Animal Mutants Commonly Studied as Models of RP

Photoreceptor Degeneration

Miniature Poodle
  Slow degeneration of outer segments in the young adult animal after full retinal maturation (PRDC)

Wag/Rij Rat
  Retina develops normally but photoreceptor cells begin to degenerate at about 1 month of age (retinal degeneration)

Photoreceptor Dysplasia

Irish Setter
  Arrested outer-segment development; outer segments degenerate as they elongate in early postnatal period; visual-cell death follows (rod–cone dysplasia I)

Collie
  Arrested outer-segment development; outer segments degenerate as they elongate; visual-cell death soon follows (rod–cone dysplasia II)

rd Mouse
  Arrested outer-segment development; pyknotic photoreceptor cell nuclei present at end of second postnatal week, photoreceptor cells lost by fourth week (retinal degeneration)

rds Mouse
  Complete arrest of outer-segment development; virtually no outer segments observed; photoreceptor cells persist for 9 to 12 months (retinal degeneration, slow)

Norwegian Elkhound
  Rod outer-segment morphogenesis abnormal; cones remain normal for sometime before degeneration (rod dysplasia)

Alaskan Malamute
  Cone outer-segment morphogenesis abnormal; subsequent cone degeneration; rods remain normal (hemeralopia)

PE–Choroid Diseases

RCS Rat
  PE-cell phagocytic defect leading to outer-segment debris accumulation in subretinal space and secondary visual-cell death (retinal dystrophy)

Dog
  PE-cell hypertrophy with accumulation of autofluorescent lipopigment and secondary retinal degeneration as in Labrador retriever (central progressive retinal atrophy)

Cat
  Chorioretinal degeneration; ornithine aminotransferase deficiency (gyrate atrophy)

Cat
  Mucopolysaccharidoses I and VI: accumulation of inclusion bodies in PE cells (Hurler's syndrome; Maroteaux–Lamy syndrome)

Unknown Etiology

Appaloosa Horse
  Rods and cones morphologically normal; rod ERG responses lack b-wave component (congenital stationary night blindness)

Pearl Mouse
  Rod and cones morphologically normal but ERG demonstrates reduced dark-adapted sensitivity

THE VISUAL PROCESS AND PHOSPHODIESTERASE ACTIVATION

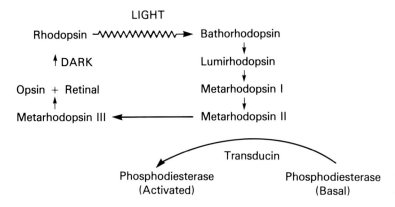

Figure 4-1. Proposed linkage of phosphodiesterase activation and the bleaching of rhodopsin.

over 90% of the total retinal cyclic GMP is concentrated in the photoreceptor cells.[62] Some years ago it was shown in simple experiments that the concentration of cyclic GMP could be reduced tenfold in dark-adapted frog rod outer segments (ROS) by bleaching.[37] Table 4-4 illustrates two important points of cyclic GMP metabolism in the ROS. First, the concentration of cyclic GMP in dark- or light-adapted ROS is very high; in most other tissues it is usually much lower than that of cyclic AMP. Second, a strong bleach either *in vivo* or *in vitro* can greatly reduce the cyclic GMP concentration.

The process by which cyclic GMP–PDE is activated is quite complex. Through the biochemical work of Bitensky and Stryer and electrophysiological studies of Miller, Cavaggioni and associates, and Liebman, a good deal is now known about the process.[18,38,56,72,82]

Cyclic GMP Metabolism in the Photoreceptor

Cyclic GMP is derived from the high-energy nucleoside triphosphate GTP through action of the enzyme guanylate cyclase, an enzyme highly active in ROS (Fig. 4-2).[48] Phosphodiesterase is the only enzyme capable of breaking the cyclic 3′-5′-bond of cyclic GMP, and in the photoreceptor it is linked to rhodopsin photolysis through a set of proteins collectively called *G-protein* or *transducin* ("T") by Stryer and his colleagues. When light strikes and activates rho-

dopsin (R*), it initiates a cycle in which transducin and GTP combine to activate the phosphodiesterase enzyme (PDE*) and reduce the cyclic GMP level. Transducin, a complex protein composed of three subunits, exhibits both GTP-binding activity and GTPase activity. Similarly the PDE enzyme has multiple subunits, one of which is now known to be an inhibitory unit; removal of this inhibitory unit appears to actually cause the increase in enzymatic activity.[80]

Table 4-4. Effect of Light on the Concentration of Cyclic GMP in Rod Outer Segments

Condition	Cyclic Nucleotide Concentration (pmol/mg protein)	
	Cyclic GMP	*Cyclic AMP*
A-adapted *in vivo*		
Dark	29	2
Light	3	3
B-adapted *in vitro*		
Dark	23	2
Light	3	2

A — ROS prepared from animals light- or dark-adapted *in vivo.* B — ROS prepared from dark-adapted frogs; a portion was exposed to light for 3 minutes prior to nucleotide determination. (Adapted from Fletcher R, Chader G: Cyclic GMP: Control of concentration by light in retinal photoreceptors. Biochem Biophys Res Commun 70:1297, 1976)

**CYCLIC GMP METABOLISM IN THE
RETINAL PHOTORECEPTOR**

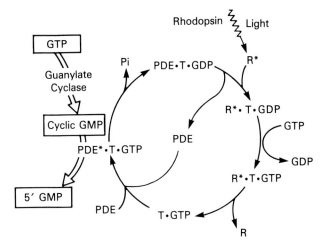

Figure 4-2. Possible sequence of steps for synthesis and degradation of cyclic GMP in the photoreceptor. R, rhodopsin; R*, light-activated rhodopsin; T, transducin (G-protein); PDE, phosphodiesterase; PDE*, activated phosphodiesterase. (Adapted from Fung B, Stryer L: Photolyzed rhodopsin catalyzes the exchange of GTP for bound GDP in retinal rod outer segments. Proc Natl Acad Sci USA 77:2500, 1980)

Cyclic GMP and Visual Transduction

Besides photon capture, the key process in visual transduction involves membrane permeability changes leading to hyperpolarization or depolarization. It is these changes in Na^+ ion flux that produce the electrophysiological signals that are ultimately perceived in the brain as a visual image. A definitive link between light activation of rhodopsin and membrane permeability changes has yet to be established.

Since most of the rhodopsin in ROS is in disc membranes that are not contiguous with the plasma membrane, it is thought that a small soluble internal messenger is probably present in the photoreceptor that could couple rhodopsin activation with the membrane changes. Mainly from the work of Yoshikami and Hagins, Ca^{2+} ion has been thought to be a prime candidate for such an internal messenger.[81] In simple form, this theory supposes that Ca^{2+} is sequestered mainly within the discs in dark-adapted vertebrate rods. Light-induced changes would allow for the movement of the ion into the cytoplasmic space, where it could block sodium channels in the rod outer-segment plasma membrane and lead to hyperpolarization.

The high concentration of cyclic GMP in ROS and the presence of a light-activated PDE enzyme, however, has made it possible to consider alternatives to the Ca^{2+} theory. Cyclic GMP could act alone in the modulation of Na^+ channels, high cyclic GMP levels in dark-adapted ROS keeping the channels open. This could involve direct action of cyclic GMP on membrane components or specific cyclic GMP-dependent phosphorylation of channel proteins. Little is known about these processes.

It is more likely that cyclic GMP and calcium act in concert to produce the visual cascade as suggested by Fatt.[35] It is yet possible that cyclic GMP acts on membranes in the dark-adapted state to maintain open channels while the Ca^{2+} is sequestered in the discs (Fig. 4-3). With light adaptation, the calcium could spill from the discs and block the channels. However a rapid Ca^{2+} reuptake mechanism would have to be present to ensure that the process could be repeated within a very short time. Cavaggioni and Sorbi and George and Hagins have reported an effect of cyclic GMP on Ca^{2+} binding to disc membranes.[20,39] So, it is possible that the primary effect of cyclic GMP could be on calcium mobilization in the discs: out of the disc in light adaptation or back into the disc in dark adaptation.

These concepts are theoretical and must be considered only as working models to test various hypotheses in a rapidly advancing field. In fact, the entire idea that a light-induced decrease in cyclic GMP concentration is of physiological importance has recently been challenged by

POSSIBLE EFFECTS OF CYCLIC GMP IN VISUAL TRANSDUCTION

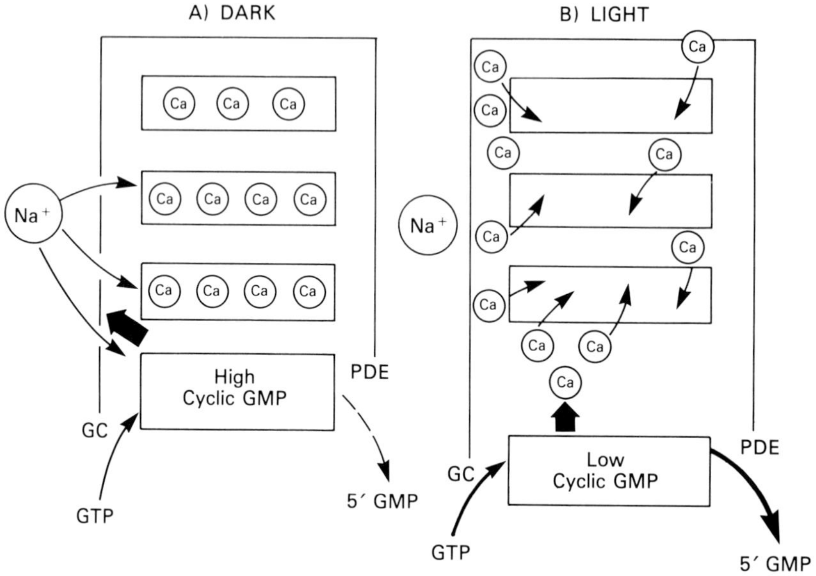

Figure 4-3. Possible modes of interaction of cyclic GMP and calcium (Ca) in controlling the photoreceptor sodium (Na$^+$) dark current.

Goldberg and associates.[41] They feel that the flux of cyclic GMP (i.e., rate of synthesis and degradation) is of greater significance than a change in the steady state level of cyclic GMP in the ROS. It is this flux that could be related to the release of calcium from disc membranes or to the inhibition of the sodium dark current. Thus, the precise role of cyclic GMP in photoreceptor metabolism has yet to be established.

PHOTORECEPTOR DEGENERATIONS

A photoreceptor degeneration is an abiotrophic process of the visual cells that occurs only after normal development. It is thought that, morphologically, electrophysiologically, and biochemically, the cells reach full maturity prior to the onset of the signs of the disease.

Miniature Poodle

The best example of a photoreceptor degeneration is progressive rod–cone degeneration (PRCD) in the miniature poodle. The retina of an affected animal develops normally, and only after the developmental period is completed do structural or functional abnormalities become evident. A clinical diagnosis can be made by ophthalmoscopy between 3 and 4 years of age; the onset of blindness varies but generally occurs in animals older than 5 years of age.

The degenerative process progresses quite differently in different retinal areas. In young animals, the disease is most severe in the posterior pole and equator; the peripheral retina is usually less involved or even normal. In older animals, the pattern is reversed, atrophic changes being most pronounced in the periphery. In the early stages of the disease the visual-cell outer segments are observed to be disoriented. Progression of the disease leads to outer and then inner segment breakdown and eventually to photoreceptor cell death. The disease affects rods more severely; cones survive for a considerably longer time.

Extensive autoradiographic and biochemical studies now seem to have identified the probable cause of the disease as a defect in the rate of outer-segment renewal. From the work of Young it is well known that rod outer-segment membranes are continually renewed by the

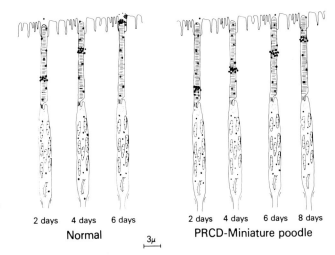

Figure 4-4. Outline of progression of radiolabeled band of protein in photoreceptor outer segments in normal miniature poodles and those affected with progressive rod-cone degeneration (PRCD).

daily addition of new discs at the base of the outer segment and the shedding of disc packets from outer-segment tips for phagocytosis and digestion by PE cells.[83] If a pulse of radiolabeled amino acids is injected intravenously or into the vitreous, much of it reaches the visual cells, where it is used for protein biosynthesis. The newly synthesized protein is thus radioactively labeled; on autoradiography, a portion of this is found to progress up the outer segment in a discrete band as new unlabeled discs are added at the base. Ultimately, the radiolabeled band disappears into the PE after being shed at the outer segment apex. To maintain a constant outer-segment length this delicately balanced process matches the rate of disc synthesis and assembly with the rate of disc shedding.

Aguirre and coworkers recently found that the renewal rate in the outer segments of miniature poodles affected with PRCD is abnormally slow (Fig. 4-4).[4] After the intravitreal injection of ^{3}H-leucine, the renewal rate (i.e., the displacement of the band of radioactivity) in control animals was found to be 2.3 μm per day; in affected animals it was significantly slower, 1.3 μm per day. Slower renewal was found both in rods that were structurally normal and in those overtly diseased. Most other biochemical parameters, including opsin biosynthesis, appeared to be normal in the early stages of the disease. How such a reduced renewal rate could result in actual photoreceptor degeneration is unknown.

As will be seen in subsequent sections, cyclic nucleotide abnormalities are apparent in retinas of several of the animal models early in the course of the disease. This does not seem to be the case in the photoreceptor degenerative diseases represented by the miniature poodle. At an early stage of the disease, when outer-segment lamellar disc changes are first observed (14 weeks of age), retinal cyclic nucleotide levels are normal (Table 4-5). Even at a somewhat later

Table 4-5. Cyclic GMP Concentration in Normal Dog Retina and in Miniature Poodles Affected with Progressive Rod–Cone Degeneration

Animal Group	Cyclic GMP Concentration (pmol/mg protein)
Control	8.7 ± 3.3
Affected	
14 weeks	8.6
23 weeks	7.9
1.5 years	4.1
2.5 years	6.4
3.5 years	3.4
5–8 years	5.9

The control retinal values were averaged from 17 phenotypically normal animals older than 7 weeks of age of the following breeds: miniature poodle, Irish setter, Norwegian elkhound, beagle and an Irish setter–Norwegian elkhound cross. (Adapted from Aguirre C, Acland G, Chader G: Hereditary retinal degenerations in the dog: Specificity of abnormal cyclic nucleotide metabolism to diseases of arrested photoreceptor development. Birth Defects: Original Article Series 18:119, 1982; by permission of March of Dimes Birth Defects Foundation) stage, when damage is more extensive (23 weeks), the cyclic GMP concentration is quite similar to that of controls. Retinal cyclic GMP does appear to decline in older affected animals, but this is to be expected as the outer segments degenerate and visual cells are lost. It thus appears that this change is a result of the disease rather than a cause of the disease.

Wag/Rij Rat

In 1975 a single report on a new, presumably hereditary, retinal degeneration in rats was published by Lai and coworkers.[50] The disease course was reported to first become apparent in the young adult (1 to 3 months) and to progress slowly until full retinal involvement was observed at about 1 year of age. The first morphological changes observed are in the nuclei of the photoreceptor cells, which become enlarged and show dispersion and margination of the heterochromatin. Subsequently, inner, and then outer, segments become involved. By 6 months of age the outer nuclear layer is reduced to about eight rows of perikarya; by 12 to 15 months, the lesions characteristic of an end-stage retinal degeneration are present. The disease course as reported is thus quite different from that observed in the poodle. Similarly, the early nuclear changes found in the Wag/Rij rat photoreceptor cells may indicate an etiology for this disease process that is fundamentally different from that in the poodle.

The extremely small number of Wag/Rij rats available for experimentation has severely limited morphological and biochemical studies on this model. Recent evidence also indicates that some of the features originally described in the disease process may no longer be observed in the current animal colony.* The presently available animals will therefore have to be thoroughly recharacterized in order to determine whether they will be useful in studies of hereditary retinal degeneration.

Abyssinian Cat

An autosomal-recessive mutation causing progressive retinal atrophy in the Abyssinian cat

* M LaVail: Personal communication

has been reported recently.[58] Although detailed histological findings have not yet been reported, ophthalmological studies reveal that the retina in affected individuals is normal until the age of approximately 1 year, when progressive retinopathy sets in. As in most of the other animal models, the disease primarily affects the photoreceptor cell layer.

PHOTORECEPTOR DYSPLASIAS

The retinal diseases that have been most extensively studied in animal models have been the photoreceptor dysplasias. Invariably in this group, degenerative changes are apparent as the outer segments develop, and normal adult morphology and function are never achieved. This group of diseases is characterized by arrested development of visual cells and has previously been reviewed.[23]

Irish Setter Dog

Irish setters carry an autosomal-recessive mutation that results in an early-onset rapidly progressive retinal degeneration in homozygous animals.[8,53,63] Electrophysiological studies in animals at 3 to 4 weeks of age demonstrate the early onset of the disease. Affected dog retinas fail to respond to a scotopic blue stimulus, while the responses to scotopic red and white stimuli are of very low amplitude and short latency. This indicates that rod-mediated ERG responses are not recordable while cone-mediated signals are present but abnormal. By the second or third week of life, morphologically, short, disorganized rod outer segments are found with stunted, diminutive inner segments. The outer segments show markedly disorganized disc membranes.[6] The PE seems normal and the process of phagocytosis appears to be unaffected in the animals. By 2 months of age, rod degeneration is extensive; cones are the predominant cell type remaining in the photoreceptor layer. Figure 4-5 compares the normal retina at 10 weeks of age with the affected retina at 8 and 12 weeks. In the normal the outer segments have fully elongated and matured. (In this micrograph, the normal PE is nonpigmented since it is

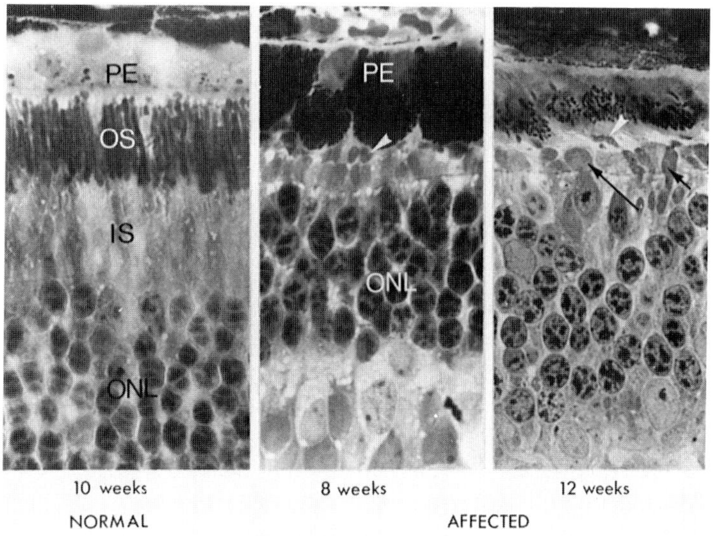

Figure 4-5. Light micrographs of retinas of normal and affected Irish setters. PE, pigment epithelium; OS, outer segments; IS, inner segments; ONL, outer nuclear layer. White arrowhead, outer segment material; black arrow, cone inner segments. (Aguirre G et al: Rod-cone dysplasia in Irish setters: a defect in cyclic GMP metabolism in visual cells. Science 201:1133, 1978; copyright 1978 by the AAAS)

from the tapetal region of the eye, an area normally not pigmented.) Even by 8 weeks, however, the photoreceptor layer of the affected retina contains little outer-segment material, and inner segments are also reduced in length and number. Although the developmental abnormality affects both rods and cones, cone damage is less severe; prominent cones are therefore present in the photoreceptor layer. The outer nuclear layer is reduced by this time, an indication of active visual-cell death.

Biochemically, a defect in cyclic GMP metabolism is observed at the time of rapid photoreceptor cell death.[5] In the neural retina, the cyclic GMP concentration was found to be ten times higher in affected retinas (102 pmol/mg protein) than in control retinas (12 pmol/mg protein). Since this was observed when virtually no outer segments remained, it must be assumed that the high concentration is present in the remaining portions of the visual cell (i.e., the inner segments, perikarya, etc.). The high cyclic GMP level is probably due to a greatly decreased phosphodiesterase (PDE) activity found in the affected retinas. In particular, one specific kinetic type of PDE appears to be missing. This high-K_m enzyme type is thought to be compartmentalized in the outer segments; decreased activity of this enzyme is thus likely to lead to the aberrantly high cyclic GMP levels characteristic of this disease.

Observing such biochemical defects late in the course of the disease may mean only that the altered cyclic GMP metabolism is a result of the disease rather than the cause. Retinas from 1- to 2-week-old setters were therefore examined, an age well before any morphological signs of the disease are observed.[6] It was found that very early in the postnatal period cyclic GMP levels were already abnormally high (Fig. 4-6). This was accompanied by a deficit in total retinal PDE activity, even at 9 days of age.[51] Not only was the PDE activity found to be low, it appeared to be of a different type, a type that could be activated by a small protein called calmodulin. In the normal adult retina PDE is calmodulin-independent; in the affected dog retina PDE remains calmodulin-dependent.[23] The original finding of calmodulin dependency in affected setter retinas used a substrate concentration of 1 μM cyclic GMP; this has been reconfirmed using a 1.0-mM substrate concentration to measure total retinal cyclic GMP–PDE activity.[23,51] No defect in general membrane protein biosynthesis was observed in the affected retinas, indicating that early in the course of the disease the genetic lesion is quite specific and localized.[6]

Figure 4-7 presents a model of possible abnormal events in affected Irish setter retinas. In control retinas at 1 week of age, outer segments have yet to develop, and the predominant cyclic

PATTERN OF CYCLIC GMP DEVELOPMENT IN
CONTROL AND AFFECTED RETINAS

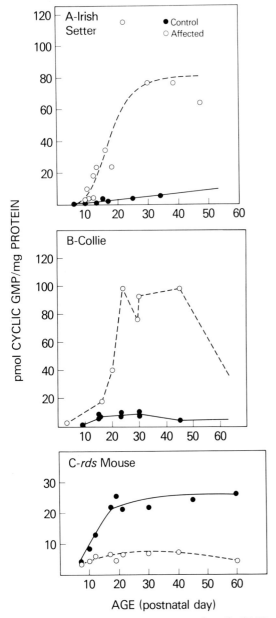

Figure 4-6. Developmental pattern of cyclic GMP concentration in retinas of *(A)* Irish setter, *(B)* collie, and *(C)* rds mouse.

GMP–PDE type present is calmodulin-dependent. As the outer segments elongate, the major PDE activity apparently switches to a calmodu-

lin-independent type, allowing for normal cyclic GMP metabolism and, thus, normal outer-segment development and function. In affected retinas, the PDE activity does not seem to switch from a calmodulin-dependent to calmodulin-independent type. This failure to change, together with the low level of calmodulin, may lead to the high cyclic GMP levels typical of the disease. It is not known, however, whether the high cyclic GMP levels are actually the primary cause of the photoreceptor membrane damage and cell death. Hollyfield and coworkers have shown in studies *in vitro* that high concentrations of cyclic GMP are toxic to rod photoreceptor cells of the human retina.[75] These results are consistent with a direct role of cyclic GMP in photoreceptor cell pathology in at least this one form of visual cell degeneration.

Collie

The collie also demonstrates an early-onset rod–cone dysplasia. As in setters, rods are more severely damaged.[79] The disease is first expressed at the time of outer-segment development, when affected photoreceptor cells produce only small, stunted outer-segment elements.[66] Figure 4-8 compares the normal 16-day retina with that of an affected animal. In normals, outer segments are already forming a discrete layer between photoreceptor inner segments and PE cells. In the affected retinas, little outer-segment material is observed; that which is present is extensively disorganized. By approximately 2 months of age, few outer and inner segments remain; extensive photoreceptor cell death is evident.

As illustrated in Figure 4-6B, cyclic GMP levels are abnormally high in the early stages of the collie disease, and PDE activity in affected retinas is low.[78] In contrast to the setter, however, the PDE in affected collie retinas is not calmodulin-dependent. So, although the major features of the metabolic defect are similar in collie and setter, the diseases in the two models are not biochemically identical. This suggests that different defects can occur at different points in the pathway that regulates the level of cyclic GMP in visual cells.

MODEL FOR ROD-CONE DYSPLASIA
IN THE IRISH SETTER

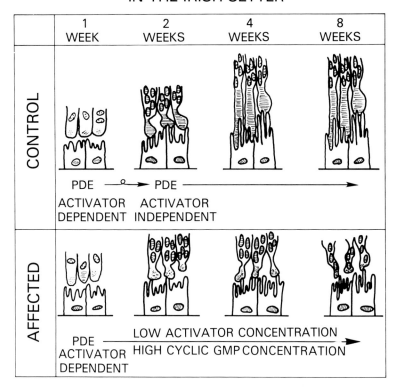

Figure 4-7. Scheme of possible events leading to normal *(control)* or abnormal *(affected)* retinal development in the Irish setter. (Liu Y et al: Involvement of cyclic GMP phospho-diesterase activator in an hereditary retinal degeneration. Nature 280:62, 1979; reprinted by permission)

rd Mouse

The retinal degeneration *(rd)* mutation in the mouse has been one of the most extensively studied types of inherited photoreceptor dysplasia.[71] The course of the disease is extremely rapid (Fig. 4-9), but, owing to the short life span of rodents, the disease progresses at a rate comparable to that in the setter and collie. Abnormal inner segments are already seen by the end of the first week of life; only small, abnormal outer segments subsequently develop.[60] The outer segments rapidly disintegrate, and visual cell nuclear pyknosis is observed. By the end of the third week, the outer nuclear layer is reduced to a single layer of nuclei; thereafter other inner-retinal neurons are affected. There is a specific spatial pattern of photoreceptor degeneration with a central-to-peripheral disease gradient.[61] Also, rods are involved much more quickly than cones. Carter-Dawson and associates found, for example, that by postnatal day 17, only about

2% of the rod nuclei remained in the peripheral retina. Yet, in the same region, 75% of the cone nuclei were still present.[19]

Biochemically, a defect in PDE activity was first described in the *rd* mouse by Schmidt and Lolley.[70] A striking accumulation of cyclic GMP was soon observed in the early postnatal period, along with an abnormally low cyclic GMP–PDE activity.[33,34] The early death and destruction of the visual cells is paralleled by a decline in the abnormally high cyclic GMP levels; by 1 to 2 months of age the levels are below those of normal control retinas.

It is interesting to note that Ferrendelli and Cohen found that heterozygous C57BL mice carrying the *rd* gene also had abnormal retinal cyclic GMP levels.[36] Instead of being higher than those of homozygous normal controls, however, the cyclic GMP levels were actually about 40% lower. If the genetic lesion in the *rd* mouse were a simple mutation affecting the PDE enzyme, one would have expected a higher

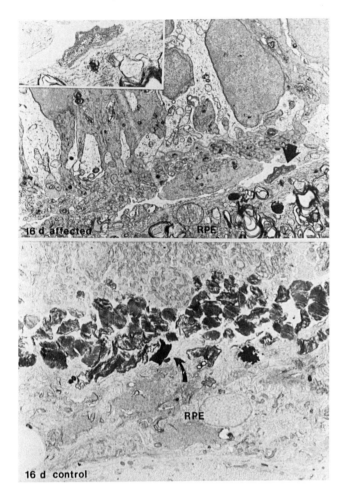

Figure 4-8. Affected *(top)* and control *(bottom)* collie retinas at 16 days of age. *Insert,* outer-segment material. (Santos-Anderson R, Tso M, Wolf D: An inherited retinopathy in collies: a light and electron microscopic study. Invest Ophthalmol Vis Sci 19:1281, 1980)

cyclic GMP level, perhaps intermediate between the homozygous-normal and homozygous-affected concentrations. That this is not the case indicates that other factors also must be involved in determining the ultimate cyclic GMP levels. In contrast to the situation in the *rd* mouse no differences in cyclic GMP levels were found between homozygous-normal and heterozygous Irish setters.[6]

rds Mouse

In this autosomal-recessive mutant, the retinal degeneration slow *(rds)* gene results in virtually no outer-segment development, and, surprisingly, a much slower photoreceptor cell death than in the *rd* retina (see Fig. 4-9).[47,67,69] The 21-day-old *rds* retina exhibits an apparent lack of outer-segment material, but the outer nuclear layer is much better preserved than in the *rd* mutant. In the *rds* retina the rods and cones are equally affected, while in the *rd* retina cones survive longer than rods. Thus, the disease in the *rds* mouse does fall into the early-onset type of photoreceptor dysplasia, but it exhibits distinct temporal differences from the *rd* mutant in the rate of visual-cell degeneration and death.

Cohen has recently confirmed and extended the general findings of Sanyal and his colleagues.[27] He reported that the 21-day *rds* retina commonly exhibits, morphologically, well-defined cilia that are normal in appearance. Biochemically, Cohen found a lower-than-normal cyclic GMP content in the 21-day retina. He did observe a fall in cyclic GMP level upon illumination of dark-adapted retinas *in vitro,* indicating that the PDE-activation mechanism is still functional in this mutant.

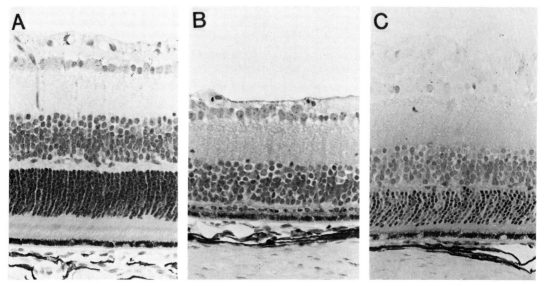

Figure 4-9. Normal and mutant mouse retinas at 21 days of age. *(A)* Normal; *(B) rd* mutant; *(C) rds* mutant.

We examined the PDE activity and cyclic GMP content in *rds* retinas from 7 through 60 days of life. PDE activity was found to be abnormally low throughout the entire period, as it was in the other photoreceptor dysplasia models.[68] The situation is quite different, however, in terms of the cyclic GMP concentration (see Fig. 4-6*C*). In control retinas the concentration of cyclic GMP (pmol/mg protein) increases in the second and third postnatal weeks, as the outer segments elongate, and reaches a plateau value of about 25 pmol/mg protein soon thereafter.[68] In the *rds* retina, the cyclic GMP concentration does not increase but remains at about 3 to 5 pmol/mg protein throughout the entire developmental period examined. This was an unexpected finding. Since the *rds* retina is morphologically of the early-onset photoreceptor-dysplasia group and since the PDE activity is abnormally low, we expected to find an abnormally high cyclic GMP level during the early developmental period, like that in the setter, collie, and *rd* mouse. Since this was not the case, it is reasonable to conclude that there are significant biochemical differences, in addition to the temporal differences cited above, that might point to an underlying genetic difference between this model and the other photoreceptor-dysplasia models.

PE–CHOROID DISEASES

It is now known that several of the so-called retinal degenerations are primarily diseases of the PE or choroid and involve the neural retina only in a secondary manner. Some of the most detailed genetic, morphological, and biochemical studies have been performed on animal mutants that fall into this category.

Rat-RCS

Rat retinal degeneration (rdy) or "dystrophy" was first described in the Royal College of Surgeons (RCS) rat strain by Bourne and coworkers.[17] This mutant appears to be different from all others in that a layer of outer-segment debris accumulates between the neural retina and the PE cells in the early postnatal period.[29] This appears to be a result of the inability of the PE cells to phagocytize shed packets of outer-segment discs.[16,46] Thanks to the pioneering work of Mullen and LaVail, it is now known that the genetic mutation is indeed expressed in the PE cell.[57] Using chimeras produced by combining embryos from normal and affected animals, they showed that photoreceptor cells degenerated only when they were in juxtaposition to PE cells derived from mutant animals.

Edwards and Szamier and Hall conducted extensive tissue culture studies on the defect in rod outer-segment phagocytosis by the PE cell.[31,43] A difference in phagocytosis between normal and affected PE cells has been confirmed as well as a light–dark difference in ROS uptake in normal PE cells. In more recent work Chaitin and Hall showed that ROS are bound to the PE-cell surface of affected animals in a normal manner but that the ingestion phase of phagocytosis is defective.[24,25] They have found that the actin contractile system appears to function properly but that the "ingestion mechanism becomes activated at only a few sites of ROS attachment." This may indicate a paucity of membrane receptors that trigger the ingestion mechanism. The singular nature of the PE-cell phagocytic defect is supported by the findings of Gery and O'Brien, who reported that macrophages from the RCS rat exhibit normal phagocytosis.[40]

Biochemically, it has been suggested that the disease may result from an inability of the affected PE cell to adequately esterify vitamin A. Berman and colleagues found that retinol esterification in the neonatal RCS rat pigment epithelium is lower than that of control tissue.[12] The block in esterification leads to a small excess of free retinol. Although free retinol is known to be a membranolytic agent, a link between this biochemical abnormality, the phagocytic defect, and the actual degenerative process in the neural retina has yet to be established. Lolley and Farber found that cyclic nucleotide metabolism in the RCS rat retina is abnormal; however, it appears that this is a secondary event as the accumulated debris exerts an inhibitory influence on retinal PDE activity.[52]

Results of an interesting series of experiments that have received too little attention point to a possible systemic defect in carbohydrate metabolism in RCS rats. DiMattio and Zadunaisky reported a defect in glucose uptake across the blood–aqueous and blood–vitreous barriers.[28] Ennis and Pautler and Stramm and Pautler also found a deranged carbohydrate metabolism in these animals, which could indicate a generalized impairment in "carbohydrate metabolism and/or transport" in RCS rat tissues.[32,73] The observed difficulty in breeding and a poor mus-cle reflex when animals are handled may indeed point to a systemic metabolic problem in the RCS animals. The high energy needs of the photoreceptor cell may make it particularly susceptible to such a lesion. Certainly, more work should be conducted in this area.

Dog PE Dystrophy

The mutation in the Labrador retriever and some other dog breeds is also in the PE and results in early PE-cell hypertrophy.[7] The condition is first localized in discrete foci but subsequently spreads to encompass most of the PE-cell layer. In more advanced stages there is PE-cell invasion of the atrophic neural retina. The PE cells contain an autofluorescent lipopigment, possibly lipofuscin or ceroid. No biochemical studies have been performed to try to identify the lesion in this condition.

Cat Gyrate Atrophy

A single report in the literature describes a feline disease that is similar to gyrate atrophy in man.[76] As in the advanced stages of the human disease, the cat was found to have only isolated patches of choriocapillaris between an atrophic retina and choroid. Biochemical studies on this animal showed abnormally high serum ornithine levels and a deficiency of the enzyme ornithine aminotransferase in tissue specimens and in cultured fibroblasts. Even though the affected cat died before it could be bred, it is probable that other such animals exist and that a truly excellent model for human gyrate atrophy could be established.

Cat Mucopolysaccharidoses

In the human, several defects in glycoprotein, glycosaminoglycan, lipid, and carbohydrate metabolism have been reported and collectively have been referred to as inborn errors of metabolism. In the cat, models for two mucopolysaccharidoses have now been reported that should be useful in gaining knowledge about their human counterparts. Haskins and coworkers recently described an excellent feline model for mucopolysaccharidosis I, (MPS I, Hurler's syndrome) and had previously reported one for mucopolysaccharidosis VI, (MPS VI, Maroteaux – Lamy syndrome).[44,45]

In both of these disease entities, the PE is severely affected. In MPS I, the PE-cell cytoplasm is rapidly filled with large blue inclusion bodies. Stramm and Aguirre identified a deficiency in the enzyme α-L-iduronidase in cultured PE cells from affected animals.* In MPS VI, a deficiency in arylsulfatase B has been pinpointed in cultured PE cells, which leads to an accumulation in dermatan sulfate.[74] Morphologically, the nonpigmented PE cells become hypertrophied and demonstrate a large number of vacuolated inclusions.[9]

As in the case of the RCS rat, it appears that the use of PE-cell tissue culture could not only afford a better understanding of the biochemical causes of these conditions but also allow for the experimental manipulation of this disease with the aim of developing new therapeutic modalities.

DISEASES OF UNKNOWN ETIOLOGY

In some animal models of retinal degeneration, the morphology of the retina remains intact but function is impaired. Two excellent examples of this phenomenon are seen in the Appaloosa horse and pearl mouse mutants.

Appaloosa Horse

In some Appaloosa horses, a recessively inherited night blindness is present which is best described as congenital stationary night blindness.[77] Although the morphology of the retina is normal and the ERG has normal a- and c-wave responses, it lacks the rod-mediated b-wave response.[65,77] The affected dark-adapted retina exhibits a distinct 510-nm absorbance peak determined by transmission densitometry and therefore has normal levels of rhodopsin.

The condition in the horse is quite similar to that observed in human hereditary night blindness, where the trait is inherited in a recessive

manner. Of interest is Ripps' finding that both the human and equine conditions are electrophysiologically similar to a case of night blindness caused by the antitumor agent vincristine.[65] This chemical apparently binds to tubulin subunits and interferes with microtubule assembly therefore affecting a number of processes including axonal transport. Ripps suggested that a possible cause of the hereditary disease may be a defect in microtubule renewal which could then affect rod synaptic-terminal function.

Pearl Mouse

As with the Appaloosa horse, this may be an excellent model for human congenital stationary night blindness. No retinal degeneration is seen in the mutant strain, but a definite decrease in dark-adapted sensitivity is observed.[10] The disease is inherited through an autosomal-recessive gene and is accompanied by general hypopigmentation, including a reduction in the number of melanosomes in retinal PE cells. In addition, Piccini and associates reported a defect in lysosome size and in the secretion of kidney lysosomal enzymes in these animals.[64] Along with the hypopigmentation, this indicates that the defect is not expressed only in the eye but rather is of a more general nature. A reduction in the number of retinal projections was also found.[10]

Balkema and coworkers found that normal sensitivity could be restored to the retina after its isolation and superfusion with a balanced salt solution.[10] Based on these results, they suggested that the retinal abnormality is caused by a "diffusable substance." Whether this substance is replenished by the salt solution, thus restoring normal sensitivity, or whether it is a blocking substance that is removed from the retina is not known at present. In any event, the intriguing finding of Balkema's group appears to have opened the door for a serious investigation of the biochemical factors responsible for the loss in retinal sensitivity. It will be interesting to see whether abnormal cyclic nucleotide concentrations, calcium concentrations, and so on are involved in the process.

* Personal communication

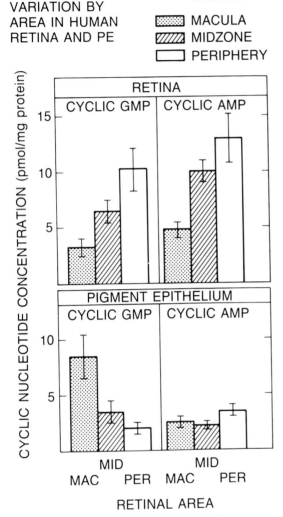

Figure 4-10. Variation in cyclic nucleotide concentration in areas of neural retina and pigment epithelium. (Adapted from Newsome D, Fletcher R, Chader G: Cyclic nucleotides vary by area in the retina and pigmented epithelium of the human and monkey. Invest Ophthalmol Vis Sci 19:864, 1980)

CONCLUSIONS

As seen in the above group of mutants, several excellent animal models are now available for the study of retinitis pigmentosa and allied hereditary retinal disorders. Many years ago when the first few of these models were being described (e.g., RCS rat) it was hoped that work on them would quickly lead to understanding *the* cause of *the* disease retinitis pigmentosa. With the diversity now known to be present in the human situation and the large number of different defects in the animal models, it is clear that there is no single cause of retinal degeneration and that it is quite possible that each of these models will be useful in studying the spectrum of retinal diseases in man, including RP.

At present, the only defect seen in more than one animal model is the cyclic nucleotide abnormality observed in some of the early-onset photoreceptor dysplasias. Although it is tempting to conclude on the surface that such a defect might be a common feature in all the photoreceptor dysplasias, there are too many temporal, biochemical, and morphological differences between the models for this to be the case. Again, each of the animal mutants described in pages 86–88 could give important information about a specific form of RP.

As yet, we have no direct biochemical evidence that cyclic nucleotide abnormalities or abnormalities in any other metabolic system are involved in any of the human types of RP. It is interesting though that the concentration of cyclic nucleotides has been found to vary by area in the retina and PE, a finding that could partially explain the highly specific regional nature of retinal degeneration observed in many cases.[59] The concentrations of cyclic GMP and cyclic AMP are much higher in the peripheral retina than in the macula, paralleling the rod distribution (Fig. 4-10). In the PE the cyclic GMP content is reversed, with the highest concentration in the macular region. No differences in cyclic AMP concentration were observed in the three areas of the PE examined. Thus, there is a specific spatial distribution of cyclic GMP in retina and in the PE. We may therefore conclude that different areas of the retina and the PE may be differentially susceptible to an underlying defect in cyclic nucleotide metabolism or another metabolic process yet to be defined.

REFERENCES

1. Adams A, Aspinall P, Hayreh S: Primary retinal pigmentary degeneration. Trans Ophthalmol Soc UK 92:233, 1972

2. Aguirre G: Inherited retinal degeneration in the dog. Trans Am Acad Ophthalmol Otolaryngol 81:667, 1976
3. Aguirre G, Acland G, Chader G: Hereditary retinal degenerations in the dog: Specificity of abnormal cyclic nucleotide metabolism to diseases of arrested photoreceptor development. Birth Defects: Original Article Series 18:119, 1982
4. Aguirre G, Alligood J, O'Brien P, et al: Pathogenesis of progressive rod–cone degeneration in the miniature poodle. Exp Eye Res 23:610, 1983
5. Aguirre G, Farber D, Lolley R, et al: Rod–cone dysplasia in Irish setters: A defect in cyclic GMP metabolism in visual cells. Science 201:1133, 1978
6. Aguirre G, Farber D, Lolley R, et al: Retinal degenerations in the dog. III. Abnormal cyclic nucleotide metabolism in rod–cone dysplasia. Exp Eye Res 35:625, 1982
7. Aguirre G, Laties A: Pigment epithelial dystrophy in the dog. Exp Eye Res 23:247, 1976
8. Aguirre G, Rubin L: Rod–cone dysplasia (progressive retinal atrophy) in Irish setters. J Am Vet Med Assoc 166:157, 1975
9. Aguirre G, Stramm L, Haskins M: Feline mucopolysaccharidosis VI: General ocular and pigment epithelial pathology. Invest Ophthalmol Vis Sci 24:991, 1983
10. Balkema G, Mangini N, Pinto L: Discrete visual defects in pearl mutant mice. Science 219:1085, 1983
11. Bennett N, Michel-Villaz M, Kuhn H: Light-induced interaction between rhodopsin and the GTP-binding protein. Metarhodopsin II is the major photoproduct involved. Europ J Biochem 127:97, 1982
12. Berman E, Segal N, Photiou S, et al: Inherited retinal dystrophy in RCS rats: a deficiency in vitamin A esterification in pigment epithelium. Nature 293:217, 1981
13. Berson EL: Retinitis pigmentosa and allied diseases: Electrophysiologic findings. Trans Am Acad Ophthal Otol 81:659, 1976
14. Berson EL, Rosen J, Simonoff EA: Electroretinographic testing as an aid in detection of carriers of X-chromosome linked RP. Am J Ophthalmol 87:460, 1979
15. Bird A, Hyman V: Detection of heterozygotes in families with X-linked pigmentary retinopathy by measurement of retinal rhodopsin concentration. Trans Ophthalmol Soc UK 92:221, 1972
16. Bok D, Hall M: The role of the pigment epithelium in the etiology of inherited retinal dystrophy in the rat. J Cell Biol 49:664, 1971
17. Bourne M, Campbell D, Pyke M: Hereditary degenerations of the rat retina. Br J Ophthalmol 22:613, 1938
18. Capovilla M, Corretta A, Cavaggioni A, et al: Metabolism and permeability in retinal rods. In Osborne N, Chader G (eds): Progress in Retinal Research, vol 1, p 233. Oxford, Pergamon Press, 1983
19. Carter-Dawson L, LaVail M, Sidman R: Differential effect of the *rd* mutation on rods and cones in the mouse retina. Invest Ophthalmol Vis Sci 17:489, 1978
20. Cavaggioni A, Sorbi R: Cyclic GMP releases calcium from disc membranes of vertebrate photoreceptors. Proc Natl Acad Sci USA 78:3964, 1981
21. Chader G, Herz L, Fletcher R: Light activation of phosphodiesterase activity in retinal rod outer segments. Biochim Biophys Acta 347:491, 1974
22. Chader G, Johnson M, Fletcher R, et al: Cyclic nucleotide phosphodiesterase of the bovine retina: Activity, subcellular distribution and kinetic parameters. J Neurochem 22:93, 1974
23. Chader G, Liu Y, Fletcher R, et al: Cyclic GMP phosphodiesterase and calmodulin in early onset inherited retinal degenerations. Current Topics Memb Transport 15:133, 1981
24. Chaitin M, Hall M: Defective ingestion of rod outer segments by cultured dystrophic rat pigment epithelial cells. Invest Ophthalmol Vis Sci 24:812, 1983
25. Chaitin M, Hall M: The distribution of actin in cultured normal and dystrophic rat pigment epithelial cells during the phagocytosis of rod outer segments. Invest Ophthalmol Vis Sci 24:821, 1983
26. Cogan D: Pathology. Am Acad Ophthalmol Otolaryngol Trans 54:629, 1949–1950
27. Cohen A: Some cytological and initial biochemical observations on photoreceptors in retinas of *rds* mice. Invest Ophthalmol Vis Sci 24:832, 1983
28. diMattio J, Zadunaisky J: Stereospecificity of ocular glucose transport in the normal and RCS rats. Invest Ophthalmol Vis Sci, Suppl 276, 1978
29. Dowling J, Sidman R: Inherited retinal dystrophy in rat. J Cell Biol 14:73, 1962
30. Duke-Elder S, Dobree J: System of Ophthalmology, vol 10, p 598. London, Kimpton, 1967
31. Edwards R, Szamier R: Defective phagocytosis of isolated rod outer segments by RCS rat retinal pigment epithelium in culture. Science 197:1001, 1977
32. Ennis S, Pautler E: Expression of the genetic defect associated with inherited retinal dystrophy in the rat. Metab Pediat Ophthal 3:11, 1979
33. Farber D, Lolley R: Cyclic guanosine monophosphate: Elevation in degenerating photoreceptor cells of the C3H mouse retina. Science 186:449, 1974
34. Farber D, Lolley R: Enzymatic basis for cyclic GMP accumulation in degenerative photoreceptor cells of mouse retina. J Cyclic Nucleotide Res 2:139, 1976
35. Fatt P: An extended Ca^{2+}-hypothesis of visual

transduction with a role for cyclic GMP. FEBS Lett 149:159, 1982

36. Ferrendelli J, Cohen A: The effects of light and dark adaptation on the levels of cyclic nucleotides in retinas of mice heterozygous for photoreceptor dystrophy. Biochem Biophys Res Commun 73:421, 1976

37. Fletcher R, Chader G: Cyclic GMP: Control of concentration by light in retinal photoreceptors. Biochem Biophys Res Commun 70:1297, 1976

38. Fung B, Stryer L: Photolyzed rhodopsin catalyzes the exchange of GTP for bound GDP in retinal rod outer segments. Proc Natl Acad Sci USA 77:2500, 1980

39. George J, Hagins W: Control of Ca^{2+} in rod outer segment discs by light and cyclic GMP. Nature 303:344, 1983

40. Gery I, O'Brien P: RCS rat macrophages exhibit normal phagocytosis. Invest Ophthalmol Vis Sci 29:675, 1981

41. Goldberg N, Ames A, Gander J, et al: Magnitude of increase in retinal cGMP metabolic flux determined by ^{18}O incorporation into nucleotide αphosphoryls corresponds with intensity of photic stimulation. J Biol Chem 258:9213, 1983

42. Gouras P, Carr R: Electrophysiological studies in early retinitis pigmentosa. Arch Ophthalmol 74:104, 1964

43. Hall M: Phagocytosis of light- and dark-adapted rod outer segments by cultured pigment epithelium. Science 202:526, 1978

44. Haskins M, Aguirre G, Jezyk P, et al: The pathology of the feline model of mucopolysaccharidosis VI. Am J Pathol 101:657, 1980

45. Haskins M, Aguirre G, Jezyk P, et al: The pathology of the feline model of mucopolysaccharidosis I. Am J Pathol 112:27, 1983

46. Herron W, Riegel B, Rubin M: Retinal dystrophy in the rat — A pigment epithelial disease. Invest Ophthalmol 8:595, 1969

47. Jansen H, Sanyal S: Development and degeneration of retina in *rds* mutant mice: Electron microscopy. J Comp Neurol 224:71, 1984

48. Krill A: Observations of carriers of X-chromosomal linked chorio-retinal degenerations. Do these support the "inactivation hypothesis"? Am J Ophthalmol 64:1029, 1967

49. Krishnan N, Fletcher R, Chader G, et al: Characterization of guanylate cyclase of rod outer segments of the bovine retina. Biochim Biophys Acta 523:506, 1978

50. Lai Y-L, Jacoby R, Jonas A, et al: A new form of hereditary retinal degeneration in Wag/Rij rats. Invest Ophthalmol 14:62, 1975

51. Liu Y, Krishna G, Aguirre G, et al: Involvement of cyclic GMP phosphodiesterase activator in an hereditary retinal degeneration. Nature 280:62, 1979

52. Lolley R, Farber D: A proposed link between debris accumulation, guanosine 3'-5' cyclic

monophosphate changes and photoreceptor cell degeneration in retina of RCS rats. Exp Eye Res 22:477, 1976

53. Lucas DR: Retinal dystrophy in the Irish setter. I. Histology. J Exp Zool 126:537, 1954

54. Merin S, Auerbach E: Retinitis pigmentosa. Surv Ophthalmol 20:303, 1976

55. Miki N, Kierns J, Freeman J, et al: Regulation of cyclic nucleotide concentrations in photoreceptors: An ATP-dependent stimulation of cyclic nucleotide phosphodiesterase by light. Proc Natl Acad Sci USA 76:3820, 1973

56. Miller W: Physiological effects of cyclic GMP in the vertebrate retinal rod outer segment. Adv Cyclic Nucleotide Res 15:495, 1983

57. Mullen R, LaVail M: Two new types of retinal degeneration in cerebellar mutant mice. Nature 258:528, 1975

58. Narfström K: Hereditary progressive retinal atrophy in the Abyssinian cat. J Hered 74:273, 1983

59. Newsome D, Fletcher R, Chader G: Cyclic nucleotides vary by area in the retina and pigmented epithelium of the human and monkey. Invest Ophthalmol Vis Sci 19:864, 1980

60. Noell W: Studies on visual cell viability and differentiation. Ann NY Acad Sci 74:337, 1958

61. Noell W: Differentiation, metabolic organization and viability of the visual cell. Arch Ophthalmol 60:702, 1958

62. Orr H, Lowry O, Cohen A, et al: Distribution of 3':5'-cyclic AMP and 3':5'-cyclic GMP in rabbit retina in vivo: Selective effects of dark and light adaptation and ischemia. Proc Natl Acad Sci USA 73:4442, 1976

63. Parry HB: Degenerations of the dog retina. II. Generalized progressive atrophy of hereditary origin. Br J Ophthalmol 37:487, 1953

64. Piccini A, Jahries G, Novak E, et al: Intracellular distribution of lysosomal enzymes in the mouse pigment mutants pale ear and pallid. Mol Cell Biochem 31:89, 1980

65. Ripps H: Night blindness revisited: From man to molecules. Invest Ophthalmol Vis Sci 23:588, 1982

66. Santos-Anderson R, Tso M, Wolf D: An inherited retinopathy in collies: A light and electron microscopic study. Invest Ophthalmol Vis Sci 19:1281, 1980

67. Sanyal S, DeRuiter A, Hawkins R: Development and degeneration of retina in *rds* mutant mice: Light microscopy. J Comp Neurol 194:193, 1980

68. Sanyal S, Fletcher R, Liu Y, et al: Cyclic nucleotide content and phosphodiesterase activity in the rds mouse (020/A) retina. Exp Eye Res 38:247, 1984

69. Sanyal S, Jansen H: Absence of receptor outer segments in the retina of *rds* mutant mice. Neurosci Lett 21:23, 1981

70. Schmidt S, Lolley R: Cyclic nucleotide phospho-

diesterase: An early defect in inherited retinal degeneration of C3H mice. J Cell Biol 57:117, 1973

71. Sidman R, Green M: Retinal degeneration in the mouse. Localization of the *rd* locus in linkage group XVII. J Hered 56:23, 1965

72. Stein P, Rasenick M, Bitensky M: Biochemistry of the cyclic nucleotide-related enzymes in rod photoreceptors. In Osborne N, Chader G (eds): Progress in Retinal Research, vol 1, p 227. Oxford, Pergamon Press, 1983

73. Stramm L, Pautler E: Glucose uptake by normal and dystrophic rat retinas and ciliary bodies. Exp Eye Res 30:709, 1980

74. Stramm L, Haskins M, Desnick R, et al: Disease expression in cultured pigment epithelium: feline mucopolysaccharidosis VI. Invest Ophthalmol Vis Sci 26:182, 1985

75. Ulshafer R, Garcia C, Hollyfield J: Sensitivity of photoreceptors to elevated levels of cGMP in the human retina. Invest Ophthalmol Vis Sci 19:1236, 1980

76. Valle D, Boison A, Jezyk P, et al: Gyrate atrophy of the choroid and retina in a cat. Invest Ophthalmol Vis Sci 20:251, 1981

77. Witzel D, Smith E, Wilson R, et al: Congenital stationary night-blindness: An animal model. Invest Ophthalmol Vis Sci 17:788, 1978

78. Woodford B, Liu Y, Fletcher R, et al: Cyclic nucleotide metabolism in inherited retinopathy in collies: A biochemical and histochemical study. Exp Eye Res 34:703, 1982

79. Wolf D, Vainisi S, Santos-Anderson R: Inherited rod-cone dysplasia in the collie. J Am Ved Med Assoc 173:1131, 1978

80. Yamazaki A, Stein P, Chernoff N, et al: Activation mechanism of rod outer segment cyclic GMP phosphodiesterase. Release of inhibitor by the GTP/GTP-binding protein. J Biol Chem 258:8188, 1983

81. Yoshikami S, Hagins W: Control of the dark current in vertebrate rods and cones. In Langer H (ed): Biochemistry and Physiology of Visual Pigments, p 245. Berlin, Springer-Verlag, 1973

82. Yee R, Liebman P: Light-activated phosphodiesterase of the rod outer segment. Kinetics and parameters of activation and deactivation. J Biol Chem 253:8902, 1978

83. Young R: Visual cells and the concept of renewal. Invest Ophthalmol Vis Sci 15:700, 1976

2

Functional Organization and Development of the Retina

5

Development of Neurotransmitter Systems in the Retina: Biochemical, Anatomical, and Physiological Correlates

Dominic Man-Kit Lam

The development of nervous systems is a complex process of cell multiplication, cell migration, cell–cell recognition, arborization of neuronal processes, synaptogenesis, and development of specific electrical activities.[19,22,33] In essence, it is a vectorial process characterized by changes in time, space, and magnitude. The precise timing of these processes and the controlling factors are at present by no means fully understood.

The vertebrate retina is an extracranial derivative of neuroectoderm originating from an outpouching of the diencephalon during early embryogenesis. The morphology and physiology of the retina have been widely examined.[4,23,44] Because of its structural simplicity and accessibility, it is a valuable model for the study of the neurochemistry, information processing, and development of the brain.[1]

There is considerable evidence that γ-amino-

The author thanks Ms. Pat Glazebrook for technical assistance and Ms. Pat Cloud for typing the manuscript. This work was supported by grants from the U.S. National Eye Institute (EY02608), Research to Prevent Blindness, Inc., N.Y., and the Retina Research Foundation (Houston).

butyric acid (GABA), glycine, and dopamine are neurotransmitters in the vertebrate retina.[3,7,8,13,26,28–32] In particular, in the rabbit retina GABA inhibits spontaneous and light-evoked activities of ganglion cells.[2] Caldwell and Daw proposed that GABAergic amacrine cells make lateral inhibitory connections in the inner plexiform layer to provide the specificity of different types of ganglion cells.[10] Glycine also has an inhibitory effect in the retina that is antagonized by strychnine.[2,47] Dopamine depresses the firing of ganglion cells in the fish retina.[39] These neurotransmitters are found in high concentrations and can be accumulated by specific high-affinity uptake mechanisms and released upon stimulation. GABA and dopamine are synthesized and metabolized in the rabbit retina.[29,30] Using transmitter-specific properties such as uptake, storage, synthesis, and release of neurotransmitters as anatomical, biochemical, and physiological probes, it is possible to characterize the temporal sequence during the differentiation of these identified neurons in the retina. In this chapter, we discuss our findings on the emergence and maturation of these properties in the rabbit retina and make correlations with other retinas.[18,26,29,30]

THE LOCALIZATION OF GABAERGIC, GLYCINERGIC, AND DOPAMINERGIC NEURONS IN THE RABBIT RETINA

Autoradiographic, histofluorescent, and immunocytochemical studies in the adult rabbit retina demonstrated that GABAergic, glycinergic, and dopaminergic neurons are localized in the inner plexiform layer, which plays an essential role in both lateral and radial information processing among bipolar and ganglion cells.[5,13,16,29,30] Both morphological and physiological studies suggest that they belong to different subpopulations of amacrine cells.

There are probably several types of GABA-accumulating amacrine cells in the rabbit retina and at least one type of GABA-accumulating ganglion cell (Fig. 5-1f).[5,6,15,17,29,51] Immunocytochemical studies of the GABA-synthesizing enzyme glutamic acid decarboxylase (GAD) show that five strata of GAD-positive processes were found in the inner plexiform layer, together with amacrine cell bodies in the innermost cell row of the inner nuclear layer.[5] In electron microscopic (EM) autoradiography, most GAD-positive processes were found to be presynaptic to amacrine and bipolar cells, and synapses to ganglion cells were seen far less often.[5]

Like the GABA-accumulating amacrine cells, the glycine-accumulating amacrine cells in the rabbit retina probably belong to several different types of amacrine cells and at least one type of bipolar cell (Fig. 5-1d).[9,26] One type of the glycine-accumulating amacrine cell may be similar to the narrow-field, bistratified (type II) amacrine cell of the cat retina.[25]

In both cat and rat retinas, GABA- and glycine-accumulating neurons are known to contact bipolar cells and ganglion cells in addition to amacrine cells.[41,49] The multiplicity of GABA- and glycine-accumulating amacrine cells is also reported in the cat retina.[41] Although neuronal populations that utilize specific amino acid transmitter substances appear capable of high-affinity uptake of those substances, it cannot be concluded that all the cells that accumulate amino acids also utilize them as neurotransmitters. Thus all the subpopulations of amacrine cells in the rabbit retina that accumulate ^{3}H-GABA and ^{3}H-glycine do not necessarily utilize these substances as transmitters. However, it is reasonable to expect that those amacrine cells that are GABAergic and glycinergic will be included among the cell types identified in our morphological studies.

The dopamine-accumulating cells in the rabbit retina belong to at least one type of amacrine cell that ramifies mainly in layer 1 of the inner plexiform layer with occasional punctate terminals deeper in the inner plexiform layer (Fig. 5-1).[27,30] Ultrastructural studies of the dopamine-accumulating neurons in this retina show that they form interamacrine connections only.[21]

THE UPTAKE OF GABA, GLYCINE, AND DOPAMINE DURING RETINAL DEVELOPMENT

Specific accumulation of exogenously applied neurotransmitters by presumed retinal neurons in rabbit retinas is first observed autoradiographically around embryonic day 22 (E22) for GABA, E25 for glycine, and E27 for dopamine.[18] This evidence suggests that the commitment for certain neurons in the rabbit retina to become GABAergic, glycinergic, or dopaminergic is made prenatally. Their uptake mechanisms emerge at different times during retinal development. The densities, position, morphology, and ramification of the GABA-, glycine-, and dopamine-accumulating cells in the newborn retina are similar to those found in the adult retina.[26,29,30] Biochemical studies of the postnatal development of the high-affinity uptake mechanism of GABA in the rabbit retina show that the activity of this system 2 days after birth is approximately 70% of the adult value, slowly increasing to adult levels by postnatal days 6 to 8.[34] These biochemical findings correlate well with the anatomical studies by Lam and coworkers.[29]

THE RELEASE OF GABA, GLYCINE, AND DOPAMINE DURING RETINAL DEVELOPMENT

Despite the fact that the uptake mechanisms of GABA, glycine, and dopamine are functional in

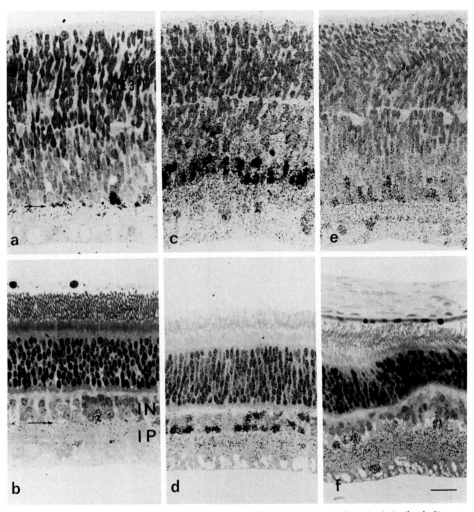

Figure 5-1. Light-microscopic autoradiographs of newborn *(a, c, e)* and adult *(b, d, f)* retinas following injections of ³H-dopamine *(a, b)*, ³H-glycine *(c, d)*, and ³H-GABA *(e, f)*, respectively into rabbit eyes *in vivo*. IN, inner nuclear layer; IP, inner plexiform layer; horizontal arrows *(a, b)*, layer 1 of the inner plexiform layer; horizontal arrows *(d)*, presumed glycine-accumulating amacrine cells; oblique arrows *(d)*, presumed bipolar cells; Arrows *(e, f)*, GABA-accumulating somata in the ganglion-cell layer; scale bar, 20 μm. (Fung SC, Kong YC, Lam DMK: Prenatal development of GABAergic glycinergic and dopaminergic neurons in the rabbit retina. J Neurosci 2:1623, 1982)

newborn rabbit retinas, there is a marked difference in the ability to release the accumulated neurotransmitters by these neurons upon K⁺-induced depolarization (Fig. 5-2). At birth, there is a small K⁺-induced Ca²⁺-dependent release of ³H-GABA. The release of ³H-glycine is negligible. However, the dopamine-accumulating neurons in the newborn retina are capable of releasing the accumulating dopamine at a rate of about 50% of the adult level. The rates of release reach 85% of the adult level on day eight after birth for ³H-GABA and ³H-dopamine, and on day twelve for ³H-glycine. For the GABAergic and glycinergic systems, the emergence of K⁺-induced, Ca²⁺-dependent release mechanisms occurs many days after the first appearance of the uptake properties. In contrast, however, the mechanisms for dopamine uptake and release emerge at approximately the same time.

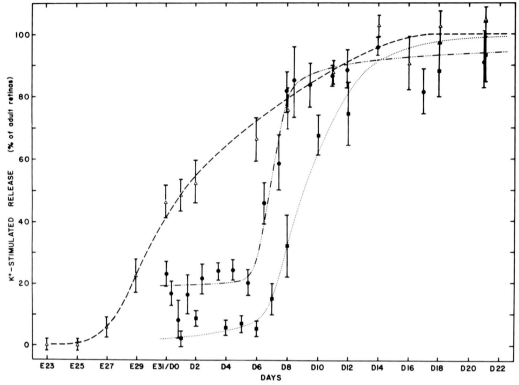

Figure 5-2. The developmental patterns of release of ^{3}H-GABA (– $\cdots$ – $\cdots$ –), ^{3}H-glycine ($\cdots\cdots\cdots$), and ^{3}H-dopamine (– – – – – –) in the rabbit retina. The releases were measured as Ca^{2+}-dependent effluxes of preloaded ^{3}H-transmitters into the medium in response to 56 mM extracellular K$^+$. (Data from Kong et al and Lam et al[26,29,30])

THE CONTENT AND BIOSYNTHESIS OF GABA AND DOPAMINE DURING RETINAL DEVELOPMENT

The endogenous contents of GABA in the rabbit retina are low at birth but increase steadily during the first 10 days after birth, reaching 80% of the adult level on day 8 or 9 (Fig. 5-3).[29] The endogenous levels of dopamine remain low for the first 6 days after birth, increasing to 35% of the adult level by about day 13 (Fig. 5-4); on day 18, there is another abrupt increase in dopamine contents, reaching 50% of the adult level on day 21, 80% on day 23, and 100% by day 25.[30]

The increase in endogenous GABA contents closely parallels the specific activity of GAD (see Fig. 5-3). Likewise, the increase in retinal dopamine levels follows the increase in the specific activity of its synthetic enzyme tyrosine hydrox-

ylase (TH). These findings suggest that during retinal development the endogenous contents of GABA and dopamine are regulated closely by the activity of their synthetic enzymes.

It is noteworthy that a similar pattern of TH activity is also observed in the rat retina using immunocytochemistry.[40] The first TH-like immunoreactive cells are observed by the third day of life. The differentiation of the neurons and the development of their processes continue until and after the opening of the eyes (day 14 or 15). The catecholaminergic system is fully developed by 3 weeks of age. The delayed development of the synthetic system is also reflected by the late augmentation of light-stimulated dopamine synthesis during development in the rat retina.[38] In the developing rabbit retina, we have recently shown that TH-immunoreactive amacrine cells and processes are first observed around day 8.

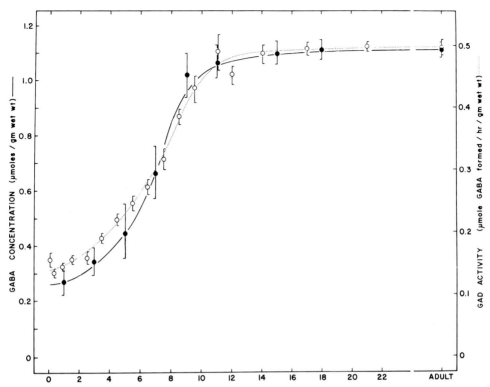

Figure 5-3. The developmental patterns of endogenous GABA concentrations (————) and specific activities of L-glutamic acid decarboxylase (··········) in the rabbit retina. (Data from Lam et al[29])

THE TEMPORAL SEQUENCE OF MATURATION OF THE RETINAL NEURONS

The findings by Lam and associates show that the commitment for certain neurons to become GABAergic, glycinergic, and dopaminergic is made prenatally; the maturation of these neurons, however, occurs postnatally.[18] The putative GABAergic neurons accumulate, synthesize, store, and release GABA at over 80% of the adult levels from about 9 days after birth. By these neurochemical criteria they may therefore be regarded as mature. Electrophysiological evidence shows that the GABAergic neurons may be functional at this stage of development.[35] The number of ganglion cells responsive to light increases from 0% on postnatal day 7 to over 80% by day 10. Visual responsiveness, concentric field organizations, and directional selectivities of ganglion cells first appear on day 10 and are

mature by about 20 days after birth in the rabbit retina. Since GABAergic amacrine cells in the rabbit retina are probably involved in the organization of direction-sensitive receptive fields of ganglion cells, these ganglion cells may possess the postsynaptic GABAergic receptors and receive functional GABAergic input at this time.[10] This notion is supported by the findings from the postnatal development of the postsynaptic GABAergic receptors in the rabbit retina.[34] The binding of GABAergic receptors is very low at birth and increases dramatically between postnatal days 7 and 12. This pattern of development is parallel to the development of electrical activity of ganglion cells and also the synaptogenesis of amacrine contacts in rabbit retina.[35,36] The synaptic density was about 20% of the adult level for the first 9 days after birth, then increased steadily to 75% by day 12 and reached the adult level by day 20.

It is interesting to note that binding of the

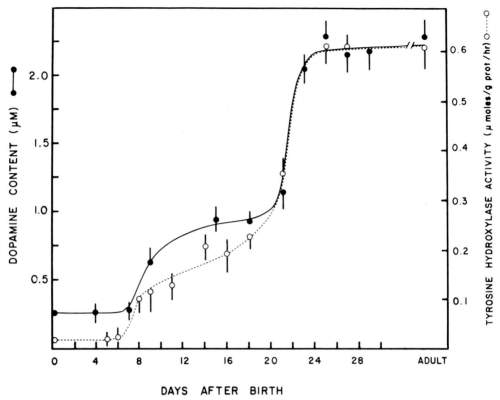

Figure 5-4. The developmental patterns of endogenous dopamine concentrations
(————) and specific activities of tyrosine hydroxylase (··········) in the rabbit retina.
(Data from Lam et al[30])

GABAergic receptor is increased by intravitreal administration of the uptake blocker nipecotic acid. This finding indicates that GABA *per se* may have a trophic effect on the development of the postsynaptic GABAergic receptor in the rabbit retina.[34] In this context, the development of GABAergic receptors follows the development of the GABA release system by 2 or 3 days.[43] The onset of presynaptic receptor activity is delayed approximately 1 to 2 days relative to the presynaptic components. These results are compatible with the possible role of presynaptic neurons in regulating the maturation of postsynaptic elements.

Although morphological and biochemical results indicate that the putative glycinergic neurons are also determined prenatally, the release mechanism for glycine does not emerge until the second week of postnatal development and is not mature until about 12 days after birth. If light-stimulated release of glycine follows a similar developmental pattern of K[+]-induced release, the results indicate that the glycinergic neurons are probably functional by about day 12 after birth, a period comparable to that required for maturation of GABAergic neurons.

Dopaminergic neurons also possess a specific uptake mechanism for dopamine before birth. However, unlike the GABA- and glycine-accumulating neurons in the newborn retina, dopamine-accumulating neurons in the newborn retina are capable of releasing a significant amount of the accumulated dopamine in response to K[+]-induced depolarization in a Ca^{2+}-dependent manner. Autoradiographic studies show that during the first few days of postnatal development, these dopamine-accumulating cells already show long and extensive arborization in the inner plexiform layer.[30] They are functionally immature at this time because they contain little endogenous dopamine and show low TH activity. The level of endogenous dopamine and TH activity increase in parallel; the reason for the biphasic pattern of development is still unknown. It is tempting to speculate that the second phase of dramatic increase in the retinal TH activities, which begins around day 18, may be related to induction by other neurons (as in the swine superior cervical ganglion and the rat adrenal chromaffin cell[46,48]) GABA and enkephalin modulate dopamine synthesis and release, respectively.[14,37] Also there may be two subpopulations of dopaminergic amacrine cells that develop at different times. The heterogeneity of dopaminergic cells in the developing rat retina has been observed using TH immunocytochemistry.[40] At present it is unclear why the endogenous dopamine content in dopaminergic amacrine cells reaches the adult level after the functional maturation of GABAergic and glycinergic amacrine cells as well as most of the ganglion cells. An understanding of the mechanism of the development of dopaminergic neurons must await the elucidation of their role in visual information processing in the retina and its wiring with other neurons.

Similar studies on the emergence and maturation of the GABAergic, glycinergic, and dopaminergic neurons have been reported in the developing retina of *Xenopus laevis*.[20,42,45] The high-affinity uptake mechanism of GABA first appears before synthesis. Synthesis is followed by the development of K^+-induced, Ca^{2+}-dependent transmitter release mechanism. Similarly, uptake of glycine appears several stages before its release. For dopamine the sequence is biosynthesis, development of the high-affinity uptake mechanism, and finally the release mechanism. The temporal sequence of emergence and maturation of these neurochemical properties in *Xenopus* is quite similar to that in the rabbit retina.

The early development of the high-affinity uptake mechanism may be of teleological significance. The neuronal system might thus ensure a fully functional reuptake mechanism for inactivation of the released neurotransmitter from the synaptic clefts; as a result, a balanced circuitry can be maintained for repeated stimulation. Our autoradiographic studies indicate that the high-affinity uptake systems for GABA, gly-

cine, and dopamine in specific neuronal types appear before synaptic specialization. This characteristic not only provides a means for the identification of specific neuronal types much earlier than was previously possible but also allows us to distinguish, on the basis of the selective uptake of different neurotransmitters, between different neurons that may share similar synaptic characteristics.

The finding that the release mechanisms of the neurons mature last in both rabbit and *Xenopus* retinas raises the possibility of using this physiological parameter as an indicator for the maturation of a particular neuron.

CONCLUSION

The present findings suggest that the commitment of certain neurons to become GABAergic, glycinergic, and dopaminergic amacrine cells is made prenatally and development occurs after birth. The emergence and maturation of neurotransmitter-specific properties are characteristic features of their differentiation. One of the puzzling questions on the process of differentiation to be answered is the identity of the triggering factors and the mechanism of timing. In this regard, it has been shown that in the histofluorescent studies of the rat retina, the initiation of retinal dopamine synthesis is independent of environmental lighting condition, but an adequate light stimulus is required for continued normal development of the dopaminergic neurons.[24] This result indicates that an as yet unidentified intrinsic factor may be essential in programming the emergence of the process.

In our studies, the rapid increase in the depolarization-induced release of GABA and glycine and also the synthesis of GABA appears to coincide with the time of eye opening of developing rabbits. These findings shed some light on the possible role of light stimulation on the maturation of these neurons. The increase in the density of conventional synapses in the inner plexiform layer of the rabbit retina also follows a similar pattern.[36] These biochemical and anatomical observations are in line with the developmental pattern of light responsiveness in the rabbit retina.[35]

Recent biochemical and anatomical studies show that apart from acetylcholine, GABA, glycine, dopamine, and perhaps an indoleamine, a large variety of neuropeptide-like substances (namely substance P, enkephalin, endorphin, somatostatin, neurotensin, thyrotropin-releasing hormone, vasoactive intestinal peptide, glucagon, and cholecystokinin) are also localized to distinct populations of amacrine cells.[7,12,50] The physiological significance for various subpopulations of a class of retinal neurons to use different transmitters is unknown. However, since the synaptic density in certain regions of the retina, especially the plexiform layers, is higher, the existence of many different transmitter-specific pathways would ensure that interactions occur only among appropriately connected neurons and decrease the probability of nonspecific stimulation by other neurotransmitters in the area due to diffusion and incomplete inactivation. Another speculation is that the diversity of transmitters within a class of retinal neurons may be of importance for guiding or specifying the precise connections between two classes of neurons during retinal development. The trophic action of GABAergic neurons on the postsynaptic elements has been suggested by Madtes and Redburn.[34] The elucidation of their possible roles as neurotransmitters or neuromodulators will provide more insights on the underlying mechanism of retinal physiology and also the factors controlling the process of morphological and biochemical differentiation from the pluripotent germinal cells both in normal and aberrant conditions.

REFERENCES

1. Ames A III, Nesbett FB: In vitro retina as an experimental model of the central nervous system. J Neurochem 37:867, 1981
2. Ames A III, Pollen DA: Neurotransmission in central nervous tissue: A study of isolated rabbit retina. J Neurophysiol 32:424, 1969
3. Bauer B: Photic release of radioactivity from rabbit retina preloaded with (^{3}H)GABA. Acta Ophthalmol(Kbh) 56:270, 1978
4. Bonting SL: Structure and mechanism of the vertebrate visual system. In Bonting SL (ed): Transmitters in the Visual Process, p 1. New York, Pergamon Press, 1976
5. Brandon C, Lam DMK, Su YYT, et al: Immunocytochemical localization of GABA neurons in the rabbit and frog retina. Brain Res Bull 5:21, 1980
6. Brandon C, Lam DMK, Wu JY: The γ-aminobutyric acid system in rabbit retina: Localization by immunocytochemistry and autoradiography. Proc Natl Acad Sci USA 76:3557, 1979
7. Brecha N: Retinal neurotransmitters: Histochemical and biochemical studies. In Emson PC (ed): Chemical Neuroanatomy, p 85. New York, Raven Press, 1983
8. Brunn A, Ehinger B: Uptake of the putative neurotransmitter glycine, into the rabbit retina. Invest Ophthalmol 11:191, 1972
9. Brunn A, Ehinger B: Uptake of certain possible neurotransmitters into retinal neurons of some mammals. Exp Eye Res 19:435, 1974
10. Caldwell JH, Daw NW: Effects of picrotoxin and strychnine on rabbit retinal ganglion cells: Changes in center surround receptive field. J Physiol 276:299, 1978
11. Caldwell JH, Daw NW, Wyatt HJ: Effects of picrotoxin and strychnine on rabbit ganglion cells: Lateral interactions for cells with more complex receptive fields. J Physiol 276:277, 1978
12. Djamgoz MBA, Stell WK, Chin CA et al: An opiate system in the goldfish retina. Nature 292:620, 1981
13. Dowling JE, Ehinger B: Synaptic organization of the dopaminergic neurons in the rabbit retina. J Comp Neurol 180:203, 1978
14. Dubocovich ML, Weiner N: Enkephalins modulate (^{3}H) dopamine release from rabbit retina in vitro. J Pharmacol Exp Ther 224:634, 1983
15. Ehinger B: Autoradiographic identification of rabbit retinal neurons that take up GABA. Experientia 26:1063, 1970
16. Ehinger B, Floren I: Quantitation of the uptake of indoleamines and dopamine in the rabbit retina. Exp Eye Res 26:1, 1978
17. Freed MA, Nakamura Y, Sterling P: Four types of amacrine in the cat retina that accumulate GABA. J Comp Neurol 219:295, 1983
18. Fung SC, Kong YC, Lam DMK: Prenatal development of GABAergic, glycinergic and dopaminergic neurons in the rabbit retina. J Neurosci 2:1623, 1982
19. Gottlieb DK, Glaser I: Cellular recognition during neuronal development. Ann Rev Neurosci 3:303, 1980
20. Hollyfield JG, Sarthy PV, Rayborn ME, et al: The emergence, localization and maturation of neurotransmitter system during development of the retina in *Xenopus laevis*. I. γ-Aminobutyric acid. J Comp Neurol 188:587, 1979
21. Holmgren–Taylor I: Ultrastructure and synapses of the (^{3}H)dopamine-accumulating neurons in the retina of the rabbit. Exp Eye Res 35:555, 1983
22. Jacobson M: Developmental Neurobiology, 2nd ed. New York, Plenum Press, 1978

23. Kaneko A: Physiology of the retina. Ann Rev Neurosci 2:169, 1979

24. Kato S, Nakamura T, Negishi K: Postnatal development of dopaminergic cells in the rat retina. J Comp Neurol 191:227, 1980

25. Kolb H: The inner plexiform layer in the retina of the cat: Electron microscopic observations. J Neurocytol 8:295, 1979

26. Kong YC, Fung SC, Lam DMK: Postnatal development of glycinergic neurons in the rabbit retina. J Comp Neurol 193:1127, 1980

27. Kramer SG: Dopamine: A retinal neurotransmission. In Bonting SL (ed): Transmitters in the Visual Process, p 165. Oxford, Pergamon Press, 1976

28. Lam DMK, Frederick JM, Hollyfield JG: Identification of putative neurotransmitters in the human retina. In Hollyfield JG (ed): The structure of the Eye, p 205. New York, Elsevier North-Holland, 1982

29. Lam DMK, Fung SC, Kong YC: Postnatal development of GABAergic neurons in the rabbit retina. J Comp Neurol 193:89, 1980

30. Lam DMK, Fung SC, Kong YC: Postnatal development of dopaminergic neurons in the rabbit retina. J Neurosci 1:1117, 1981

31. Lam DMK, Steinman L: The uptake of γ-aminobutyric acid in the goldfish retina. Proc Natl Acad Sci USA 68:2777, 1971

32. Lam DMK, Su YYT, Swain L et al: Immunocytochemical localization of L-glutamic acid decarboxylase in the goldfish retina. Nature 278:565, 1979

33. Lund RD: Development and plasticity of the brain. New York, Oxford University Press, 1978

34. Madtes PC Jr, Redburn DA: Synaptic interactions in the GABA system during postnatal development in retina. Brain Res Bull 10:741, 1983

35. Masland RH: Maturation of function in the developing rabbit retina. J Comp Neurol 175:275, 1977

36. McArdle CB, Dowling JE, Masland H: Development of outer segments and synapses in the rabbit retina. J Comp Neurol 175:253, 1977

37. Morgan WW, Kamp CW: A GABAergic influence on the light-induced increase in dopamine turnover in the dark-adapted rat retina in vivo. J Neurochem 34:1082, 1980

38. Morgan WW, Kamp CW: Postnatal development of light response of dopaminergic neurons in the rat retina. J Neurochem 39:283, 1982

39. Negishi K, Drujan BD: Reciprocal changes in center and surround S-potentials of the fish retina in response to dopamine. Neurochem Res 4:313, 1979

40. Nguyer-Legros J, Vigny A, Gay M: Postnatal development of TH-like immunoreactivity in the rat retina. Exp Eye Res 37:23, 1983

41. Pourcho RG: Uptake of (^{3}H)glycine and (^{3}H)GABA by amacrine cells in the cat retina. Brain Res 198:333, 1980

42. Rayborn ME, Sarthy PV, Lam DMK et al: The emergence, localization and maturation of neurotransmitter systems during development of the retina in *Xenopus laevis*. II Glycine. J Comp Neurol 195:585, 1981

43. Redburn DA, Mitchell CK: ^{3}H-musicmol binding in synaptosomal fractions from bovine and developing rabbit retina. J Neurosci Res 6:387, 1981

44. Rodieck RW: Visual pathways. Ann Rev Neurosci 2:193, 1979

45. Sarthy PV, Rayborn ME, Hollyfield JG, et al: The emergence, localization and maturation of neurotransmitter system during development of the retina in *Xenopus laevis*. III. Dopamine. J Comp Neurol 195:595, 1981

46. Stanton HC, Phinney G, Mueller RL: Ontogenesis of choline acetyltransferease, tyrosine hydroxylase, monoamine oxidase and catechol-O-methyltransferase in the superior cervical ganglion of swine. Biochem Pharmacol 23:3423, 1974

47. Strachill M: Actions of drugs on single neurons in cat retina. Vision Res 8:35, 1968

48. Thoenen H: Induction of tyrosine hydroxylase in peripheral and central adrenergic neurons by cold exposure of rats. Nature 228:861, 1970

49. Vaugh JE, Famiglietti EV Jr, Barber R, et al: GABAergic amacrine cells in rat retina: Immunocytochemical identification and synaptic connectivity. J Comp Neurol 197:113, 1981

50. Watt CB, Su YYT, Lam DMK: Enkephalins in the vertebrate retina. Prog Ret Res 4:221–242, 1985

51. Yu BCY, Watt CB, Lam DMK, Fry KR: GABAergic ganglion cells in the rabbit retina. ARVO Abstracts 349, 1987

6

Electrical Interactions Between the Neuronal Cells of the Retina: Encoding of Visual Images in the Vertebrate Retina

Samuel M. Wu

The vertebrate retina is a thin layer of nervous tissue, embryologically derived from the brain (neuroectoderm), lining the back of the eye where the image is formed (Fig. 6-1). Its primary function is to absorb light and to encode visual images as patterns of nerve impulses that can be conveyed to and understood by the brain.

Visual objects of various brightness, colors, shapes, and motions are projected onto the retina by the lenses. Each human retina contains about 100 million receiving elements (photoreceptors) — rods and cones, each of which detects a tiny part of the image that is projected on it and produces a small electrical signal.[13] These discrete electrical signals are the first representation of the visual world in a neuronal language encoded by the retina. Photoreceptor signals are further processed when they are transmitted through the retinal network consisting of hundreds of millions of higher-order neurons and billions of synapses. The cell bodies are restricted to two nuclear layers, and the synapses are confined to two plexiform

layers. Retinal signals in their final form are gathered in ganglion cells and conveyed to the brain via the axons of these cells.

The concept of vision can probably be divided into two parts: encoding and decoding. Encoding processes start in the retina and continue in the lateral geniculate nucleus and the visual cortex.[8,9] Visual images are encoded in electrical signals that in no way resemble the images they represent. Retinal signals representing the image of a red rose, for example, have neither the color nor the shape of the flower. Yet when the brain receives these signals, it decodes them and interprets them as a red rose. At present, we have no idea how the decoding processes occur, nor even where exactly in the brain they take place. It is quite likely that we do not understand the brain well enough to even formulate the right question about the decoding of visual signals.

The aims of this chapter are to examine the encoding processes of visual images in the vertebrate retina and to address the question of how and in what form the electrical signals are used to represent elements of visual images.

Electrical signals in the nervous system are mediated by ionic currents as they flow through individual channel proteins in the membrane of

This work was supported by grants from the U.S. National Eye Institute (EY04446), Research to Prevent Blindness, Inc., N.Y., and the Retina Research Foundation (Houston).

112

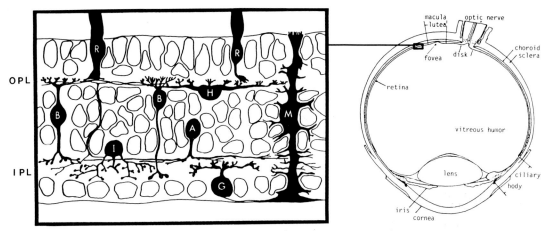

Figure 6-1. Structure of the vertebrate retina *(left)* and its relative location in the eye *(right)*. The retina consists of six types of neurons—photoreceptors (R), horizontal cells (H), bipolar cells (B), amacrine cells (A), interplexiform cells (I), and ganglion cells (G)—and a primary type of glial cells—the Müller fibers (M). Processes of retinal cells are confined in the outer and inner plexiform layers (OPL, IPL). (Modified from Wu SM: Physiological and pharmacological properties of the cyprinid fish retina, Doctoral dissertation, Harvard University, 1979)

individual neurons. These current flows result in voltage change across the cell membrane. The opening and closing of individual ionic channels determine the magnitude and kinetics of membrane currents and the shape of the electrical signals in individual cells.

Ionic channels in the cell membrane can be controlled (or gated) either by the transmembrane voltage or by ligands. Ligand molecules gate these channels either from the intracellular or the extracellular side of the membrane. In the vertebrate photoreceptors, when a photon is absorbed the level of intracellular ligand molecules in the cytoplasm is altered and it causes a net outward flow of current across the membrane.[7] Photoreceptors are therefore hyperpolarized (inside more negative) by illumination (Fig. 6-2).

The light-evoked photoreceptor signals are transmitted to other retinal neurons in two ways: they spread laterally to other photoreceptors via electrical synapses and travel proximately to second-order cells via chemical synapses. Electrical synapses are specialized regions of the cell membrane where channel molecules reside and through which ionic currents can flow directly from one cell to another. Chemical synapses involve relays of voltage signals from one cell to another via chemical transmitters. Transmitter molecules are released when a depolarizing signal reaches the presynaptic cell; these molecules act as extracellular ligands for membrane channels and generate voltage signals in the postsynaptic cell.

Higher-order retinal neurons (horizontal cells, bipolar cells, amacrine cells, and ganglion cells) also transmit and process their signals via electrical and chemical synaptic synapses.[6] A summary diagram of major synaptic connections and electrical responses of individual cells in the retina is shown in Figure 6-3.

ENCODING OF ELEMENTS OF VISUAL IMAGES IN THE RETINA

Visual scenes consist of objects in the visual field that emit or reflect light. These objects of different shapes, located at different positions in the visual field, send out light of different intensities and wave lengths. Some of them are stationary, and others are moving. A few basic elements of visual images can be defined: brightness (intensity), color, shape, and motion. The former two describe the properties of light (i.e., the number and wave length of photons), the latter two de-

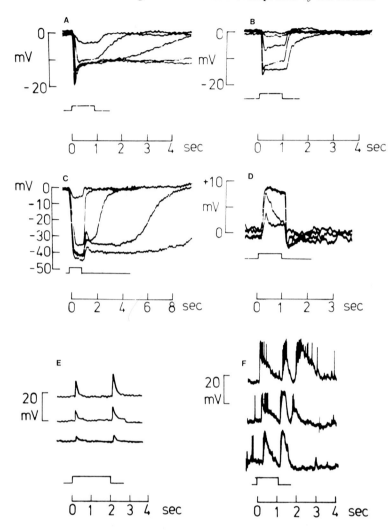

Figure 6-2. Voltage responses recorded intracellularly from a rod *(A)*, a cone *(B)*, a horizontal cell *(C)*, a depolarizing bipolar cell *(D)*, an amacrine cell *(E)*, and a ganglion cell *(F)* to various intensities of light flashes. In *A, B,* and *C,* the lowest traces are responses to flashes of highest intensity; in *D, E,* and *F* the uppermost traces are responses to flashes of highest intensity. Light intensities are at increments of log units. Only ganglion cells exhibit action potentials; other cells exhibit graded potentials.

scribe the geometry of light patterns. *Shape,* in this contex, includes spatial patterns that are stationary in the visual field, and *motion* information includes the changes of spatial patterns with respect to time. These parameters obviously do not cover every aspect of vision. For example, depth vision, which is probably mediated by the higher centers in the brain, will not be discussed in this chapter.[2]

Brightness

In the vertebrate retina, most neurons, except the ganglion cells, exhibit graded voltage responses to light stimuli. The amplitude of these signals is proportional to the intensity of light

flashes. The ganglion cells, on the other hand, generate action potentials in response to light. The amplitude of the action potentials remains the same, but the frequency of the action potentials is proportional to flash intensity. The intracellular voltage responses to various intensities of light stimuli are shown in Figure 6-2. Within a certain intensity range, the voltage changes are proportional to the light intensity. The voltage responses of these cells are plotted against stimulus intensity in Figure 6-4. It is a convention of retinal physiology to plot the fractional voltage change (V/Vmax) against the logarithm (base 10) of the light intensity; such plots are called V–log I curves. The V–log I plots of all retinal neurons can be approximated by sigmoid-

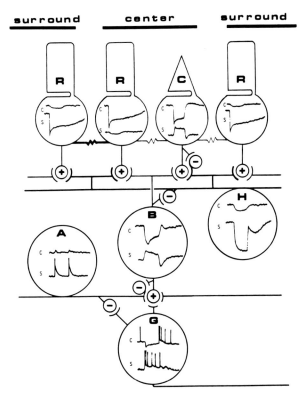

Figure 6-3. Summary of major synaptic connections and light responses in the vertebrate retina. R, rod; C, cone; B, bipolar cell; H, horizontal cell; A, amacrine cell; and G, ganglion cell. ⌁, electrical synapse; ⊕ sign-preserving chemical synapse; ⊖ sign-inverting chemical synapse. The upper trace in each cell is the actual voltage response recorded intracellularly from the cell to a spot of light falling on the central region of this piece of retina *(center bar)*, and the lower trace is the voltage response to light stimuli falling on the peripheral region *(surround bars)*. Note that the cone, the bipolar cell, and the ganglion cell exhibit center-surround antagonistic light responses.

shaped curves that can be described by

$$V/V_m = 0.5[1 + \tanh 1.15N (\log I - \log \sigma)]$$

where V is the voltage response of the cell at the light intensity I; V_m is the maximum voltage response; σ is the intensity at which half maximum response is elicited; and N is a constant that determines the intensity span, or dynamic range, of the cell. The dynamic range of a cell is defined as the span of light intensities, in log units, that corresponds to the response range from $0.05V_{max}$ to $0.95V_{max}$. It is easy to show from the given equation that the dynamic range of a cell is equivalent to

$$\log I_{0.95} - \log I_{0.05} = 2.65/N.^{[14]}$$

The V–log I curves of the rod, the cone, and the bipolar cell shown in Figure 6-2A,B,D are plotted in Figure 6-4. The dynamic ranges for both photoreceptors are about 4.5 log units, although the rod is about 2 log units more sensitive than the cone, as reflected by their positions along the log I axis. The dynamic range for bipolar cells, when directly illuminated, are markedly narrower (about 2 log units). Similarly narrow dynamic ranges for amacrine cells and ganglion cells have been reported.[17]

The principle of brightness (or intensity) encoding appears quite simple: the intensity of flashes is proportional to the amplitude of voltage responses in individual cells. The only exception is ganglion cells, which encode the intensity of flashes into the frequency of action potentials. Based on everyday experience we know that the human retina is not a good brightness detector. For instance, if one uses a light meter to measure the amount of light reflected from a piece of newspaper under the sun and under room light, one will find that the light reflected from the black words under the sun is much more intense than that reflected from the white page of paper under room light. Yet, everyone who looks at this newspaper under the two conditions will see *black* words on *white* paper.

Another example is demonstrated in Figure 6-5. Two identical gray discs reflecting the same amount of light are surrounded by different

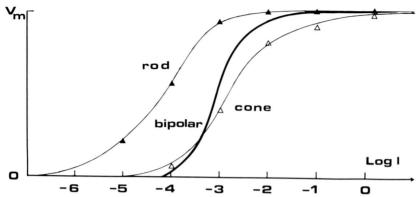

Figure 6-4. V-log I plots for the rod, the cone, and the bipolar cell shown in Figure 6-3; ▲, rod; △, cone; thick solid line, bipolar cell. Note that the dyamic range for the bipolar cell is much narrower than those for the rod and the cone. Logarithm is base 10; V_m is the normalized membrane voltage change in each cell.

backgrounds. The background on the left is black and the one on the right is white. The disc on the right appears to everyone's eyes darker than the left disc. This psychophysical phenomenon is called *simultaneous contrast*.[4] We shall describe one possible mechanism in the retina that may mediate this visual phenomenon. Bipolar cells receive synaptic input from the cone

photoreceptors; the V−log I curves for a cone and a bipolar are shown in Fig. 6-6. As mentioned earlier, the dynamic range of the bipolar cell is much narrower along the log I axis than that of the cone. Therefore the voltage range of synaptic transmission in cones does not cover the full light response range. A window of voltage in the cone is probably used to mediate the

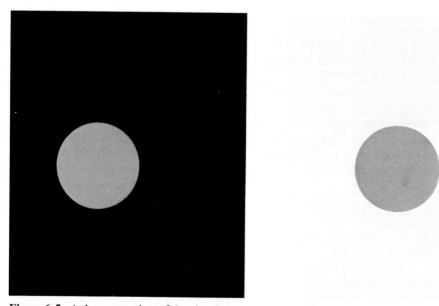

Figure 6-5. A demonstration of the simultaneous contrast phenomenon. The two circular discs were made with the same gray paper pasted on black *(left)* and white *(right)* background. The right disc appears darker although the amount of light reflected from the two disc regions to the reader's eyes is identical.

cone-to-bipolar synaptic transmission.[20] When an object is surrounded by a bright background, as is the gray disc on the right (Fig. 6-5), the cone photoreceptors "looking" at the disc are depolarized by the feedback synapse from horizontal cells to cones (see Fig. 6-3), because the horizontal cells have long lateral processes that can transmit signals from the bright surrounding region to the central (gray disc) region. This feedback depolarization reduces the amplitude of the hyperpolarizing light responses of the cone and results in a downward shift of the V – log I curve (*dashed curve,* Fig. 6-6, upper portion). The V – log I curve of the bipolar cell, under this condition, shifts to the right (dashed curve, Fig. 6-6, bottom) because cone inputs can be transmitted only within the "window" voltage range. Therefore, retinal bipolar cells "looking" at the two gray discs should exhibit different voltage responses, although the absolute intensities of light reflected from the two disc regions are identical. Bipolar cells responding to the left disc follow the solid V – log I curve, while those responding to the right disc follow the dashed V – log I curve (Fig. 6-6, lower portion). If the intensity of the two gray discs is about − 5 log units, the bipolars on the left will be polarized much more than those on the right. (Compare the heights of the intersecting point between the vertical line at − 5 log units and the solid curve, and that between the vertical line and the dashed curve.) The left bipolar cells would tell the brain that they see a brighter disc than the right bipolar cells.

Color

There is a common misconception about color vision that implies that the cones can discriminate color while the rods cannot. In fact, neither the cones nor the rods can discriminate color; they merely have different sensitivities to photons of different wave lengths. In a human retina there are three types of cones and one type of rod; each of these cell types contains a different photopigment. The peak sensitivities for cones are at 419 nm, 531 nm, and 559 nm in wave length; that for rods is at 496 nm.[2] In the salamander retina, the rod spectral absorbance curve peaks at 520 nm, and that of the cone peaks at 620 nm. Take the salamander cone as an example: it is about three times more sensitive to 650-nm (red) light than to 520-nm (green) light.[1] However, if one increases the intensity of green light so that it is three times more intense than the red light, the cone would

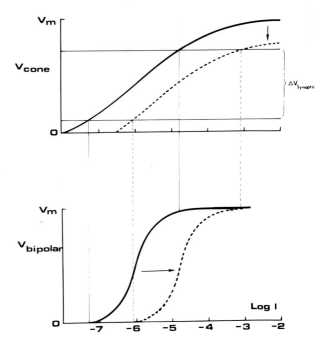

Figure 6-6. A possible explanation of the phenomenon shown in Figure 6-5. V-log I curves for a cone *(upper portion)* and a bipolar cell *(lower portion)* are plotted as solid lines when no background illumination is present. The two horizontal lines in the upper plot indicate the voltage window for cone-to-bipolar-cell synaptic transmission. Dashed curves are the V-log I plots for the cone and bipolar cell in the presence of background illumination. The amplitude of cone responses is reduced by sign-inverting feedback signals from the horizontal cells. The V-log I curve of bipolar cell is shifted to the right. The arrows indicate the transition from dark background to bright background illumination.

not be able to distinguish the green flashes from red. This principle was first recognized by Rushton, who called it *the principle of univariance:* the voltage response of a photoreceptor depends only on the number of photons absorbed, not on the wave length of photons absorbed.[12] This principle was demonstrated by Attwell, Wilson, and Wu in the tiger salamander retina (Fig. 6-7).[1] Isolated rods and cones from the salamander retina were impaled with microelectrodes, and the voltage responses to red and green flashes were measured. The light intensity was adjusted according to the absorption spectra, so that the probability of absorption of red photons and green photons by the pigments is approximately the same. Under such conditions, isolated rods or cones showed identical light responses to red and green flashes, both in amplitude and in time course. In other words, photoreceptors cannot discriminate the wave length of photons they absorb. Information carried by ensembles of photons of different wave lengths is determined by the probability of photon absorption (sensitivity) of the photopigments, whereas the information carried by the energy of a single absorbed photon (h/λ) is lost in photoreceptors.

Retinal neurons discriminate different colors by using opposite voltage polarities of their light responses (Fig. 6-8). This process starts at the second-order cell level.[15] A population of horizontal cells, for example, gives hyperpolarizing voltage responses to blue and green light flashes with hyperpolarization but depolarizes to red flashes. Another population of horizontal cells hyperpolarizes to blue and red flashes but depolarizes to green flashes. It is important to note that these cells can indeed discriminate color. No matter how one adjusts the relative intensities of the light stimuli, the voltage responses generated by red photons are always of opposite polarity to those generated by green photons.

Shape

The shape of an object is outlined by its contour, which consists of dots, lines, and curves. The simplest form of shape encoding is to register spots or dots of light. A series array of dots can form a line or a curve; lines and curves of various lengths, widths, and orientations can form contours of an object.

In the vertebrate retina, cones, bipolar cells, and ganglion cells exhibit center-surround receptive field organization: spots of light falling on the center of the receptive field of a cell elicit voltage response of opposite polarity to those falling on the periphery of its receptive field.[19] This receptive field organization is used by cells in the visual system to register light spots of limited size: light spots of the same size as the

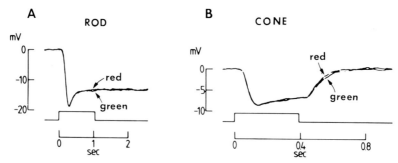

Figure 6-7. Voltage responses recorded from an isolated rod *(A)* and an isolated cone *(B)* from the tiger salamander retina to a red and a green flash. The intensities of light flashes were adjusted according to the spectral absorbances of the visual pigments in each cell so that the number of red photons absorbed was equal to the number of green photons absorbed. Note that for both the rod and the cone, the voltage responses to the adjusted red and green flashes are superimposeable, not only in peak amplitude but also in time course. (Modified from Attwell D, Wilson M, Wu SM: A quantitative analysis of interactions between photoreceptors in the salamander (Ambystoma) retina. J Physiol 352:703–737, 1984)

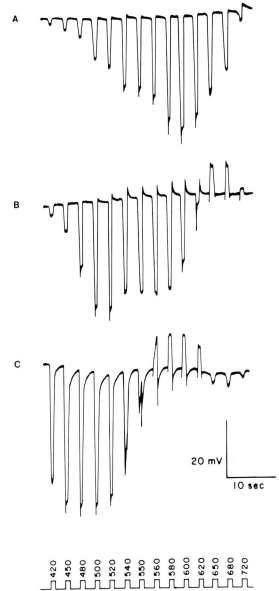

Figure 6-8. Voltage responses recorded intracellularly from a luminosity (L-type) horizontal *(A)*, a biphasic chromaticity (C-type) horizontal cell *(B)*, and a triphasic C-type horizontal cell *(C)* in carp retina. The bottom trace shows the wave lengths of light stimuli used to elicit the voltage responses of these cells. The L-type cell responded to flashes of all wave lengths with hyperpolarization and thus it is not a color-coded cell. The C-type cells *(B, C)* respond to flashes of different wave lengths with two voltage polarities, and they are regarded as color-coded cells. (Wu SM: Physiological and pharmacological properties of the cyprinid fish retina, Doctoral dissertation, Harvard University, 1979)

receptive field center produce optimal response, larger spots produce less response because of the antagonistic surround. The center responses are mediated by direct synaptic inputs of the light–photoreceptor–bipolar cells–ganglion cell pathway. In Figure 6-2, only the off-center (or hyperpolarizing) bipolar and ganglion cells are shown, and the synaptic connections are all sign-preserving (+). For on-center cells, on the other hand, sign-inverting synapses are involved between the photoreceptors and bipolar cells.[5] The antagonistic surround responses in cones and bipolar cells are probably mediated by horizontal cells. Light falling on the photoreceptors peripheral to the central cone excites the horizontal cells. Horizontal cells carry the signals laterally to the central cone via their long horizontal processes and a sign-inverting feedback synapse.[3] These signals result in an antagonistic, depolarizing response in the cone. The antagonistic surround responses in bipolar cells are mediated in a similar way, by the horizontal cells via either a direct sign-inverting synapse or the feedback sign-inverting synapse. Ganglion cells receive input from bipolar cells. Therefore their antagonistic surround responses are partially mediated by horizontal cells. In addition to bipolar cell input, ganglion cells also receive signals from amacrine cells via sign-inverting synapses.[11,18] These signals provide additional surround input to ganglion cells because amacrine cells have long lateral processes in the inner plexiform layer of the retina.

The antagonistic surround responses in retinal cells are primarily mediated by lateral sign-inverting synapses. This may be the general strategy used by the visual system to enhance spatial contrast and to encode spatial information such as spots, lines, and shapes.

Motion

The detection of motion in the visual system is very complicated. In principle, any time-dependent signal in the visual pathway can be part of a motion-detecting system. For example, a time-dependent membrane current that shapes the wave form of the light responses in rods can be responsible for registering movement of an edge in the retina.[1] Time delays of synaptic transmission can also be used to mediate time-dependent events or motion detection. In the vertebrate retina, a population of ganglion cells are directional sensitive (i.e., they respond differently to spots of light moving in opposite directions).[16] One of the possible mechanisms underlying these directional-sensitive cells is shown in Figure 6-9. If the ganglion cell receives synaptic input as illustrated in Figure 6-9, a spot of light moving in the null direction would activate an inhibitory synaptic input to the central bipolar cell before it moves to the center to excite that bipolar cell. If the time taken for the inhibitory signal to reach the central bipolar cell (due to synaptic delays) equals the time taken for the spot moving from the left bipolar to the central bipolar, then two signals cancel each other and cause no excitation in the ganglion cells (or cause an inhibitory hyperpolarization). On the other hand, when the same spot moves in the preferred direction, no inhibition on the central bipolar cell occurs, and the ganglion cell is depolarized and excited.

GENERAL STRATEGY OF IMAGE ENCODING

In the vertebrate retina, visual images are encoded and represented by individual cells as electrical signals, the messengers carrying information in the nervous system. All retinal neurons (except ganglion cells) use graded potentials to encode visual information. Elements of visual images are stored as amplitudes of voltage signals. Antagonistic voltage polarities are used to discriminate different colors, locations (center/surround), or directions of motion. An amplitude-modulated, antagonistic signaling system is used by the retina (except ganglion cells) to encode visual images. This system is translated into frequency-modulated signals by ganglion cells so that they can be transmitted to the brain in the form of action potentials.

If one compares the retina with a computer, these signaling systems resemble the software: different input generates different sets of signals in the same system. The "hardware" of the retina is then the cellular and synaptic organization. "Hard" synaptic pathways, such as the sign-inverting synapses between HC and cones, are formed during development to carry and process visual signals. These synaptic connections are relatively permanent, and they stay the same when visual scenes are switched.

There are hundreds of millions of neurons in a human retina. These cells are arranged in layers of two-dimensional arrays, and they are interconnected to one another by synapses. A

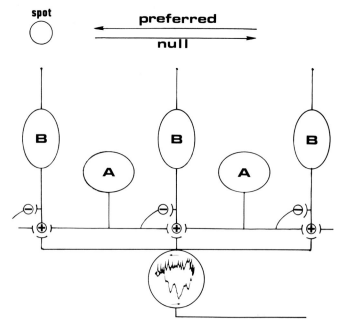

Figure 6-9. A possible synaptic mechanism mediating the direction-sensitive ganglion cell (lowest cell in the figure). A, amacrine cell; B, bipolar cell; ⊕ sign-preserving synapse; ⊖ sign-inverting synapse. The upper trace in the ganglion cell is the voltage response to the light spot moving in the preferred direction, and the lower trace is that to the spot moving in the null direction. (Ganglion cell responses adapted from Werblin[16])

point in the visual field is topologically mapped onto a point in the retina, and the interactions among different regions are mediated by lateral synapses. It is thus apparent that visual information is carried not only by electrical signals (software) but also by the cellular and synaptic organization (hardware). This dual representation of visual images does not occur only in the retina; it has been observed in the lateral geniculate nucleus and in the visual cortex.

REFERENCES

1. Attwell D, Wilson M, Wu SM: A quantitative analysis of interactions between photoreceptors in the salamander *(Ambystoma)* retina. J. Physiol 352:703–737, 1984
2. Barlow HB Mollon JD: The Senses. New York, Cambridge University Press, 1982
3. Baylor D, Fourtes MG, O'Bryan P: Receptive fields of single cones in the retina of the turtle. J Physiol 214:265–294, 1971
4. Cornsweet T: Visual Perception. New York, Academic Press, 1970
5. Dacheux RF, Miller RF: Photoreceptor-bipolar cell transmission in the perfused retina eyecup of the mudpuppy. Science 191:963–964, 1976
6. Dowling JE: Information processing by local circuits: The vertebrate retina as a model system. In Schmitt FO, Worden FG (eds): The Neuroscience Fourth Study Program, pp 161–181. Cambridge, MA, MIT Press, 1979
7. Hagins WAR, Penn RD, Yoshikami S: Dark current and photocurrent in retinal rods. Biophys J 10:380–412, 1970
8. Hubel DH, Wiesel TN: Integrative action in the cat's lateral geniculate body. J Physiol 155:385–398, 1961
9. Hubel DH, Wiesel TN: Receptive fields, binocular interaction and functional architecture in the cat's visual cortex. J Physiol 160:106–154, 1962
10. Kaneko A: Receptive field organization of bipolar and amacrine cells in the goldfish retina. J Physiol 235:133–153, 1973
11. Miller RF: The neuronal basis of ganglion cell receptive field organization and the physiology of amacrine cells. In Schmitt FO, Worden FG (eds): The Neuroscience Fourth Study Program, pp 227–245. Cambridge, MA, MIT Press, 1979
12. Naka KI, Rushton WAH: S-potentials from color units in the retina of fish *(Cyprinidae)*. J Physiol 185:536–555, 1966
13. Osterberg G: Topography of the layer of rods and cones in the human retina. Acta Ophthalmol (Suppl)6:8, 1935
14. Thibos LN, Werblin FS: The response properties of the steady antagonistic surround in the mudpuppy retina. J Physiol 278:79–99, 1978
15. Tomita T: Electrophysiological study of the mechanisms subserving color coding in the fish retina. Cold Spring Harbor Sympos Quantit Biol 30:559–566, 1965
16. Werblin FS: Response of retinal cells to moving spots: Intracellular recording in *Necturus maculosus*. J Neurophysiol 33:342–350, 1970
17. Werblin FS: Integrative pathways in local circuits between slow potential cells in the retina. In The Neuroscience Fourth Study Program, pp 193–211. Cambridge, MA, MIT Press, 1979
18. Werblin FS, Copenhagen D: Control of retinal sensitivity, III. Lateral interactions at the inner plexiform layer. J Gen Physiol 63:88–110, 1974
19. Werblin FS, Dowling JE: Organization of the retina of the mudpuppy, *Necturus maculosus*. II. Intracellular recording. J Neurophysiol 32:339–335, 1969
20. Werblin FS, Skrzypek J: Formation of receptive fields and synaptic inputs to horizontal cells. In Drujan JH, Laufer FJ (eds): New York, Alan R Liss Inc, 1982
21. Wu SM: Physiological and pharmacological properties of the cyprinid fish retina, Ph.D. dissertation, Harvard University, 1979

3

Retinal and Choroidal Circulatory Regulation and Vascular Diseases

7

Regulatory Mechanisms of the Choroidal Vasculature in Health and Disease

J. Terry Ernest

The control of the choroidal blood flow is different from that of the retina or the optic nerve. The retinal circulation is autoregulated (see Chap. 8), and there is considerable evidence that the optic nerve circulation is also.[20] The choroidal circulation is not autoregulated because of important anatomic differences.[3,16,41] The choroidal vasculature is innervated by the sympathetic nervous system; because these nerves stop at the lamina cribrosa, the optic disc and the retinal vasculature are not under sympathetic control.[30,45]

While not autoregulated the choroidal blood flow is a high-flow system that, to some extent, does not require adaptation to ocular pressure and oxygen changes. Indeed, the choroidal blood flow appears to be the highest in the body; as a result, the amount of oxygen extracted from the blood is far less than that for other tissues.[19] Retinal metabolism is high, but the choroidal blood flow is still greater than local tissue requirements. It may be that the high flow is a necessity either for delivering heat to the retina to maintain its temperature or for removing heat generated by incident light. One result of the high choroidal blood flow is that the inspiration of 100 percent oxygen will result in normal oxygenation of the inner retina following occlusion of the retinal arteries.[29] This may be important in patients with retinal artery occlusions, although there obviously are other metabolically important factors. At any rate, the fact that the choroidal circulation lacks autoregulation does not usually present a metabolic problem since the high-flow system with its low oxygen extraction can easily be decreased in pathologic conditions without compromising the retinal pigment epithelium (RPE) or outer retina. Indeed, the problems are at the other extreme with a high-flow, high-pressure system, which must be carefully regulated by the autonomic nervous system. When this regulation breaks down, as it appears to in hypertensive cardiovascular disease and in the late stages of diabetes mellitus, leakage from the vasculature and retinal edema may result.

The choroidal vasculature, which is heavily innervated, is regulated in the classical fashion by the autonomic nervous system.[9,37,42] The autonomic nervous system actually may protect the choroidal vasculature from systemic hypertension. We know that if the normal sympathetic tonus breaks down, there may be leakage of fluid into the retina.[21] We also know that acute hyperglycemia can overcome choroidal sympathetic tone.[26] A relationship may exist among hyperglycemia, systemic hypertension, and retinal leakage that could contribute to the macular edema associated with these retinopathies.

The entire ocular circulation responds, to one degree or another, to epinephrine, angiotensin, and the prostaglandins.[17,35] It has been hypothesized that circulating vasoconstrictors may play a role in the pathogenesis of ocular disease, but there is thus far little hard evidence of this.[5] Unfortunately, the choroidal blood flow varies with changes in the systemic blood pressure. In general, it appears that vasoconstrictive agents that raise the systemic blood pressure also increase peripheral resistance in the choroidal circulation; this effect, however, is overwhelmed by the increased blood pressure, so the result is simply a greater choroidal blood flow. The same appears to be true in the other direction, with a reduction in systemic blood pressure not being compensated by a decrease in choroidal vascular resistance, resulting in a decrease in choroidal blood flow. The situation is further complicated by the fact that the administration of the powerful vasodilator carbon dioxide has only minimal effect on the choroidal blood flow.[3,25,44] Moreover, local administration of vasodilators has little effect on the choroid.[34,38] It is evident, then, that the sympathetic nervous system exerts the primary control over the choroidal circulation.

REGULATION

In the strict sense, autoregulation is defined as the intrinsic tendency of an organ to maintain constant blood flow despite changes in perfusion pressure.[28] The choroidal circulation, then, is not ordinarily considered capable of autoregulation.[1–3,10,41] Several factors must be considered, however. First, the inverse relationship between choroidal blood flow and perfusion pressure is not perfectly linear. Our work using the microsphere impaction method and intraocular pressure elevation revealed a nonlinearity in the middle range of ocular hypertension.[42] These results are different from those of other investigators, but we also found, using our indocyanine dye clearance method, that elevated intraocular pressure changes choroidal vascular resistance. (Fig. 7-1).[39] We believe that this may be due to an increase in vortex vein resistance as the veins exit through the oblique scleral canal when the intraocular pressure is atmospheric.

Second, in theory the choroidal circulation does not need to be autoregulated because the blood flow is so high. While local changes in metabolic need may thus be ignored, it may be that the choroidal circulation is regulated by

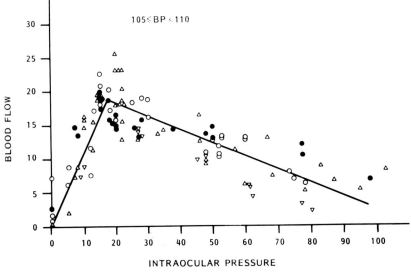

Figure 7-1. Choroidal blood flow (ml/min/ml choriocapillaris) measured by indocyanine green dye washout decreases with intraocular pressures below approximately 20 mm Hg.

light or heat.[8,32,33] We have not been able to confirm that either factor affects choroidal blood flow in cats, but the response may be species specific.[39] Nonetheless, an autoregulatory mechanism based on light or heat rather than perfusion pressure is reasonable and should be carefully considered. In fact, the initial damage to the choriocapillaris done by photocoagulation might be more serious than heretofore believed if the remaining retina loses its heat regulation.[14]

The third factor in the regulation of choroidal blood flow is a sympathetic tonus.[9,42] Stimulation of the cervical sympathetic chain decreases choroidal blood flow, and sympathectomy increases the circulation. The presence of this tonus is now thought to be more important than previously believed. In 1966 Potts speculated that if all neural control of the choroidal arterioles was abolished, the vessels would be exposed to a high pressure resulting in leakage.[36] This does occur in the cat uvea and the monkey choroid.[11,21] We have recently extended our studies on rhesus monkeys with Tso.[39] We injected horseradish peroxidase as a protein tracer following sympathectomy and induced systolic hypertension. There was diffuse leakage into the retina plus exaggerated multiple focal areas of retinal leakage in the macular area. We now believe that the autonomic nervous system normally protects the ocular circulation from systemic hypertension.

The choroidal circulation is regulated by the autonomic nervous system and perhaps intrinsically by heat and light. Just as we are concerned that diabetes may break down retinal circulation autoregulation (see Chap. 8), we are equally concerned that a combination of diabetes and hypertension may break down the regulatory mechanisms of the choroidal circulation. In both cases there may be vasodilation and leakage through the inner and outer blood–retinal barriers.

OCULAR VASCULAR DISEASES

Diabetes Mellitus

Ocular complications of diabetes have devastating effects for many citizens of the United States. Systemic hypertension is equally serious, affecting some 60 million in the U.S.[26] Moreover, in one study, 50% of over a thousand patients with juvenile-onset diabetes were hypertensive by age 30.[43] Clinicians have long appreciated the fact that diabetic retinopathy progresses more rapidly in patients who develop renal failure and hypertension. It may be that diabetic patients with high systemic blood pressures are more likely to have proliferative retinopathy than are those with normal blood pressures.[18] We examined 84 consecutive patients from our Early Treatment Diabetic Retinopathy Study center.[13] Juvenile- and maturity-onset diabetes patients were classified from their ocular fundus photographs as having no (n=26), mild (n=13), moderate (n=19), or severe (n=26) macular edema. The groups with no macular edema and severe macular edema had significantly different (p <0.03) systolic blood pressures. The patients with background diabetic retinopathy but no macular edema had systolic blood pressures of 139±4 mm Hg, while the patients with macular edema had systolic blood pressures of 152±4 mm Hg. We believe we may know some of the reasons for a possible correlation between the macular edema of diabetic retinopathy and systemic hypertension.

The normal sympathetic tonus of the choroidal circulation is eliminated by sympathectomy, but it can also be inhibited by the rapid infusion of intravenous mannitol or glucose.[23,26] The rapid intravenous infusion of glucose causes a decrease in choroidal vascular resistance and an increase in blood flow (Fig. 7-2). The mechanisms by which mannitol and glucose dilate the choroidal vasculature and increase blood flow is not known, but changes in osmolarity do decrease arterial resistance.[40] Osmotic stress is also known to break down the RPE barrier while the retinal vessels remain unaffected.[31] Dodge and colleagues have demonstrated that the RPE is disrupted and leaky in experimental diabetes.[15] Another factor may be that hyperglycemia stimulates cells to metabolize glucose by the polyol and sorbitol pathways, resulting in intracellular accumulation of sorbitol- and fructose-producing osmotic effects.[39] Should the ocular vascular endothelium or retinal pigment epithelium be similarly affected,

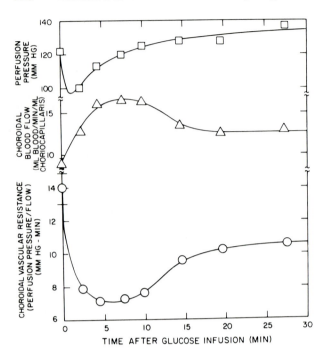

Figure 7-2. The rapid infusion of glucose (3 ml/kg) results in a decrease in choroidal vascular resistance and an increase in blood flow. Perfusion pressure is the difference between the systemic arterial blood pressure and the intraocular pressure.

there might be osmotic stress with ion shifts involving vascular smooth muscle cells and altering vasomotor tone and vascular regulation.[4]

We have hypothesized that episodes of hyperglycemia that occur in patients with diabetes may result in increased blood flow and pressure in the submacular choroidal circulation as well as changes in the RTE. These could result in leakage of fluid into the retina and contribute to macular edema. Leakage of fluid from the submacular choroidal circulation could be exacerbated by elevation of the systemic blood pressure. Moreover, diabetic patients may have autonomic-nervous-system defects that predispose them to labile blood pressure and perhaps even ocular sympathetic nerve dysfunction.[12] There is no evidence for the latter, but it seems a reasonable hypothesis for diabetic patients. We have recently recorded an increase in the ocular pulse pressure in diabetic patients with macular edema, suggesting a defect in the ocular sympathetic control of these patients.

Retrolental Fibroplasia (Retinopathy of Prematurity)

The choroidal circulation appears to have a role in retinopathy of prematurity. In general, the circulation and its relationship to such diseases as diabetes and hypertension are discussed in Chapter 8. For purposes of this discussion, however, it would appear that the choroidal circulation brings about sufficiently high retinal oxygen tensions during oxygen breathing to cause retinal vascular obliteration. This is evident in the kitten retina, where the vaso-obliterative effect of elevated oxygen on vasculature is prevented if the retina is detached and moved away from the choroid.[6] In the normal kitten exposed to oxygen, the choroidal circulation furnishes excessive oxygen, resulting in the obliteration of the retinal vasculature. Indeed, it has been postulated that retinal vasoconstriction may be a normal physiologic mechanism to protect the immature retina from the damaging effects of high blood oxygen levels. If retinal detachment is induced in a kitten breathing room air, however, the apparently hypoxic retina stimulates retinal vessels to proliferate throughout the retina and into the vitreous.[7] Under these conditions, the retinal neovascularization is similar to that seen in the retinopathy of prematurity that follows chronic oxygen exposure. Without an adequate choroidal circulation the neonatal retinal circulation will proliferate abnormally.

In the retinopathy of prematurity the choroidal circulation is initially deleterious because it furnishes excessive concentrations of oxygen to the inner retina, resulting in constriction and obliteration of the retinal vasculature. Later, on return to room air, the choroidal circulation is not adequate to provide the metabolic needs of the inner retina and thus the process (or processes) that induces neovascularization is stimulated.

REFERENCES

1. Alm A, Bill A: Blood flow and oxygen extraction in the cat uvea at normal and high intraocular pressure. Acta Physiol Scand 80:19, 1970
2. Alm A, Bill A: The oxygen supply to the retina. II. Effects of high intraocular pressure and of increased arterial carbon dioxide tension on uveal and retinal blood flow in cats. Acta Physiol Scand 84:306, 1972
3. Alm A, Bill A: Ocular and optic nerve blood flow at normal and increased intraocular pressures in monkeys (Macaca irus): A study with radioactively labelled microspheres including flow determinations in brain and some other tissues. Exp Eye Res 15:15, 1973
4. Altura BT, Altura BM: Factors affecting vascular responsiveness. In Kaley G, Altura B (eds): Microcirculation, vol II, p 547. Baltimore, University Park Press, 1978
5. Anderson DR: The mechanisms of damage of the optic nerve. In Leydhecker W (ed): Symposium, Glaucoma Committee, International Congress of Ophthalmology, p 89. Berlin, Springer-Verlag, 1983
6. Ashton N, Cook C: Direct observation of the effect of oxygen on developing vessels. Br J Ophthalmol 38:433, 1954
7. Ashton N, Cook C: Studies on developing retinal vessels. I. Influence of retinal detachment. Br J Ophthalmol 39:449, 1955
8. Auker CR, Parver LM, Doyle T, et al: Choroidal blood flow. I. Ocular tissue temperature as a measure of flow. Arch Ophthalmol 100:1323, 1982
9. Bill A: Autonomic nervous control of uveal blood flow. Acta Physiol Scand 56:70, 1962
10. Bill A: Intraocular pressure and blood flow through the uvea. Arch Ophthalmol 67:336, 1962
11. Bill A, Linder J: Sympathetic control of cerebral blood flow in acute arterial hypertension. Acta Physiol Scand 96:114, 1977
12. Christlieb AR: Diabetes and hypertensive vascular disease. Am J Cardiol 32:592, 1973
13. Deutsch TA, O'Riordan JF, Ernest JT, et al: Systemic blood pressure and diabetic macular edema (abstr). Invest Ophthalmol Vis Sci (Suppl) 24:80, 1983
14. Diddie KR, Ernest JT: The effect of photocoagulation on the choroidal vasculature and retinal oxygen tension. Am J Ophthalmol Vis Sci 84:62, 1977
15. Dodge JT, Blair NP, Tso MOM: Retinal pigment epitheliopathy in the spontaneously diabetic BB rat (abstr). Invest Ophthalmol Vis Sci (Suppl) 22:173, 1982
16. Dollery CT, Henkind P, Kohner EM, et al: Effect of raised intraocular pressure on the retinal and choroidal circulation. Invest Ophthalmol Vis Sci 7:191, 1968
17. Dollery CT, Hill DW, Hodge JV: The response of normal retinal blood vessels to angiotensin and noradrenaline. J Physiol 165:500, 1963
18. Drury PL, Bodansky HJ, Oddie CJ, et al: Increased plasma renin activity in type I diabetes with microvascular disease. Clin Endocrinol 16:453, 1982
19. Elgin SS: Arteriovenous oxygen difference across the uveal tract of the dog eye. Invest Ophthalmol Vis Sci 3:417, 1964
20. Ernest JT: Autoregulation of the optic disk oxygen tension. Invest Ophthalmol Vis Sci 13:101, 1974
21. Ernest JT: The effect of systolic hypertension on rhesus monkey eyes after ocular sympathectomy. Am J Ophthalmol 84:341, 1977
22. Ernest JT, Goldstick TK: The effect of perfusion pressure on uveal blood flow (abstr). Invest Ophthalmol Vis Sci (Suppl) 19:83, 1980
23. Ernest JT, Stern WH, Trimble JL: The effect of mannitol infusion on retinal function and oxygen tension. Invest Ophthalmol Vis Sci 16:670, 1977
24. Flower RW, Blake DA, Wajer SD, et al: Retrolental fibroplasia: Evidence for role of the prostaglandin cascade in the pathogenesis of oxygen-induced retinopathy in the newborn beagle. Pediatr Res 15:1293, 1981
25. Friedman E, Chandra SR: Choroidal blood flow. III. Effects of oxygen and carbon dioxide. Arch Ophthalmol 87:70, 1972
26. Goldstick TK, Ernest JT: The effect of glucose, oxygen and carbon dioxide on choroidal blood flow (abstr). Invest Ophthalmol Vis Sci (Suppl) 22:194, 1982
27. Hayes AH Jr: Food and Drug Administration letter, June 24, 1982
28. Johnson PC: Review of previous studies and current theories of autoregulation. Circulation Res (Suppl) 14:15, 1964
29. Landers MB III: Retinal oxygenation via the choroidal circulation. Trans Am Ophthalmol Soc 76:528, 1978
30. Laties AM, Jacobowitz D: A comparative study of the autonomic innervation of the eye in monkey, cat and rabbit. Anat Rec 156:383, 1966

31. Laties AM, Rapoport S: The blood–ocular barriers under osmotic stress: Studies on the freeze-dried eye. Arch Ophthalmol 94:1086, 1976

32. Parver LM, Auker C, Carpenter DO: Choroidal blood flow as a heat dissipating mechanism in the macula. Am J Ophthalmol 89:641, 1980

33. Parver LM, Auker C, Carpenter DO, et al: Choroidal blood flow. II. Reflexive control in the monkey. Arch Ophthalmol 100:1327, 1982

34. Paul SD, Leopold IH: The effect of vasodilating drugs on choroidal circulation. Am J Ophthalmol 42:899, 1956

35. Peyman GA, Bennett TO, Vlchek J: Effects of intravitreal prostaglandins on retinal vasculature. Ann Ophthalmol 7:279, 1975

36. Potts AM: An hypothesis on macular disease. Trans Am Acad Ophthalmol Otolaryngol 70:1058, 1966

37. Schachar RA, Weiter JJ, Ernest JT: Control of intraocular blood flow. III. Effect of chemical sympathectomy. Invest Ophthalmol Vis Sci 12:848, 1973

38. Stein HA, Wakim KG, Rucker CW: In vivo studies on the choroidal circulation of rabbits. Arch Ophthalmol 56:726, 1956

39. Varma SD, Kinoshita JH: Sorbitol pathway in diabetic and galactosemic rat lens. Biochim Biophys Acta 338:632, 1974

40. Wahl M, Kuschinsky W, Bosse O, et al: Dependency of pial arterial and arteriolar diameter on perivascular osmolarity in the cat: A microapplication study. Circ Res 32:162, 1973

41. Weiter JJ, Schacher RA, Ernest JT: Control of intraocular blood flow. I. Intraocular pressure. Invest Ophthalmol Vis Sci 12:337, 1973

42. Weiter JJ, Schacher RA, Ernest JT: Control of intraocular blood flow. II. Effects of sympathetic tone. Invest Ophthalmol Vis Sci 12:332, 1973

43. White P: Natural course and prognosis of juvenile diabetes. Diabetes 5:445, 1956

44. Wilson TM, Strang R, MacKenzie ET: The response of the choroidal and cerebral circulations to changing arterial PCO_2 and acetazolamide in the baboon. Invest Ophthalmol Vis Sci 16:576, 1977

45. Wolter JR: Nerves of the normal human choroid. Arch Ophthalmol 64:120, 1960

8

Regulatory Mechanisms of the Retinal Vasculature in Health and Disease

J. Terry Ernest

There is persuasive evidence that the retinal circulation is normally regulated by intrinsic factors unrelated to the autonomic nervous system. Moreover, we know that the failure of autoregulation is part of the pathophysiology of all ocular vascular disease. Indeed the loss of normal vascular reactivity is one of the earliest changes, if not the earliest change, in ocular vascular disorders. If vascular disease and its complications are to be avoided, treatment must begin before leakage, obstruction, and neovascularization occur. Once these changes take place, there are few methods of treatment currently available that do not result in even more destruction.

Ocular vascular reactivity decreases with age; also, a number of eye diseases manifest a premature loss of autoregulation. In patients with diabetic retinopathy, ocular vascular reactivity is impaired and may be one of the earliest signs, occurring even before background changes appear. Indeed both hyperglycemia and diabetes impair vascular reactivity, which together with increased blood flow may cause an intermittent stress that results in permanent vascular damage. This may be one of the earliest pathogenetic events in diabetic retinopathy. Because of the association between impaired vascular reactivity and age, the assessment of autoregulation in diabetic patients must be made carefully, with attention to age-matching of patients. Because

hyperglycemia inhibits vascular reactivity, marked fluctuations in the blood glucose of diabetic patients may result in the loss of normal ocular vascular reactivity, with the loss of the ability to adapt to even normal changes in blood pressure and arterial oxygen tension. On the other hand, after the development of diabetic retinopathy, the retinal circulation, while compromised, might nonetheless be maintained by the intermittent hyperglycemic increases in blood flow. If the latter assumption is true, then patients with diabetic retinopathy who are suddenly well controlled (e.g., with an insulin pump) might actually have decreased blood flow, resulting in areas of retinal ischemia and possibly even infarction.

Ocular vascular reactivity appears to be decreased in patients with hypertensive retinopathy, which compounds circulation problems by eliminating the mechanism that normally protects the capillaries from destructive pressure levels. At the other extreme are the effects of hypotony, in which the loss of vascular adaptation to the abnormally low intraocular pressures may be detrimental. This is important because the intraocular pressure is very low or equal to atmospheric pressure during some intraocular surgical procedures and in eyes after surgery or trauma.

In retrolental fibroplasia, immature retinal

vessels apparently respond to oxygen by severe constriction with vaso-obliteration. While the normal adult retinal circulation responds to oxygen by vasoconstriction, the immature vessels apparently have an exaggerated response, resulting in a collapse of the circulation followed by catastrophic vasoproliferation. It appears that the vascular reactivity of immature retinal vessels is excessive and at the opposite pole from the impaired (or absent) vascular reactivity of aging and retinopathies associated with diabetes and systemic hypertension. At any rate the result is an avascular retina that must be relatively hypoxic and dominated by anaerobic metabolism, at least in the inner layers. Retinal neovascularization may be due to hypoxia and either the products of, or the enzymes accounting for, the anaerobic metabolism may diffuse through the vitreous and stimulate formation of new vessels.

AUTOREGULATION

Autoregulation is defined as the maintenance of constant blood flow with changes in perfusion pressure. Blood flow is primarily controlled by the metabolic needs, mainly for oxygen, of tissues. Oxygen autoregulation has also been used to describe the local homeostatic regulation aimed at providing a constant metabolic environment. Autoregulation is a complex physiologic function of the microcirculation. A spontaneous activity of the vascular smooth muscle appears to create a tonus that can be modified by both myogenic and metabolic factors.

In the retina the myogenic vascular response can be demonstrated by experimentally occluding a venule. This increases peripheral resistance and causes a stretching and immediate vasoconstriction of the associated arteriole. Change in the metabolic status of the retina also produces a compensatory change in vascular tonus and blood flow. Indeed the same eye that has had the experimental occlusion of a venule with resultant vasoconstriction of the arteriole will after several minutes show dilation of that vessel. This is presumably due to the buildup of the products of metabolism that causes a vaso-

dilation that overwhelms the initial myogenic vasoconstrictive response. The retinal circulation is most sensitive to changes in oxygen tension, but elevation in carbon dioxide, decrease in pH, and accumulation of metabolites, all, to some extent, decrease vascular tone.

The ocular circulation autoregulates to acute changes in oxygen tension and perfusion pressure. Because of the relatively high ocular tissue hydrostatic pressure present with normal intraocular pressure, perfusion pressure is defined as the blood pressure minus the intraocular pressure. Autoregulation of the ocular circulation to pressure changes may thus be studied by altering the intraocular pressure. Systemic blood pressure changes can be evaluated, of course, but this brings into play the autonomic nervous system, which is separate from local tissue autoregulation. Long-term oxygen *deficiency* increases tissue vascularity with the development of collaterals and neovascularization. Long-term oxygen *excess* causes the obliteration of blood vessels (at least in immature retinas). This inverse relationship between tissue vascularity and oxygen concentration is a form of long-term autoregulation.

The earliest evidence of oxygen autoregulation in the retinal circulation was furnished in the early 1960s by Hickam and coworkers, who showed that increased inspiratory oxygen resulted in marked vasoconstriction.[14,19,20] In the early 1970s Russel and Ffytche and colleagues demonstrated that elevation of the intraocular pressure resulted in dilation of the retinal vessels.[13,34] At about the same time we demonstrated that while visual function was compromised by ocular hypertension, after about a minute vision returned. This was important because, although previous investigators had shown that thresholds in the visual field could be elevated by raising the intraocular pressure, they had not waited long enough to test recovery. We maintained the intraocular pressure at an elevated level and discovered that for the first 30 seconds there was little change in threshold; however, this was followed by an abrupt elevation that slowly returned to normal. The time course of this phenomenon could be explained by an initial period when oxygen was being consumed, leading to hypoxia, autoregulation, and recovery. This seemed reasonable evidence of ocular circulation autoregulation.

In two studies using the microsphere impaction method to measure blood flow in animals, Bill demonstrated autoregulation of the retinal circulation to changes in perfusion pressure.[1,15] In humans, Riva and colleagues showed that the retinal circulation autoregulates within physiologic levels of the intraocular pressure.[7,31,33] These investigators used the blue-field entopic phenomenon, which allows individuals to "see" their own leukocytes, to study the effect of changes in intraocular pressure on retinal blood velocity. This group also used the technique to demonstrate the marked vasoconstrictive effect of oxygen breathing on the retinal circulation.[24] We demonstrated, using computer processing of digitized television images, that oxygen breathing constricts retinal vessels while 5-percent carbon dioxide has little effect.[7,8] Riva and coworkers used a laser Doppler technique to show that the velocity of blood in retinal vessels is decreased with oxygen breathing.[30] Using this technique both Riva and associates and Feke and others have shown that retinal blood velocity increases in the dark.[12,32] They believe this reflects autoregulation due to increased retinal oxygen utilization in the dark. Measuring preretinal oxygen tensions in cat and monkey using a micro-oxygen electrode, we found no difference in light and dark conditions. Our findings suggest that the change in retinal oxygen consumption under conditions of different light intensities may be compensated by a change in blood flow.

All of these data bespeak the existence of a sensitive retinal vascular autoregulatory system that is able to adapt within minutes to changes in perfusion pressure and oxygen tension. This system breaks down with age and disease and may be abnormal in premature infants.

OCULAR VASCULAR DISEASE

Diabetes

A consequence of the extension of life expectancy of patients with diabetes by insulin therapy is an increase in diabetic retinopathy. It is the leading cause of blindness and disability in the United States.[19] While a good deal is known about the anatomic changes in the vasculature there is less information about the physiology of the abnormal circulation.[18] Hickam and Sieker demonstrated over 20 years ago that retinal vascular reactivity was reduced in patients with diabetes.[21,35] These investigators photographed the retinal vessels before and after oxygen breathing and showed that diabetic patients with and without retinopathy had less vasoconstriction than the control group.

More recently, studies in the brain by Bentsen and colleagues and in the retina by Rhie and coworkers showed that diabetic patients had an impairment of autoregulation.[5,29] These investigators varied the perfusion pressure by systemic infusion of angiotensin. Brain blood flow was evaluated by measuring the arteriovenous oxygen difference and applying the Fick principle. The diameter of the retinal vessels was measured photographically. Kohner and others measured retinal fluorescein transit times to estimate blood flow in diabetic patients both with and without retinopathy. The transit times were lower with the same retinal vascular volume (implying higher blood flow) in the diabetic patients than in normal control subjects. The technique has serious problems relating to concentration changes due to leakage as well as fluorescein return in veins not measured. Nonetheless, the implication is that the increased blood flow is an attempt, possibly only partially effective, at autoregulatory adaptation to disease by the circulation.

Sinclair and associates studied the retinal vascular autoregulatory response to acute changes in intraocular pressure in diabetic patients.[36] The patients compared the blue-field entopic perception of capillary leukocyte speeds between eyes. They found that leukocyte speeds decrease in the diabetic patients at intraocular pressures below those of normal subjects, suggesting a loss of autoregulation in the former.

We believe that the retinal circulation of diabetic patients loses its normal autoregulatory capacity early in the course of the disease. We are not certain if this takes place before the development of ophthalmoscopically visible retinopathy, but our guess is that the defect occurs very early. The relationship between the loss of autoregulation and leakage is not clear. Leakage is present in experimental background retinopathy and may be present in humans.[6,40] The important focus for research, however, is the mechanism or mechanisms that act to destroy the autoregulatory capacity of the retinal circulation. We know from our early studies of mannitol infusion in monkeys that hyperosmotic agents cause vasodilation and an increase in retinal blood flow.[11] Atherton and others have shown that the infusion of glucose increases the retinal blood flow in the normal cat.[4]

We have studied the effect of acute hyperglycemia in both alloxan diabetic dogs and normal human volunteers.[16,27] In the experimental animals we monitored blood flow using a preretinal oxygen microelectrode. Glucose infusion resulted in an immediate albeit transient (approximately 10-min) increase in retinal oxygen tension (Fig. 8-1). This might have been due to an inverse Pasteur or Crabtree effect (the ability of glucose to inhibit the use of oxygen), which has been demonstrated in the brain.* Our human studies, however, suggest that hyperglycemia can dilate retinal vessels. For these studies, we used computer image processing of television pictures of ocular fundus fluorescein angiograms that were coupled with the inhalation of oxygen, which normally causes vasoconstriction. Glucose infusion decreased the oxygen-induced vascular constriction. It is important to note that hyperoxia itself may impair autoregulation.[37]

We believe that there may be chronic osmotic or metabolic factors that disrupt retinal vascular autoregulation in diabetics. We know that there is a loss of pericytes, a proliferation of endothelial cells, and a thickening of the basement membrane. We do not know how these changes relate to the loss of autoregulation or to hyperglycemia. The hyperosmolality that accompanies the acute hyperglycemia is short lived but may shrink precapillary vascular smooth muscle, inhibit vascular myogenic pacemaker activity, release vasodilating humoral factors, decrease tissue levels of vasodilators, affect Na-K active transport, or decrease blood viscosity.[26]

* A Gjedde: Personal communication

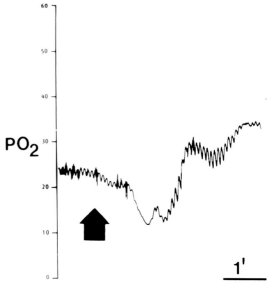

Figure 8-1. The intravenous infusion of glucose (3 ml/kg) at the arrow resulted in an initial decrease in preretinal oxygen tension (mm Hg) followed by an increase when the systemic blood pressure returned to normal.

Hyperglycemia may have a direct cytotoxic effect on the vascular endothelium.[39] We have recently shown that the infusion of isotonic glucose inhibits autoregulation, implying that glucose affects the circulation independent of osmotic effects. We do not have extensive evidence at this time, but hyperglycemia may change extra- and intracellular potassium and calcium so that they in turn might affect the autoregulatory processes. If this turns out to be true, calcium blockers might help restore normal vascular reactivity in the diseased eye.

Retrolental Fibroplasia (Retinopathy of Prematurity)

The incidence of retrolental fibroplasia has now increased to a level similar to that during the 1940s epidemic.[25] This unfortunate state of affairs is partly due to better medical care for low-birth-weight premature infants. Vitamin E therapy looks promising, but it is evident that the disease is still and again a major health problem in the United States.[22] Space limitations prevent an extensive review of the fascinating history and voluminous literature on retrolental fibroplasia, but the reports of the 1978 Academy Symposium and the Washington Conference are fairly comprehensive.[28,38]

In retinopathy of prematurity there is an exaggerated oxygen response of the immature retinal vessels, which begins as marked vasoconstriction and progresses to vaso-obliteration.[3] We have accepted the explanation that the vasoproliferative phase in retrolental fibroplasia follows capillary closure just as it does in diabetic retinopathy and sickle-cell disease.[2] In these diseases, it is hypothesized that biochemical changes associated with vasoproliferative substances are responsible for new vessel formation. A low oxygen tension promoting hypoxic metabolism is one part of this theory, but, surprisingly, direct measurements have never been made. Indeed, in the study we carried out on intraretinal neovascularization following experimental branch retinal vein obstruction, retinal oxygen tensions were normal.[10] This was because the retina was atrophic and thin enough in the areas of capillary dropout that the choroidal circulation could furnish adequate oxygen. Nonetheless, new intraretinal vessels grew into the nonperfused areas of the retina.

It is persuasive that hyperoxia constricts and eventually obliterates immature retinal vessels, but the mechanisms involved in the proliferative stages during air breathing are less clear. Tso and Yoneya have described five types of retinal and vitreal new vessels in kittens exposed to oxygen.[41] The investigators point out that there is a tremendous variability not only between litter mates of equal weight and oxygen exposure but between areas within the same eye. Their five types of retinal and vitreal new vessels are categorized according to geographic location. We have compared retinal oxygen tensions and blood flows in different areas of the same eyes of

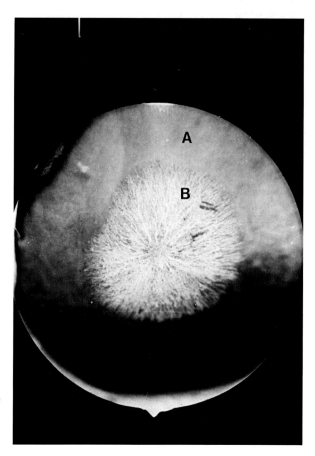

Figure 8-2. Retinal vascular cast from a 4-week-old kitten that had been exposed to pure oxygen. Preretinal oxygen tensions were close to zero in the retinal avascular area, A, but were in the normal range (10 to 15 mm Hg) in the neovascular area, B.

these kittens to see if there are areas of relative hypoxia or abnormalities in autoregulation of the circulation. We discovered that preretinal oxygen tensions in the areas of avascular retina caused by chronic oxygen exposure were close to zero (Fig. 8-2). Surprisingly, however, the administration of oxygen seemed to change retinal oxygen utilization but apparently not choroidal blood flow. Recently, Tso and colleagues showed an increase in the total number of large retinal vessels in adult cats that had been exposed to oxygen as kittens.* It may be that these eyes have overcompensated for the early retinal vascular obliteration. Surprisingly, however, these vessels have a normal autoregulatory response to hyperoxemia. It is evident that more work needs to be done before we will understand the many factors involved in the pathogenesis of retinal vascular disease.

REFERENCES

1. Alm A, Bill A: Ocular and optic nerve blood flow at normal and increased intraocular pressure in monkeys: A study of radioactively labelled microspheres including flow determinations in brain and some other tissues. Exp Eye Res 15:15, 1973
2. Ashton N: Retinal vascularization in health and disease. Am J Ophthalmol 44:7, 1957
3. Ashton N: The pathogenesis of retrolental fibroplasia. Trans Am Acad Ophthalmol 86:1695, 1979
4. Atherton A, Hill DW, Keen H, et al: The effect of acute hyperglycemia on the retinal circulation of the normal cat. Diabetologia 18:233, 1980
5. Bentsen N, Larson B, Lassen NA: Chronically impaired autoregulation of cerebral blood flow in long-term diabetics. Stroke 6:497, 1975
6. Cunha-Vaz J, Faria de Abreu JR, Campos AJ, et al: Early breakdown of the blood-retinal barrier in diabetes. Br J Ophthalmol 59:649, 1975
7. Deutsch RA, Read JS, Ernest JT, et al: Effects of oxygen and carbon dioxide on the retinal circulation in man (abstr). Invest Ophthalmol Vis Sci (Suppl) 22:195, 1982
8. Deutsch TA, Read JS, Ernest JT, et al: Effects of oxygen and carbon dioxide on the retinal vasculature in humans. Arch Ophthalmol 101:1278, 1983
9. The Diabetic Retinopathy Study Research Group: Preliminary report on effect of photoco-
agulation therapy. Am J Ophthalmol 81:383, 1976
10. Ernest JT, Archer DB: Vitreous body oxygen tension following experimental branch retinal vein obstruction. Invest Ophthalmol Vis Sci 18:1025, 1979
11. Ernest JT, Stern WH, Trimble JL: The effect of mannitol infusion on retinal function and oxygen tension. Invest Ophthalmol Vis Sci 16:670, 1977
12. Feke GT, Zuckerman R, Green GJ, et al: Response of human retinal blood flow to light and dark (abstr). Invest Ophthalmol Vis Sci (Suppl) 22:195, 1982
13. Ffyche TJ, Bulpitt CJ, Kohner EM, et al: Effect of changes in intraocular pressure on the retinal microcirculation. Br J Ophthalmol 58:514, 1974
14. Frayser R, Hickam JB: Retinal vascular response to breathing increased carbon dioxide and oxygen concentrations. Invest Ophthalmol Vis Sci 3:427, 1964
15. Geijer C, Bill A: Effect of raised intraocular pressure on retinal, prelaminar and retrolaminar optic nerve blood flow in monkeys. Invest Ophthalmol Vis Sci 18:1030, 1979
16. Goldstick TK, Ernest JT, Engerman RL: Impaired retinal vascular reactivity in diabetic dogs (abstr). Invest Ophthalmol Vis Sci (Suppl) 20:92, 1981
17. Gruwald JE, Sinclair SH, Riva CE: Autoregulation of the retinal circulation in response to decrease of intraocular pressure below normal. Invest Ophthalmol Vis Sci 23:124, 1982
18. Henkind P: The eye in diabetes mellitus: Signs, symptoms and their pathogenesis. In Mausolf F (ed): The Eye and Systemic Diseases, p 195. St Louis, CV Mosby, 1975
19. Hickam JB, Frayser R: Studies of the retinal circulation in man: Observations of vessel diameter, arteriovenous oxygen differences, and mean circulation time. Circulation 33:302, 1966
20. Hickam JB, Frayser R, Ross JC: A study of retinal venous blood-oxygen saturation in human subjects by photographic means. Circulation 27:375, 1963
21. Hickman JB, Sieker HO: Retinal vascular reactivity in patients with diabetes mellitus and with atherosclerosis. Circulation 22:243, 1960
22. Hittner HM, Godio LB, Rudolph AJ, et al: Retrolental fibroplasia: Efficacy of vitamin E in a double-blind clinical study of preterm infants. N Engl J Med 305:1365,1981
23. Kohner EM, Hamilton AM, Saunders SJ, et al: The retinal blood flow in diabetes. Diabetologica 11:27, 1975
24. Petrig BL, Riva CE, Sinclair SH, et al: Quantification of changes in leukocyte velocity in retinal macular capillaries during oxygen breathing (abstr). Invest Ophthalmol Vis Sci (Suppl) 22:194, 1982

* MOM Tso: Personal communication

25. Phelps DL: Retinopathy of prematurity: An estimate of vision loss in the United States–1979. Pediatrics 67:924, 1981

26. Raizner AE, Costin JC, Croke RP, et al: Reflex systemic, and local hemodynamic alterations with experimental hyperosmolality. Am J Physiol 224:1327, 1973

27. Read JS, Ernest JT, Goldstick TK, et al: Hyperglycemia and the retinal circulation in man (abstr). Invest Ophthalmol Vis Sci (Suppl) 19:168, 1980

28. Retinopathy of Prematurity Conference, Washington DC, Dec 4–6, 1981. Columbus, OH, Ross Laboratories, vols 1 and 2

29. Rhie FH, Christlieb AR, Aiello LM, et al: Retinal vascular reactivity to angiotensin II and norepinephrine in diabetic subjects. Diabetes (Suppl) 28:387, 1979

30. Riva CE, Grunwald JE, Petrig BL, et al: Effect of breathing pure oxygen on human retinal blood flow measured by laser Doppler velocimetry, abstracted. Invest Ophthalmol Vis Sci (Suppl) 22:194, 1982

31. Riva CE, Loebl M: Autoregulation of blood flow in the capillaries of the human macula. Invest Ophthalmol Vis Sci 16:586, 1977

32. Riva CE, Grunwald JE, Petrig BL: Reactivity of the human retinal circulation to darkness: A laser Doppler velocimetry study. Invest Ophthalmol Vis Sci 24:737, 1983

33. Riva CE, Sinclair SH, Grunwald JE: Autoregulation of retinal circulation in response to decrease of perfusion pressure. Invest Ophthalmol Vis Sci 21:34, 1981

34. Russel RW: Evidence for autoregulation in human retinal circulation. Lancet 2:1048, 1973

35. Sieker HO, Hickman JB: Normal and impaired retinal vascular reactivity. Circulation 7:79, 1953

36. Sinclair SH, Grunwald JE, Riva CE, et al: Retinal vascular autoregulation in diabetes mellitus. Ophthalmology 89:748, 1982

37. Sullivan SM, Johnson PC: Effect of oxygen on blood flow autoregulation in cat sartorius muscle. Am J Physiol 241 H807–H815, 1981

38. Symposium on retrolental fibroplasia. Trans Am Acad Ophthalmol 86:1685, 1979

39. Tripathi BJ, Tripathi RC: Human retinal vessels in tissue culture: A preliminary report of the effect of acute glucose poisonings on cultured vascular cell. Ophthalmology 89:858, 1982

40. Wallow IHL, Engerman RL: Permeability and patency of retinal blood vessels in experimental diabetes. Invest Ophthalmol Vis Sci 16:447, 1977

41. Yoneya S, Tso MOM: A SEM study of retinal neovascularization in retrolental fibroplasia (abstr). Invest Ophthalmol Vis Sci 19 (Suppl):139, 180

9

Vascular Diseases of the Retina

Robert N. Frank

Many disorders that appear to be localized to the eye as well as those that attack organs and tissues elsewhere in the body affect the blood vessels of the retina. In searching for means to treat the ocular lesions of these diseases, it is useful to attempt to discover the cellular and biochemical mechanisms by which these lesions are produced. We are aided in this effort by the fact that, although the pattern and location of the vascular lesions in the retina differ in various diseases, the individual lesions are often similar. So it may be possible to deduce the mechanisms by which different pathological stimuli act to create a specific morphological or functional result. In this chapter, I shall illustrate a number of the individual abnormalities that occur during the course of several retinal vascular diseases as a means of demonstrating that, in these diseases, different pathological processes may produce similar anatomic results, likely through similar mechanisms.

ALTERATIONS OF RETINAL BLOOD FLOW

Because direct measurement of flow rates in retinal vessels has become possible only recently, detailed studies of retinal blood flow in various diseases are, to date, extremely limited. Among methods that may have value for the quantitation of retinal blood flow are the densitometric analysis of rapid sequence fluorescein angiograms using either photographic images or television ophthalmoscopy, the measurement of the Doppler shift using laser light reflected from flowing erythrocytes (both of which techniques are limited to the largest retinal vessels near the optic disc), and the semiquantitative evaluation of capillary flow using the entoptic visualization of white blood cells in the perifoveal circulation produced by gazing at a bright blue background.[17,37,42,52] Because of the lack of quantitative data, the discussion in this section cannot yet be documented by actual measurements, but there appears to be good clinical reason to suggest that the lesions described here are caused by alterations in blood flow.

The best evidence that *dilation* of retinal veins is related to flow is found in the rapid dilation that may be observed upstream from the lesion if one constricts or occludes a retinal vein by photocoagulation.[25] The dilated vessel may also become increasingly *tortuous*. In such cases, the dilation and tortuosity are caused by a local constricting lesion. Similar abnormalities may be observed clinically in retinal vein occlusions (Fig. 9-1, 9-2), where a solitary constricting lesion is presumed to be present, or in "venous stasis retinopathy" where, presumably, the constriction is not so severe.[26] However, other disease processes also cause venous dilation and tortuosity, possibly by other mechanisms. For example, these abnormalities may also be present in diabetic retinopathy, perhaps as a result of the increased blood viscosity; in the dysproteinemias, in which increases in serum viscosity are present; and in disorders in which there are increased cellular elements in the blood (Fig. 9-3).[43]

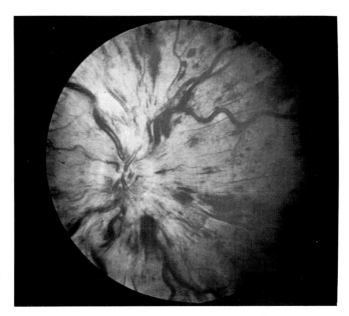

Figure 9-1. Marked venous dilation and tortuosity and profuse intraretinal hemorrhages and disc edema in a patient with an acute central retinal vein occlusion.

In all of these conditions constrictive lesions of the retinal veins or increased blood viscosity produces venous dilation and tortuosity by slowing the flow of blood. However, a similar result may occur when the flow is markedly increased. Examples are the racemose angioma of the retina in the Wyburn–Mason syndrome and the massive dilation and tortuosity of both the feeding arteriole and the draining venule to the large peripheral retinal angioma seen in von

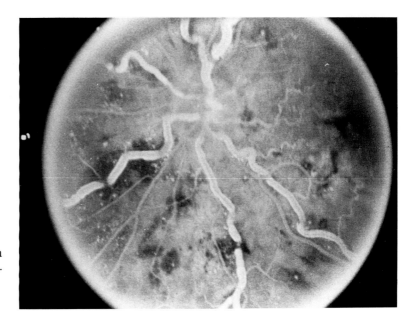

Figure 9-2. Arteriovenous phase of the fluorescein angiogram in a patient with a central retinal vein occlusion. Again, marked dilation and tortuosity of the veins are present.

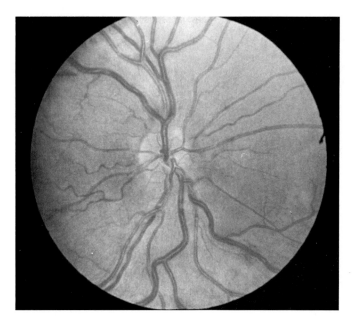

Figure 9-3. Moderate dilation and tortuosity of the retinal veins in a patient with chronic myelocytic leukemia and a massively elevated white cell count. This patient, whose retinal findings were described in detail by Frank and Ryan,[55] also had peripheral retinal neovascularization bilaterally and an extensive vitreous hemorrhage in the fellow eye.

Hippel–Lindau disease (Fig. 9-4, 9-5). The mechanisms by which dilation and tortuosity of retinal veins, vessels with few smooth muscle elements in their walls, occur are probably largely mechanical, related to blood flow, blood viscosity, and transmural pressure. A recent paper attempts to analyze these factors theoretically.[54]

Certain alterations in retinal arterial caliber may also relate to increases in transmural pressure. These include the sudden narrowing ("nicking") of venous caliber at arteriovenous crossing points in hypertensive patients and retinal arterial macroaneurysms (Fig. 9-6, 9-7). Arteriovenous nicking doubtless results from the partial collapse of the adjoining thin-walled

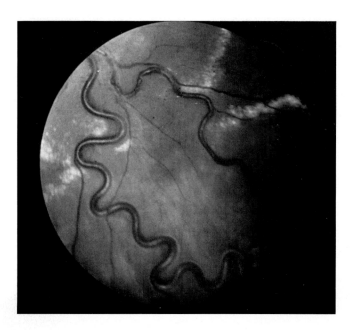

Figure 9-4. Massive dilation and tortuosity of the feeding artery and the draining vein leading to a very large peripheral retinal angioma in a 19-year-old woman. In this situation, the dilation and tortuosity is attributed to extremely high blood flow, while in the cases illustrated in Figures 9-1 to 9-3 the dilation and tortuosity are attributed to decreased flow, related either to an occlusive lesion or to elevated whole blood viscosity.

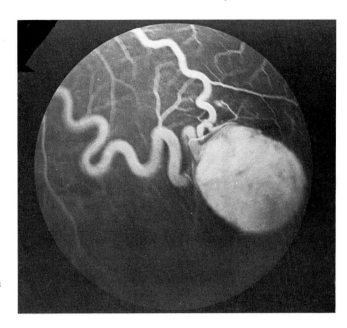

Figure 9-5. A frame from the arteriovenous phase of the fluorescein angiogram of the patient shown in Figure 9-4, demonstrating the angioma itself.

vein, or venule, by the high pressure in the adjoining muscular artery or arteriole. Macroaneurysms may be the result of a defect in the muscular wall of an arteriole, perhaps caused by the continued stress of hypertension.

A peculiar abnormality of caliber of the retinal veins that appears to be unique to diabetic retinopathy is "beading" or "sausaging" (Fig. 9-8). It is difficult to determine the cause for such an abnormality, involving as it does marked irregularity in the venous caliber. Alterations in blood flow seem an unlikely mechanism. Regional differences in the ability of the sparse smooth-muscle cells of the retinal veins

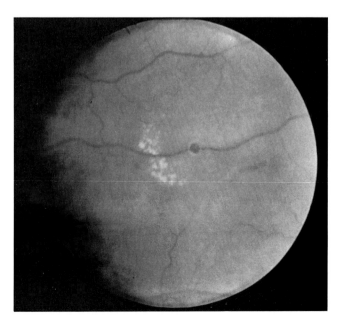

Figure 9-6. A retinal arterial macroaneurysm in a 60-year-old hypertensive woman. Note also the small amount of lipid exudate surrounding the lesion.

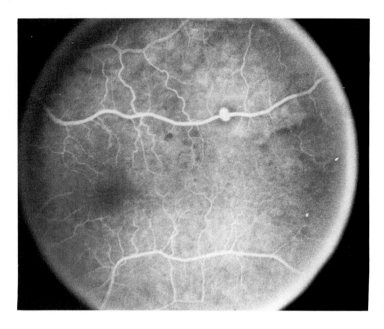

Figure 9-7. A frame from the fluorescein angiogram of the patient shown in Figure 9-6.

to contract, induced by the metabolic disturbances of diabetes, seem to be the most likely cause of this unusual lesion.

BREAKDOWN OF THE BLOOD–RETINA BARRIER

Normally, the retina is protected against the influx of many foreign substances by the blood–retina barrier (BRB), which is formed by the layer of retinal pigment epithelial (RPE) cells and their junctional complexes and by the endothelial cells of the retinal blood vessels, which are joined to one another by tight junctions (*zonulae occludentes*). A discussion of this barrier at the RPE cell level is beyond the scope of this chapter. The barrier may be breached at the level of the retinal vessels in a number of dis-

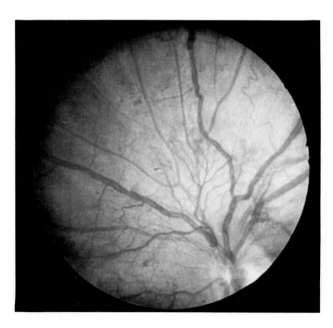

Figure 9-8. Marked irregularity of venous caliber (beading or sausaging) in a patient with proliferative diabetic retinopathy. Multiple areas of flat neovascularization are also present.

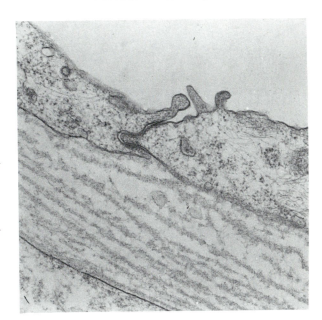

Figure 9-9. An electron micrograph of a newly formed vessel arising from the optic nerve head in a patient with panuveitis due to sarcoidosis. Note that there is no junctional complex between the endothelial cells, as would normally be observed in retinal vascular endothelium, and hence, the blood–retina barrier is not intact at this point. (Frank KW, Weiss H: Unusual clinical and histopathological findings in ocular sarcoidosis. Br J Ophthalmol 67:8–16, 1981; original magnification ×20,000)

eases, and the mechanisms by which this occurs have been of interest to many cell biologists. Among these are *breakdown of the cell junctions* permitting the efflux of many substances from the vascular lumina that would normally be confined intraluminally. Such junctional abnormalities have been observed by electron microscopy in humans with diabetic retinopathy as well as in the experimental disease in animals.[56] The vessel illustrated in Figure 9-9 was taken from a neovascular tuft arising from the optic nerve head in an eye enucleated as a consequence of severe uveitis due to sarcoidosis.[20]

Another way in which the BRB may break down at the level of the retinal vessels is by attenuation of the endothelial cell cytoplasm with the formation of *fenestrae*, through which, presumably, material from the intraluminal space may

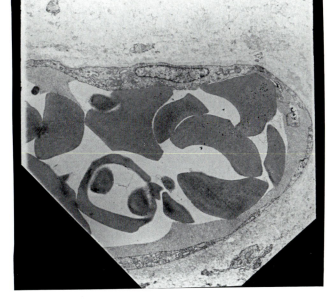

Figure 9-10. Marked thinning of vascular endothelium with appearance of fenestrae in another portion of the neovascular network in the case shown in Figure 9-9. Intravascular contents may also leak out of the lumen at these sites. (Frank KW, Weiss H: Unusual clinical and histopathological findings in ocular sarcoidosis. Brit J Ophthalmol 67:8–16, 1981; original magnification ×2400)

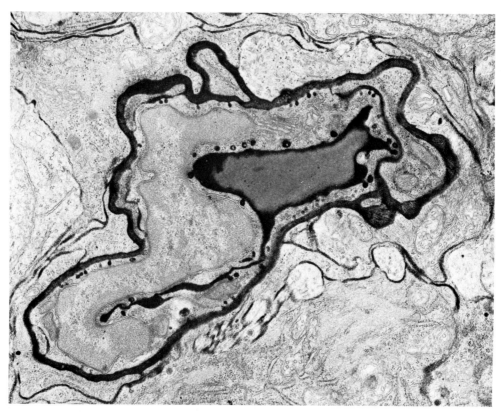

Figure 9-11. Electron micrograph of a capillary from a rat of the RCS strain with a hereditary retinal dystrophy. The animal was injected intravenously with horseradish peroxidase before sacrifice, and the thin sections were treated so as to produce electron-dense granules in the places where the peroxidase molecules are located. Note the heavy reaction in the vascular lumen, in the extravascular space, and in particular in the vesicles traversing the cell cytoplasm. In normal animals, the peroxidase reaction is restricted to the vascular lumen. Hence, this is an example of abnormal vesicular transport, another mechanism by which the blood–retina barrier may break down. (Essner E, Pino RH, Griewski RA: Breakdown of blood retinal barrier in RCS rats with inherited retinal degeneration. Lab Invest 43:418–426, 1980; original magnification ×26,000)

pass (Fig. 9-10). Finally, a presumably normal mechanism for the passage of substances from the intraluminal space (in capillaries) into the retina, and *vice versa*, is *vesicular transport* via pinocytotic vesicles that traverse the endothelial cell cytoplasm. While vesicles are normally seen in the cytoplasm of retinal capillary endothelial cells, experiments with electron-dense tracers rarely show these imbibing their contents at the luminal surface of the endothelial cell or discharging them at the abluminal side. However, in the outermost layer of retinal capillaries of RCS rats (that have an inherited retinal dystrophy) Essner and associates showed a marked increase in vesicular transport of both horseradish peroxidase and microperoxidase (Fig. 9-11).[16] Although this mechanism has not yet been shown to account for BRB breakdown in human disease, the possibility that it contributes to the barrier breakdown at least in some situations is entirely plausible.

MANIFESTATIONS OF BRB BREAKDOWN

Experimentally, breakdown of the BRB may be demonstrated by the passage of labelled molecules, including fluorescein and fluoresceinated proteins, microperoxidase, peroxidase, various heme proteins, dextrans, ferritin, and radiolabelled molecules, through the RPE or the retinal vessels. Clinically, the process may also be shown in its earliest stages by the "leakage" of fluorescein dye through retinal microaneurysms or other vascular abnormalities, using the photographic technique of intravenous fluorescein angiography (Fig. 9-12). An even more sensitive technique is that of vitreous fluorophotometry, which may demonstrate a barrier breakdown even before lesions detectable by ophthalmoscopy, fundus photography, or fluorescein angiography are present.[8] However, vitreous fluorophotometry cannot distinguish between fluorescein leakage through the retinal vessels and that through the RPE, and there is at

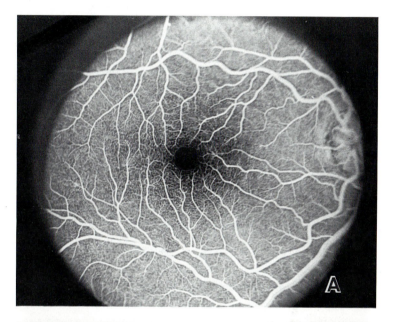

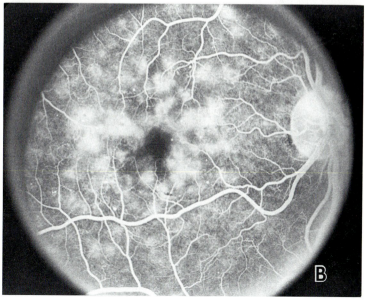

Figure 9-12. *(A)* A frame from a fluorescein angiogram showing the macular circulation of the normal retina. When the blood–retina barrier is intact, all of the vessels, down to the smallest capillaries, show sharp outlines, and no fluorescein leaks outside the vascular lamina. *(B)* Breakdown of the BRB in a diabetic patient with multiple microaneurysms. Note the diffuse haze of fluorescein which has leaked into the neural retina.

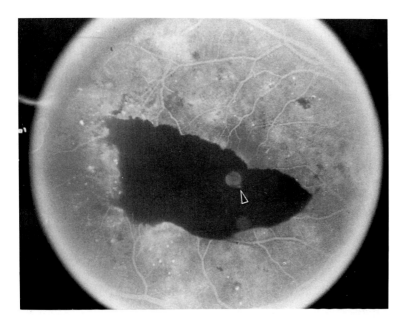

Figure 9-13. A preretinal hemorrhage in a diabetic patient. In this fluorescein angiogram, the hemorrhage blocks fluorescein and appears as a sharply demarcated, dark silhouette. The sharp demarcation is typical of preretinal hemorrhages, which are limited either by the internal limiting membrane of the retina or by the posterior face of the vitreous. In this case, the hemorrhage must be bounded by the vitreous because it is also limited by the attachment of the vitreous to the fovea, which leaves a hole in the hemorrhage *(arrow)* through which this patient could see with 20/60 (6/18) acuity, despite the fact that the hemorrhage otherwise covers almost the entire macula.

least some evidence that the earliest functional and morphological abnormalities in diabetic rats are actually at the RPE level.[23,35]

More advanced breakdown of the BRB may be demonstrated by hemorrhages, which may occur in a wide variety of diseases and may be located within the retinal substance (intraretinal), between the retinal neurons and glia and the internal limiting membrane of the retina, between this membrane and the posterior face of the vitreous (preretinal, Fig. 9-13), or within the vitreous substance (vitreal). While the mechanisms by which hemorrhages from the retinal vessels occur in many diseases may be easy to comprehend (for example, marked increase in transmural venous pressure in retinal

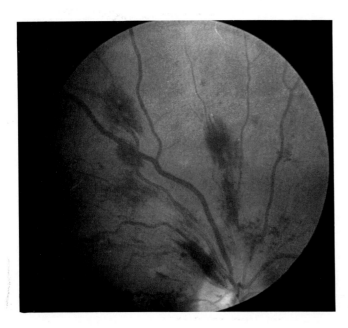

Figure 9-14. Multiple intraretinal hemorrhages in a patient with profound anemia (hematocrit 15%) and multiple myeloma.

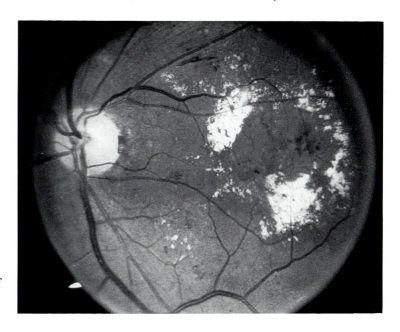

Figure 9-15. A ring of lipid exudates in the macula of a diabetic patient. Note the cluster of vascular abnormalities in the center of the ring.

vein occlusion with damage to endothelial cells or junctional complexes, or metabolic damage to vascular endothelial cells, pericytes, and smooth-muscle cells in diabetic retinopathy), in some disorders, such as severe anemia, it is difficult to understand why retinal hemorrhages occur (Fig. 9-14).

Lipid exudates may also occur in a wide variety of retinal vascular disorders. Presumably, these result from the precipitation of lipid or lipoprotein material within the retinal substance following escape of plasma from the retinal vessels. These may be diffuse but they often have a circular ("circinate retinopathy") pattern, in which the "leaking" vascular abnormality producing the lipid exudate is located in the center of the circle (Fig. 9-15). Finally, lipid deposited (for unknown reasons) within Henle's fiber layer of the macula may produce a star-shaped pattern (the so-called macular star) in severe hypertensive retinopathy and occasionally in other disorders (Fig. 9-16). Lipid precipitates are not irreversible. They may appear and disappear without therapeutic intervention in the course of a disease and may also respond to therapy. A study from Great Britain demonstrated that when diabetic patients with lipid exudates in the retina were placed on a diet low in saturated fats, the exudates diminished but

visual acuity did not improve.[34] Similarly, it is a widely held clinical impression that argon laser photocoagulation of the vascular abnormalities in the center of lipid rings causes the prompt disappearance of these rings (Fig. 9-17). Since one may assume that the leaking vascular lesion produces a constant efflux of plasma from which the lipid precipitates and that the precipitated lipid material is continuously being removed by wandering phagocytic cells, a beneficial effect of photocoagulation in this circumstance implies that the lipid precipitate is produced by a dynamic equilibrium between deposition and removal.

When lipid is present in the retina in any quantity there is almost surely also edema (i.e., retinal thickening by the presence of serous fluid either intercellularly, intracellularly, or both). Of course, retinal edema may also be present in the absence of lipid exudates. Particularly when vascular leakage in the macula is widespread, the edema may be diffuse. In the presence of lipid rings, edema may be localized to the centers of the rings. A particularly interesting form of macular edema is so-called cystoid macular edema in which fluid-filled cysts form in the extracellular space within Henle's fiber layer, producing a pattern like petals on a flower ("petaloid" pattern). Cystoid macular edema

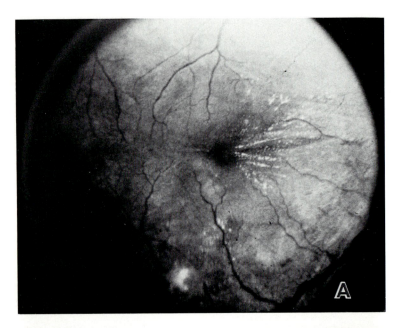

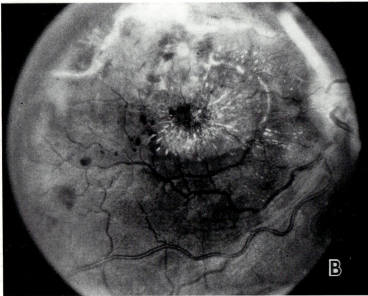

Figure 9-16. *(A)* A macular star figure of lipid exudates located in Henle's fiber layer of the retina in a patient with malignant hypertension. *(B)* A similar macular star in a normotensive patient with retinal vasculitis of unknown cause. This patient also later developed a severe granulomatous uveitis.

may frequently be visualized by slit-lamp ophthalmoscopy, using the Hruby lens or fundus contact lens, but in many cases the abnormality is subtle and fluorescein angiography may be required (Fig. 9-18). In cystoid macular edema the vessels that leak are those of the perifoveal capillary network, but the mechanisms by which this particular edema pattern is produced in a variety of disorders are unclear. Cystoid macular edema may occur in diabetic retinopathy, following both central and branch retinal vein occlusions, following prolonged uveitis, as a familial syndrome and, interestingly, in aphakic eyes (Fig. 9-18).[11] While cystoid macular edema has been observed following uncomplicated cataract surgery, it has also been associated with complicated procedures in which vitreous has been lost or a vitreous strand to the surgical incision is present, or in glaucomatous eyes treated with topical epinephrine

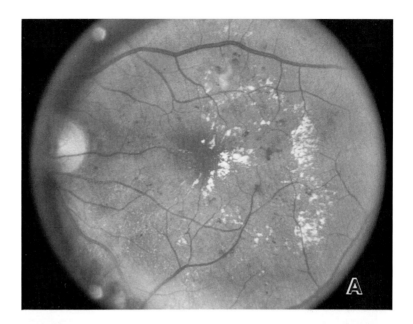

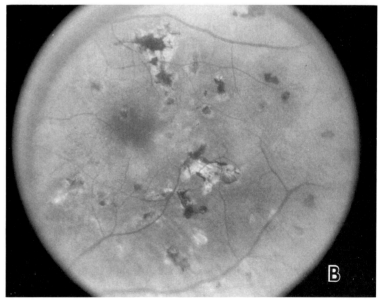

Figure 9-17. *(A)* Lipid exudates in the macula of a diabetic patient before laser treatment. *(B)* The same patient 1 year after focal laser treatment to the macula. Note disappearance of the lipid.

following cataract extraction. One report that cystoid macular edema occurs less frequently after extracapsular than after intracapsular cataract extraction and another that its incidence is reduced when patients are treated with topical indomethacin following cataract surgery suggest a relationship of vitreous traction and of postoperative inflammation, most likely in the anterior segment, to this disorder.[30,40]

Although retinal (in particular, macular) edema occurs most frequently in the presence of vascular disease localized to the edematous area, it may also occur in the macula as a result of a lesion in the retinal periphery.[59] Figure 9-19 shows such a situation in the macula of the eye with the large peripheral angioma shown in Figures 9-4 and 9-5. Extensive edema was present with visual acuity reduced to 20/50 (6/15). The

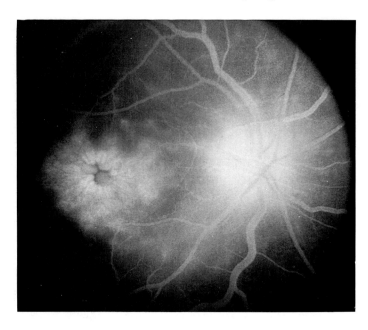

Figure 9-18. A fluorescein angiogram showing cystoid macular edema in an aphakic patient.

cause of such an event is unknown, but it may in some way be the result of the enormous increase in blood flow in the nearby vessels feeding and draining the tumor. Why this should selectively involve the macula is unclear, but it suggests that changes in flow in the major vessels near the macula in patients with macular edema should be monitored with newer techniques of measurement such as laser Doppler velocimetry.

OCCLUSIVE PHENOMENA

Occlusive disease of the larger retinal vessels may be produced in the arterial circulation by emboli, often from atheromatous plaques in the carotid system. These may produce the disastrous consequences of a central retinal arterial occlusion (Fig. 9-20). Often a small island of central vision is spared because a cilioretinal ar-

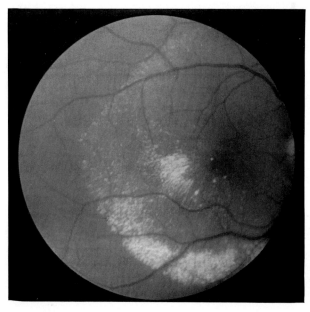

Figure 9-19. The macula of the same eye shown in Figures 9-4 and 9-5, with a large, peripheral retinal angioma. Note the extensive lipid exudation. Retinal edema was also present, and visual acuity was reduced to 20/50 (6/15).

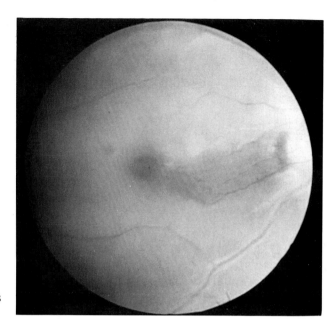

Figure 9-20. Gray edema of the retina acutely following occlusion of the central retinal artery. An island of normal retinal tissue extends temporally from the optic nerve head, where a cilioretinal artery has preserved retinal function.

tery arising from a different portion of the ophthalmic artery remains patent. Smaller emboli may be visualized ophthalmoscopically as glistening white plaques, usually located at a bifurcation of the retinal arterial tree (Fig. 9-21). This finding requires a search for atherosclerotic disease of the great vessels in the hope that surgical correction may forestall a major cerebrovascular embolic episode.

Venous occlusive disease in the retina is usually thrombotic. In its acute stages it produces the typical hemorrhagic appearance of the fundus. Retinal venous occlusions may occur anywhere from the central retinal vein (in which

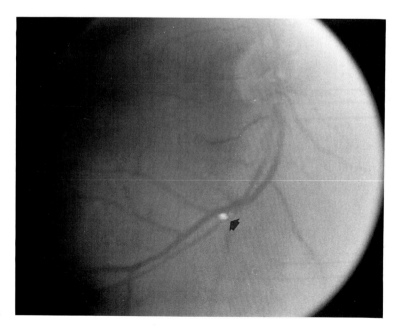

Figure 9-21. A cholesterol embolus at the bifurcation of two retinal arterioles *(arrow)*. This patient later underwent carotid endarterectomy for atheromatous plaques partially occluding the common carotid artery on the side of this lesion.

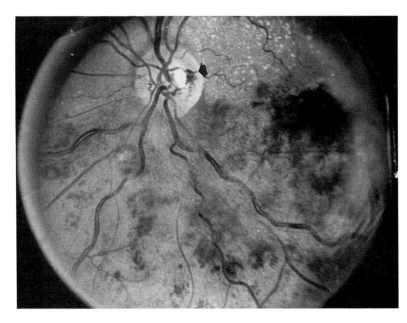

Figure 9-22. The posterior retina of an eye with a hemiretinal vein occlusion. Note the hemorrhages, sharply demarcated at the horizontal meridian of the retina, extending both rostrad and temporally from the optic disc. Note also the dilated collateral vessels on the disc *(arrow).*

case the hemorrhages occur in all four quadrants of the fundus, surrounding the optic disc) to the smallest branch veins. In branch vein occlusions, the occlusion nearly always occurs at an arteriovenous crossing point that forms the apex of a triangle of hemorrhage extending peripherally into the retina. Although the central retinal artery and vein usually have four major branches, on occasion the central vessel initially bifurcates, and occlusion at one of these two branches produces the picture of "hemiretinal vein occlusion," recently emphasized by Hayreh (Fig. 9-22, 9-23).[28] Neovascularization of the retina and iris may follow central retinal vein occlusion. Neovascularization of the iris often leads to neovascular glaucoma when the

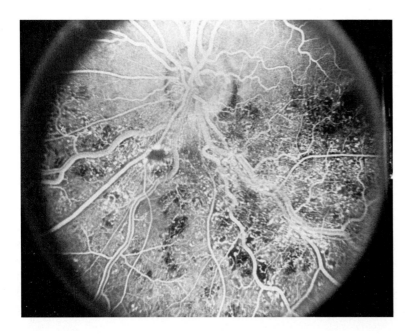

Figure 9-23. A frame from the fluorescein angiogram of the patient shown in Figure 9-22.

vessels grow into the anterior chamber angle. At present, it is widely believed that neovascularization of the retina or iris is most likely to occur when there is extensive nonperfusion of the retinal capillary bed.[44] Retinal neovascularization may also follow branch vein occlusion, but neovascularization of the iris rarely occurs in this situation. The prognosis for the development of new vessels on the iris following hemiretinal vein occlusion is still not clear. The visual prognosis following central retinal vein occlusions is rather poor; few patients recover vision to better than 20/200 (6/60). Following branch vein occlusion at least 60 percent of patients recover to 20/40 (6/12) or better visual acuity within a year of the event, even without therapy.[24,47] Though the prognosis for individuals with hemiretinal vein occlusions has not been determined it probably is intermediate between the two extremes. Because of the gravity of sequelae such as neovascularization and macular edema, and the possibility that retinal photocoagulation might be beneficial, the National Eye Institute sponsored a multi-institutional, controlled clinical trial of photocoagulation in retinal branch vein occlusion. This study demonstrated a clear benefit of "grid" argon laser photocoagulation in areas of macular edema secondary to retinal branch vein occlusion and of "scatter" photocoagulation to the involved quadrant for the prevention of retinal neovascularization and resultant vitreous hemorrhage.[4,5]

A variety of systemic and ocular causes of retinal venous occlusive diseases have been postulated—diabetes mellitus, systemic hypertension, systemic atherosclerosis, hyperlipoproteinemias, dysproteinemias and other "hyperviscosity syndromes," glaucoma and "ocular hypertension."[36] As none has been proved, specific therapeutic and preventive measures cannot be recommended. Photocoagulation appears to markedly reduce the incidence of neovascular glaucoma in central retinal vein occlusion but does not ultimately improve visual acuity. Anticoagulants are ineffective in retinal venous occlusive disease, as is intravenous streptokinase, a fibrinolytic enzyme.[39,45] A small controlled clinical trial of streptokinase demonstrated a modest benefit to

the final visual acuity in patients who received this agent. However, those treated with streptokinase suffered a larger number of vitreous hemorrhages than did the control subjects. A clinical trial of a different fibrinolytic, tissue plasminogen activator (TPA) is planned. TPA is endogenous in humans and can be produced by recombinant DNA techniques for intravascular administration in larger quantities. Currently, many physicians treat retinal vein occlusions with agents to lower the blood pressure, agents to lower the intraocular pressure when it is elevated, even when no glaucomatous optic nerve head changes are present, and drugs such as aspirin, dipyridamole, and sulfinpyrazone to inhibit platelet aggregation, even though there is no evidence of beneficial effects from these agents.

Opacified retinal arterioles appear as white threadlike vessels that usually do not carry blood, as demonstrated by their nonperfusion on fluorescein angiography (Fig. 9-24, 9-25). These may occur in many diseases, including diabetic and hypertensive retinopathy, the collagen vascular diseases, and following retinal vasculitides. The vascular pathology includes fibrinoid necrosis of the vessel wall with obliteration of the lumen. When the involved area includes the macular retina severe and irreversible visual loss may occur. Occluded cilioretinal arteries on the optic disc have a similar white, threadlike appearance (Fig. 9-26), and when the choroidal blood supply to portions of the disc is interrupted, severe visual field defects occur.

Occlusion of smaller arterioles produce cotton-wool spots (Fig. 9-27), small areas of infarction in the inner retina that appear microscopically as swollen retinal ganglion cell axons resulting from the ischemia. These may occur in hypertensive retinopathy, diabetic retinopathy, the collagen vascular disorders, and retinal vein occlusions, all without evidence of hypertension.

In all of the vascular occlusive disorders, collateral vessels may develop if the occlusion is sufficiently chronic. These collaterals may occur on the optic nerve head in retinal vein occlusions (see Fig. 9-22) and may be confused with disc neovascularization, which they closely

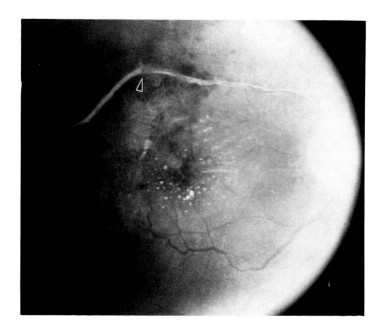

Figure 9-24. Fundus photograph of the patient with retinal vasculitis shown in Figure 9-16*B*. The vessels are "sheathed" with white exudates of inflammatory cells, though at least some of the white appearance is probably due to fibrinoid necrosis of the vessel walls. The arrow indicates the vessel that will be shown to be occluded in Figure 9-25.

resemble. However, disc collaterals are of greater caliber than new vessels and, most important, they do not leak fluorescein.[29]

MICROVASCULAR DISEASE

Abnormalities of the smallest vessels are also a feature of many retinal vascular diseases. Cer-

tain features may be relatively specific to particular diseases, for example, capillary pericyte dropout in diabetic retinopathy.[1,7,53,60] Capillary microaneurysms occur in many other diseases. They have been described in the retinal periphery in leukemic retinopathy, and they sometimes occur in the posterior retina in other blood disorders (Fig. 9-28) and in retinal vein occlusion.[15] The pathogenetic events leading to

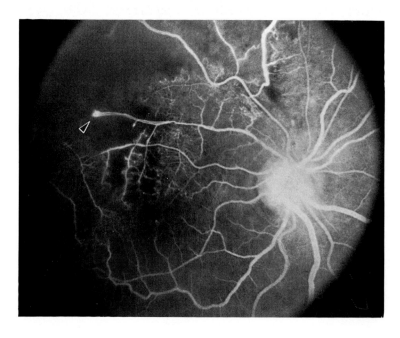

Figure 9-25. A frame from a fluorescein angiogram of the patient shown in Figure 9-24, showing obstruction of a major arteriole *(arrow).*

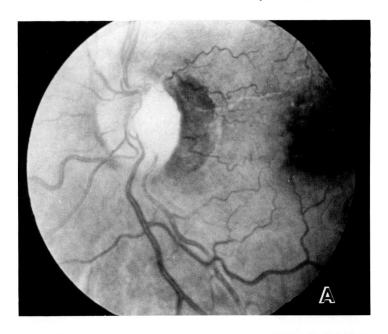

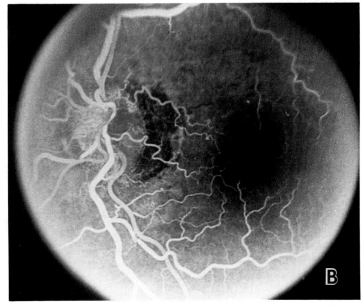

Figure 9-26. *(A)* An old cilio-retinal artery occlusion, shown as a white, threadlike vessel on the temporal side of the disc. Note the pallor of the optic disc. *(B)* In a fluorescein angiogram of this patient, the white vessel does not fill, and the temporal half of the disc is dark, indicating nonperfusion of its capillaries.

the formation of microaneurysms are unclear because their structure, as seen microscopically, may vary. They may be saccular, like small grapes bulging out of the capillary wall connected to the main capillary lumen only by a small stalk, or they may be simply fusiform dilations of the capillary. Microaneurysms may be highly cellular (perhaps resulting from localized regions of endothelial cell proliferation) or they

may be totally acellular. Perhaps the different types of microaneurysms are produced by different causes, including local weakening of the capillary wall due to loss or malfunction of pericytes or endothelial cells, and foci of endothelial cell proliferation.

Capillary endothelial cells may be lost selectively in the aging retina, but most often they degenerate in the same disorders that cause loss

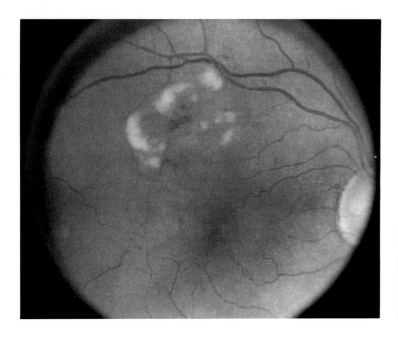

Figure 9-27. A ring of cotton wool spots, indicating small infarctions of the nerve fiber layer due to arteriolar occlusions from retinal vasculitis in a patient with systemic lupus erythematosus.

of pericytes.[41] When a capillary has lost both pericytes and endothelial cells, what remains is an empty tube of basement membrane. Clinicopathological studies combining fluorescein angiography and postmortem trypsin digest preparations show that these empty tubes are not capable of carrying blood.[12,38] Examples of such vessels are shown in a trypsin-digest preparation from the retina of a rat with experimental diabetes (Fig. 9-29) and in an electron micrograph from a similar animal (Fig. 9-30). (I do not wish to suggest by this example that diabetes produced the acellular capillaries in this animal. We have not observed such changes commonly in

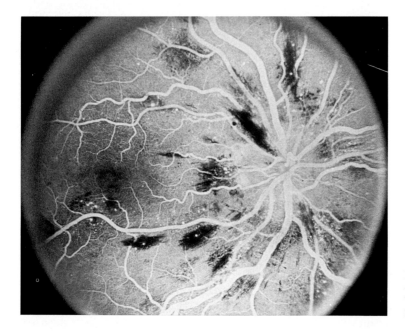

Figure 9-28. A frame from the fluorescein angiogram of the patient with multiple myeloma and anemia shown in Figure 9-14. Note the mutliple microaneurysms.

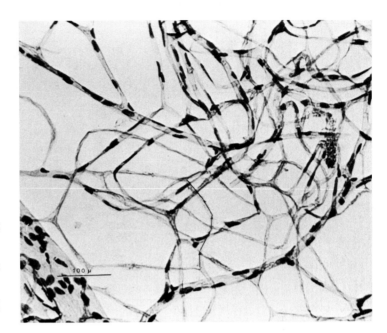

Figure 9-29. A trypsin digest preparation of the retinal vessels from a rat that had diabetes induced by injection of the antibiotic streptozotocin and was then maintained for 18 months without insulin treatment. Note the many capillaries that appear as empty tubes, devoid of cellular nuclei. On a fluorescein angiogram, these vessels would be "nonperfused." (Periodic acid-Schiff stain; original magnification ×400)

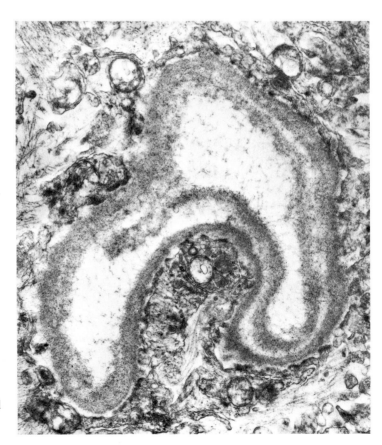

Figure 9-30. Electron micrograph of an acellular capillary from a diabetic rat retina. Note the abnormal appearance of the basement membrane with feathery borders, the empty spaces where cellular elements were present, and the copious surrounding fibrillar collagen.

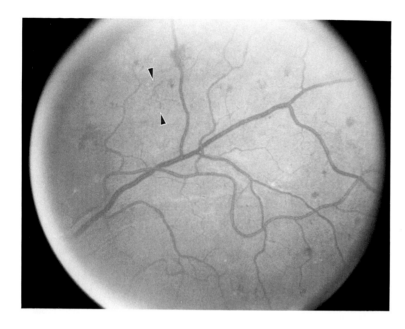

Figure 9-31. Small, dilated vascular sprouts (intraretinal microvascular abnormalities or IRMA) in a diabetic patient *(arrows)*. These probably represent new vessel formation at an early stage in which the vessels are still confined within the retina.

diabetic rats, and they may sometimes occur in older animals without diabetes. The vessels illustrated here were chosen because they provided a particularly photogenic example, and they happened to come from a diabetic rat.)

NEOVASCULARIZATION

Retinal neovascularization has long been a subject of intense interest.[27,46,51,58] Current thinking on the pathogenesis of this lesion is discussed in Chapter 10. I will limit this discussion to a brief description of the development of new blood vessels in the retina. Their earliest appearance may be as tiny, intraretinal loops, often protruding from venules (Fig. 9-31). Because of the controversy over whether these formations were actually intraretinal new vessels or simply dilated pre-existing shunt vessels, the term *intraretinal microvascular abnormalities* (IRMA) was used to describe them.[10] However, in an important clinicopathologic study, DeVenecia and associates showed that vessels that appeared clinically and by fluorescein angiography to be IRMA were, on microscopic examination of the trypsin-digest preparation of the retinal vascular bed, early neovascular networks demonstrating proliferation of endothelial cells.[13] Larger neo-

vascular proliferations may break through the internal limiting membrane of the retina and lie flat on its surface. Since the internal limiting membrane is a collagenous basement membrane, and since there is evidence that proliferating endothelial cells elaborate collagenase activity one can readily understand how the growing vessels can accomplish this.[2,33] Still later, new vessels may arborize on the posterior surface of the vitreous and, as the vitreous retracts, they may be drawn anteriorly into the vitreal cavity.[9] With posterior vitreous detachment the neovascular proliferations may regress.[6] This also happens not infrequently following surgical vitrectomy in diabetic patients. Sometimes, new vessels actually penetrate into the vitreous itself, an occurrence that is somewhat puzzling in view of the current hypothesis that a substance in vitreous inhibits retinal neovascularization.[6] Although accompanying fibrous or glial proliferations usually are not visible with the ophthalmoscope in early retinal neovascularization, they are probably almost universally present at this stage of the disease. Their occurrence late in the course of neovascular proliferation in many retinal diseases is well recognized.[9] Following spontaneous regression of the new vessels or successful photocoagulation the fibroglial scaffolding is all that remains

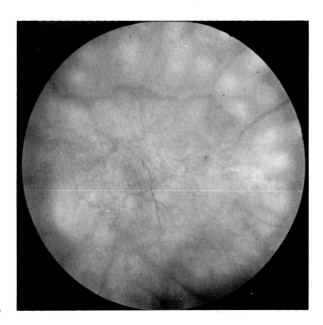

Figure 9-32. Extensive neovascularization on the optic nerve head of a diabetic patient. Argon laser treatment has just been performed.

(Fig. 9-32, 9-33). The traction on the retina caused by this fibroglial tissue may cause disturbances of vision that are often extreme (Fig. 9-34).

The locus of retinal neovascularization is frequently typical of a particular disease process. In diabetic retinopathy new vessels are most common in the posterior retina arising (in descending order of frequency) from the optic nerve head, the superior temporal vessels, the inferior temporal vessels, the nasal vascular arcades, and locations in the retina unassociated wth major branches of the central retinal trunks.[55] In considering the causes of retinal neovascularization in diabetic retinopathy, it may be interesting to speculate on this frequency distribution of the

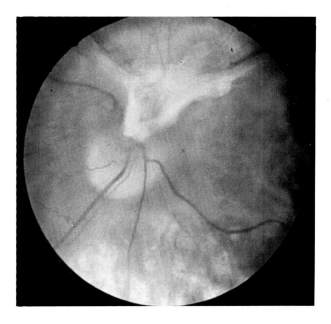

Figure 9-33. The patient shown in Figure 9-32, 6 weeks after laser treatment. The vessels have now completely regressed, and only fibrous tissue remains. Because of its attachment to the retina, however, this tissue exerts traction that has decreased vision.

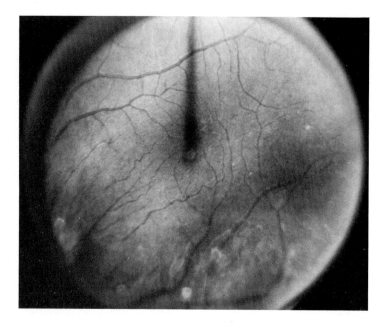

Figure 9-34. Ectopic dislocation of the fovea superiorly in a patient with regressed retrolental fibroplasia and extensive vitreous traction.

lesions. The predilection of retinal neovascularization in proliferative sickle retinopathy and in retinopathy of prematurity (retrolental fibroplasia) for the temporal periphery is well known, and it happens that the two published cases of proliferative retinopathy complicating chronic myelogenous leukemia also had lesions arising in this location.[19,49] The possible reasons for the

location of the vasoproliferative lesions in these locations has been discussed.[19,22,50] Sarcoidosis as well as some other disorders occasionally produce neovascularization in the peripheral retina.[32]

Although the current leading hypothesis holds that retinal hypoxia is a major pathogenic factor in retinal neovascularization, other

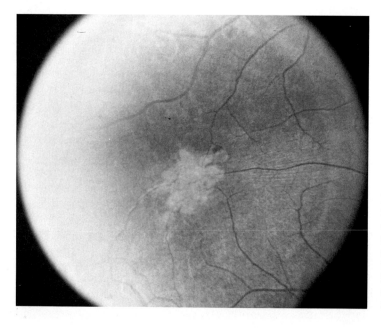

Figure 9-35. A white, cheesy-looking epiretinal mass with vessels extending into it in a 52-year-old man with carcinoma of the breast and skeletal and cerebral metastases. Vision was still 20/20 (6/6) in this eye but reduced with a choroidal metastasis involving the fovea in the fellow eye.

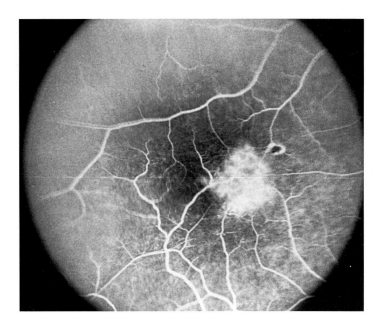

Figure 9-36. A frame from a fluorescein angiogram of the patient shown in Figure 9-35, demonstrating extensive fluorescence due to new vessels in this lesion. This probably represents a retinal metastasis, although we were unable to examine the eyes at autopsy to confirm this clinical impression.

causes may sometimes play a part. Folkman suggested that malignant tumors elaborate an "angiogenesis factor," and it has been demonstrated that when a homologous malignant tumor is implanted in the vitreous of a rabbit in contact with the epiretinal vessels of the visual streak the tumor rapidly becomes vascularized.[10,21] An analogous situation in a human patient, illustrated in Figure 9-35 and 9-36, probably represents a highly vascularized tumor that has metastasized to the retina.[61]

END STAGES

Retinal disease may regress spontaneously at any stage or it may progress to an end stage of severe loss of vision with marked anatomic derangement of the retina. The prognosis varies with the particular disease process. For example, Beetham reported[59] that only about 10 percent of individuals with proliferative diabetic retinopathy undergo spontaneous regression.[3] Although there are no detailed statistics, regression of proliferative sickle retinopathy appears to be more common.[48] Like the highly favorable results of photocoagulation in proliferative diabetic retinopathy, results of a small clinical trial

of photocoagulation in proliferative sickle retinopathy showed a modest benefit from argon laser treatment in reducing vitreous hemorrhage in this disease.[14,31] Xenon arc photocoagulation appears to be somewhat less useful, and both techniques carry a risk of producing choroidovitreal neovascularization. (However, treatment techniques in these two studies differed; proliferative diabetic retinopathy was treated by panretinal scatter photocoagulation using either the argon laser or the xenon arc; proliferative sickle lesions were treated focally, using the feeder vessel technique.) A newer study is investigating the effects of panretinal photocoagulation on proliferative sickle retinopathy.

The most severe end stages of retinal vascular disease are traction detachment of the retina produced by fibroglial bands, neovascular glaucoma produced (it is thought) by an angiogenic substance diffusing forward from the retina to the iris, and marked ischemia of the retinal (and sometimes, choroidal) circulation (Fig. 9-37). By understanding the cellular events that produce the earlier stages of these diseases, we may hope to find methods of preventing them or of treating them before they reach these severely disabling later forms.

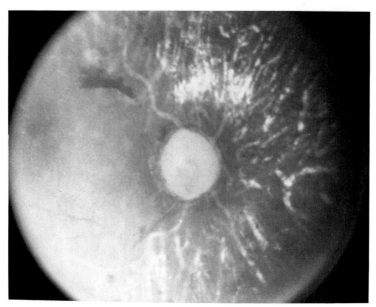

Figure 9-37. Severe ischemia of the retinal and choroidal vessels of a patient who underwent panretinal photocoagulation for rather mild preproliferative diabetic retinopathy with macular edema as a part of the Early Treatment in Diabetic Retinopathy Study (ETDRS). However, rubeosis iridis and neovascular glaucoma appeared despite the apparent mildness of the retinopathy and despite additional photocoagulation. Although the intraocular pressure was not observed to go above 38 mm Hg and was usually in the mid-20s, visual acuity decreased over several weeks to no light perception. Cerebral arteriography revealed bilateral occlusion of the internal carotid arteries, although the patient had no other signs or symptoms of cerebrovascular disease. Note the pale disc, the opacified vessels coming from the disc, and the absence of visible vessels elsewhere.

REFERENCES

1. Addison DJ, Garner A, Ashton N: Degeneration of intramural pericytes in diabetic retinopathy. Br Med J 1:264–266, 1970
2. Ausprunk DH, Folkman J: Migration and proliferation of endothelial cells in preformed and newly formed blood vessels during tumor angiogenesis. Microvasc Res 14:53–65, 1977
3. Beetham WP: Visual prognosis of proliferating diabetic retinopathy. Br J Ophthalmol 47:611–619, 1963
4. The Branch Vein Occlusion Study Group: Argon laser photocoagulation for macular edema in branch vein occlusion. Am J Ophthalmol 98:271–282, 1984
5. The Branch Vein Occlusion Study Group: Argon laser scatter photocoagulation for prevention of neovascularization and vitreous hemorrhage in branch vein occlusion. Arch Ophthalmol 104:34–41, 1986
6. Brem S, Preis I, Langer R, et al: Inhibition of neovascularization by an extract derived from vitreous. Am J Ophthalmol 84:323–328, 1977
7. Cogan DG, Toussaint D, Kuwabara T: Retinal vascular patterns. IV. Diabetic retinopathy. Arch Ophthalmol 66:366–378, 1961
8. Cunha-Vaz JG: Vitreous fluorophotometry. In Cunha-Vaz JG (ed): The Blood-Retinal Barriers, pp 195–210. New York, Plenum Press, 1980
9. Davis MD: Vitreous contraction in proliferative diabetic retinopathy. Arch Ophthalmol 74:741–751, 1965
10. Davis MD, Norton EWD, Myers FL: The Airlie classification of diabetic retinopathy. In Goldberg MF, Fine SL, (eds): Symposium on the Treatment of Diabetic Retinopathy, pp 7–22. USPHS Publication No 1890. Washington: US Government Printing Office, 1969
11. Deutman AF, Pinckers AJLG, Aan de Kerk AL: Dominantly inherited cystoid macular edema. Am J Ophthalmol 82:540–548, 1976

12. DeVenecia G, Davis MD: Histology and fluorescein angiography of microaneurysms in diabetes mellitus. Invest Ophthalmol 6:555, 1967
13. Devenecia G, Davis M, Engerman R: Clinicopathologic correlations in diabetic retinopathy. I. Histology and fluorescein angiography of microaneurysms. Arch Ophthalmol 94:1766–1773, 1976
14. The Diabetic Retinopathy Study Research Group: Photocoagulation treatment of proliferative diabetic retinopathy. Ophthalmology 88:583–600, 1981
15. Duke JB, Wilkinson CP, Sigelman S: Retinal microaneurysms in leukemia. Br J Ophthalmol 52:368–374, 1968
16. Essner E, Pino RM, Griewski RA: Breakdown of blood retinal barrier in RCS rats with inherited retinal degeneration. Lab Invest 43:418–426, 1980
17. Feke GT, Riva C: Laser Doppler measurements of blood velocity in human retinal vessels. J Opt Soc Amer 68:526–531, 1978
18. Finkelstein D, Brem S, Patz A, et al: Experimental retinal neovascularization induced by intravitreal tumors. Am J Ophthalmol 83:660–664, 1977
19. Frank RN, Ryan SJ Jr.: Peripheral retinal neovascularization with chronic myelogenous leukemia. Arch Ophthalmol 87:585–589, 1972
20. Frank KW, Weiss H: Unusual clinical and histopathological findings in ocular sarcoidosis. Br J Ophthalmol 67:8–16, 1981
21. Folkman J: The vascularization of tumors. Sci Amer 234:58–73, 1976
22. Goldberg MF: Classification and pathogenesis of proliferative sickle retinopathy. Am J Ophthalmol 71:649–665, 1971
23. Grimes PA, Laties AM: Early morphological alteration of the pigment epithelium in streptozotocin-induced diabetes: Increased surface area of the basal cell membrane. Exp Eye Res 30:631–640, 1980
24. Gutman FA, Zegarra H: The natural course of temporal retinal branch vein occlusion. Trans Am Acad Ophthalmol Otolaryngol 78:OP-178–OP-192, 1974
25. Hamilton AM, Kohner EM, Rosen D, Bowbyes JA: Experimental retinal venous occlusion. Proc Roy Soc Med 67:1045–1048, 1974
26. Hayreh SS: So-called central retinal vein occlusion. II. Venous stasis retinopathy. Ophthalmologica 172:14–37, 1976
27. Hayreh SS, Hayreh MS: Hemiretinal central retinal vein occlusion. Arch Ophthalmol 98:1600–1609, 1980
28. Henkind P: Ocular neovascularization. Am J Ophthalmol 85:287–301, 1978
29. Henkind P, Wise GN: Retinal neovascularization, collaterals, vascular shunts. Br J Ophthalmol 58:413–422, 1974
30. Jaffe NS, Clayman HM, Jaffe MS: Cystoid macular edema following intracapsular and extracapsular cataract extractions with and without an intraocular lens. Ophthalmology, 89:25–29, 1982
31. Jampol LM, Condon P, Farber M, et al: A randomized clinical trial of feeder vessel photocoagulation of proliferative sickle cell retinopathy. Ophthalmology 90:540–545, 1983
32. Jampol LM, Goldbaum MH: Peripheral proliferative retinopathies. Surv Ophthalmol 25:1–14, 1980
33. Kalebic J, Garbisa S, Glaser B, Liotta LA: Basement membrane collagen: Degradation by migrating endothelial cells. Science 221:281–283, 1983
34. King RC, Dobree JA, Kok D'A, et al: Exudative diabetic retinopathy: Spontaneous changes and effects of a corn oil diet. Br J Ophthalmol 47:666–672, 1963
35. Kirber WM, Nichols CW, Grimes PA, et al: A permeability defect of the retinal pigment epithelium. Arch Ophthalmol 98:725–728, 1980
36. Kohner EM, Cappin JM: Do medical conditions have an influence on central retinal vein occlusion? Proc Roy Soc Med 67:1052–1054, 1974
37. Kohner EM, Hamilton AM, Saunders SJ, et al: The retinal blood flow in diabetes. Diabetologia 11:27–33, 1975
38. Kohner EM, Henkind P: Correlation of the fluorescein angiogram and retinal digest in diabetic retinopathy. Am J Ophthalmol 69:403–414, 1970
39. Kohner EM, Pettit JE, Hamilton AM, et al: Streptokinase in central retinal vein occlusion: a controlled clinical trial. Br Med J 1:550–553, 1976
40. Kraff MC, Sanders DR, Jampol LM et al: Prophylaxis of pseudophakic cystoid macular edema with topical indomethacin. Ophthalmology 89:885–890, 1982
41. Kuwabara T, Carroll JM, Cogan DG: Studies of retinal vascular pattern III. Age, hypertension, absolute glaucoma, injury. Arch Ophthalmol 65:708–716, 1961
42. McCormick BH, Read JS, Borouec RT, et al: Image processing in television ophthalmoscopy. In Preston K, Onoe E (eds): Digital Processing of Biomedical Images, pp 399–415. New York, Plenum Press, 1976
43. McMillan DE: Plasma protein changes, blood viscosity, and diabetic microangiopathy. Diabetes 25:858–864, 1976
44. Magargal LE, Donoso LA, Sanborn GE: Retinal ischemia and risk of neovascularization following central retinal vein occlusion. Ophthalmology 89:1241–1245, 1982
45. May DR, Klein ML, Peyman GA: A prospective study of xenon arc photocoagulation for central

retinal vein occlusion. Br J Ophthalmol 60:816–818, 1976

46. Michaelson IC: The mode of development of the retinal vessels and some observations of its significance in certain retinal diseases. Trans Ophthalmol Soc UK 68:137–180, 1948

47. Michels RG, Gass JDM: The natural course of retinal branch vein obstruction. Trans Am Acad Ophthalmol Otolaryngol 78:OP-166–OP-177, 1974

48. Nagpal KC, Patrianakos D, Asdourian GK, et al: Spontaneous regression (autoinfarction) of proliferative sickle retinopathy. Am J Ophthalmol 80:885–892, 1975

49. Morse PH, McCready JL: Peripheral retinal neovascularization in chronic myelocytic leukemia. Am J Ophthalmol 72:975–978, 1971

50. Patz A: The role of oxygen in retrolental fibroplasia. Trans Am Ophthalmol Soc 66:940–985, 1968

51. Patz A: Studies on retinal neovascularization. Invest Ophthalmol Vis Sci 19:1133–1138, 1980

52. Riva CE, Petrig B: Blue field entoptic phenomenon and blood velocity in the retinal capillaries. J Opt Soc Amer 70:1234–1238, 1980

53. Speiser P, Gittelsohn AM, Patz A: Studies on diabetic retinopathy III. Influence of diabetes on intramural pericytes. Arch Ophthalmol 80:332–337, 1968

51. Stelson KA, Blackshear PL, Jr, Wirtschafter JD: On the tortuosity of the veins of the retina. Microvasc Res 26:126–128, 1983

55. Taylor E, Dobree JH: Proliferative diabetic retinopathy. Site and size of the initial lesions. Br J Ophthalmol 54:11–18, 1970

56. Wallow IHL, Engerman RL: Permeability and patency of retinal blood vessels in experimental diabetes. Invest Ophthalmol 16:447–461, 1977

57. Wallow IHL, Geldner DS: Endothelial fenestrae in proliferative diabetic retinopathy. Invest Ophthalmol Vis Sci 19:1176–1183, 1980

58. Wise GN: Retinal neovascularization. Trans Am Ophthalmol Soc 54:729–826, 1956

59. Wise GN, Dollery CT, Henkind P: The Retinal Circulation, pp 236–238; 492–493. New York, Harper & Row, 1971

60. Yanoff M: Diabetic retinopathy. N Engl J Med 274:1344–1349, 1966

61. Young SE, Cruciger M, Lukeman J: Metastatic carcinoma to the retina: Case report. Ophthalmology 86:1350–1354, 1979

10

Studies in Diabetic Retinopathy

Robert N. Frank

Thanks to new developments in clinical ophthalmology and in basic laboratory research, our knowledge of diabetic retinopathy has advanced considerably in the last few years. Although it would have seemed presumptuous not long ago, we can now propose reasonable hypotheses about the pathogenesis of this common, often terribly disabling, but also puzzling and fascinating disease. Like any scientific hypotheses, they will have value only if they meet certain criteria. First, they must explain the clinical and laboratory observations that have been made and confirmed by skilled observers over the years. Second, they must advance the state of research by suggesting experiments to confirm or deny the hypotheses. Third, they may suggest therapeutic or preventive measures that we may employ to the benefit of our patients.

The following observations are particularly relevant to the pathogenetic mechanisms I wish to propose.

Diabetic retinopathy is observed only in patients with diabetes mellitus; its prevalence increases with the duration of the systemic disease.

The laboratory research at the Kresge Eye Institute cited in this chapter has been supported by grants RO1 EY-01857 and EY-02566 from the National Eye Institute, and by grants from the Juvenile Diabetes Foundation. The author is indebted to Dr. Karni W. Frank for her many useful discussions of this work, and to Gail Keirn, Richard Keirn, Alexander Kennedy, Janet Khoury, Michael Mancini, Kevin Mikus, and Ann Randolph for their valuable assistance in the laboratory.

This apparently self-evident statement has, in fact, been questioned by several investigators. There have been descriptions of so-called diabetic retinopathy in nondiabetic individuals, some of whom have diabetic parents or siblings.[52,73] These reports have been criticized, and I believe that the burden of proof still rests with those who claim that they have seen diabetic retinopathy in a nondiabetic subject.[24] In an ongoing clinical study my colleagues and I performed fundus photography and fluorescein angiography according to the protocol established by the nationwide Diabetic Retinopathy Study.[36,37] Our study populations were 173 diabetic children and adolescents ranging in age from 6 to 21 years and 75 normal children of comparable age, race, and sex distribution, most of whom were siblings of the diabetic patients. The photographic and angiographic studies were evaluated independently by five ophthalmologists subspecializing in retinal disease, and who were masked to the names and diagnoses of the subjects. We determined that retinopathy was present if three of the five readers judged the photograph, the angiogram, or both, to be positive. None of the control children showed signs of retinopathy. In fact, the agreement among the five observers on this point was impressive. This statement still leaves room for argument, for instance, by someone who claims that there is a gene for retinopathy that is closely linked to that for diabetes but may on rare occasions segregate independently. To disprove the hypothesis of a purely genetic basis for diabetic retinopathy at this time would require evaluating an impossi-

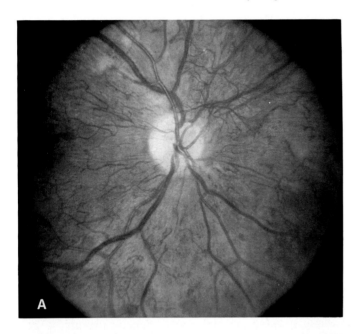

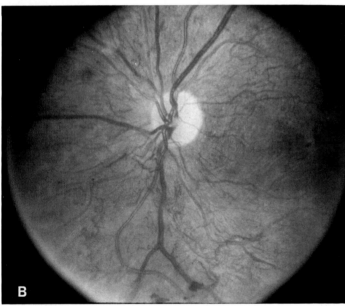

Figure 10-1. This 19-year-old girl had extremely brittle, insulin-dependent diabetes mellitus, growth failure, delayed puberty, and fatty liver (Mauriac syndrome). After she was brought under rigorous blood-sugar control she was noted rapidly to develop severe proliferative retinopathy in both eyes. A single field of each eye is shown, demonstrating extensive flat neovascular proliferations. One episode of argon laser photocoagulation was carried out, but the patient did not return for follow-up. This patient was one of a series described in detail by Daneman et al.[47]

bly large number of nondiabetic subjects for the presence of diabetic retinopathy. While the hypothesis cannot yet be absolutely refuted, I think that it is unlikely to be true.

A number of studies indicate that, at least in juvenile-onset diabetic subjects, retinopathy is infrequent during the early years of the disease, but becomes increasingly prevalent with longer duration.[12,70,101] More recently, this has been confirmed using standardized, stereoscopic fundus photography and fluorescein angiography in addition to the usual ophthalmoscopic examination to detect retinopathy.[29,36,37,65,84,95] There has also been strong disagreement with this conclusion by several investigators who claim that when fluorescein angiography is used for diagnosis, 50% or more of children with diabetes of less than 5 years' duration—often with less than 1 year's duration—show evidence of retinopathy.[9,10,77] Failure to use stereoscopic photography or angiography, and lack of evidence of observer masking are serious flaws in these studies. Our own results, and those of Palmberg and coworkers and of Klein and associates agree that there is virtually no retinopathy within 5 years of the diagnosis of insulin-dependent diabetes in children and adolescents, a sharp increase in prevalence between years 5 and 9, and a prevalence of 60% to 80% at year 10 and beyond.[36,37,65,84] The effect of diabetes duration on the development of retinopathy is consistent with (though it does not prove) the hypothesis that hyperglycemia is critical for the development of diabetic retinopathy.

Age and diabetes duration influence the prevalence of diabetic retinopathy, and severe retinopathy is more prevalent in young men than in young women. Palmberg's, Klein's, and our group each found that the duration of the diabetes and the age of the patient correlated with the presence of retinopathy.[36,66,84] There was little retinopathy prior to the mid-teen years, approximately the time of puberty. In a much smaller study, Nanda and coworkers demonstrated this point directly by showing that retinopathy was rare before puberty and increased in frequency after puberty, regardless of diabetes duration.[81] This observation suggests that hormonal influences may be important for the development of diabetic retinopathy, including, perhaps, growth hormone, the somatomedins (or insulinlike growth factors), and the sex hormones. Several other results bear on this point. First, while the earliest stages of retinopathy in young, insulin-dependent diabetic subjects are equally prevalent in males and females, proliferative retinopathy develops significantly more frequently in males.[6,30,36,37,65] Moreover, blindness from diabetic retinopathy occurs much more frequently in males than in females before the age of 45 (approximately the age of menopause), but equally in the two sexes thereafter.[107] Also, in three cases of the Mauriac syndrome (a disorder of extremely brittle insulin-dependent diabetes, delayed growth and pubescence, and an enlarged, fatty liver), no retinopathy was observed prior to the establishment of excellent blood glucose control. Once such control was achieved, physical growth and puberty occurred; in addition, florid diabetic retinopathy developed (Fig. 10-1).[23] These cases suggest that one or more of the hormones newly released in quantity to initiate the delayed adolescent development may also have stimulated retinal vasoproliferation. A recent study that appears to have bearing on this same point indicates that in young, Type-I (insulin-dependent) diabetic subjects, plasma levels of insulinlike growth factor I (somatomedin C) are elevated in persons with proliferative retinopathy.[79] Since the insulinlike growth factors are released by the action of growth hormone, it would appear that several hormones may be closely connected to the development of at least certain stages of retinopathy.

Diabetic retinopathy is primarily a disease of the posterior portion of the retina. The location of the vascular lesions in different types of retinal blood vessel diseases is a clue to their pathogenesis. In diabetic retinopathy, most of the abnormalities are clustered around the posterior pole of the eye, within a few disc diameters of the optic nerve head and the macula.* This is a unique situation. Among other retinal vascular diseases, for example, sickle-cell retinopathy and retrolental fibroplasia predominantly affect the temporal periphery. Retinal vein occlusions demonstrate capillary abnormalities and neovascularization in the circulatory bed distal to the occlusion. Retinal vasculitides and blood dyscrasias may demonstrate diffuse involvement.

* Some recent work using fluorescein angiographic surveys of large areas of the fundus has suggested that many diabetic subjects may have extensive capillary nonperfusion in the midperipheral retina.[89] Although I have not performed similar angiographic studies, I believe that it is possible to suspect such extensive areas of nonperfusion clinically, using indirect ophthalmoscopy, by the presence of multiple blot hemorrhages or cotton wool spots. I have not observed such lesions in the midperipheral retina early in diabetic retinopathy, and even in more advanced cases, the most severe involvement, in my experience, is virtually always seen posteriorly. I therefore cannot explain the cases presented by Shimizu's group in the context of my own observations and will await with interest the appearance of more such cases, perhaps from other countries. Could this represent an unusual diabetic retinopathy syndrome?

What is special about the posterior retina? In humans, its major portion is the highly specialized macula, with a large proportion of cone receptors and multiple layers of ganglion cells. The retina is a tissue with tremendous metabolic activity. The German biochemist Otto Warburg demonstrated in the 1920s that the retina has an extremely high oxygen consumption, and later work has shown it to be higher per unit weight than any other tissue in the body, including the cerebral cortex.[98,100] The retinas used in these experiments were from species lacking a specialized macula or area centralis. No one has compared the metabolic activities of different areas of human retina, but it would not be surprising if the macula were much more active in terms of oxygen or glucose consumption or carbon dioxide production than other portions of the neural retina. The glucose metabolism of most cells of the retina (unlike muscle cells or adipose tissue) is not sensitive to insulin.[17] (An exception appears to be the cells of the retinal blood vessels themselves. This point will be discussed below.) Therefore, at least up to the point at which the various enzyme systems that use glucose are saturated, the more glucose that is available, the greater will be the metabolic activity of the tissue and the greater the requirement for oxygen. It may well be this increased metabolic activity in the diabetic macula during the frequent periods of hyperglycemia coupled with the increased oxygen requirement that provides the biochemical basis for diabetic retinopathy.

In general, the development and progression of diabetic retinopathy is associated with poor control of blood glucose levels. However, there are outstanding exceptions in the experience of most clinicians. I recognize that this is a controversial point, although I suspect that if a poll were taken of clinicians involved in the care of diabetic patients, far more would argue the value of good control than would oppose it. Certainly, none of the many studies on this point is flawless.[67] At least until recently there was no rigorous definition of good control that satisfied all critics. The sheer bulk of the studies and expert opinion in support of the argument that good control is the cornerstone of management of the diabetic patient is impressive. The references cited here are only a few of those that concern themselves with this controversy.[16,32,53,55,90,102] Nevertheless some of them, in particular Engerman's study of diabetic dogs, make impressive reading.[32]

Conversely, there are some strong arguments that can be used in rebuttal. How, for example, can one account for the patients with apparently good diabetic control who develop severe retinopathy or other complications while others whose control is obviously poor seem to escape difficulty? It is now widely accepted that the concentration of glycosylated hemoglobins, in particular hemoglobin A_{1C}, expressed as a fraction of the total hemoglobin concentration, reliably estimates the integrated blood glucose level in an individual over the preceding 4 to 8 weeks.[11,44,68] Periodic measurements of glycosylated hemoglobin levels may, therefore, be a better monitor of long-term control in the diabetic patient than sporadic blood or urine glucose determinations. There are now three reports indicating that, if patients with diabetes of long duration are separated into groups according to the presence and severity of retinopathy, the glycosylated hemoglobin concentrations in all groups are substantially higher than those in comparable controls but do not differ one from another.[20,76,88] This might indicate that control of blood sugar in the diabetic has no influence on the development of retinopathy. By contrast, a recent study by Rand and coworkers strongly correlates elevated glycosylated hemoglobin levels and severity of retinopathy in insulin-dependent diabetics.[86] A second paper from the same group suggests that development of proliferative retinopathy in insulin-dependent diabetics is correlated with recent poor blood-glucose control but not with poor control in the first 5 years of diabetes.[71]

To account for those patients whose severe complications (or lack of same) seem at odds with their blood glucose control, I suggest that there are other genetic factors at work. To give a hypothetical example, we know that in diabetic and galactosemic animals (and, presumably, in humans), cataracts develop as a result of the accumulation of sugar alcohols in the lens cells, resulting from the action of the enzyme aldose reductase.[40,41,64] This enzyme has a low affinity for glucose, hence, in normoglycemic individuals, it has a minimal metabolic effect. Only when the blood (and aqueous humor) glucose concentrations are sufficiently elevated to saturate the normal pathways of glucose metabolism, whose activity in lens cells is very low, will aldose reductase produce substantial amounts of sorbitol, the sugar alcohol of glucose. To make matters more complicated, aldose reductase requires as a cofactor the reduced form of nicotinamide adenine dinucleotide phosphate (NADPH, formerly called TPNH). This is produced largely by the pentose shunt pathway, one of the alternate pathways of glucose metabolism. If this pathway is relatively inactive in a tissue, the NADPH concentration will be low, and the aldose reductase system will be less effective. Hence, diabetic cataract formation is a good example of a complication of diabetes that requires hyperglycemia but whose development can be hindered (or accelerated) by variations in the activity of several enzymes or metabolic pathways, each of which is presumably controlled by genetic loci separate from those that control the development of diabetes mellitus itself. An individual with low or absent aldose-reductase activity, or whose pentose shunt is inactive, will not develop diabetic cataracts no matter how poor is his diabetic control. We have investigated this point with regard to the enzyme glucose-6-phosphate dehydrogenase (G6PD), the first enzyme in the pentose shunt pathway. G6PD deficiency is relatively common, particularly in black males, in whom it has a prevalence of roughly 10% to 15% of the population. These men (who have the so-called A-variant of G6PD deficiency) have only a mild enzyme defect. More severe variants, such as the chronic hemolytic and the Mediterranean types, have almost no G6PD activity in their erythrocytes or somatic cells.

We have incubated cultured skin fibroblasts from individuals with the A- and Mediterranean variants of G6PD deficiency in media enriched in glucose and galactose. In high-glucose media the sorbitol levels in cells were no different from those of normal controls, probably because, in fibroblasts, aldose-reductase activity is low, the intracellular hexose levels are regulated by a membrane pump, and the small amounts of sorbitol produced are oxidized to fructose by the enzyme sorbitol dehydrogenase. However, in high-galactose media, fibroblasts from individuals with the Mediterranean variety of G6PD deficiency accumulated significantly less galactitol (the sugar alcohol of galactose) than did those of the control subjects or those with the A-variant of the disorder. We interpret this to mean that severe G6PD deficiency protects against excessive sugar alcohol accumulation produced by aldose reductase by sharply reducing the amount of NADPH required for aldose reductase activity.[60] Because individuals with the A-variant do not have severe G6PD deficiency, and because NADPH levels must be very low to reduce aldose reductase activity (the Michaelis constant, or K_m, for NADPH for bovine-lens aldose reductase is $10^{-6}M$),[50] these individuals are not similarly protected.

These experiments provide a model for the biochemical pathogenesis of complications of diabetes caused by the interaction of hyperglycemia (or an analog, galactosemia) and a particular enzyme system, the "sorbitol pathway." Similar models might be developed for other biochemical systems that might be responsible for the production of retinopathy and other complications of diabetes.

The most important point of this discussion is that all of these enzyme pathways will not lead to vascular complications in normoglycemic individuals. Thus, we may hypothesize that poor blood glucose control is the critical factor in the development of the late complications of diabetes but that some individuals may be more susceptible to these complications and some less so, based on independent genetic determinants of the activity of certain critical biochemical pathways.

The conflicting results using either blood-glucose measurements or glycosylated hemoglobin data to evaluate the influence of blood glucose control on diabetic retinopathy may simply reflect the fact that all of these studies are *retrospective.*[20,70,76,86,88] That is, patients who already had long-term diabetes and retinopathy (or lack of same) then had a single glycosylated-hemoglobin determination, which was correlated with the diabetic complication whose presence or absence was already known. Alternatively, individuals with a known retinopathy status were evaluated with reference to a series of recent blood-glucose determinations. A single glycosylated-hemoglobin determination measures, at best, the average blood-glucose levels for the past *2 months,* but what we really need to know are the average levels for at least the past *5 years or more,* the minimum duration of diabetes required for the onset of retinopathy in insulin-dependent, juvenile-onset subjects.[36,37,65,84] To obtain these figures and relate them meaningfully to diabetic retinopathy or other complications of diabetes will require long-term prospective studies of blood-glucose control and the development of retinopathy and other complications of diabetes in much larger populations. One such study, the Diabetes Control and Complications Trial (DCCT) sponsored by the U.S. National Institute of Diabetes, Digestive Diseases, and Kidney (NIDDK) and involving 27 institutions in the United States and Canada, is currently (1987) in its recruiting phase.

An early histopathologic finding in diabetic retinopathy is loss of intramural pericytes from the retinal capillaries with relative preservation of the endothelial cells. This observation has been well documented and is the most nearly pathognomonic anatomic abnormality in diabetic retinopathy.[1,18,91,105] It clearly implies that there is a specific defect, presumably biochemical, that affects the pericytes but not the endothelial cells. What are the metabolic and functional differences between these two types of cells? Is the defect that results in pericyte loss intrinsic to the pericyte, or does it result from metabolic disturbances in the surrounding neuronal and glial elements of the retina? What is the functional result of pericyte loss? Since the development of a system for growing retinal capillary cells in tissue culture, we have been investigating the properties of these cells in several ways.[13] The cells that we were initially able to culture appeared to be pericytes, but there is now evidence that one can also culture well-differentiated retinal microvessel endothelial cells.[7,15,39,42] Hence, it should be possible to study the biochemical properties of endothelial cells as well as of pericytes in isolation. Our biochemical investigations thus far have involved, in part, studies of aldose reductase and of the

overall activities of the glycolytic and pentose-shunt pathways in retinal microvessel fragments and in cultured retinal microvessel cells.[14,59] In addition, we have studied extracellular matrix macromolecules secreted by these cells in culture.[57,58] We have been able to show that an aldose reductase-like activity is present in the cultured pericytes and endothelial cells, not only by direct assay, but also because the cells accumulate sorbitol or galactitol in excess when they are incubated for 3 to 5 weeks in the presence of a fivefold increase in the glucose or galactose concentrations.[14,59] When we assay isolated calf retinal microvessels quantitatively for aldose reductase we find activity, although the kinetic constants suggest that both aldose reductase and a similar enzyme, L-hexonate dehydrogenase, are present together.[40,41] A puzzling finding is that the aldose reductaselike activity measured in freshly isolated retinal microvessels is no different from that in cerebral microvessels, and that measured in cultured retinal pericytes is indistinguishable from that in retinal endothelial cells.[59] Since the microvascular complications of diabetes have been observed in the human retinal, but not in the cerebral, microcirculation a simple relationship of aldose reductaselike activity to diabetic retinopathy does not appear to be present.[25]

Also puzzling is the failure of some investigators to find any aldose reductase, immunocytochemically, in retinal microvessels of rat or dog, while others have recently reported its presence exclusively in the pericytes of the human retinal microcirculation.[2,61,75] I cannot explain these results. One possibility is that there are several enzymes, collectively known as aldehyde reductases that may have similar activities, but are immunologically distinct.[21] These enzymes may also be inhibited by similar drugs in which case they would all respond to identical pharmacologic methods to prevent the complications of diabetes.[92]

Should aldose-reductase activity, and sugar alcohol accumulation, be responsible all or in part for the production of diabetic retinopathy, its mechanism of action is unclear. The production of so-called sugar cataracts in diabetic and galactosemic animals is related to osmotic decompensation of the lens epithelial cells due to sugar-alcohol accumulation. The sorbitol pathway also appears to have an important role in the production of diabetic autonomic and sensory neuropathy in humans but this may not involve an osmotic mechanism, since it is not clear that the Schwann cells of peripheral nerve (where the aldose reductase is located) accumulate osmotically damaging sugar alcohol concentrations in diabetes or galactosemia.[54,56,106]

Recently, we and also Robison and coworkers have noted dramatic thickening, as well as pathologic degeneration, of retinal capillary basement membranes in rats fed a 30 percent galactose diet for prolonged periods (Fig. 10-2).[38,87] The abnormalities did not occur in animals that also received the aldose-reductase inhibitor Sorbinil (Pfizer). Although glucose and galactose are both involved in several aspects of the biosynthesis of basement-membrane macromolecules, their sugar alcohols do not appear to have a direct role in these processes. So further studies of the biochemistry of retinal-capillary basement-membrane synthesis and degradation and of the role of the sorbitol pathway in this process must be conducted. We have recently demonstrated that isolated retinal microvessel basement membranes contain collagen Types I and IV, and that cultured retinal pericytes and endothelial cells synthesize the same collagen types.[58] Also, these cell types are capable of synthesizing heparan sulfate and chondroitin sulfate.[57] Thus, it would appear that our cell culture system is quite suitable for studying the physiology and pathology of retinal-capillary basement-membrane production.

Other evidence suggesting an important role for the sorbitol pathway in the production of diabetic retinopathy has been suggested by Kern and Engerman.[33] In two nondiabetic dogs maintained for 5 years on a diet containing 30

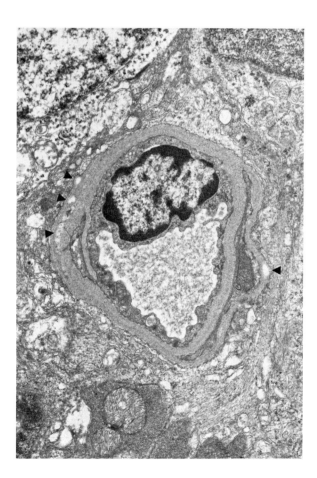

Figure 10-2. Electron micrograph of a retinal capillary from a rat that had received a diet containing 30 percent (by weight) galactose for 21 months before sacrifice. The rat was nondiabetic. Note marked thickening of the capillary basement membrane and the Swiss-cheese vacuolizations *(arrows)*. (Original magnification ×18,000)

percent galactose, they found typical capillary microaneurysms, pericyte loss, and acellular capillaries, all typical lesions of diabetic retinopathy. The role of the sorbitol pathway in this animal model is not clearly established, however, because as yet there have been no animals on the galactose diet, together with an aldose reductase inhibitor to demonstrate that the diabeticlike lesions can be prevented by this regimen.

Another way in which retinal pericytes might be disturbed initially by diabetes has been suggested by King and coworkers.[63] These investigators have reported that cultured retinal pericytes have specific cell membrane receptors for insulin and a specific requirement for insulin, which may be present at very low (nanomolar) concentrations, for proliferation in culture. Retinal endothelial cells, as well as aortic smooth-muscle and endothelial cells, do not have such a requirement. Moreover, although an effect of insulin on membrane transport of glucose and other sugars has not been demonstrated in pericytes, King's group have shown that insulin stimulates the incorporation of glucose into glycogen in these cells.[63] However, when pericytes are cultured in high-glucose medium, their rate of proliferation is depressed.[62,72] While these results are of great interest, their relationship to

diabetic retinopathy is still unclear. Beyond fetal life in humans and the neonatal period in some animals, the cells of the retinal microvessels are an extremely stable population, only rarely demonstrating cell division.[34,104] It is not easy to see how to apply these experimental results on cell proliferation *in vitro* to the properties of nonproliferating cells *in vivo.*

The new blood vessels that form in proliferative diabetic retinopathy are most frequently associated with the venous side of the circulation. They occur more commonly in younger patients with juvenile-onset diabetes, while individuals with maturity-onset disease often lose vision from background retinopathy. There is now good clinical evidence that retinal hypoxia is a stimulus to retinal neovascularization. The suggestion that hypoxia is a major factor in the development of retinal new vessels was first made some years ago and has subsequently been emphasized by several authors.[45,51,69,80,103] An argument frequently heard in support of the hypoxic theory is that neovascularization often occurs at the borders of ischemic areas of the retina, as demonstrated by fluorescein angiograms in a number of retinal vascular diseases, including diabetic retinopathy, sickle cell retinopathy, and retinal vein occlusions. (Fig. 10-3, 10-4, 10-5). Not so frequently pointed out, but

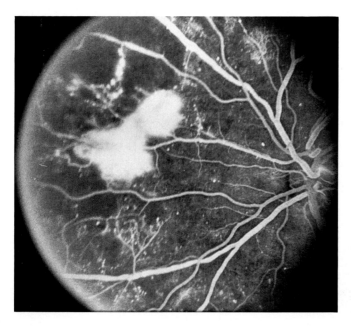

Figure 10-3. A frame from a fluorescein angiogram of a 30-year-old woman with long-standing insulin-dependent diabetes mellitus. Note the neovascular tuft, demonstrated by profuse fluorescein leakage forming at the edge of a zone of capillary nonperfusion, which appears black.

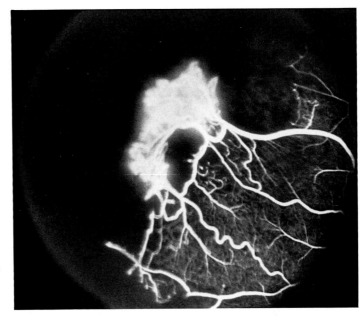

Figure 10-4. Frame from a fluorescein angiogram of the peripheral retina of a 32-year-old woman with hemoglobin SC disease and proliferative sickle retinopathy. Note the abrupt border between perfused and nonperfused retina, with the neovascular tuft occurring at the border zone.

in my view equally important, is the converse: that in retinal areas that are adequately oxygenated from other sources capillaries do not grow. For example, trypsin-digest preparations of the human retinal vascular bed demonstrate an avascular zone alongside the retinal arteries and arterioles, but none on the venous side of the vascular network.[104] Retinal vessels in humans are normally found only in the inner layers of the retina, never external to the inner nuclear layer, probably because oxygen that penetrates from the choroidal circulation is sufficient to supply the cells of the outer retina as far as this level. The foveal avascular zone probably exists for the same reason: the only cells present in the fovea are photoreceptors, which receive suffi-

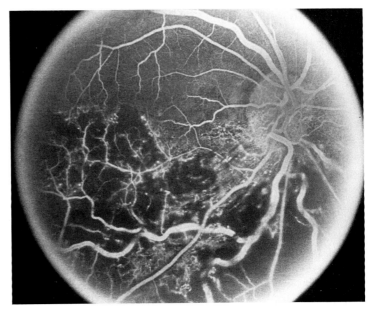

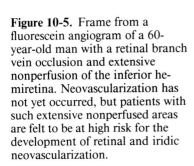

Figure 10-5. Frame from a fluorescein angiogram of a 60-year-old man with a retinal branch vein occlusion and extensive nonperfusion of the inferior hemiretina. Neovascularization has not yet occurred, but patients with such extensive nonperfused areas are felt to be at high risk for the development of retinal and iridic neovascularization.

cient oxygen from the choriocapillaris and do not need the retinal vascular supply.

The pathogenesis of retinal neovascularization in diabetes mellitus, then, may well be as follows. The primary metabolic disease, most likely acting through biochemical abnormalities in the posterior retina resulting from chronic hyperglycemia, damages the cells of the retinal capillaries. When there has been sufficient damage, capillaries in large areas of the retina can no longer carry blood, and these areas become hypoxic, being supplied only minimally by diffusion of oxygen laterally from retinal areas that have an adequate oxygen supply. The hypoxic retina sends out a signal, whose chemical nature is still unknown, that initiates neovascularization. Since hypoxia is the major stimulus for new vessel formation, it is reasonable that the venous side of the circulation, where the oxygen tension is lowest, will be the most severely affected.[94]

Hypoxia need not be the only factor to influence retinal neovascularization. There are a variety of hormones and other circulating factors, some of which may be produced locally in the retina and some at more distant sites, that may act independently of hypoxia, or they may have an additive effect. Hypophysectomy is now used by only a few institutions to treat proliferative diabetic retinopathy, and its efficacy has never been convincingly demonstrated. However, there have been a sufficient number of favorable observations on hypophysectomy in proliferative diabetic retinopathy to suggest that there probably is some beneficial effect of this treatment. This indicates that some factor produced in the pituitary may stimulate vascular growth in the retinas of certain diabetic individuals. The possibility that somatotropin (growth hormone) is the responsible agent has been suggested by others, and I have already presented evidence suggesting a role for the insulinlike growth factors (somatomedins), which are polypeptides released from liver through the action of growth hormone. Still another polypeptide that has been isolated from the bovine pituitary and that is capable of stimulating endothelial cell proliferation in culture has been called *fibroblast growth factor.*[46-49] Other agents may also be important, such as prostaglandins and

cyclic nucleotides.[5,97] Finally, particular interest has recently arisen from the report of a factor (presumably a polypeptide) extractable from bovine retina in aqueous medium that stimulates proliferation of cultured aortic endothelial cells.[22,43] It appears likely that this "retinal-derived growth factor" is a form of fibroblast growth factor. The demonstration of a biological role for this substance will require showing that it can stimulate proliferation of retinal microvessel cells as well as those from aortic endothelium. It is perplexing that such a substance should be present in normal adult retina, whose microvascular cells normally demonstrate so little tendency to proliferate.

The possible role of hormonal agents and the importance of the extremely high rates of glucose and of oxygen utilization in the posterior retina may help to explain why proliferative diabetic retinopathy is more common in younger diabetic patients than in those with maturity-onset disease. The activity of many biochemical pathways tends to decline with age, and it is possible, too, that appropriate hormonal agents are produced in lower concentrations. Alternatively, the target tissues, the cells of the retinal capillaries, may become less responsive to these stimuli with increasing age. (In the same way, cells from fetuses and from younger animals proliferate much more rapidly in tissue culture than do those from older creatures.) Conversely, changes in the metabolism of the retinal microvasculature with age may explain the increasing incidence of diabetic macular edema in the older diabetic population.

Photocoagulation by the so-called panretinal technique of multiple burns throughout the fundus is often effective in arresting proliferative diabetic retinopathy. Photocoagulation of macular edema using small, focal laser burns to leaking microvessels or microaneurysms is also successful in slowing the progress of this complication. The favorable results of the U.S. Diabetic Retinopathy Study (DRS) and of the British Multicentre Photocoagulation Trial are now well known.[9,26,27,28] Why does this treatment work? A widely accepted theory holds that extensive photocoagulation reduces the concentration of some angiogenesis factor that is produced by the hypoxic diabetic retina. Perhaps

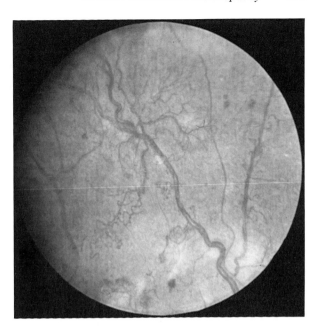

Figure 10-6. Fundus photograph of the right eye of a 24-year-old woman with extensive proliferative diabetic retinopathy. Despite panretinal photocoagulation, begun at this point, the retinopathy progressed and neovascular glaucoma developed, eventually causing loss of the eye.

so, but I do not believe that the effect is due to the destruction of the cells that are producing this mysterious factor itself. First of all, it appears that panretinal photocoagulation as it is now applied, usually covers at most about 20% of the total area of the retina.* [82,93] Second, photocoagulation when applied at intensities within the range usually employed for this treatment and when not directed at the retinal vessels themselves destroys only the cells of the outer layers of the retina: the retinal pigment epithelium and photoreceptors as well as segments of

---

* These conclusions were based on calculations or on actual measurements of the area covered by photocoagulation treatment.[82,93] I have claimed that the treated area is larger, as much as 40% of the retina, based on the fractional reduction of the electroretinographic b-wave following panretinal photocoagulation.[35] The assumption was that the b-wave amplitude is directly proportional to the area of functioning retina. While this may be true, for example, in cases of retinal detachment, Dr. Werner Noell has suggested to me that the assumption may not hold for photocoagulated retina, since the treatment destroys the retinal pigment epithelial cells and disrupts the junctional complexes between them. These complexes form an electrical resistance barrier (at one time called the *R-membrane*), whose disruption may diminish the b-wave amplitude out of proportion to the total area of treated retina.[19]

the choriocapillaris.[3,82,85,96] Since retinal blood vessels usually do not grow in these layers, which are normally supplied by the choriocapillaris, there is no reason why they should produce a "retinal angiogenesis factor." What these outer retinal layers actually do that is relevant to our discussion is to use a very great deal of oxygen.[99] Destruction of retinal receptors and pigment epithelial cells by photocoagulation therefore may substantially reduce the consumption of oxygen (supplied by the ample blood flow through the choriocapillaris) by the outer layers of the retina, permitting the oxygen to diffuse to the inner retina for use by the hypoxic cells of these inner retinal layers. Destruction of pigment epithelial cells with their junctional complexes may also decrease the diffusional barriers and atrophy of the photoreceptors may shorten the distance for diffusion between the choriocapillaris and the inner retina, but these are probably relatively minor effects.

Owing to space limitations this discussion of retinal neovascularization is necessarily oversimplified. The reader will quickly recognize that I have not touched on many of the complexities of the subject. For example, does hypoxia play a role in neovascularization arising from the optic disc? What, if any, is the role of the vitreous? Can it serve as a chemical inhibitor

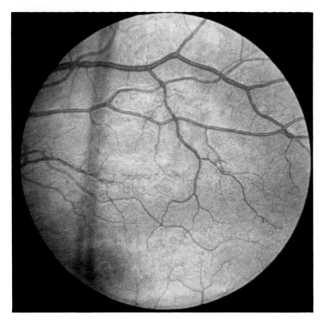

Figure 10-7. Photograph of the left eye of the patient in Figure 10-6. There is minimal diabetic retinopathy, and the visual acuity is 20/20 (6/6). Retinoscopy at the outset of treatment revealed no substantial difference in refractive error in the two eyes; initially intraocular tensions were practically equal and in the normal range, and there were no carotid bruits or evidence of intracranial vascular disease. Subsequently, early neovascular lesions were detected in the right eye, and panretinal photocoagulation was carried out with complete regression of the new vessels. No further lesions have developed in over 5 years of follow-up, and visual acuity remains 20/20 in this eye. The marked asymmetry of the retinopathy in this patient remains unexplained.

of neovascularization?[8] Is iris neovascularization related in a causal way to retinal neovascularization, as suggested by the frequent clinical observation of rapid growth of iris new vessels following surgical vitrectomy and lensectomy for complications of proliferative diabetic reti-

nopathy, and also by the observation that pan*retinal* photocoagulation can prevent or cause the regression of *iridic* neovascularization?[74,78] How can one explain many cases of unilateral proliferative diabetic retinopathy where known predisposing factors (unilateral

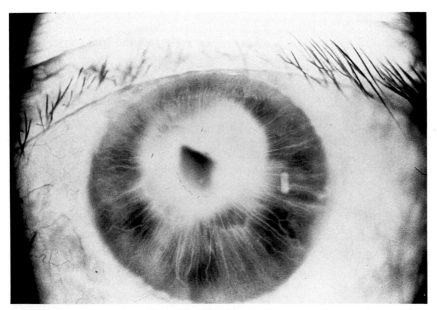

Figure 10-8. Iris angiogram from the right eye of this patient. Note leakage of dye from the new vessels; it was not present in the left eye.

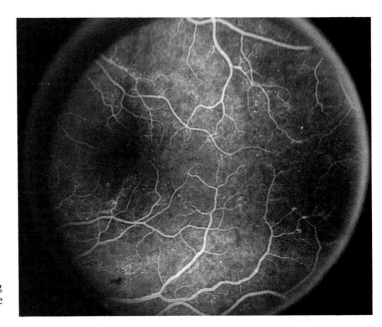

Figure 10-9. Fluorescein angiogram from the left eye of the patient in Figure 10-8 taken during the same sequence. Note that there is only minimal retinopathy.

high myopia, retinal artery occlusion, glaucoma, chorioretinitis affecting the eye less severely involved by retinopathy, or unilateral carotid occlusive disease) are absent (Fig. 10-6–10-9)? What is the explanation for cases of proliferative diabetic retinopathy that are resistant to massive photocoagulation? At the present time, our general hypothesis cannot satisfactorily deal with these questions. Similarly, the successful treatment of diabetic macular edema by laser photocoagulation, recently reported by the Early Treatment Diabetic Retinopathy Study (ETDRS) Research Group, lacks a theoretical explanation.[31] In the ETDRS, macular edema was treated by small (50- to 100-micron diameter) focal argon laser burns applied directly to areas of fluorescein leakage, demonstrated angiographically. The success of this method suggests that sealing off these leaking sites is effective because physiologic mechanisms for resorbing intraretinal fluid, which are continuously in operation, can then dry up the edema. However, Olk has recently suggested that photocoagulation of macular edema by a grid pattern of argon laser burns, in which no attempt is made to treat leaking areas directly, is equally effective.[83] While the efficacy of this method has not been demonstrated in a large-scale randomized, controlled trial, Olk's report suggests that the mechanism by which laser photocoagulation reduces diabetic macular edema may not be obvious.

REFERENCES

1. Addison DJ, Garner A, Ashton N: Degeneration of intramural pericytes in diabetic retinopathy. Br Med J 1:264–266, 1970
2. Akagi Y, Kador PF, Kuwabara T, et al: Aldose reductase localization in human retinal mural cells. Invest Ophthalmol Vis Sci 24:1516–1519, 1983
3. Apple DJ, Goldberg MF, Wyhinny G: Histopathology and ultrastructure of the argon laser lesion in human retinal and choroidal vasculatures. Am J Ophthalmol 75:595–609, 1973
4. Barta L, Brooser L, Molnar M: Prognostic value of fluorescein angiography of the fundus in diabetic children. Acta Diabetol Latina 15:24–28, 1978
5. Ben Ezra D: Neovasculogenic ability of prostaglandins, growth factors, and synthetic chemoattractants. Am J Ophthalmol 86:455–461, 1978
6. Bodansky HJ, Wolf E, Cudworth AT, et al: Genetic and immunologic factors in microvascular disease in type I insulin-dependent diabetes. Diabetes 31:70–74, 1982
7. Bowman PD, Betz, AL, Goldstein GW: Primary culture of microvascular endothelial cells

from bovine retina: Selective growth using fibronectin-coated substrate and plasma-derived serum. In Vitro 18:626–632, 1982

8. Brem S, Preis I, Langer R, et al: Inhibition of neovascularization by an extract derived from vitreous. Am J Ophthalmol 84:323–328, 1977

9. The British Multicentre Photocoagulation Trial: Proliferative diabetic retinopathy: Treatment with xenon-arc photocoagulation. Br Med J 1:739–741, 1977

10. Brooser G, Barta L, Anda L, Molnar M: Frühdiagnose der Mikroangiopathie bei kindlichem Diabetes. Klin Mbl Augenheilk 166:233–236, 1975

11. Bunn HF, Gabbay KH, Gallop PM: The glycosylation of hemoglobin: Relevance to diabetes mellitus. Science 200:21–27, 1978

12. Burditt AF, Caird FI, Draper GJ: The natural history of diabetic retinopathy. Quart J Med 37:303–317, 1968

13. Buzney SM, Frank RN, Robison WG Jr: Retinal capillaries: Proliferation of mural cells *in vitro.* Science 190:985–986, 1975

14. Buzney SM, Frank RN, Varma SD, et al: Aldose reductase in retinal mural cells. Invest Ophthalmol Vis Sci 16:392–396, 1977

15. Buzney SM, Massicotte SJ: Retinal vessels: Proliferation of endothelium *in vitro.* Invest Ophthalmol Vis Sci 18:1191–1194, 1979

16. Cahill GF Jr, Etzwiler DD, Freinkel N: "Control" and diabetes. N Engl J Med 294:1004–1005, 1976

17. Caird FI, Pirie A, Ramsell TG: Diabetes and the Eye, p 62. Oxford, Blackwell, 1968

18. Cogan DG, Toussaint D, Kuwabara T: Retinal vascular patterns. IV. Diabetic retinopathy. Arch Ophthalmol 66:366–378, 1961

19. Cohen AI: A possible cytological basis for the "R" membrane in the vertebrate eye. Nature 205:1222–1223, 1965

20. Coller BS, Frank RN, Milton RC, et al: Plasma cofactors of platelet function: Correlation with diabetic retinopathy and hemoglobins A_{1a-c} Ann Int Med 88:311–316, 1978

21. Crabbe MJ, Pecker CO, Halder AB, et al: Erythrocyte glyceraldehyde-reductase levels in diabetes with retinopathy and cataract. Lancet 2:1268–1270, 1980

22. D'Amore PA, Glaser BM, Brunson SK, et al: Angiogenic activity from bovine retina: Partial purification and characterization. Proc Natl Acad Sci USA 78:3068–3072, 1981

23. Daneman D, Drash AL, Lobes LA, et al: Progressive retinopathy with improved control in diabetic dwarfism (Mauriac's syndrome). Diabetes Care 4:360–365, 1981

24. Davis MD: Discussion of paper by Hutton et al. Trans Am Acad Ophthalmol Otolaryngol 76:978–979, 1972

25. DeOliveira F: Pericytes in diabetic retinopathy. Br J Ophthalmol 50:134–143, 1966

26. The Diabetic Retinopathy Study Research Group: Preliminary report on the effects of photocoagulation therapy. Am J Ophthalmol 81:383–396, 1976

27. The Diabetic Retinopathy Study Research Group: Photocoagulation treatment of proliferative diabetic retinopathy. The second report of Diabetic Retinopathy Study findings. Ophthalmology 85:82–105, 1978

28. The Diabetic Retinopathy Study Research Group: Photocoagulation treatment of proliferative diabetic retinopathy. Ophthalmology 88:583–600, 1981

29. Dorchy H, Toussaint D, Devroede M, et al: Diagnostic de la retinopathie diabetique infantile par angiographie fluoresceinique. Nouv Presse Med 6:345–347, 1977

30. Dornan TL, Ting A, McPherson CK, et al: Genetic susceptibility to the development of retinopathy in insulin-dependent diabetes. Diabetes 31:226–231, 1982

31. Early Treatment Diabetic Retinopathy Study Research Group: Photocoagulation for diabetic macular edema. Early Treatment Diabetic Retinopathy Study Report Number 1. Arch Ophthalmol 103:1796–1806, 1985

32. Engerman RL, Bloodworth JMB Jr, Nelson S: Relationship of microvascular disease to metabolic control. Diabetes 26:760–769, 1977

33. Engerman RL, Kern TS: Experimental galactosemia produces diabetic-like retinopathy. Diabetes 33:97–100, 1984

34. Engerman RL, Pfaffenbach D, Davis MD: Cell turnover of capillaries. Lab Invest 17:738–743, 1967

35. Frank RN: Visual fields and electroretinography following extensive photocoagulation. Arch Ophthalmol 93:591–598, 1975

36. Frank RN, Hoffman WH, Podgor MJ, et al: Retinopathy in juvenile-onset diabetes of short duration. Ophthalmology 87:1–9, 1980

37. Frank RN, Hoffman WH, Podgor MJ, et al: Retinopathy in juvenile-onset type I diabetes of short duration. Diabetes 31:874–882, 1982

38. Frank RN, Keirn RJ, Kennedy A, et al: Galactose-induced retinal capillary basement membrane thickening: Prevention by Sorbinil. Invest Ophthalmol Vis Sci 24:1519–1524, 1983

39. Frank RN, Kinsey VE, Frank KW, et al: *In vitro* proliferation of endothelial cells from kitten retinal capillaries. Invest Ophthalmol Vis Sci 18:1195–1200, 1979

40. Gabbay KH: The sorbitol pathway and the complications of diabetes. N Engl J Med 288:831–836, 1973

41. Gabbay KH: Hyperglycemia, polyol metabolism, and the complications of diabetes mellitus. Ann Rev Med 26:521–536, 1975

42. Gitlin JD, D'Amore PA: Culture of retinal capillary cells using selective growth media. Microvasc Res 26:74–80, 1983

43. Glaser BM, D'Amore PA, Michels RG, et al: Demonstration of vasoproliferative activity from mammalian retina. J Cell Biol 84:298–304, 1980

44. Glycosylated haemoglobin and diabetic control (editorial). Br Med J 1:1373–1374, 1978

45. Goldberg MF: The role of ischemia in the production of vascular retinopathies. In Lynn JT, Snyder WB, Vaiser A (eds): Diabetic Retinopathy, pp 47–63. New York, Grune and Stratton, 1974

46. Gospodarowicz D: Purification of a fibroblast growth factor from bovine pituitary. J Biol Chem 250:2515–2520, 1975

47. Gospodarowicz D, Bialecki H, Greenburg G: Purification of the fibroblast growth factor activity from bovine brain. J Biol Chem 253:3736–3743, 1978

48. Gospodarowicz D, Brown KD, Birdwell CR, et al: Control of proliferation of human vascular endothelial cells. J Cell Biol 77:774–788, 1977

49. Gospodarowicz D, Moran JS, Braun DL: Control of proliferation of bovine vascular endothelial cells. J Cell Physiol 91:377–386, 1977

50. Hayman S, Kinoshita JH: Isolation and properties of lens aldose reductase. J Biol Chem 240:877–882, 1965

51. Henkind P: Ocular neovascularization. Am J Ophthalmol 85:287–301, 1978

52. Hutton WL, Snyder WB, Vaiser A, et al: Retinal microangiopathy without associated glucose intolerance. Trans Am Acad Ophthalmol Otolaryngol 76:968–978, 1972

53. Ingelfinger FJ: Debates on diabetes. N Eng J Med 296:1228–1230, 1977

54. Jaspan J, Maselli R, Herold K, et al: Treatment of severely painful diabetic neuropathy with an aldose reductase inhibitor: Relief of pain and improved sensory and autonomic nerve function. Lancet 2:758–761, 1983

55. Job D, Eschwege E, Guyot-Argenton C, et al: Effect of multiple daily insulin injections on the course of diabetic retinopathy. Diabetes 25:463–469, 1976

56. Judzewitsch RG, Jaspan JB, Polonsky KS, et al: Aldose reductase inhibition improves nerve conduction velocity in diabetic patients. N Eng J Med 308:119–125, 1983

57. Kennedy A, Frank RN: *In vitro* production of glycosaminoglycans by retinal microvascular cells and lens epithelium. Invest Ophthalmol Vis Sci 27:746–754, 1986

58. Kennedy A, Frank RN, Mancini MA, et al: Collagens of the retinal microvascular basement membrane and of retinal microvascular cells *in vitro*. Exp Eye Res 42:177–199, 1986

59. Kennedy A, Frank RN, Varma SD: Aldose reductase activity in retinal and cerebral microvessels and cultured vascular cells. Invest Ophthalmol Vis Sci 24:1250–1258, 1983

60. Kennedy A, Frank RN, Varma SD: Galactitol accumulation by glucose-6-phosphate deficient fibroblasts: A cellular model for resistance to the complications of diabetes mellitus. Life Sci 33:1277–1284, 1983

61. Kern TS, Engerman RL: Distribution of aldose reductase in ocular tissues. Exp Eye Res 33:175–182, 1981

62. King GL, Buzney SM: Modulation of growth in retinal capillary cells by insulin and hyperglycemia: possible roles in the development of early diabetic retinopathy. Invest Ophthalmol Vis Sci 24 (ARVO Suppl.):14, 1983

63. King GL, Buzney SM, Kahn CR, et al: Differential responsiveness to insulin of endothelial and support cells from micro- and macrovessels. J Clin Invest 71:974–979, 1983

64. Kinoshita JH: Mechanisms initiating cataract formation. Invest Ophthalmol 13:713–724, 1974

65. Klein R, Klein BEK, Moss SE: The Wisconsin epidemiologic study of diabetic retinopathy. II. Prevalence and risk of diabetic retinopathy when age at diagnosis is less than 30 years. Arch Ophthalmol 102:520–526, 1984

66. Klein R, Klein BEK, Moss SE, et al: Retinopathy in young-onset diabetic patients. Diabetes Care 8:311–315, 1985

67. Knowles HC: The control of diabetes mellitus and the progression of retinopathy. In Goldberg MF, Fine SL (eds): Symposium on the Treatment of Diabetic Retinopathy. US Public Health Service Publication No 1890, pp 115–118. Washington DC: US Government Printing Office, 1968

68. Koenig RJ, Peterson CM, Jones RL, et al: Correlation of glucose regulation and hemoglobin A_{1C} in diabetes mellitus. N Engl J Med 295:417–420, 1976

69. Kohner EM, Shilling JS, Hamilton AM: The role of avascular retina in new vessel formation. Metabolic Ophthalmol 1:15–24, 1976

70. Kornerup T: Studies in diabetic retinopathy: An investigation of 1,000 cases of diabetes. Acta Med Scand 153:81–101, 1955

71. Krolewski AS, Warram JH, Rand LI, et al: Risk of proliferative diabetic retinopathy in juvenile-onset type I diabetes: A 40-yr. follow-up study. Diabetes Care 9:443–452, 1986

72. Li W, Shen S, Khatami M, et al: Stimulation of retinal capillary pericyte protein and collagen synthesis in culture by high-glucose concentration. Diabetes 33:785–789, 1984

73. Linner E, Svanborg A, Zelander T: Retinal and renal lesions of diabetic type without obvious disturbance of glucose metabolism in a patient

with a family history of diabetes. Am J Med 39:298–304, 1965

74. Little HL, Rosenthal AR, Dellaporta A, et al: The effect of pan-retinal photocoagulation on rubeosis iridis.. Am J Ophthalmol 81:804–809, 1976

75. Ludvigson MA, Sorenson RL: Immunohistochemical localization of aldose reductase. II. Rat eye and kidney. Diabetes 29:450–459, 1980

76. Malone JI, Simons CA, Van Cader TC: Correlation of Hb A₁ and diabetic microvascular disease. Diabetes 27:434, 1978

77. Malone JI, Van Cader TC, Edwards WC: Diabetic vascular changes in children. Diabetes 26:673–679, 1977

78. May DR, Klein ML, Peyman GA: A prospective study of xenon arc photocoagulation for central retinal vein occlusion. Br J Ophthalmol 60:816–818, 1976

79. Merimee TJ, Zapf J, Froesch ER: Insulin-like growth factors: Studies in diabetics with and without retinopathy. N Engl J Med 309:527–529, 1983

80. Michaelson IC: The mode of development of the retinal vessels and some observations of its significance in certain retinal diseases. Trans Ophthalmol Soc UK 68:137–180, 1948

81. Nanda M, Murphy RP, Plotnick L, et al: The effects of puberty on the prevalence of diabetic retinopathy. Invest Ophthalmol Vis Sci (Suppl) 27:5, 1986

82. Ogden TE, Riekhof FT, Benwith SM: Correlation of histologic and electroretinographic changes in peripheral retinal ablation in the rhesus monkey. Am J Ophthalmol 81:272–279, 1976

83. Olk RJ: Modified grid argon (blue-green) laser photocoagulation for diffuse diabetic macular edema. Ophthalmology 93:938–950, 1986

84. Palmberg P, Smith M, Waltman S, et al: The natural history of retinopathy in insulin-dependent, juvenile-onset diabetes. Ophthalmology 88:613–618, 1981

85. Powell JO, Bresnick GH, Yanoff M, et al: Ocular effects of argon laser radiation. II. Histopathology of chorioretinal lesions. Am J Ophthalmol 71:1267–1276, 1971

86. Rand LI, Krolewski AS, Aiello LM, et al: Multiple factors in the prediction of risk of proliferative diabetic retinopathy. New Engl J Med 313:1433–1438, 1985

87. Robison WG Jr, Kador PF, Kinoshita JH: Retinal capillaries: Basement membrane thickening by galactosemia prevented with aldose reductase inhibitor. Science 221:1177–1179, 1983

88. Schanzlin D, Jay WH, KJ, et al: Hemoglobin A₁ and diabetic retinopathy. Am J Ophthalmol 88:1032–1038, 1979

89. Shimizu K, Kobayashi Y, Muraoka K: Midperipheral fundus involvement in diabetic retinopathy. Ophthalmology 88:601–612, 1981

90. Siperstein MD, Foster DW, Knowles HC Jr, et al: Control of blood glucose and diabetic vascular disease. N Engl J Med 296:1060–1063, 1977

91. Speiser P, Gittelsohn AM, Patz A: Studies on diabetic retinopathy. III. Influence of diabetes on intramural pericytes. Arch Ophthalmol 80:332–337, 1968

92. Srivastava SK, Petrash M, Sadana IJ, et al: Susceptibility of aldehyde and aldose reductases of human tissues to aldose reductase inhibitors. Curr Eye Res 2:407–410, 1983

93. Taylor E: Proliferative diabetic retinopathy: Regression of optic disc neovascularization after retinal photocoagulation. Br J Ophthalmol 54:535–539, 1970

94. Taylor E, Dobree JH: Proliferative diabetic retinopathy. Site and size of initial lesions. Br J Ophthalmol 54:11–18, 1970

95. Toussaint D, Quaetaert M, Dorchy H, et al: Early diagnosis of retinopathy in juvenile diabetes by fluorescein angiography. Acta Paediat Belg 29:177–180, 1976

96. Tso MOM, Wallow IHL, Powell JO: Differential susceptibility of rod and cone cells to argon laser. Arch Ophthalmol 89:228–234, 1973

97. Waitzman MB: Prostaglandins and diabetic retinopathy. Exp Eye Res 16:307–313, 1973

98. Warburg OH: The Metabolism of Tumors, pp 237–238, 322–324. New York, RR Smith, 1931

99. Weiter JJ, Zuckerman R: The influence of the photoreceptor-RPE complex of the inner retina. An explanation for the beneficial effects of photocoagulation. Ophthalmology 87:1133–1139, 1980

100. White A, Handler P, Smith EL: Principles of Biochemistry, 5th ed, p 364. New York; McGraw-Hill, 1973

101. White P: Childhood diabetes. Diabetes 9:345–355, 1960

102. Winternitz WW, Gorelick DA, Feldman N, et al: Letters to the editor. N Engl J Med 295:509–512, 1976

103. Wise GN: Retinal neovascularization. Trans Am Ophthalmol Soc 54:729–826, 1956

104. Wise GN, Dollery CT, Henkind P: The Retinal Circulation, pp 2–18; 34–54. New York, Harper & Row, 1971

105. Yanoff M: Diabetic retinopathy. N Engl J Med 274:1344–1349, 1966

106. Young RJ, Ewing DJ, Clarke BF: A controlled trial of Sorbinil, an aldose reductase inhibitor, in chronic painful diabetic neuropathy. Diabetes 32:938–942, 1983

107. Yuen KK, Kahn HA: The association of female hormones with blindness from diabetic retinopathy. Am J Ophthalmol 81:820–822, 1976

4

Degenerative Diseases of the Macula and Retina

11

Submacular Neovascularization

Koichi Shimizu

Submacular neovascularization is one of the few macular diseases that can be arrested effectively by timely photocoagulation. Since the late 1960s, submacular neovascularization has become easy to identify accurately with fluorescein angiography of the fundus.

CLINICAL MANIFESTATIONS

Submacular neovascularization denotes a neovascular net located at either the inner or outer aspect of the retinal pigment epithelium (RPE) that is fed by the choroidal vasculature. The newly formed vessels under the macula often arise as a whitish-yellow net posterior to the sensory retina and can appear "hard," simulating a fibrous scar, or "soft," like an exudative focal lesion. Occasionally, the neovascular net is associated with hemorrhagic patches.

Fluorescein angiography provides clues to the diagnosis of submacular neovascularization. In the early phase of the angiogram, the neovascular net appears as a network of fine vessels surrounded by a nonfluorescent halo. These fine vessels fill with dye sooner than the retinal vessels, indicating that they are fed by the choroidal vascular system. A closer look sometimes reveals one or more vascular stalks feeding the net from behind. Since the neovascular network is highly permeable, prompt dye leakage follows the early phase of the angiogram (Fig. 11-1, 11-2). Clinical conditions under which submacular neovascularization occurs as the main pathologic feature are shown in Table 11-1.

PATHOGENETIC FACTORS

Because submacular neovascularization occurs in diverse conditions, it may be worthwhile to explore the pathogenetic features common to these cases. The best known instance of submacular neovascularization is high myopia, clinically known as Fuchs' spot. Fuchs (1901) described a peculiar lesion that may occur as a pigmented net or as a grayish or whitish patch following or preceding the formation of submacular hemorrhage in the fovea of highly myopic eyes. Usually less than one-fifth the diameter of the disc, the foveal lesion is frequently associated with extensive atrophy of the choroid, particularly in the posterior fundus. A "lacquer-crack" lesion, located at the level of Bruch's membrane, often accompanies this condition.

The triggering mechanism leading to senile disciform macular degeneration remains controversial. Gass claimed initially that new vessels grow into the sub-RPE space following hemorrhagic detachment of the RPE.[1] He later modified this view and said that neovascular ingrowth under the RPE may occur without prior sub-RPE hemorrhage. In a series of elegant papers based on histopathologic studies in humans, Sarks has convincingly demonstrated that drusen appear to be one of the precursors leading to senile disciform macular degeneration and that neovascular ingrowth may occur in drusen as well as in degenerated Bruch's membrane.[3]

A common pathogenetic factor appears to exist for submacular neovascularization in these

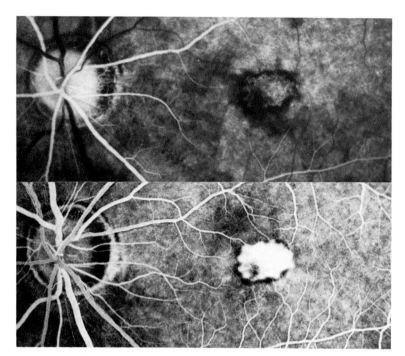

Figure 11-1. Subfoveal neovascularization in high myopia. Early-phase angiogram *(top)* shows the scalloped appearance of the neovascular mass. The lesion fills with fluorescein earlier than the retinal vessels and is surrounded by a dark halo. Diffuse extravasation of dye occurs in a later angiogram *(bottom)*.

lesions: blunt ocular trauma, angioid streaks, and inadequate ocular photocoagulation, all of which exhibit "breaks" or degenerative defects in Bruch's membrane. The overlying retina must be fairly intact for submacular neovascularization to develop. In an eye with angioid streaks or blunt ocular trauma, submacular neovascularization frequently fails to arise in an atrophic macular area.

Submacular neovascularization can be induced in experimental animal models with laser photocoagulation if the laser beam is sufficiently intense in energy, small in diameter, and

Table 11-1. Clinical Conditions Associated with Submacular Neovascularization

Senile disciform macular degeneration
High myopia (Fuchs' spot)
Angioid streaks
Presumed ocular histoplasmosis
Inadequate photocoagulation
Central exudative chorioretinopathy
Hemorrhagic detachment of RPE

of short duration (Fig. 11-3). Ideally, a miniscule explosion occurs at the level of the RPE producing a break at the level of Bruch's membrane while preserving the overlying retina. Unintentional submacular neovascularization in the photocoagulation therapy of macular lesions may be avoided by using a laser beam of relatively low intensity with a relatively large diameter and long duration (preferably more than 0.1 second).

The Japanese literature is limited concerning a precise pathogenetic mechanism in submacular neovascularization occurring in so-called ocular histoplasmosis, since this is a rare condition in our country. It appears the selective destruction of Bruch's membrane is necessary for new vessels to develop.

Little is known about the role of submacular neovascularization in hemorrhagic detachment of the RPE, but its presence appears to be a precursor, not a consequence. We failed to detect new vessel growth into the detached sub-RPE space after a hemorrhagic episode in our study of 24 cases.

We have observed some of the pathologic features leading to the formation of submacular

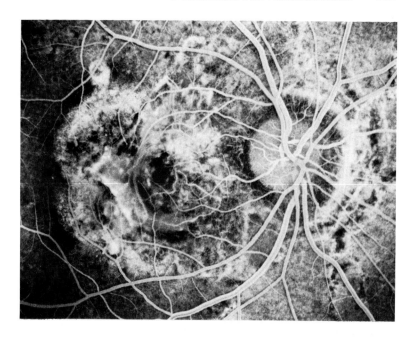

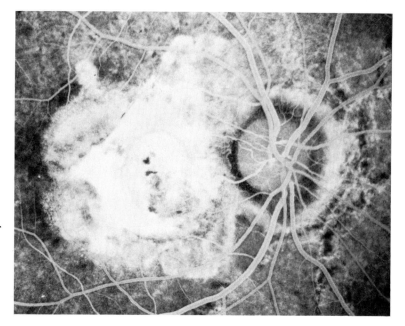

Figure 11-2. Submacular neovascularization in an eye with angioid streaks. A pair of feeder vessels appears medial to the fovea *(top)*. A large, triangular fibrovascular membrane, surrounded by an atrophic area, becomes visible in a later angiogram *(bottom)*.

neovascularization. First, Bruch's membrane or the RPE must be damaged in an acute or subacute manner. Second, the overlying retina must be more or less intact. It appears that new vessel ingrowth does not develop unless both of these prerequisites are present.

Retinitis pigmentosa is a striking example in which RPE degeneration is seen but is not associated with submacular neovascularization. Even with extensive degeneration of the RPE, new vessel growth fails to develop because the neuroretina is extensively involved in the dis-

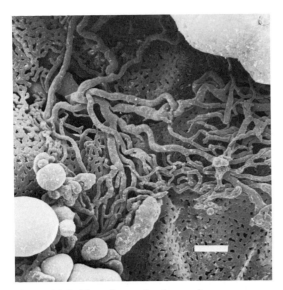

Figure 11-3. Experimental submacular neovascularization in a monkey eye induced by photocoagulation. This corrosion-cast specimen shows a break in the RPE through which newly formed vessels invade the subretinal space. The spherical bodies in the upper right and lower left corners are artifacts. (Bar = 100μ)

ease process and is not intact. Submacular neovascularization also fails to develop in proliferative diabetic retinopathy. It is generally agreed that the main factor inducing retinal or disc neovascularization is "hypoxia" secondary to capillary nonperfusion, particularly in the midperipheral retina.[4] A similar pathogenetic mechanism seems to be at work in retinal neovascularizations that occur in branch retinal vein occlusion.[2]

The consistent absence of submacular neovascularization in proliferative diabetic retinopathy and branch retinal vein occlusion seems to indicate that the stimulus for neovascularization from the retinal or optic disc vessels does not apply to submacular neovascularization. Degeneration of RPE in the macular region in diabetic retinopathy or branch retinal vein occlusion may occur as a late event and secondarily to the impaired neuroretina in the macular area, another example of the validity of the two prerequisites for submacular neovascularization.

TREATMENT

Based on the pathogenetic mechanisms proposed herein, it is possible to plan a rational therapeutic approach. Medical treatment seems to be of no value after submacular neovascular tissue has attained a certain size. A relatively favorable prognosis may be expected in an eye with a diseased neuroretina such as one with high myopia or central exudative chorioretinopathy.

At present, photocoagulation seems to be the only effective treatment for submacular lesions. The whole neovascular net must be destroyed in addition to photocoagulation of the neuroretina overlying the lesion. An eye with a serous detachment of the macula is a poor candidate for effective photocoagulation.

If the submacular neovascular lesion is located outside the central fovea, early detection and timely treatment by photocoagulation are essential to save vision. While no therapeutic approach has been established to treat an eye with submacular neovascularization on the central fovea, one may consider treating the macular area surrounding the neovascular lesion with photocoagulation applied in a grid pattern. Final evaluation of this approach cannot be made until more has been learned about the prognosis in individual cases and until better clinical evidence has been accumulated.

REFERENCES

1. Gass JDM: Pathogenesis of disciform detachment of the neuroepithelium. IV. Fluorescein angiographic study of senile disciform macular degeneration. Am J Ophthalmol 63:645–659, 1967
2. Patz A: Clinical and experimental studies on retinal neovascularization. Am J Ophthalmol 94:715–743, 1982
3. Sarks SH: Aging and degeneration in the macular region: Clinicopathologic study. Br J Ophthalmol 60:324–341, 1976
4. Shimizu K, Kobayasi Y, Muraoka K: Midperipheral fundus involvement in diabetic retinopathy. Ophthalmology 88:601–621, 1981

12

Photic Injury to the Retina and Pathogenesis of Age-Related Macular Degeneration

Mark O.M. Tso

The primary function of the retina is light perception. Yet in the past 70 years, photic injury to the retina had not attracted much interest. This was due partly to the landmark manuscript of 1916 by Verhoeff and Bell in which they reported that the retina was impervious to environmental light under normal circumstances.[88] However, research in the past two decades has shown that the photoreceptor cells are fragile and can be easily damaged by environmental or artificial lighting.[46,47,58-62] As photoreceptor cells are neurons of the central nervous system, they do not regenerate once destroyed. Research on photic injury to the retina has increasingly assumed primary importance in clinical ophthalmology and visual sciences. Indeed, photic injury to the retina has wide socioeconomic implications.[14] Safety standards must be set for environmental lighting in homes, offices, and public buildings, as well as for the intensity of light from ophthalmic instruments. In addition, the efficacy of protective devices, such as sunglasses and goggles, must be evaluated. The cumulative effects of prolonged photic injury to the retina as a pathogenetic factor of age-related macular degeneration should also be explored. This chapter examines the damage to photoreceptor cells by light and the pathogenetic mechanisms of photic injury.

Radiant energy damages retinal tissue in three ways. Retinal tissues may be disrupted mechanically by a microexplosion with acoustic transients or gaseous formation generated by short pulses of energy, such as that from a YAG laser. Thermal coagulation of the retinal proteins may be produced by laser energy of continuous wave length that raises the temperature of the retina to 10 degrees above body temperature. Photochemical injury inflicts damage without significantly raising the temperature of the retinal tissues or mechanically disrupting the cells. In recent years, most environmental light damage, including solar retinitis, has been ascribed to photochemical injury rather than to thermal coagulative insult.[28-33,89] The discussion in this chapter will be confined to photochemical injuries of the retina.

The phototransduction process starts at the receptor element of the photoreceptor cells, where a small number of photons are instantly transformed into a physiologic visual impulse. The mechanism by which photoreceptor cells and associated cellular systems remove exces-

Supported in part by Research Grant EY 1903, EY 06761 (Dr. Tso); Core Grant EY 1792 and Training Grant EY 7038 from the National Eye Institute.
Dr. Tso is the recipient of the Research to Prevent Blindness, Inc., Senior Scientific Investigator's Award, 1987.

sive light energy received by the retina is not fully understood. A portion of the light energy is absorbed by melanin granules of the retinal pigment epithelium (RPE) and dissipated into surrounding structures. It has been proposed that the blood flow of the choriocapillaris has a cooling effect and removes excessive energy absorbed by the RPE.[36,68] In recent years, it has been suggested that cytoplasmic photosensitizers such as riboflavin, rhodopsin, and retinol may also absorb excessive light energy and generate a primary photodynamic reaction that results in the production of free radicals that will attack retinal tissues, causing photoreceptor cell damage.[59] These radicals, however, are quickly quenched by naturally occurring antioxidants such as supraoxide dismutase, catalase, ascorbate, and tocopherol. Other associated responses to photic injury include reactive and reparative changes of the RPE, the Müller cells, and the choroidal vascular system. Clearly, photochemical injury is not an isolated event but a cascade of reactions involving a number of pathogenetic mechanisms, each with a different action spectrum. The complexity of retinal photic injury has begun to unfold.

The possible relationships between chronic photic insult and retinal degenerative diseases also need investigation. Indeed, chronic cumulative damage produced by low-intensity light may provide a clue to the senescence of photoreceptor cells. Young, Bok, and coworkers have pointed out that the photoreceptor elements of both rods and cones are renewed continuously.[5,95–97] They have described how amino acid precursors in rough endoplasmic reticulum of photoreceptor cell inner segments are synthesized into proteins that pass through the connecting cilia to the outer segments. Photoreceptor outer segment discs are continuously produced at the tip of the cilia and are phagocytosed by the RPE. If this physiologic renewal system becomes defective from excessive light exposure, cumulative photic injury may lead to irreversible photoreceptor cell damage.[95] Interestingly, photoreceptor cells in rhesus monkeys that have suffered photic injury have persistent shortened outer segments 5 years after light exposure.[83] Since light damage is probably the

most common injury to photoreceptor cells, it seems important to investigate whether chronic exposure to light of low intensity may cause gradual degeneration of photoreceptor cells during the aging process. Age-related macular degeneration may be associated with chronic repeated mild photic injury to the retina over a lifetime. Indeed, Gartner and Henkind have noted that photoreceptor cells in the aging human eye decrease in number.[24] In this chapter, the pathogenetic mechanisms of aging macular degeneration will be discussed in relationship to photic injury to the retina.

EFFECTS OF ENVIRONMENTAL LIGHTING ON THE HUMAN RETINA

A number of reports have described the effects of environmental lighting on vision. Clark and associates observed that Navy personnel who were exposed to sunlight for 3 to 4 hours a day for 2 weeks had markedly elevated night vision thresholds.[13] The effect was, however, temporary, and thresholds returned to normal after their eyes were protected from sunlight for 1 day. Personnel wearing protective polarizing sunglasses with 12% transmission had significantly lower night vision thresholds than those who were unprotected.

Hecht and coworkers compared subjects who had been exposed to the bright sky for periods ranging from 4 minutes to an hour with those who had been exposed to the sun at sandy beaches for 4 hours a day for 2 weeks.[35] The authors concluded that repeated daily exposure to sunlight resulted in delayed dark adaptation, which could persist overnight. The elevated thresholds correlated significantly with deterioration of visual acuity, range of visibility, and contrast sensitivity and discrimination.

Smith reported gradually decreased visual acuity and macular pigmentary changes in military personnel who were stationed on a tropical island in the Pacific Ocean during World War II and worked outdoors for 4 months or longer.[72] Such pigmentary changes were not found in yeomen and pharmacists, who worked indoors under similar conditions.

PHOTIC MACULOPATHY AS A CONSEQUENCE OF GAZING AT THE SUN

The sun and its eclipses have fascinated mankind since ancient times, and direct gazing at the sun or an eclipse has long been reported to result in photic maculopathy (Fig. 12-1).[15,69,80] In recent years, Cordes described 23 patients from San Francisco who suffered from eclipse retinitis as having "central angioplastic retinopathy," and noted that some patients showed remarkable recovery of visual acuity with time.[15] A form of foveomacular retinitis has been observed in military personnel by Ewald and Ritchey.[14] Sun gazing in the form of self-inflicted injury associated with drug abuse, has been considered the cause of the disease. In the acute stage, a yellow "exudate" appeared deep in the fovea. Two weeks later, the fovea showed a deep red holelike defect with finely granular pigmentation and a ring of coarse pigment aggregate. The inner retinal layers appeared intact. In the late stage, macular lamellar or full-thickness holes in a honeycomb pattern were visible. Fluorescein angiography was unremarkable in the late stage. During the acute stage, however, localized leakage occurred at the site of the yellowish "exudate."

We conducted clinical and histopathologic studies of the effects of sun gazing on the human fovea with four patients who had malignant melanoma of the choroid in one eye and were

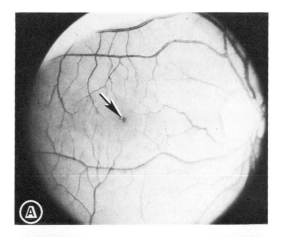

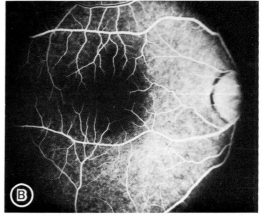

Figure 12-1. *(A)* Photic maculopathy in a patient who admitted that he had been gazing at the sun. Note a small macular hole *(arrow)* in the foveal area. *(B)* Fluorescein angiography shows no leakage or staining of the macular area.

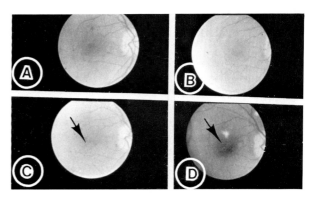

Figure 12-2. Fundus photographs of a patient who had gazed at the sun for a half hour. *(A)* Before gazing. *(B)* One hour after gazing; note the absence of macular change. *(C)* Minimal foveal edema *(arrow)* is manifested 2 days later. *(D)* A discrete pigmented lesion is seen 9 days after gazing at the sun.

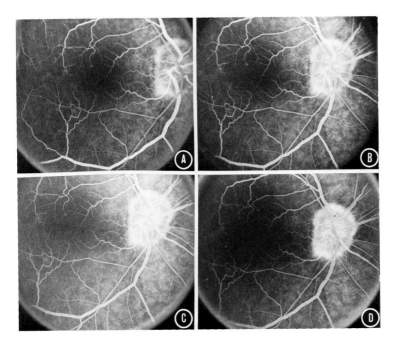

Figure 12-3. Fluorescein angiograms, taken before sun grazing, of the patient whose fundus photographs appeared in Fig. 12-2 demonstrate no macular abnormalities.

scheduled for enucleation.[80] The maculas were normal, and central visual acuity ranged from 20/30 to 20/15. All four agreed to sun gaze for 1 hour before enucleation (Fig. 12-2). The refractive error of the affected eye was corrected with lenses, and the contralateral eye was covered

during the sun gazing experiment.

All patients were free of pain during exposure, and none had difficulty fixating on the sun. They described the sun initially as a bright red ball that turned black with a pink halo. The two patients who gazed at the sun with undilated

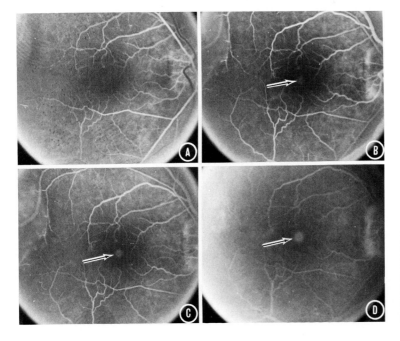

Figure 12-4. There is distinct foveal leakage *(arrows)* 48 hours after gazing at the sun that increases in intensity in the later venous phase of the fluorescein angiogram of the patient shown in Fig. 12-2.

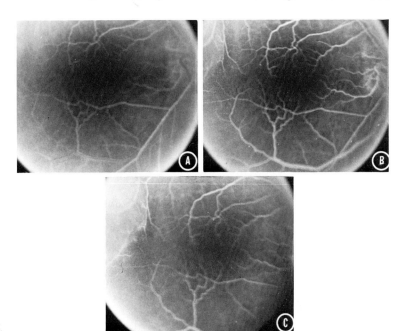

Figure 12-5. Nine days after gazing at the sun, the foveal leakage seen in Fig. 12-4 has disappeared in all phases of fluorescein angiography, suggesting healing of the RPE.

pupils detected no scotoma on tangent-screen and Amsler-grid testing, and their visual acuity was unchanged. The two with dilated pupils described a relative central scotoma, and one of them had mild loss of visual acuity from 20/20 to 20/25. However, recovery times on the photostress test for all exposed eyes were markedly prolonged. All foveas appeared mildly swollen and minimally discolored. Three eyes were enucleated within 2 days after sun gazing. The fourth was delayed until 12 days after exposure. During this time, the latter patient suffered a continuous loss of visual acuity, which deteriorated from 20/20 to 20/40. A definitive discoid yellowish-white foveal lesion surrounded by a pigmented ring was seen. Fluorescein angiography showed that all foveas leaked dye in the late venous phase 24 hours after exposure (Fig. 12-3, 12-4). The foveal leakage of the patient whose enucleation was delayed for 12 days was healed by 10 days after sun gazing (Fig. 12-5).

On histopathologic study, the foveas of the four patients showed a spectrum of changes. In the mildest case, the RPE demonstrated irregular pigmentation with margination of nuclear chromatin (Fig. 12-6, 12-7). Ultrastructurally, the RPE had moderate intracellular edema, but no cellular necrosis was observed. The cytoplasm contained abundant phagosomes, some of which had engulfed mature melanin granules and photoreceptor outer segments.

In the more severe cases, the RPE sloughed into the subretinal space and exhibited necrosis, with densified cytoplasm and disrupted plasma membrane (Fig. 12-8). At the edge of the lesion, the RPE cells had flattened and slid over the bare Bruch's membrane at the foveal region. The pericytes of the choriocapillaris appeared to have been activated, and some had migrated into Bruch's membrane. A shallow serous retinal detachment was observed, but the photoreceptor cells appeared unremarkable by light microscopy.

By electron microscopy, the photoreceptor cells overlying the pigment epithelial lesions disclosed irregularly arranged outer segments associated with mild vesicular changes (Fig. 12-9). Densified tubular structures aggregated in the inner segments (Fig. 12-10). However, no pyknosis of the photoreceptor nuclei was noted.

The patient whose eye was enucleated 12 days after sun gazing showed a different histopathologic picture. A thinned and flattened RPE relined Bruch's membrane. Pigment-laden mac-

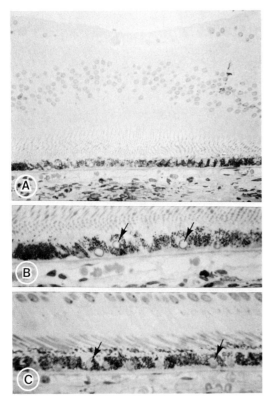

Figure 12-6. *(A)* Foveal lesion in a patient who gazed at the sun with undilated pupils for 1 hour. The eye was enucleated 24 hours later. Note the irregular pigmentation of the RPE and the integrity of the photoreceptor cells and elements in the foveal region. *(B)* Under high power, the RPE in the center of the fovea has swollen cytoplasm and margination of the nuclear chromatin *(arrows)*. The pigment epithelial cells are irregularly pigmented. *(C)* In contrast, the RPE in the perifoveal region shows normal nuclei *(arrows)* and regular pigmentation of the cells. (Original magnifications, *A* × 165; *B, C* × 350) (Tso MOM, LaPiana FG: The human fovea after sungazing. Trans Am Acad Ophthalmol Otol 79:788, 1985)

rophages appeared in the subretinal space, clustering around damaged photoreceptor elements. The fovea disclosed a distinct loss of photoreceptor nuclei and elements (Fig. 12-11).

This study on sun gazing suggested that direct exposure to the sunlight may produce foveal damage affecting the RPE and photoreceptor cells. Because the patients experienced no pain, there had been no signals to warn them of any injury. The earliest pathologic changes appeared in the RPE, which necrosed and sloughed into the subretinal space. Initially, the photoreceptor outer segments were only mildly affected by tubulovesicular changes. Early degenerative changes in the photoreceptor cells consisted of microtubular aggregates in the cytoplasm of the inner segments. Severe changes evolved several days later as the photoreceptor cell bodies gradually degenerated and an influx of macrophages in the subretinal space occurred. The RPE regenerated rapidly, and by 2 weeks, the small foveal lesion was relined with depigmented RPE and no longer leaked fluorescein on fluorescein angiography. Degenerative changes in the human retina started soon after light exposure and deteriorated progressively, even though photic exposure had been discontinued. The absence of pain and the delayed degeneration of photoreceptor cells after exposure to light make it very hazardous, as patients are unaware of injury until days after the insult.

The pathogenetic mechanisms of solar retinitis were not well understood previously. In 1916, Verhoeff and Bell believed that solar retinal lesions were photocoagulative in nature, as heat was being absorbed.[88] They also thought that the retina was impervious to normal envi-

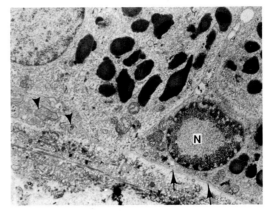

Figure 12-7. Electron micrograph of the RPE in a patient who had gazed at the sun with an undilated pupil. Note the margination of the chromatin material of the pigment epithelial nucleus (N), the abundant lipofuscin granules within the RPE cells, loss of infolding of the basal plasmalemma *(arrows)*, and the increased curvilinear profiles in Bruch's membrane *(arrowheads)*. (Original magnification, × 3500).

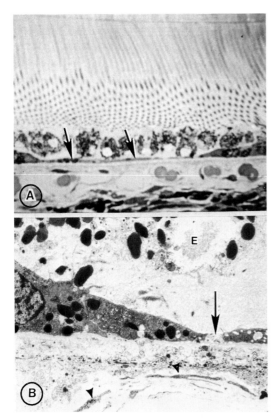

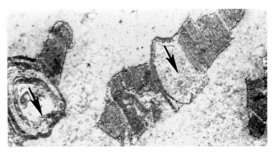

Figure 12-9. Photoreceptor elements in a patient who gazed at the sun with dilated pupils. Note the tubulovesicular disruption *(arrows)* of the photoreceptor lamellae in the foveal region. (Original magnification × 7000)

Figure 12-8. *(A)* The foveal region of a patient who had gazed at the sun with a dilated pupil demonstrates sloughing of the RPE cells in the subretinal region. The neighboring RPE cells have flattened *(arrows)* and spread to cover bare Bruch's membrane. *(B)* The flattened pigment epithelial cells have attempted to cover bare Bruch's membrane, but gaps *(arrow)* are still present. Necrotic pigment epithelial cells (E) are seen in the subretinal space. Pericytes *(arrowheads)* of the choriocapillaris have migrated into the outer layers of Bruch's membrane. (Original magnifications, *A* × 350; *B* × 7000) (*A*, Tso MOM, LaPiana FG: The human fovea after sungazing. Trans Am Acad Ophthalmol Otol 79:788, 1985)

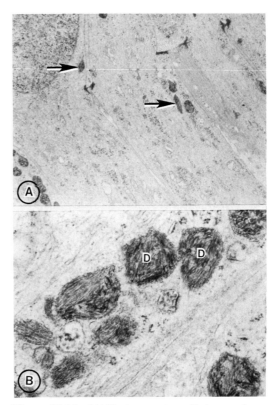

Figure 12-10. *(A)* Photoreceptor cells in a patient who had gazed at the sun appear unremarkable on light microscopy in Fig. 12-8. Under the electron microscope, however, dense bodies *(arrows)* are observed in the inner segments and perikaryon of the photoreceptor cells. *(B)* Under high power, the dense bodies (D) consist of densified tubular elements appearing in aggregates, an early feature of photoreceptor degeneration. (Original magnifications, *A* × 10,000; *B* × 40,000)

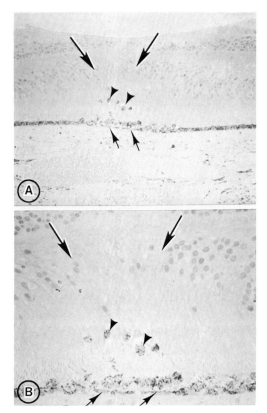

Figure 12-11. *(A)* Fovea of the patient shown in Fig. 12-2 who gazed at the sun with a dilated pupil. The eye was enucleated 12 days later. The foveal region shows a distinct loss of photoreceptor cells *(black and white arrows)*. Pigment-laden macrophages *(arrowheads)* are scattered in the subretinal space and clustered around the damaged photoreceptor elements. The RPE *(small arrows)* at the foveal region is flattened and has migrated to cover bare Bruch's membrane. *(B)* Under high power, the loss of photoreceptor cells *(black and white arrows)*, the infiltration of subretinal pigment laden macrophages *(arrowheads)*, loss of photoreceptor elements, and thinning of the RPE cells *(small arrows)* are clearly seen. (Original magnifications, *A* × 100; *B* × 225)

ronmental lighting and that excessive visible and infrared radiation produced thermal burns. However, Vos studied solar retinitis and determined that retinal temperature rose only 2 degrees (centigrade) during sun gazing.[89] Ham undertook detailed studies of retinal sensitivity to radiation damage and concluded that solar retinitis was primarily a photochemical event, because the temperature rise in the retinal lesion was insufficient to produce photocoagulative

damage.[28-33] He proposed that the short wave length component of the solar spectrum was the major source of injury, while the infrared component played only a minor role in producing retinal lesions. Most contemporary investigators have agreed with Ham that solar retinitis is a form of photochemical injury.

PHOTIC MACULOPATHY AFTER CATARACT EXTRACTION

Since solar retinitis is a relatively rare clinical entity, the significance and the prevalence of photic retinopathy in the practice of clinical ophthalmology were not recognized until McDonald and Irvine first described photic maculopathy in six patients who had extracapsular cataract extraction with posterior chamber lens implantation.[56] These authors believed that a standard ceiling-mounted Zeiss operating microscope with a 30-watt bulb was responsible for the retinal lesions. Each of the patients underwent an anterior lens capsulotomy, expression of the lens nucleus, and removal of the cortical material with a close microsurgical approach using an automated infusion-aspiration instrument. The posterior capsule was polished with a diamond-coated irrigating cannula, and the lens implant was inserted under an air bubble. The operating time varied from 1 hour and 30 minutes to 1 hour and 50 minutes. Each of these patients showed a characteristic paramacular lesion with retinal edema and discrete disturbances of the RPE. Scotomas were demonstrated on tangent screen perimetry. Fluorescein angiography exhibited a sharply defined elliptical area of fluorescein staining of the RPE.

Subsequently, Boldrey and coworkers reported 12 additional cases that showed paramacular and macular changes allegedly induced by a Zeiss OP MI IV operating microscope with a tungsten bulb or a Weck ceiling-mounted operating microscope (Model 108) with a halogen fiberoptic illumination system.[6] These patients had extracapsular cataract extractions with peripheral iridectomy. Operating time varied from 55 to 175 minutes. The visual acuity of one patient improved to 20/30 from 20/200 after a 3-month recovery period, while the visual acuity of another remained at 20/200. Symptomatic central or paracentral scotomas were present in four cases, but four patients were unaware of their symptoms. The ophthalmoscopic and fluorescein angiographic appearance of the lesions in this series appeared to be identical to those seen by McDonald and Irvine.[56] A number of measures to prevent these retinal burns from the operating microscope were applied during surgery. Ultraviolet (UV) filters were placed on the operating microscopes for 9 of the 12 cases, and air was introduced into the anterior chamber to deflect light. One case had a piece of gel-foam placed on the cornea after lens implantation, to shield the retina. The pupils were constricted with Miochol in all 12 cases. In spite of these preventive measures, all patients developed photic retinopathy after cataract extraction.

Robertson and coworkers experimented with an operating microscope by focusing its light for 30 minutes on the posterior pole of the totally blind eye of a patient who had clear ocular media and a normal-looking retina.[71] The authors observed a distinct retinal lesion showing retinal pigment epithelial edema. Later, a striking mottled pigmentary pattern developed. Fluorescein angiography showed a well-defined mottled hyperfluorescent area, similar to that reported by McDonald and Irvine and Boldrey and coworkers.[56] A second patient, who had malignant melanoma of the peripheral choroid, consented to stare at the light of an operating microscope for 30 minutes. A Zeiss OP MI VI operating microscope was used, which gave a retinal irradiance of 0.37 W/cm^2. Sixty-three hours after light exposure, visual acuity decreased from 20/20 to 20/25, and the patient complained of blurred vision and micropsia. The results of an Amsler-grid test showed a dense paracentral scotoma, and the fundus examination exhibited a grayish lesion located in the macular area temporal to the fovea. Histopathologic study of the enucleated eye showed a sharply demarcated macular lesion. There was extensive degeneration of the RPE with loss of basal infolding and apical villi. The endothelial cells of the choriocapillaris were edematous. The photoreceptor lamellae of the outer segments of the photoreceptor cells appeared mildly disrupted. These histopathologic changes were comparable to those seen in a patient who had sun gazed with an undilated pupil and strongly suggested that the pathogenetic mechanism of sun gazing may be similar to that of looking at the light of an operating microscope!

PATHOLOGIC PROCESS OF PHOTOCHEMICAL RETINAL INJURY

Since only a few retinal photic lesions have been studied in human patients, a number of animal models have been established to examine the clinical course, the physiologic parameters, the pathologic processes, and the physical characteristics of damaging light on the retina.

The clinical and pathologic changes of the human retina preceding exposure to light from the operating microscope after cataract extraction were comparable to those seen in rhesus monkeys whose maculas were exposed to the light of an indirect ophthalmoscope for 60 to 120 minutes with a +20D lens.[77,79,81,83] The animals were administered general anesthesia and the pupils were dilated with drops containing 1% atropine and 10% phenylephrine. The clinicopathologic changes were classified into three phases. In phase 1, no ophthalmoscopic changes were noted in the retina immediately following light exposure. Approximately 6 to 24 hours later, mild edema and swelling of the retina developed. Fluorescein angiography at this time showed diffuse leakage from the RPE (Fig. 12-12). Surprisingly, fluorescein leakage at the macula, where abundant xanthophyll pigment was present, was frequently less intense (Fig. 12-13). Histopathologically, the RPE appeared edematous, with discontinuous plasma membrane (Figs. 12-14, 12-15), but the junctions between adjacent cells were occasionally intact, suggesting that disruption of the blood–retina barrier was due to the decompensation of the plasma membrane rather than to the separation of the cell junctions. The photoreceptor elements showed marked tubulovesicular degeneration. Also observed were focal pyknosis of the photoreceptor cells and marked swelling of the Müller-cell cytoplasm between adjacent photoreceptor cells (Fig. 12-16). The inner layers of the retina were unremarkable.

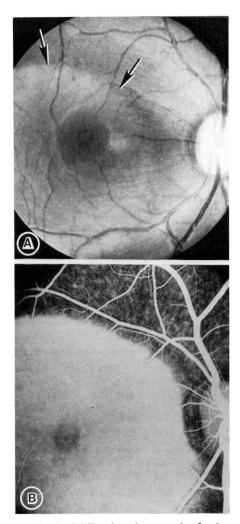

yellowish-white scar. Histologically, the RPE appeared depigmented. Pigment-laden macrophages clustered around the damaged photoreceptor outer segments (Fig. 12-18), accounting for the spotty pigmentation seen ophthalmo-

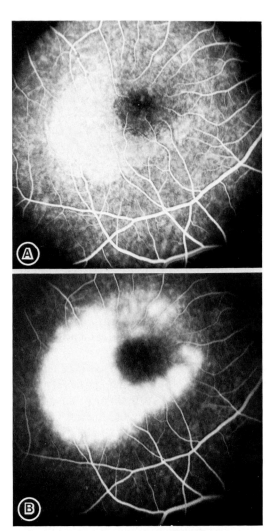

Figure 12-12. *(A)* Fundus photograph of a rhesus monkey that has been exposed to the light of an indirect ophthalmoscope for 1 1/2 hours. Note edema *(arrows)* of the posterior pole and macular area. *(B)* Fluorescein angiogram of the macula shown in *A* exhibits diffuse leakage of fluorescein from the RPE. (Tso MOM, Woodford BJ: Effect of photic injury on the retinal tissues. Ophthalmology 90(8): 952–963, 1983)

In phase 2, during the first month after exposure, the retinal edema gradually subsided. Clinically, the macula appeared spottily pigmented (Fig. 12-17). Fluorescein angiography showed irregular and granular staining of the RPE. The pigmented areas gradually diminished in size after the first month and some disappeared entirely after 3 to 5 months, leaving a

Figure 12-13. *(A)* Fluorescein angiogram of photic maculopathy in a rhesus monkey after exposure to the light of an indirect ophthalmoscope directed at the macular area. *(B)* Even in the late venous phase of the fluorescein angiogram, leakage in the perimacular area is diffuse, while the macula appears to be less affected, suggesting possible protection from photic injury by xanthophyll pigment of the macula. (Tso MOM: Retinal phototoxicity in ocular surgery. In Sears M, Tarkkanen A (eds): Surgical Pharmacology of the Eye, pp 205–219. New York, Raven Press, 1985)

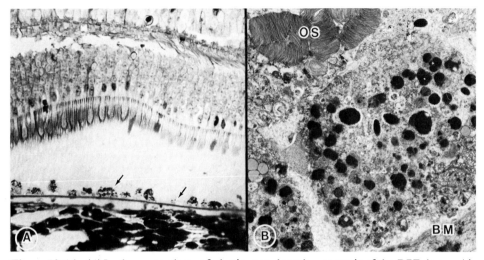

Figure 12-14. *(A)* In the acute phase of photic maculopathy, necrosis of the RPE *(arrows)* is seen in the macular area. *(B)* The degenerated RPE cells show disruption of the plasmalemma and densification of the cytoplasm. The outer segments (OS) anterior to the RPE cells disclose disorganization without evidence of coagulation necrosis. Bruch's membrane: BM. (Original magnifications, *A* × 320; *B* × 8500) (Tso MOM, Woodford BJ: Effect of photic injury on the retinal tissues. Ophthalmology 90(8): 952–963, 1983)

scopically. In focal areas, the RPE proliferated into three or four layers (Fig. 12-19). The pyknotic nuclei of the photoreceptor cells had dropped out, and the outer nuclear layer was thinned.

Phase 3 included follow-up of 2 months to 5 years after light exposure. The macula demonstrated a yellowish, irregularly pigmented raised lesion (Fig. 12-20). The foveal area was frequently less severely affected, even though the

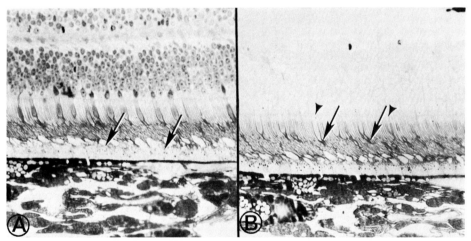

Figure 12-15. *(A)* The RPE cells *(arrow)* at the periphery of a lesion of photic maculopathy are swollen but the photoreceptor cells and elements appear relatively intact. *(B)* Horseradish peroxidase study (unstained) shows leakage of tracer *(arrows)* through the RPE into the subretinal space. The tracer, however, is stopped by the external limiting membrane *(arrowheads)* of the retina. (Original magnifications, *A, B* × 320) (Tso MOM, Woodford BJ: Effect of photic injury on the retinal tissues. Ophthalmology 90(8): 952–963, 1983)

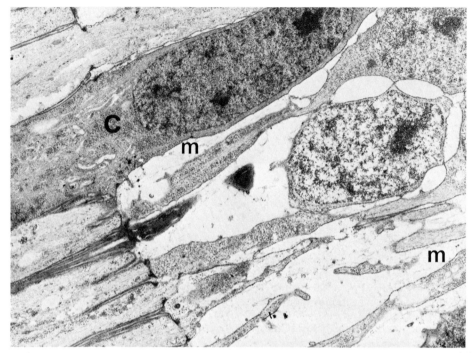

Figure 12-16. Photoreceptor cells in the acute phase of photic maculopathy showing densification of the cytoplasm (C) and marked edema of the Müller cells (m). (Original magnification × 6200) (Tso MOM, Woodford BJ: Effect of photic injury on the retinal tissues. Ophthalmology 90(8): 952–963, 1983)

entire macula had been directly exposed. A raised depigmented scar was commonly observed in the perimacular area and persisted up to 5 years after injury without much alteration. Fluorescein angiography disclosed that the lesion exhibited irregular hypofluorescence in the early arterial phase but late diffuse staining and leakage in the late venous phase.

Histopathologically, the proliferated RPE assumed a spindle shape and formed a placoid lesion posterior to a layer of cuboidal pigment epithelium (Fig. 12-21). In horseradish peroxidase tracer study, the anterior pigment epithelium leaked tracer material into the subretinal space and diffused anteriorly to the external limiting membrane. Electron microscopy disclosed the proliferated spindle pigment epithelial cells to be entirely surrounded by basement membrane. Occasionally, these cells had joined adja-

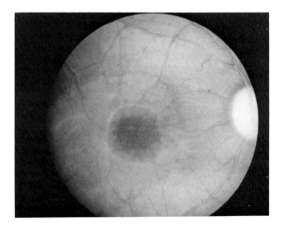

Figure 12-17. Photic maculopathy in the reparative phase demonstrates irregular pigmentation of the macular area. The edema around the macula has begun to subside. (Tso MOM, Woodford BJ: Effect of Photic injury on the retinal tissues. Ophthalmology 90(8): 952–963, 1983)

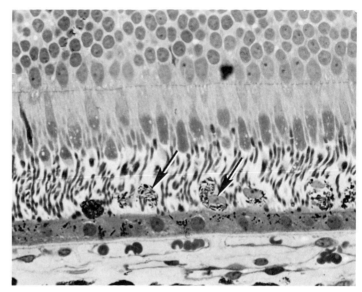

Figure 12-18. Photic maculopathy in the reparative phase. Macrophages *(arrows)* laden with pigment granules cluster around the damaged photoreceptor cells. The RPE remains depigmented. Notice that the photoreceptor nuclei appear intact. (Original magnification × 660) (Tso MOM, Fine BS, Zimmerman LE: Photic maculopathy produced by indirect ophthalmoscope. I. A clinical and histopathologic study, 1970. Am J Ophthalmol 73: 686–699, 1972; published with permission from The American Journal of Ophthalmology)

cent pigment epithelial cells by junctional complexes. The abundant basement membrane gave the proliferated RPE an appearance of "fibroblastic metaplasia," but ultrastructurally the cells had retained their epithelial characteristics. Choroidal neovascularization sometimes ex-

tended to the retinal pigment epithelial plaque (Fig. 12-22). In focal areas of the macula, the outer nuclear layer was reduced in thickness to one to two nuclei (Fig. 12-23). The inner segments appeared very plump, and the outer segments remained one third this original length 5

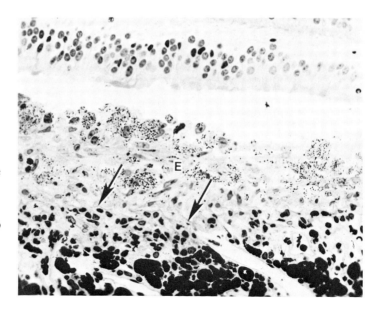

Figure 12-19. In the reparative phase of photic maculopathy, plaque of irregularly proliferated RPE cells (E) is present between the retina and Bruch's membrane *(arrows)*. Note the extensive loss of photoreceptor outer segments. (Original magnification × 305) (Tso MOM: Retinal phototoxicity in ocular surgery. In Sears M, Tarkkanen A (eds): Surgical Pharmacology of the Eye, pp 205–219. New York, Raven Press, 1985)

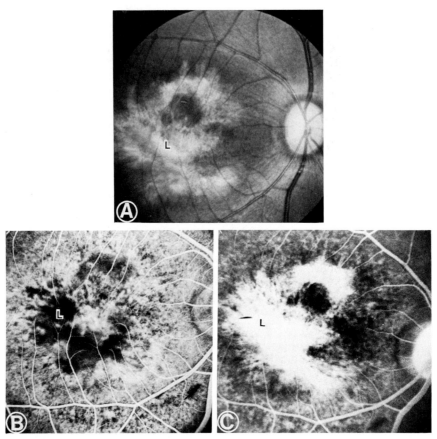

Figure 12-20. Chronic degenerative phase of photic maculopathy in rhesus monkey. *(A)* Fundus photograph showing a raised yellowish lesion (L) in the macular area. *(B)* Fluorescein angiogram in the arteriovenous phase demonstrates that the yellowish patches (L) are hypofluorescent while surrounding areas are hyperfluorescent. *(C)* Fluorescein angiogram in the late venous stage reveals that the yellowish patches (L) are hyperfluorescent. (Tso MOM, Woodford BJ: Effect of photic injury on the retinal tissues. Ophthalmology 90(8): 952–963, 1983)

years after exposure. The RPE was thin and atrophic (Fig. 12-24). The shortening of the outer segments probably derived from the impaired production of outer segment discs by photoreceptor cells. The exact metabolic disturbance the photoreceptor cells undergo by photic insult needs further investigation. Interestingly, shortening of the photoreceptor cell outer segments is common in people with age-related macular degeneration.

Physiologic Factors Affecting Retinal Light Toxicity

Photic injury to the retina involves complicated physiologic mechanisms. Many of the factors

that influence photic injury are derived from animal experiments with rats, rabbits, cats, dogs, pigeons, and nonhuman primates. Only some of them may apply to human photic insult; others are species specific. Different regions in the retina exhibit different susceptibilities to injury.

Howell, Rapp, and Williams have described the central superior region of the hooded rat retina as being highly susceptible to light injury.[40] Noell has noted that photoreceptor cells around the optic disc and the ora serrata seem to be especially resistant to light damage.[59] Sprague-Dawley rats exposed to green fluorescent light exhibited considerable individual variation in severity of injury.[54] In general, the

Figure 12-21. Chronic degenerative phase of photic maculopathy in the rhesus monkey. A plaque of proliferated RPE cells (E) is present in the subretinal region, accounting for the elevated yellowish lesion observed ophthalmoscopically (Fig. 12-20). The anterior layer of cuboidal pigment epithelium *(arrows)* is irregularly depigmented. Scattered macrophages *(arrowhead)* are still present in the subretinal space. (Original magnification × 195) (Tso MOM, Fine BS, Zimmerman LE: Photic maculopathy produced by indirect ophthalmoscope. I. A clinical and histopathologic study, 1970. Am J Ophthalmol 73:686–699, 1972; published with permission from The American Journal of Ophthalmology)

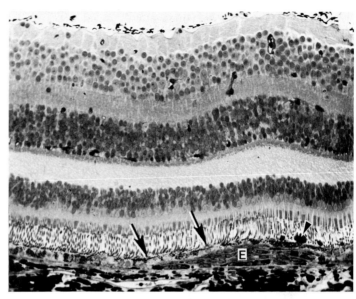

superior and temporal areas appeared to be the two most susceptible quadrants. Carter-Dawson and coworkers have shown that the inferonasal region of the retina in both normal and vitamin A–deficient rats appears more readily damaged by light.[10]

A second factor affecting retinal photic toxicity is dark and light adaptation.[58] Rats maintained in cyclic light are much more resistant to photic injury than rats that were dark-adapted for 2 days before light exposure. Also, increased body temperature during light exposure re-

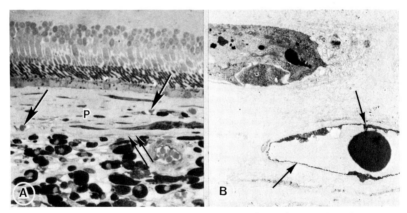

Figure 12-22. *(A)* Chronic degenerative phase of photic maculopathy. A plaque of proliferated RPE (P) is present anterior to Bruch's membrane. The most anterior layer of the proliferated pigment epithelium has assumed a cuboidal shape while the cells in the plaque have a spindly appearance. New vessels *(single arrows)* infiltrate into the plaque. *Double arrows* indicate Bruch's membrane. *(B)* Electron micrograph of the subretinal pigment epithelial neovascularization showing fenestrated endothelial cells *(arrows)* in both the anterior and posterior surfaces of the capillaries. (Original magnifications *A* × 170; *B* × 3000) (*A*, Tso MOM, Woodford BJ: Effect of photic injury on the retinal tissues. Ophthalmology 90(8): 952–963, 1983; *B*, Tso MOM: Pathogenetic factors of aging macular degeneration. Ophthalmology 92:628–635, 1985)

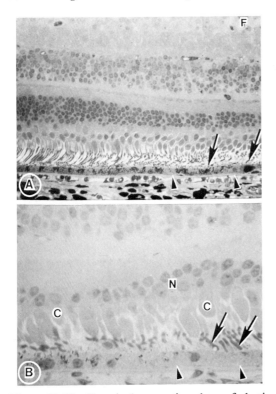

Figure 12-23. Chronic degenerative phase of photic maculopathy in a monkey that has been exposed to the light of an indirect ophthalmoscope. Note the decrease of the photoreceptor nuclei toward the fovea (F). The photoreceptor elements *(arrows)* are shortened and thinned, and the irregular pigmentation of the RPE *(arrowheads)* is apparent. *(B)* At the foveal area, the nuclei (N) of the photoreceptor cells are reduced to one to two nuclei thick. The inner segments of the cone cells (C) show moderate hypertrophy and the outer segments are shortened *(arrows)*. The RPE *(arrowheads)* is largely depigmented. (Original magnifications, *A* × 140; *B* × 420)

sulted in severe retinal degeneration in rodents and monkeys after photic injury.[57,61] This observation may account in part for the frequent complaint of photophobia in patients with high fever.

Pigmentation may affect susceptibility to retinal photic toxicity as well.[49,74] It has long been suspected that albino patients, who frequently are photosensitive and have a central scotoma, may be more susceptible to photic injury than normally pigmented persons. However, when Rapp and Williams exposed albino and pig-

mented rats with dilated pupils to light that was controlled to produce equal steady-state bleaching in both strains of rats, they observed comparable retinal degeneration in both.[70] The authors believe that the pigmented rat appeared less susceptible to light damage because iris pigmentation lowered retinal irradiance. However, it is difficult to compare rats of different strains and draw conclusions about the effects of pigmentation.

Rats, rabbits, frogs, pigeons, dogs, and humans exhibit marked differences in susceptibility to photic injury. Rabbits, monkeys, and humans have much higher thresholds to photic injury than rats. Hamsters suffer more damage when exposed to light when compared to cats or rabbits.[53]

Genetic makeup also affects susceptibility to light damage among different strains of the same species.[18] LaVail and colleauges demonstrated variations in photic susceptibility among albino mice of different strains.[50] Mice of the C57 B1/6J-c2J strains were more resistant to light damage than those of the Balb/c strain. Genetic crosses between these strains produced offspring that exhibited an intermediate response to light damage.

Susceptibility to light damage in rats appears to increase with age.[3,48] O'Steen and coworkers observed that rats 7 weeks of age were more likely to suffer light damage than those 3 to 4 weeks old.[62,63] However, Messner and associates studied photic injury in the retinas of newborn rhesus monkeys and observed increased susceptibility.[57]

Vitamin A–deficient rats have shown more resistance to light damage than rats fed a normal diet.[59,60] This observation supports the hypothesis that photic injury in rats is rhodopsin dependent. On the other hand, vitamin E deficiency does not produce more severe light damage in rodents.[74] Vitamin C–deficient guinea pigs showed an exaggerated response to photic injury of the retina.[93] Furthermore, monkeys deficient in ascorbic acid appeared to exhibit a more severe reaction to photic injury than animals fed a normal diet.

Short wave lengths in the visible spectrum appear to produce more severe retinal injury than long wave length light.[30,73] In general, the

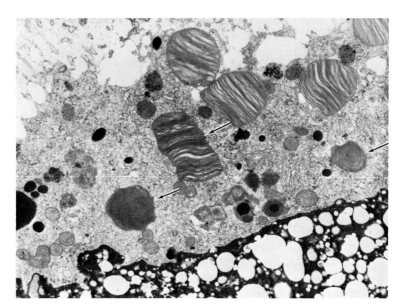

Figure 12-24. Atrophic pigment epithelium in chronic degenerative phase of photic maculopathy. The cells are thinned and have few melanin granules. Numerous outer segments *(arrows)* of the photoreceptor cells in different stages of degradation are engulfed in the cytoplasm. Basal plasmalemmal infolding of the RPE cells is absent. (Original magnification × 10,000) (Tso MOM, Woodford BJ: Effect of photic injury on the retinal tissues. Ophthalmology 90(8): 952–963, 1983)

action spectrum of the damaging light is a decreasing function of the wave length. The higher the intensity of the inflicting light, the more severe the retinal lesion. Similarly, a dilated pupil allows more damaging light into the retina during exposure and produces increased photic insult.

Sperling and coworkers have observed that intermittent blue or green light produced damage to the blue- and green-responsive cone cells in monkeys.[34,73] Continuous exposure created more severe damage to the RPE than did intermittent exposure under similar conditions.

In human patients, a cataractous lens or an implanted intraocular lens may filter light of different wave lengths from the retina. Since photic injury varies with wave length, the lenticular changes in the cataractous state will affect the degree of damage.

Physical Parameters of Light From Ophthalmic Instruments

Some ophthalmic instruments are capable of producing retinal photic injury. Calkins, Delori, Mainster, and others have examined the physical parameters of light from indirect and direct ophthalmoscopes, slit lamps, operating microscopes, overhead surgical lamps, fundus cameras, and other instruments.[7–9,11,16,17,37,55] The severity of damage is affected by the area of retina exposed, the duration of the exposure, the transmittal of light through the ocular media, the spectral characteristics of the light source, and the retinal irradiance.

While standards for white incoherent light sources have not been developed, most investigators use standards established for coherent laser sources (ANSI Z-136.1-1980) to define the maximum permissible exposure (MPE) of white light to the retina. The average retinal irradiance from an indirect ophthalmoscope is about 69 to 125 mW per cm^2 when the transformer is at the maximum setting. Conversely, direct ophthalmoscopes, such as the American Optical Gianscope and the Welch-Allyn ophthalmoscope with a standard bulb, produce a retinal irradiance of 29 mW per cm^2, approximately half that of the indirect ophthalmoscope. Overhead surgical lamps are comparable with the direct ophthalmoscope; they emit light in the range of 25 mW per cm^2. The slit-lamp bimicroscope delivered a retinal irradiance three times higher than that of an indirect ophthalmoscope. The most striking finding has been the operating microscope, such as the Zeiss OP MI I with external fiberoptic sources, which produces a retinal irradiance of about 100 to 970 mW per cm^2 in phakic patients. Thus, the operating microscope may emit two to five times more light than the indirect ophthalmoscope. Calkins and colleagues have calculated that the operating microscope light would be unsafe after an exposure of only 1 minute! They have also ascertained that the maximum permissible exposure from the binocular indirect ophthalmoscope with a 20-diopter lens is between 20 and 40 seconds. Delori has also assessed fundus cameras and found the maximum permissible exposure ranged from 5 to 53 minutes, suggesting little risk of photic injury from the light of the fundus camera.[16]

Proposed Mechanisms in Retinal Photic Injury

As outlined, many physiologic factors influence the severity of photic injury. The pathogenic mechanisms involved probably consist of a cascade of reactions that finally result in damage to the photoreceptor cell–pigment epithelium complex. In his pioneer study of photic injury to rat retinas, Noell suggested there were two kinds of photic injury.[59] The first was characterized by loss of RPE associated with necrosis of the photoreceptor nuclei. This response was dramatically exaggerated by increased body temperature. Lesions could be produced in rats by exposure to 50- to 200-foot candle light for 8 to 48 hours, and were exaggerated when the animals were fully dark-adapted because of the sensitization of the retina to photic injury. Rats maintained in daily cyclic lighting might not be affected by similar exposures.

A second kind of damage was described by Noell in rats younger than 24 days that were exosed to continuous light for 8 to 50 days. The damage produced was characterized by widespread photoreceptor cell death, but the RPE was preserved. In contrast to the first type of light damage, constant dark-adaptation provided apparent resistance to insult in the young rats.

Noell postulated that the first kind of photic damage is rhodopsin mediated, although as a primary mechanism, this appears inconsistent with widespread necrosis of the RPE. A modification of this hypothesis is that primary damage

occurs in the pigment epithelium and secondary changes result in photoreceptor cell death. However, it may be argued that even when the RPE is wiped out by iodate poisoning, the photoreceptor cells can still survive.

Noell also suggested that photo-oxidation may be an important mechanism for photic damage. Transformation of the physiologic response of photoreceptor cells to light may be magnified by photosensitization reactions and may result in retinal photic injury. However, he believed that the lytic effect of retinol on the membrane is probably not the major pathogenetic mechanism involved.

Feeney-Burns and coworkers studied lipofuscin and melanin granules in the human RPE in various age groups and observed an increase in lipofuscin pigment with advancing age.[20,21] They proposed that photic exposure causes a univalent reduction in oxygen, which produces a series of free radicals that react with polyunsaturated fatty acids in the photoreceptor–RPE complex to produce various breakdown products of lipid peroxidation. These investigators suggested that lipofuscin in the RPE results from insufficiency of protective mechanisms against free radicals, and that vitamin E is a powerful antioxidant that may quench free radicals and, so, is the major protective antioxidant in the eye. Indeed, monkeys and rats given a vitamin E–deficient diet accumulate abundant fluorescent lipofuscin granules in the RPE. However, Organisciak and coworkers showed that the level of vitamin E or glutathione did not decrease after rats were exposed to light.[65] Stone and coworkers noted that rats deficient in vitamin E and selenium did not have exaggerated light injury.[74] In spite of the uncertain role of vitamin E in retinal photic injury, lipid peroxidation must be an important process. This hypothesis is supported by the work of Anderson and others, who showed an increase in lipid hydroperoxide and a decrease in the relative ratio of docosahexanoic acid to total lipids in the retina after photic injury.[1,2,42,92]

Lawwill summarized three pathophysiologic mechanisms of retinal photic injury.[52,53] The first was rhodopsin specific, similar to that described in rodents by Noell. He believed that rat retinas are particularly susceptible to rhodopsin-dependent photic injury, but asserted that this mechanism may not be as important in primates. The second mechanism, which was cone pigment specific, was observed in primates after long-term repeated spectral exposure resulting in damage to red- or green-sensitive cone populations. The third mechanism occurred in primates after continuous exposure and involved an action spectrum with maximum damage in blue light. Lawwill proposed that the direct action of blue light on the mitochondria of the retinal tissues could result in damage to all layers of the retina.

In our study of photic injury in humans, monkeys, guinea pigs, and rats, we proposed that the disease process may be classified into three phases, each of which elicits a different pathogenetic mechanism. In phase I, shortly after photic injury, the predominant pathologic changes include disruption and vesiculation of photoreceptor outer segments, vacuolization of mitochondria, and swelling of the RPE. The primary mechanism may be photodynamic in nature, induced by light photosensitizers and tissue oxygen. When light hits the transparent retina, some energy is absorbed by the photopigments in the phototransduction process, creating a nerve impulse. The excess energy must then be disposed of. A portion of the energy is absorbed by the melanin granules and dissipated into the surrounding cytoplasmic components. Some excess energy activates photosensitizers in the retina and the RPE into a triplet state. At this juncture, two major reactions may take place. In the type 1 reaction, activated photosensitizers react with reducing substances in retinal tissue to produce free radicals. In the type 2 reaction, activated photosensitizers react with oxygen, which is abundant in the outer layers of retinal tissue, to form singlet oxygen. The type 2 response accounts for the predominant quenching effect in the photosensitizer triplet state. In either reaction, free radicals and singlet oxygen may further react with polyunsaturated fatty acids in retinal tissues resulting in lipid peroxidation and tissue damage.

The phase II photic injury is characterized by an invasion of macrophages from the systemic circulation into the subretinal area to remove the pigment epithelial and photoreceptor debris. Different pathogenetic mechanisms are activated with the arrival of macrophages. Activated macrophages undergo a respiratory burst, in which 10 to 20 times more oxygen is consumed, producing a series of oxygen-free radicals including superoxide radicals and hydrogen peroxide. The hydroxyl groups are also generated through the well-known Haber-Weis and Fenton reactions. The macrophages engulf and digest cellular debris with the assistance of these free radicals. Excessive free radicals attack the surrounding retinal tissues and cause degeneration.

A number of defense mechanisms against these free radicals have been identified in the retina. Superoxide dismutase, catalase, peroxidase, and glutathione in the RPE and in the subretinal space may be activated to eliminate the excess free radicals. However, macrophages linger in the subretinal space for as long as 5 years after the photic exposure, continuing to generate free radicals and resulting in progressive photoreceptor cell degeneration.

In phase III, photoreceptor cell death and pigment epithelial necrosis are followed by a reparative process. The RPE surrounding the light-exposed area flattens and migrates to replace the necrotic cells. The blood–retina barrier is disrupted with necrosis of the RPE but is reformed as the pigment epithelial cells proliferate. At times, disruption of the blood–retina barrier persists 5 years after the initial photic injury, but does not necessarily result in the death of photoreceptor cells or RPE. As necrotic photoreceptor cells drop out, remaining photoreceptor cells slide over and regenerate the photoreceptor elements to some extent. The regenerative potential probably varies with species. The regenerative process is frequently incomplete, resulting in short and stubby outer segments, and thin, atrophic, and depigmented RPE, which may be more vulnerable to subsequent photic insult.

Since photic injury involves a cascade of pathogenetic mechanisms, many factors may alter the injurious effects. Some mechanisms are primary, such as light absorption by rhodopsin, cone pigments, or melanin granules and activation of photosensitizers. Other reactions are secondary, such as the macrophagic response to damaged retinal tissues. The reparative process may be species specific and may affect the severity of retinal degeneration.

PHOTIC INJURY AND AGE-RELATED MACULAR DEGENERATION

The causal relationship between photic injury and various forms of retinal degeneration has aroused much interest.[78,95] The possible linkage between age-related macular degeneration and photic insult has been diligently pursued, but only circumstantial evidence has been gathered. As yet, there has been no direct implication of photic injury in the pathogenesis of hereditary retinal degeneration or age-related macular degeneration.

Even though age-related macular degeneration is one of the most common causes of blindness in the United States, there is no effective therapy because definitive pathogenetic mechanisms have not been established. Age-related macular degeneration has been associated with sex, age, iris pigmentation, refractive errors, hereditary factors, and family history, but none of these can be altered.[22] If photic injury exerts a pathogenetic influence on age-related macular degeneration, therapeutic regimens can be developed for patients in the early stage of the disease.

Judging from the many factors influencing its pathogenesis, age-related macular degeneration must be a syndrome in which many etiologic factors converge on a common pathway. Hereditary influences, photic injury, nutritional deficiency, toxic insult, cardiovascular and respiratory disturbances, and pre-existing eye diseases may be involved. Individually or synergistically, these factors may predispose the macula to senescent changes, resulting in a set of clinical manifestations that are defined as age-related macular degeneration. Some of the pathogenetic factors that are directly or indirectly ascribed to photic injury are discussed below.

Age

Of the many pathogenetic factors in senile macular degeneration, age is the most closely corre-

lated.[22,41] The prevalence of macular degeneration in men and women aged 52 to 64 is 1.6%. It increases dramatically to 11% for ages 65 to 74, and reaches 27.9% for people over 75 years of age.[22] Since the primary function of the photoreceptor cells is light perception, it may be assumed that the cumulative effects of light exposure may inflict degenerative changes in the photoreceptor cells in the macula with increasing age. There is definite evidence that photoreceptor elements regenerate after mild photic insult, including sun gazing. Experiments in animals, however, have shown that the reparative process is incomplete and imperfect. The cumulative effects of retinal photic insult may lead to eventual photoreceptor cell death. In a study of the human macula, Gartner and Henkind have observed that the number of photoreceptor cells in the macula decreases with age.[24]

Race and Pigmentation

Some epidemiologic studies have reported a lower incidence of macular degeneration in blacks than in whites of comparable age. Gregor and Joffe[27] compared blacks in two South African hospitals with whites in Moorfield Eye Hospital in London and observed that drusen and pigment epithelial changes occurred twice as often in whites.[27] Chumbley also found a low incidence (1%) in adults over age 65 suffering from macular degeneration in Rhodesian blacks.[12] Clinical impressions described by Schatz also suggested that age-related macular degeneration is uncommon in blacks in the United States. Conversely, Klein and Klein examined data from the National Health and Nutritional Survey and showed comparable instances of age-related macular degeneration in whites and blacks.[45]

Hyman and associates reported that patients with brown iris coloration are less likely to develop age-related macular degeneration than those with light irides.[41] Weiter and coworkers compared 650 white patients with age-related macular degeneration with a control group of 363.[90] As many as 76% of the patients with age-related macular degeneration had light-colored irides compared with 30% of the control group. Fundus pigmentation was similarly related. These authors suggested that dark ocular pigmentation tends to decrease the risk of developing age-related macular degeneration. They further demonstrated an inverse relationship between melanin and lipofuscin in the human RPE with age. Lipofuscin granules, they found, increase with age and are more abundant in the RPE of whites than blacks. They hypothesized that the accumulation of lipofuscin in the RPE is related to photic damage and that melanin would provide protection by absorbing excessive light in the retina as well as by scavenging light-induced free radicals. Feeney-Burns and Berman also examined lipofuscin in human RPE and proposed that it was a product of phototoxic reactions in the retina.[21]

Central Location of Retinal Photic Lesion and Macular Degeneration

Young proposed that the optical system of the eye focuses light in the macula, producing more damage there than in the retinal periphery.[95] Sykes and coworkers studied injury to the monkey eye from diffuse fluorescent light and observed that most damage occurred in the photoreceptor cells in the macula.[75] The central superior region of the hooded rat retina has also been described as being more susceptible to photic injury. The distribution of photoreceptor degeneration in age-related macular degeneration appeared to coincide with the central location of diffuse photic exposure to the retina.

COMPARISON OF PATHOLOGIC CHANGES IN RETINAL PHOTIC INJURY AND AGE-RELATED MACULAR DEGENERATION

In general, age-related macular degeneration may be classified in two pathologic patterns: alveolar pigment epithelial atrophy, or atrophic maculopathy, and subretinal pigment epithelial neovascularization resulting in transudative, hemorrhagic, and (eventually) disciform macular degeneration.[26] Alveolar pigment epithelial atrophy is characterized ophthalmologically by irregular depigmentation in the macula, thinning of the central retina, and loss of the foveal light reflex. Fluorescein angiography shows irregular window defects without leakage. Histo-

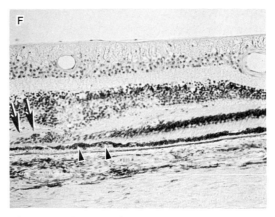

Figure 12-25. Atrophic maculopathy in a human patient. Note the gradual loss of photoreceptor nuclei *(arrows)* toward the fovea (F). The photoreceptor cell elements are shortened. RPE cells appear irregular. The subretinal pigment epithelial region is filled with drusenoid material *(arrowheads)*. (Original magnification × 156)

pathologically, the RPE is flattened and filled with lipofuscin granules. Progressive thinning of the outer nuclear layer of the retina also is observed as the photoreceptor cells gradually drop out (Fig. 12-25, 12-26). The remaining photoreceptor cells have short outer segments. In advanced cases, the photoreceptor cells and the RPE disappear, and the inner nuclear layer approximates Bruch's membrane.

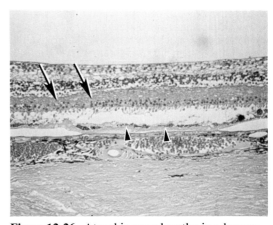

Figure 12-26. Atrophic maculopathy in a human patient showing marked loss of photoreceptor nuclei *(arrows)*, shortening of the photoreceptor elements, and irregular thinning and loss of the RPE. Drusenoid material *(arrowheads)* is present in the subpigment epithelial region. (Original magnification × 90)

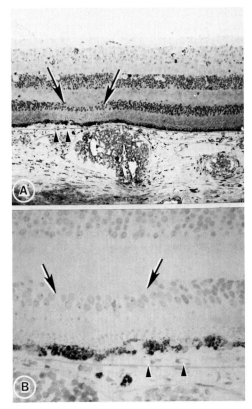

Figure 12-27. *(A)* Subpigment epithelial neovascularization in a human. Note the focal loss of photoreceptor nuclei *(arrows)* in the region of neovascularization. The RPE is elevated, and new blood vessels *(arrowheads)* are lying anterior to Bruch's membrane in the subretinal pigment epithelial region. *(B)* Under high power, the new vessels *(arrowheads)* have infiltrated into the subretinal pigment epithelial region. Note the loss of photoreceptor nuclei *(arrows)* and staining of the photoreceptor elements. (Original magnifications, *A* × 100; *B* × 250)

In subretinal pigment epithelial neovascularization, new vessels break through Bruch's membrane into the subretinal pigment epithelial space (Fig. 12-27). A transudative detachment of the RPE may result. As the disease progresses, hemorrhage occurs posterior to the RPE. Ophthalmoscopically, the blood appears as a raised greenish lesion. Later, the blood extends into the subretinal space and stimulates the proliferation of RPE and retinal glial cells and the invasion of organizing fibrovascular tis-

sue. The proliferated RPE and glial cells form a disciform scar. At times, the neovascular net remains transudative for months or years, resulting in a persistent serous cystoid macular detachment and a yellowish transudative lipoidal reaction.

Similar atrophic maculopathy and subretinal pigment epithelial neovascularization were produced in rhesus monkeys after the maculas were exposed to the light of an indirect ophthalmoscope for 1 to 2 hours at one sitting.[78,81,85] Between 5 and 12 months later atrophic maculopathy developed. It was characterized by the depigmentation of pigment eithelium and thinning of the photoreceptor cell layer. The outer segments of the remaining photoreceptor cells frequently were shortened or absent, suggesting incomplete regeneration. In a few instances, new capillaries insinuated into the proliferated RPE. These new capillaries had focally attenuated endothelial cells in both the anterior and posterior walls and were surrounded by poorly developed pericytes. The subretinal pigment epithelial neovascularization closely resembled that in humans. Thus, the two forms of age-related macular degeneration, atrophic maculopathy and subretinal pigment epithelial neovascularization, can be reproduced by subjecting monkeys to photic injury.

Vitamin C and Light Damage

While ascorbate is ubiquitous in body tissues, the level of retinal ascorbate is approximately 20 times more than that in plasma, suggesting a special role for the vitamin in the metabolism and function of the retina. Recent biochemical studies suggest that ascorbate may act as a superoxide radical scavenging agent in ocular tissues.[64-66,81,95] It has been hypothesized that photosensitizers, such as riboflavin and retinal cytochrome C, among others, are present in the retina and may be activated by excess energy from light exposure. A photodynamic reaction takes place, resulting in singlet oxygen, hydroxyl radicals, hydrogen peroxide, and other free radicals, and ascorbate may act as an antioxidant to ameliorate photic insult.

We have noted that in the neuroretina of guinea pigs and baboons, reduced ascorbate is

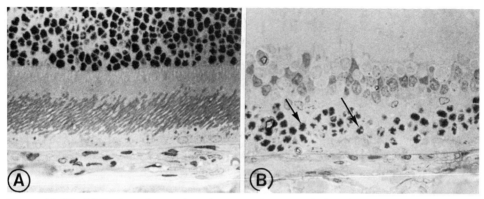

Figure 12-28. *(A)* Retina of a rat given large supplements of vitamin C discloses relatively intact photoreceptor cells and RPE after exposure to fluorescent light for 24 hours. *(B)* Retina of a rat fed with normal diet with no vitamin C supplement shows marked loss of photoreceptor cell elements and nuclei *(arrows)* after exposure to the same light. (Toluidine blue: original magnifications *A* × 370; *B* × 320) (Tso MOM: Pathogenetic factors of aging macular degeneration. Ophthalmology 92:628–635, 1985)

present as 97% and 93% of the total ascorbate, respectively.[84,94] After mild photic insult in both species, the reduced ascorbate descreases in the neuroretina while oxidized ascorbate increases. Organisciak and coworkers exposed normal rats to fluorescent light for 24 hours and observed that retinal ascorbate in the neuroretina may be oxidized during excessive light exposure and may act to scavenge free radicals.[64,66] Furthermore, the authors compared photic injury in rats fed a normal diet and those fed a diet supplemented with vitamin C and noted that ascorbate reduced the loss of rhodopsin after photic injury in rats fed the ascorbate-supplemented diets.[66] L-ascorbate, sodium ascorbate, and dehydroascorbate were equally effective in preserving rhodopsin after photic injury, while D-ascorbate was not. In addition, the protective action of rhodopsin loss by ascorbate was dose dependent. Ascorbate was effective when administered before light exposure, but not afterward. We studied the loss of photoreceptor cells in retinal photic injury in rats and noted significantly less damage in those given an ascorbate supplement (Fig. 12-28).[54] We next examined photic injury in normal and scorbutic guinea pigs and monkeys and observed that the scorbutic animals suffered more photic injury than normal animals.[93] It appeared that retinal pho-

tic injury may indeed by ameliorated by ascorbate.

Choroidal Vascular Changes in Age-Related Macular Degeneration

The role that the choriocapillaris plays in atrophic and disciform macular degenerations has been controversial. Klein noted choroidal vascular insufficiencies in age-related macular degeneration, while Hogan described a relatively normal choriocapillaris in senile maculopathies.[38,39,44] Green and Key observed that the choriocapillaris is relatively intact in macular degeneration.[26] One main reason for this dispute has been the difficulty of studying aging changes in the choriocapillaris. According to Kerschbaumer, senile changes in the choriocapillaris consisted of loss of cellularity, increased hyalinization of the capillary walls, narrowing and obliteration of the lumen, and atrophy of the capillary bed.[43] However, Friedman and Smith could not confirm these observations in their study of senile changes in the choroidal choriocapillaris of the posterior pole by flat preparation.[23] They noted that changes in the aging choriocapillaris were relatively mild and consisted of decreased cellularity and prominent staining of vessel walls in periodic acid-

Schiff preparation and increased intercapillary pillars of connective tissue. They described atrophic choriocapillaris and capillary dropout as being related to large choroidal vessels, but found no choriocapillaris atrophy resulting from obliteration of the choroidal arteries.

We studied the choriocapillaris by flat preparation and noted that in the normal adult, the posterior pole consisted of a network of sinusoidal capillaries arranged in a lobular pattern with a central feeding arteriole and peripheral draining venules.[76,82] In a patient with atrophic age-related macular degeneration, the sinusoidal choriocapillaris was replaced by a tubular capillary network that was definitely pathologic in the macular area. Whether this abnormal pattern in the choriocapillaris was a primary change in age-related macular degeneration or a secondary reaction to a primary insulting agent needs investigation.

Parver and coworkers have postulated that the rapidly flowing choroidal circulation in the posterior pole has a temperature-regulating function.[68] The retina may become overheated by radiant energy from light perception. In age-related macular degeneration, sclerosis of the choriocapillaris may impede the choroidal circulation and result in increased susceptibility to photic injury when excessive light exposure to the retina is not removed.

Smoking and Age-Related Macular Degeneration

Paetkau and colleagues observed that the mean age for the onset of blindness due to age-related macular degeneration in smokers was 64 years compared with 71 years in nonsmokers.[67] Hyman and coworkers showed a positive association between smoking and macular degeneration in men.[41] Smokers have been observed to be relatively scorbutic and require large doses of vitamin C. It is possible that the relative scurvy in smokers may make them more susceptible to photic injury than nonsmokers.

Cataracts and Age-Related Macular Degeneration

Van der Hoeve suggested that opacification of the lens provides partial protection against age-

related macular degeneration.[85-87] In his series of 1,336 patients over 60 years of age, twice as many patients with cataracts were free of age-related macular degeneration as patients who had no cataracts. In 1953 Gjessing from Norway examined 4088 men and 4606 women over 55 years of age.[25] He observed that 27.84% of the men had cataracts, 7.5% had macular changes, and only 1.86% had both. Of the women, 27.17% had cataracts, 9% had macular changes, and 3.2% had both. Gjessing believed that the lenticular opacities protected the patients from the developement of age-related macular degeneration.

Elastotic Degeneration of Skin and Age-Related Macular Degeneration

Blumenkranz and colleagues compared the elastosis in the dermis of sun-exposed and sun-protected areas of the arm in 26 patients.[4] Age, white-cell blood count, and the extent of elastosis in sun-protected dermis were all predictive of age-related macular degeneration. Patients with disciform macular degeneration were more than twice as likely to develop moderate to severe elastotic degeneration in sun-protected areas. Substantial differences were observed in skin exposed to the sun. These investigators suggested that patients with disciform macular degeneration may have a generalized systemic suceptibility to photic injury.

CONCLUSION

Light damage cannot be solely responsible for the pathogenesis of age-related macular degeneration. For example, drusen precedes most forms of age-related macular degeneration, but none has been observed with photic injury. Furthermore, while photic injury may bring about subretinal pigment epithelial neovascularization in an experimental model, it is soon followed by a reparative healing process. In disciform aging macular degeneration, the neovascular net is relentless, resulting in total destruction of the macula. Even repeated photic injury in nonhuman primates failed to induce the aggressive extension of subretinal pigment epithelial neovascularization of age-related macular degeneration.

Despite sporadic reports of photic injury in certain areas of the world, no epidemiologic data confirm that certain lifestyles or increased exposure to environmental lighting is more conducive to age-related macular degeneration. However, in an ongoing research project, the maculas of full-time seamen in Maryland are being compared with those in seamen who go to sea occasionally. More epidemiologic research is needed in this area.

Factors other than photic injury may contribute to disease, such as hyperopia, systemic hypertension, respiratory diseases, or toxic exposure. These were prevalent among patients with age-related macular degeneration. The possibility that photic injury is one of the contributing factors must be explored, because most of the other associated factors in age-related macular degeneration, such as hereditary features, ocular characteristics, and systemic diseases are immutable. Photic injury, however, may be ameliorated through the use of antioxidants such as vitamin C and protective lenses.

REFERENCES

1. Anderson RE, Maude MB, Nielsen JC: Effect of lipid peroxidation on rhodopsin regeneration. Curr Eye Res 4:65–71, 1985
2. Anderson RE, Rapp LM, Wiegand RD: Lipid peroxidation and retinal degeneration. Curr Eye Res 3:223–227, 1983
3. Ballowitz L, Dammrich K: Ratinaschaden bei Ratten nach einer Fototherapie. Z Kinderheilkd 42:113, 1972
4. Blumenkranz MS, Russell S, Robey M, et al: Risk factors in age-related maculopathy complicated by choroidal neovascularization. Ophthalmology 93:552–558, 1986
5. Bok D: Retinal photoreceptor–pigment epithelium interactions. Invest Ophthalmol Vis Sci 26:1659, 1985
6. Boldrey EE, Ho BT, Griffith RD: Retinal burns occurring at cataract extraction. Ophthalmology 91:1297–1302, 1984
7. Calkins JL, Hochheimer BF: Retinal light exposure from operating microscopes. Arch Ophthalmol 97:2363, 1979
8. Calkins JL, Hochheimer BF: Retinal light exposure from ophthalmoscopes, slit lamps and overhead surgical lamps: An analysis of potential hazard. Invest Ophthalmol Vis Sci 19:1009, 1980
9. Calkins JL, Hochheimer BF, D'Anna SA: Potential hazards from specific ophthalmic devices. Vision Res 20:1039–1053, 1980
10. Carter-Dawson L, Kuwabara T, Bieri JG: Intrinsic, light-independent, regional differences in photoreceptor cell degeneration in vitamin A–deficient rat retinas. Invest Ophthalmol Vis Sci 22:249–255, 1982
11. Cavonius CR, Elgin S, Robbins DO: Thresholds for damage to the human retina by white light. Exp Eye Res 19:543, 1974
12. Chumbley LC: Impressions of eye diseases among Rhodesian blacks in Moshonaland. S Afr Med J 52:316–318, 1977
13. Clark B, Johnson ML, Dreher RE: The effect of sunlight on dark adaptation. Am J Ophthalmol 29:828–836, 1946
14. Cogan DC: Light and health hazards. Arch Ophthalmol 79:2, 1968
15. Cordes FC: Eclipse retinitis. Am J Ophthalmol 31:101–103, 1948
16. Delori FC, Parker JS, Mainster MA: Light levels in fundus photography and fluorescein angiography. Vision Res 20:1099–1104, 1980
17. Delori FC, Parker JS, Mainster MA: Light levels in ophthalmic diagnostic instruments. Proc Soc Photo-Optical Instrum Eng 229:154–160, 1980
18. Emig MD, Ando H, Braniecki MA, et al: A genetic factor in retinal light damage of the rat. Invest Ophthalmol Vis Sci (suppl)27:55, 1986
19. Ewald RA, Ritchey CI: Sun gazing as the cause of foveomacular retinitis. Am J Ophthalmol 70:491–497, 1970
20. Feeney L, Berman ER: Oxygen toxicity membrane damage by free radicals. Invest Ophthalmol Vis Sci 15:1789, 1976
21. Feeney-Burns L, Berman ER, Rothman H: Lipofuscin of human retinal pigment epithelium. Am J Ophthalmol 90:783–791, 1980
22. Ferris FL III: Senile macular degeneration: Review of epidemiologic features. Am J Epidemiol 118:132–51, 1983
23. Friedman E, Smith TR: Senile changes of the choriocapillaris of the posterior pole. Trans Am Acad Ophthalmol Otolaryngol 69:652–661, 1965
24. Gartner S, Henkind P: Aging and degeneration of the human macula. I: Outer nuclear layer and photoreceptors. Br J Ophthalmol 65:23–28, 1981
25. Gjessing HGA: Gibt es einen Antagonismus zwischen Cataracta senilis und Haabscher seniler Makulaveränderungen? Acta Ophthalmol 31:401–421, 1953
26. Green RW, Key SN III: Senile macular degeneration: A histopathologic study. Trans Am Ophthalmol Soc 75:180–254, 1977
27. Gregor Z, Joffe, L: Senile macular changes in the black African. Br J Ophthalmol 62:547–550, 1978

28. Ham WT Jr: Ocular hazards of light sources: Review of current knowledge. J Occup Med 25:101–103, 1983

29. Ham WT Jr, Mueller HA, Ruffolo JJ, Jr, et al: Solar retinopathy as a function of wavelength: Its significance for protective eyewear. In William TP, Baker BN (eds): The Effects of Constant Light on Visual Processes, pp 319–346. New York, Plenum Press, 1980

30. Ham WT Jr, Mueller HA, Ruffolo JJ Jr, et al: Sensitivity of the retina to radiation damage as a function of wavelength. Photochem Photobiol 29:735–743, 1979

31. Ham WT Jr, Mueller HA, Sliney DH: Retinal sensitivity to damage from short wavelength light. Nature 260:153–155, 1976

32. Ham WT Jr, Mueller HA, Williams RC, et al: Ocular hazard from viewing the sun unprotected and through various windows and filters. Appl Optics 12:2122–2129, 1973

33. Ham WT Jr, Ruffolo JJ, Jr, Mueller HA, et al: The nature of retinal radiation damage: Dependence on wavelength, power level and exposure time. Vision Res 20:1105–1111, 1980

34. Harwerth RS, Sperling HG: Effects of intense visible radiation on the increment-threshold spectral sensitivity of the rhesus monkey eye. Vision Res 15:1193–1204, 1975

35. Hecht S, Hendley CD, Ross S, et al: The effect of exposure to sunlight on night vision. Am J Ophthalmol 31:1573–1580, 1948

36. Henkind P, Hansen RE, Szalay J: Ocular circulation. In Duane TD, Jaeger EA (eds): Biomedical Foundations of Ophthalmology, vol 2, pp 1–54. Philadelphia, Harper & Row, 1986

37. Hochheimer BF, D'Anna SA, Calkins JL: Retinal damage from light. Am J Ophthalmol 88:1039, 1979

38. Hogan MJ: Role of the retinal pigment epithelium in macular diseases. Trans Am Acad Ophthalmol Otolaryngol 76:64–80, 1972

39. Hogan MJ, Alvarado JA: Studies on the human macular. IV: Aging changes in Bruch's membrane. Arch Ophthalmol 77:410–420, 1967

40. Howell WL, Rapp LM, Williams TP: Distribution of melanosomes across the retinal pigment epithelium of a hooded rat: Implications for light damage. Invest Ophthalmol Vis Sci 22:139–144, 1982

41. Hyman LG, Lilienfeld AM, Ferris FL III et al: Senile macular degeneration: A case-control study. Am J Epidemiol 118:213–27, 1983

42. Kagan VE, Shvedova AA, Norikou KN, et al: Light induced free radical oxidation of membrane lipids in photoreceptors of frog retina. Biochem Biophys Acta 330:76, 1973

43. Kerschbaumer R: Über Alters-veränderungen der Uvea. Arch Ophthalmol 38:127–148, 1892

44. Klein BA: Some aspects of classification and differential diagnosis of senile macular degeneration. Am J Ophthalmol 58:927–939, 1964

45. Klein BE, Klein R: Cataracts and macular degeneration in older Americans. Arch Ophthalmol 100:571–573, 1982

46. Kuwabara T, Gorn RA: Retinal damage by visible light: An electron microscopic study. Arch Ophthalmol 79:69–78, 1968

47. Lai YL, Jacoby RO, Jonas AM: Age-related and light-associated retinal changes in Fischer rats. Invest Ophthalmol Vis Sci 17:634–638, 1978

48. Lanum J: The damaging effects of lights on the retina: Empirical findings, theoretical and practical implications. Surv Ophthalmol 22:221–249, 1978

49. LaVail MM: Survival of some photoreceptor cells in albino rats following long-term exposure to continuous light. Invest Ophthalmol 15:64–70, 1976

50. LaVail MM, Battelle BA: Influence of eye pigmentation and light deprivation on inherited retinal dystrophy in the rat. Exp Eye Res 21:167–192, 1975

51. LaVail MM, Gorrin GM, Ginsberg HM, et al: Evidence for genetic regulation of light damage. Invest Ophthalmol Vis Sci (suppl)27:55, 1986

52. Lawwill T: Three major pathologic processes caused by light in the primate retina: A search for mechanisms. Trans Am Ophthalmol Soc 80:517–579, 1982

53. Lawwill T, Crockett S, Currier G: Retinal damage secondary to chronic light exposure, thresholds and mechanisms. Doc Ophthalmol 44:379–402, 1977

54. Li Z-Y, Tso MOM, Wang H, et al: Amelioration of photic injury in the rat retina by ascorbic acid. Invest Ophthalmol Vis Sci 26:1589–1598, 1985

55. Mainster MA: Spectral transmittance of intraocular lenses and retinal damage from intense light sources. Am J Ophthalmol 85:167–170, 1978

56. McDonald HR, Irvine AR: Light-induced maculopathy from the operating microscope in extracapsular cataract extraction and intraocular lens implantation. Ophthalmology 90:945–951, 1983

57. Messner KH, Maisels MJ, Leure-dePree AE: Phototoxicity to the newborn primate retina. Invest Ophthalmol Vis Sci 17:178–182, 1978

58. Noell WK: Effects of environmental lighting and dietary vitamin A on the vulnerability of the retina to light damage. Photochem Photobiol 29:717–723, 1979

59. Noell WK: Possible mechanisms of photoreceptor damage by light in mammalian eyes. Vision Res 20:1163–1171, 1980

60. Noell WK, Albrecht R: Irreversible effects of visible light on the retina: Role of vitamin A. Science 172:76–80, 1971

61. Noell WK, Walker VS, Kang BS, et al: Retinal

damage by light in rats. Invest Ophthalmol 5:450–473, 1966

62. O'Steen WK, Anderson KV: Photoreceptor damage after exposure of rats to incandescent illumination. Zellforsch Anat 127:306–313, 1972

63. O'Steen WK, Anderson KV, Shear CR: Photoreceptor degeneration in albino rats: Dependency on age. Invest Ophthalmol 13:334–339, 1974

64. Organisciak DT, Wang HM: Ascorbic acid as a probe to study light damage in rats. Invest Ophthalmol Vis Sci (Suppl)26:130, 1985

65. Organisciak DT, Wang HM, Kou AL: Ascorbate and glutathione levels in the developing normal and dystrophic rat retina: Effect of intense light exposure. Curr Eye Res 3:257, 1984

66. Organisciak DT, Wang HM, Li Z-Y, et al: The protective effect of ascorbate in retinal light damage of rats. Invest Ophthalmol Vis Sci 26:1580–1588, 1985

67. Paetkau ME, Boyd TAS, Grace M, et al: Senile disciform macular degeneration and smoking. Can J Ophthalmol 13:67–71, 1978

68. Parver LM, Auker C, Carpenter DO: Choroidal blood flow as a heat dissipating mechanism in the macula. Am J Ophthalmol 89:641–646, 1980

69. Penner R, McNair JN: Eclipse blindness. Am J Ophthalmol 61:1452, 1966

70. Rapp LM, Williams TP: The role of ocular pigmentation in protecting against retinal light damage. Vision Res 20:1127–1131, 1980

71. Robertson DM, Feldman RB: Photic retinopathy from the operating room microscope. Am J Ophthalmol 101:561–569, 1986

72. Smith HE: Actinic macular retinal pigment degeneration. US Naval Med Bull 42:675–680, 1944

73. Sperling HG, Johnson C, Harwerth RS: Differential spectral photic damage to primate cones. Vision Res 20:1117, 1126, 1980

74. Stone WL, Katz ML, Lurie M, et al: Effects of dietary vitamin E and selenium on light damage to the rat retina. Photochem Photobiol 29:725–730, 1979

75. Sykes SM, Robison EG Jr, Waxler M, et al: Damage to the monkey retina by broad-spectrum fluorescent light. Invest Ophthalmol Vis Sci 20:425–434, 1981

76. Torczynski E, Tso MOM: The architecture of the choriocapillaris at the posterior pole. Am J Ophthalmol 81:428, 1976

77. Tso MOM: Photic maculopathy in rhesus monkey: A light and electron microscopic study. Invest Ophthalmol 12:17–34, 1973

78. Tso MOM: Pathogenetic factor of aging macular degeneration. Ophthalmology 92:628–635, 1985

79. Tso MOM, Fine BS, Zimmerman LE: Photic maculopathy produced by the indirect ophthalmoscope. I: Clinical and histopathologic study. Am J Ophthalmol 73:686–699, 1972

80. Tso MOM, La Piana, FG: The human fovea after sungazing. Trans Am Acad Ophthalmol Otolaryngol 79:788–795, 1975

81. Tso MOM, Robbins DO, Zimmerman LE: Photic maculopathy: A study of functional and pathologic correlation. Mod Probl Ophthalmol 12:220–228, 1974

82. Tso MOM, Torczynski E: Architecture of the choriocapillaris and macular edema. In Shimizu K, Oosterhuis JA (eds): International Congress Series 450 XXIII Concilium Ophthalmologicum, Kyoto 1978, pp 239–241. Amsterdam-Oxford Excerpta Medica.

83. Tso MOM, Woodford, BJ: Effects of photic injury on the retinal tissues. Ophthalmology 90:952–963, 1983

84. Tso MOM, Woodford BJ, Lam KW: Distribution of ascorbate in normal primate retina and after photic injury: A biochemical morphological correlated study. Curr Eye Res 3:181–191, 1984

85. van der Hoeve J: Senile Maculadegeneration und senile Linsentrübung. von Graefes Arch Ophthalmol 98:1–6, 1918

86. van der Hoeve J: Eye lesions produced by light rich in ultraviolet rays: Senile cataract, senile degeneration of the macula. Am J Ophthalmol 3:178–194, 1920

87. van der Hoeve J: Der Antagonismus zwischen seniler Katarakt und seniler Makuladegeneration (HAAB) und die Frequenz der senilen Makuladegeneration unmittelbar nach Staroperation. Augenheild 63:127–136, 1927

88. Verhoeff FH, Bell L: The pathological effects of radiant energy on the eye. Proc Am Acad Arts Sci 51:628–759, 1916

89. Vos JJ: Digital computations of temperature in retinal burn problems. Inst for Perception, RVO-TNO Report 12F, 19650-16. Soesterberg, The Netherlands, 1963

90. Weiter J, Delori FC, Wing CF, et al: Relationship of senile macular degeneration to ocular pigmentation. Am J Ophthalmol 99:185–187, 1985

91. Wiegand RD, Giusto NM, Rapp LM, et al: Evidence for rod outer segment lipid peroxidation following constant illumination of the rat retina. Invest Ophthalmol Vis Sci 24:1433-1435, 1983

92. Wiegand RD, Giusto NM, Anderson RE: Lipid changes in albino rat rod outer segments following constant illumination. In Clayton R, Haywood J, Reading H, et al (eds): Problems of Normal and Genetically Abnormal Retinas, pp 121–128. New York, Academic Press, 1982

93. Woodford BJ, Tso MOM: Exaggeration of photic injury in scorbutic guinea pig retinas. Invest Ophthalmol Vis Sci (suppl)25:90, 1984

94. Woodford BJ, Tso MOM, Lam K-W: Reduced

and oxidized ascorbates in guinea pig retina under normal and light-exposed conditions. Invest Ophthalmol Vis Sci 24:862–867, 1983

95. Young RW: A theory of central retinal disease. In Sears ML (ed): New Directions in Ophthalmic Research, pp 237–270. New Haven, Yale University Press, 1981

96. Young RW, Bok D: Metabolism of the pigment epithelium. In Zimm KM, Marmor MF (ed): The Retinal Pigment Epithelium, pp 103. Cambridge, Harvard University Press, 1979

97. Young RW, Droz B: The renewal of protein in retinal rods and cones. J Cell Biol 39:169–184, 1968

13

Cystoid Macular Edema

Mark O. M. Tso

Cystoid macular edema (CME) is a syndrome comprising a set of clinical manifestations that exhibits macular edema as the major feature.[16,22,24] CME is seen in a wide variety of ocular and systemic diseases. It is associated with hereditary, metabolic, vascular, and neoplastic diseases of the vitreous, retina, and uvea; is observed in patients suffering from systemic disease such as hypertension, diabetes mellitus, and nicotinic acid poisoning; and also occurs secondary to a number of intraocular procedures. That so many different disease processes exhibit this common manifestation in the macula is fascinating. Conceptually, CME illustrates how intimately the macular tissues are related to the physiologic functions of other ocular tissues and organ systems in the body. Because the pathogenesis of CME remains unclear and most suggested therapy is ineffective, the exploration of this syndrome has attracted many investigators.[22]

CLINICAL MANIFESTATIONS OF CME

Patients with CME complain of blurred central vision and occasionally of flashes of light. Visual acuity varies from 20/200 to 20/25 and may

Supported in part by Research Grant EY 1903, EY 06761 (Dr. Tso); Core Grant EY 1792 and Training Grant EY 7038 from the National Eye Institute.
Dr. Tso is the recipient of the Research to Prevent Blindness, Inc., Senior Scientific Investigator's Award, 1987.

fluctuate from day to day. Slit-lamp biomicroscopy shows a swollen macula with a shallow foveal depression. The silhouette of the cystoid spaces may be seen against a background of macular pigment epithelium. The retina in the entire posterior pole may be edematous, and the optic disc may also be swollen. The vitreous, retinal pigment epithelium (RPE), and choroid may show other changes, depending on associated ocular or systemic diseases.

The characteristic fluorescein angiographic pattern of CME discloses an accumulation of dye around the fovea in a petalloid fashion. The pointed ends of the petals face the center of the fovea and the rounded ends are directed toward the retinal periphery. Cystoid spaces may extend to the perimacular area well beyond the capillary free zone. In many patients, abnormalities in the retinal capillary bed develop around the macula. These consist of retinal capillary dilation (Fig. 13-1), leakage from the perifoveal capillaries, widening of the capillary free zone, microaneurysms (Fig. 13-2), or small hemorrhages. Other patients may not reveal retinal capillary abnormalities in the early phase of fluorescein angiography, but the petalloid leakage pattern may emerge in the late venous phase (Fig. 13-3). Patients may exhibit the typical angiographic changes without having severe visual impairment. The angiographic changes frequently improve spontaneously and resolve with time (Fig. 13-4). Few patients, however, exhibit persistent angiographic findings and progressively deteriorating central vision. In some patients, the rapid leakage of fluorescein

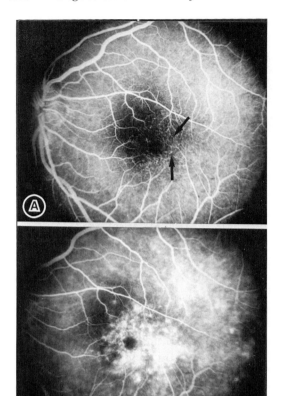

Figure 13-1. *(A)* Aphakic patient with CME shows retinal capillaries *(arrows)* that are dilated more extensively on the temporal than on the medial side of the fovea. *(B)* In the venous phase of the fluorescein angiogram, more extensive leakage occurs on the temporal side of the fovea than on the medial side.

into the vitreous produces a haze. Swelling of the optic nerve head and leakage of fluorescein from the peripapillary capillaries may also be noted.

CME AFTER CATARACT EXTRACTION AND OTHER INTRAOCULAR SURGICAL PROCEDURES

Most commonly, CME is seen in patients who have had complicated cataract extractions associated with either vitreous loss, iris prolapse, or extensive surgical manipulation.[15,18,19,24] A high

incidence of CME has been described with the implantation of an iris clip intraocular lens.[54–56,75] The recent popularity of planned extracapsular cataract extraction with the implantation of posterior chamber intraocular lens has appeared to reduce the incidence of this complication.[24,25,54,55] CME has also been observed in patients after penetrating keratoplasty, glaucoma filtering procedures, repair of retinal detachment, or pars plana vitrectomy. Although CME may occur as early as the 3rd postoperative week, it most commonly develops between the 4th and 12th week, with a peak incidence at the 6th week. However, CME has developed months or even years after an initially uneventful postoperative course. The variable delay between lens extraction and the onset of CME may be caused by a parallel delay in posterior vitreous detachment and degeneration after cataract extraction. Direct vitreous adhesion to the macula has not been seen in the majority of cases. Patients with hypertensive or diabetic vascular diseases are more likely to develop CME after intraocular procedures.

Patients with aphakic CME have abnormally high values of fluorescein leakage by vitreous fluorophotometry, ranging from 6 x 10^{-8} g/ml to 15 x 10^{-8} g/ml.[5] On follow-up, vitreous fluorescein values frequently decrease, preceding clinical improvement observed by fluorescein angiography. Fluorescein concentration in the posterior vitreous is most often elevated in patients who had vitreous loss after cataract extraction. Two mechanisms may be involved in these high fluorophotometric findings: disruption of the blood–retina barrier at the macular area with increased vitreous leakage and increased diffusion of fluorescein from the anterior chamber, causing higher values in the posterior vitreous. In most cases, both factors probably contribute to the increased levels of fluorescein in the vitreous.

Pathologically, maculae with CME exhibit cystoid spaces in Henle's fiber layer, extending into the inner nuclear layer (Fig. 13-5).[1,2,38,45,46,62–64] The central pointed ends of the petaloid leakage pattern observed in the fluorescein angiogram correspond to the cystoid spaces in Henle's fiber layer, while the rounded ends of the petals correlate with cysts in the inner nu-

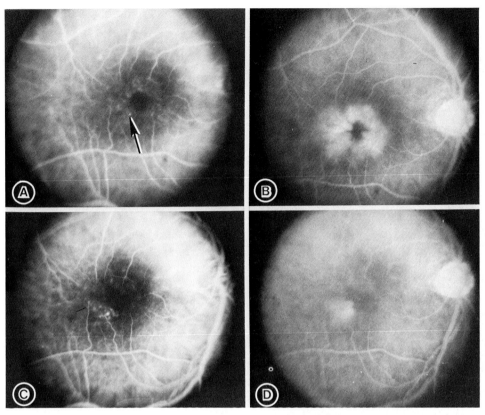

Figure 13-2. *(A)* Patient with CME exhibits capillary leakage and a microaneurysm *(arrow)* at the 7 o'clock position of the macula. *(B)* In the late venous phase of the fluorescein angiogram, a petalloid leakage pattern is seen. *(C)* Four months later, CME is moderately improved, but the fluorescein angiogram demonstrates persistence of the microaneurysm *(arrow)* at the 7 o'clock position, associated with focal capillary dilation. Capillary leakage in the rest of the perimacular area has improved greatly. *(D)* In the late venous stage of the same fluorescein angiogram shown in C, only petalloid leakage persists around the 7 o'clock position.

clear layer. Frequently, the cystic fluid does not stain in histologic preparations, suggesting that it is watery and contains little protein. Photoreceptor nuclei drop out, and the remaining inner and outer segments are shortened. Occasionally, cysts in the inner nuclear layer extend to the ganglion cell and nerve fiber layers of the retina. RPE changes are variable, ranging from mild proliferative changes to vacuolization and atrophy (Fig. 13-6).

The clinical course of CME after cataract extraction varies. Most frequently, the edema gradually subsides over a 6- to 12-month period, and visual acuity improves from 20/100 to 20/25. If the clinical course is prolonged, pa-

tients may show irregular pigmentation of the macula and progressive loss of central vision to 20/200. Patients with vitreous prolapse often have a worse prognosis. Patients who have CME after lens extraction in one eye tend to develop CME in the other eye.

CME ASSOCIATED WITH SYSTEMIC AND RETINAL VASCULAR DISEASES

Often, CME is associated with retinal vascular diseases such as central or branch retinal vein occlusion (Fig. 13-7), retinal telangiectasia, radiation retinopathy, and others.[20,21] These

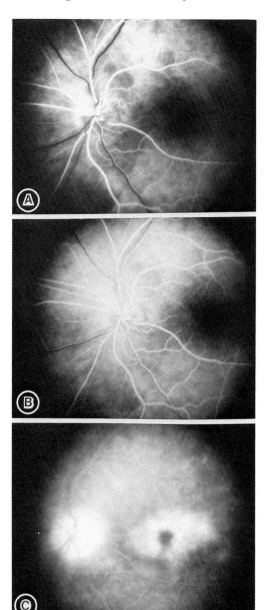

Figure 13-3. Patient with aphakic CME shows no capillary leakage or dilation in the arterial *(A),* or arteriovenous *(B)* phase of the fluorescein angiogram, but the petalloid leakage pattern of CME is seen in the late venous phase (C).

diseases tend to produce conspicuous retinal capillary abnormalities, such as dilated or nonperfused retinal capillaries, leaking microaneurysms, and intraretinal microvascular abnormalities or hemorrhages.

Histopathologically, the macula shows cystoid spaces, extending from the outer nuclear layer to the nerve fiber layers (Fig. 13-8 – 13-10).[61-63] The fluid is proteinaceous and stains positively with hematoxylin and eosin. When stained with phosphotungstic acid hematoxylin, fibrinous deposits may be seen. Extensive cell loss is noted in different layers of the retina. The pathologic features differ considerably from those of CME after cataract extraction and are consistent with liquefaction necrosis secondary to infarction. Furthermore, CME secondary to ischemic retinal vascular disease is more frequently accompanied by permanent visual loss. Ischemic necrosis in the retina seen in pathologic studies is consistent with a poorer visual prognosis when compared with CME after lens extraction.

Some systemic vascular diseases involve both the retinal and choroidal vasculatures and result in CME. For example, young patients suffering from acute systemic hypertension, such as is seen in toxemia of pregnancy, renal hypertension, pheochromocytoma, and systemic diseases of connective tissue may develop CME in the early stages of their disease without typical features of hypertensive retinopathy.[69,73] In these patients, CME may be seen associated with hard exudate forming a macular star (Fig. 13-11). In addition, focal bullous detachment of the retina and focal RPE lesions, known as Elschnig spots, may result. Fluorescein angiography shows minimal retinal vascular leakage but there is ample evidence of hypertensive choroidopathy, and there are focal areas of hypoperfusion of the choriocapillaris and staining of the RPE. CME in acute systemic hypertension is primarily due to hypertensive choroidopathy. The retinal vasculature is autoregulated, while the choroidal vasculature is under sympathetic control. Young patients with pliable blood vessels who have developed acute hypertension show mild vasoconstriction of the blood vessels, partially compensated by autoregulation. Under sympathetic control, the choroidal vasculature develops severe constriction, leading to choroidal ischemia, hypertensive

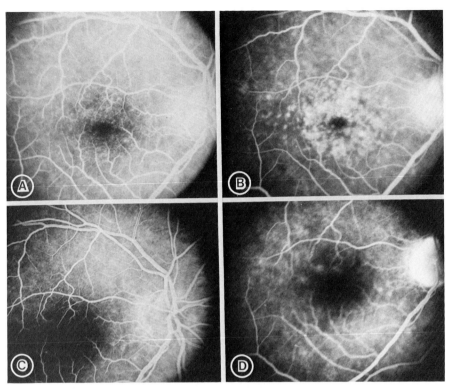

Figure 13-4. *(A)* Patient with CME shows capillary dilation in the early arterial phase of the fluorescein angiogram, and exhibits moderate CME in the late venous phase *(B)*. After 18 months, the patient shows spontaneous improvement in the CME, with relatively normal perimacular capillary filling *(C)* and minimal capillary leakage in the late venous phase *(D)*.

choroidopathy, and CME. If hypertension persists, typical features of hypertensive retinopathy will develop. Hard exudate, cotton wool spots, marked arterial narrowing, macroaneurysms, branch retinal artery, or retinal vein occlusion may evolve in the exudative and sclerotic phases of hypertensive retinopathy. It should be noted that CME is not a prominent feature in hypertensive retinopathy or in essential hypertension in middle-aged or elderly patients who have developed generalized vascular sclerosis secondary to prolonged hypertension.

Histopathologically, patients with acute hypertension show fibrinoid necrosis of the choroidal arteries and arterioles which leads to occlusion of the choriocapillaris. Necrosis of the RPE brings about a shallow serous retinal de-

tachment. Cystoid spaces form in the outer plexiform layer and fill with proteinaceous fluid (Fig. 13-12). Therefore, hypertensive choroidopathy may lead to CME.

CME ASSOCIATED WITH DIABETES MELLITUS

Patients with diabetic retinopathy may suffer from CME with retinal changes comparable to the ischemic findings described in association with retinal vascular disease.[7] In addition, these patients have a microangiopathic retinopathy (Fig. 13-13) consisting of scattered microaneurysms and proteinaceous and fibrinous exudate in the outer plexiform and inner layers of the

(Text continues on p. 222).

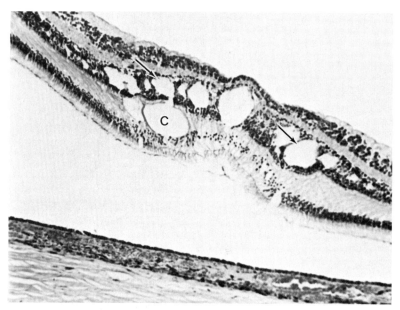

Figure 13-5. CME in an aphakic patient. Cysts are seen in Henle's fiber layer (C) and extend into the inner nuclear layer *(arrows)*. Note the loss of photoreceptor cells in the foveal area. (Hematoxylin and eosin, original magnification × 88) (Tso MOM: Pathology of cystoid macular edema. Ophthalmology 89(8): 902–915, 1982)

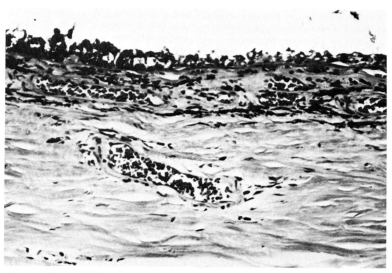

Figure 13-6. RPE in the macula of an aphakic CME patient reveals moderate proliferative changes. (Hematoxylin and eosin, original magnification × 220) (Tso MOM: Pathology of cystoid macular edema. Ophthalmology 89(8):902–915, 1982)

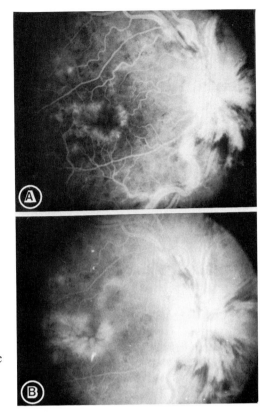

Figure 13-7. *(A)* Central retinal venous occlusion demonstrates marked venous congestion, optic disc edema, and hemorrhage. The perimacular capillaries leak markedly. *(B)* The petalloid pattern of CME occurs in the late venous phase.

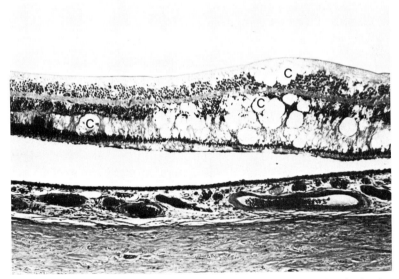

Figure 13-8. CME in a diabetic patient associated with central retinal vein occlusion. The cystoid degeneration (C) extends from the outer plexiform layer, through the inner nuclear layer to the ganglion cell layer. All retinal layers show cell loss. (Hematoxylin and eosin, original magnification × 60) (Tso MOM: Pathology of cystoid macular edema. Ophthalmology 89(8): 902–915, 1982)

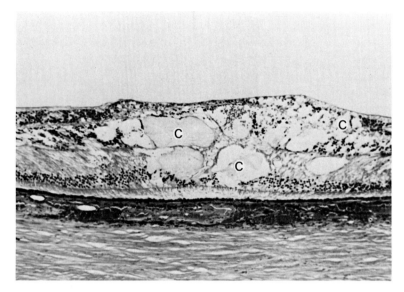

Figure 13-9. CME in a patient with retinal vein occlusion. Note the extensive cystoid degeneration (C) in all layers of the retina, including the outer and inner nuclear and ganglion cell layers. Extensive cell loss in all layers is reminiscent of liquefaction necrosis secondary to infarction. Patient shows marked loss of central vision and has a poor prognosis. (Tso MOM: Pathology of cystoid macular edema. Ophthalmology 89(8): 902–915, 1982)

retina (Fig. 13-14, 13-15). Preretinal membranes may be observed with wrinkling of the internal limiting membrane.

Diabetic macular edema may be associated with retinal vascular and choroidal vascular changes and with retinal pigment epithelial abnormalities. Diabetic choroidopathy with sclerotic changes in the choroidal vasculature may be seen histopathologically.[23] In a study of streptozotocin-induced diabetes in rats and monkeys, we demonstrated that the experimental diabetic retinopathy showed leakage of horseradish peroxidase tracer from the choroidal circulation through the RPE into the subretinal space.[64,66] In a recent study of photocoagulation treatment of diabetic macular edema, it was demonstrated that the application of a grid pattern of light to moderate laser burns to the macular area improves the macular edema.[6] It is possible that this treatment regimen provides a surgical de-

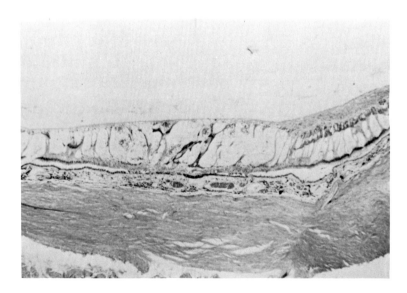

Figure 13-10. Cystoid degeneration of the retina extending along the entire posterior pole in a patient with retinal vein occlusion demonstrates extensive ischemic necrosis. (Hematoxylin and eosin, original magnification × 2) (Tso MOM: Pathology of cystoid macular edema. Ophthalmology 89(8): 902–915, 1982)

bridement of the diseased RPE, leading to the proliferation of a more healthy population of cells, the reestablishment of the blood–retina barrier, and improvement of the CME.[6]

CME ASSOCIATED WITH CHOROIDAL AND RETINAL PIGMENT EPITHELIAL DISEASE

Patients with small hemangioma or malignant melanoma of the choroid or a subretinal neovascular net of age-related macular degeneration (Fig. 13-16) show decompensation of the outer blood–retina barrier at the RPE and frequently exhibit CME. [61–63,73] In such cases, retinal capillary leakage may not be conspicuous on fluorescein angiography. In some patients, the massive disruption of the outer blood–retina barrier, diffuse leakage of fluorescein from the choroid, and intense background hyperfluorescence may mask a petalloid pattern of fluorescein leakage.

Pathologically, large cystoid spaces occur mostly in the outer nuclear and outer plexiform layers, extending into the inner nuclear layer (Fig. 13-17), but frequently sparing the gan-

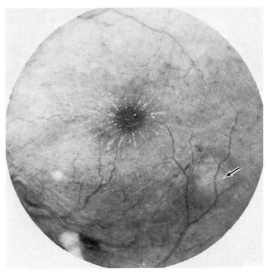

Figure 13-11. Hypertensive choroidopathy in a 37-year-old woman with a blood pressure reading of 230/140 mm Hg. Note CME associated with a macular star, showing perimacular leakage of hard exudate. Focal serous detachment of the retina is present in the posterior pole *(arrow)*. (Tso MOM, Jampol LM: Pathophysiology of hypertensive retinopathy. Ophthalmology 89(10): 1132–1145, 1982)

Figure 13-12. Hypertensive choroidopathy with CME. *(A)* Cystoid spaces *(arrows)* are present in the outer plexiform layer of the macula. Proteinaceous exudate is present in the subretinal space. The macula is artifactitiously detached. *(B)* Fibrinoid necrosis is observed in the choroidal arterioles with choriocapillary occlusion and retinal pigment epithelial necrosis *(arrows)*. (Tso MOM, Torczynski E: Architecture of the choriocapillaris and macular edema. Ed. K. Shimizu, International Congress Series No. 450 XXIII Concilium Ophthalmologicum, Kyoto, 1978)

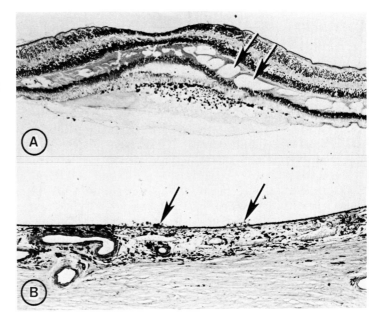

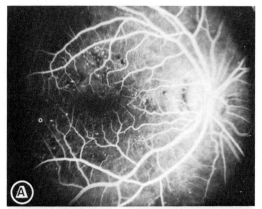

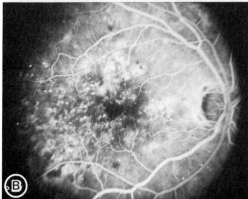

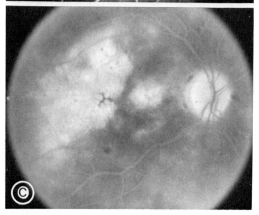

Figure 13-13. Diabetic microangiopathy and CME. Abundant microaneurysms and retinal hemorrhages are revealed in the arteriovenous phase *(A)* of the fluorescein angiogram. Vascular leakage from the microaneurysms is observed in the venous phase *(B)*. A petalloid pattern is seen in the macular area in the late venous phase *(C)*.

glion-cell and nerve-fiber layers of the retina. The RPE shows depigmentation, vacuolization,

disruption, atrophy, or papillary proliferation, and "fibrous metaplasia."

Sometimes when a malignant melanoma develops in the peripheral choroid, CME may be seen in the posterior pole. The pathologic changes and the pathogenetic mechanisms of this condition have been a subject of controversy. Fine and Brucker have viewed intracytoplasmic swelling of Müller cells as an important feature of CME.[8] They believe extracellular cystic formation is a late change following prolonged intracellular edema. More recently, Gass, Anderson, and Davis have studied a patient with CME and peripheral choroidal melanoma but failed to observe intracellular edema of Müller cells.[17] Additional investigation is required to define the early pathologic changes in CME in these patients.

The contribution of RPE and choroidal diseases to aphakic CME is not defined, but experimental lens extraction in monkeys demonstrates that retinal pigment epithelial leakage is a component of aphakic CME.[60,64,72] This mechanism of CME will be discussed in more detail later in this chapter. Better clinical methods to demonstrate retinal pigment epithelial seepage must be developed to define further its contribution to CME.

In recent years, CME has been observed in patients with retinitis pigmentosa. These patients not only show angiographic evidence of CME but exhibit generalized abnormalities in the blood–retina barrier by vitreous fluorophotometry.[5] Since retinitis pigmentosa predominantly affects the RPE and photoreceptor cells, this observation further implicates the involvement of the outer blood–retina barrier in the pathogenesis of CME.

CME ASSOCIATED WITH TRAUMA AND TRACTION

Undoubtedly, physical traction on the macula will lead to CME. In idiopathic preretinal fibrosis or cellophane retinopathy, a preretinal membrane develops and pulls on the retina, producing CME (Fig. 13-18). Patients who suffer blunt ocular injuries may also develop macular cysts. Fluorescein angiographic patterns in

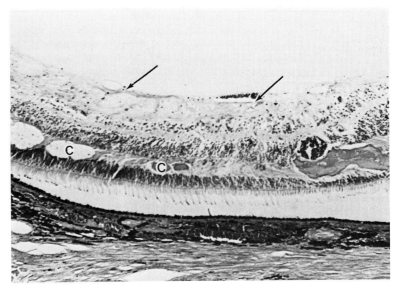

Figure 13-14. CME in a diabetic patient exhibiting exudate in the cystoid spaces (C) in the outer plexiform layer. The exudate stains intensely with eosin to show its proteinaceous nature. A preretinal membrane *(arrows)* overlies a wrinkled internal limiting membrane. (Hematoxylin and eosin, original magnification × 100) (Tso MOM: Pathology of cystoid macular edema. Ophthalmology 89(8): 902–915, 1982)

such cases vary greatly. In the acute stage, the RPE may leak. In chronic cases, it stains, but a petalloid pattern of fluorescein leakage is not seen.

Histopathologic changes range from atrophy of the RPE, occlusion of the choriocapillaris, and focal loss of photoreceptor cells to localized cysts in the outer plexiform layer and outer layers of the retina with cell loss in all retinal layers (Fig. 13-19).[62] Vitreous degeneration and traction may lead to serous retinal detachment and cysts.

The pathogenesis of cystoid degeneration of the retina following blunt trauma is not clearly defined. Cogan proposed that trauma may disrupt the RPE and liberate proteolytic en-

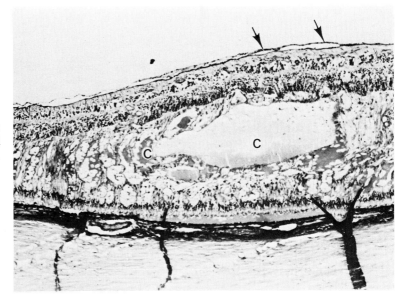

Figure 13-15. Marked CME in a diabetic patient. The exudate in the outer plexiform layer coalesces to form cystoid degeneration (C). There is cell loss in all layers of the retina. A preretinal membrane *(arrows)* lies on the anterior surface of the retina. (Hematoxylin and eosin, original magnification × 60) (Tso MOM: Pathology of cystoid macular edema. Ophthalmology 89(8): 902–915, 1982)

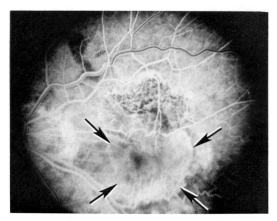

Figure 13-16. Patient with age-related macular degeneration showing a subretinal neovascular net *(arrows)* resulting in marked CME.

ula. In most cases of aphakic CME, however, direct vitreous traction to the macula cannot be seen clinically. Vitreous disease may be a contributing factor, but is probably not the primary pathogenetic mechanism. Schepens further postulated that vitreous traction creates a local inflammatory reaction around the macula and disc, resulting in capillary dilation and leakage. Most histologic studies of maculas with CME do

zymes from these cells.[4] The latter may digest the retinal tissues, resulting in traumatic retinopathy. Quigley, Sipperly, and Gass studied traumatic retinopathy in an experimental model in monkeys and observed photoreceptor and pigment epithelial degeneration without extracellular exudative edema.[53] They believed that disrupted photoreceptor cells may account for the loss of vision and whitening of retina known as Berlin's edema, but did not attempt to explain the pathogenesis of macular cysts and holes seen in the later stages of traumatic maculopathy.

CME AND PATHOLOGY OF THE VITREOUS

Disturbance of the vitreous after cataract extraction and vitreous adherence to the wound leads to CME. Tolentino, Schepens and coworkers and Sebag and associates have suggested that vitreous degeneration is a primary mechanism for the pathogenesis of CME.[50,52,57–59] They describe two types of vitreous traction to the macula: narrow traction bands connecting the macula to the partially detached posterior hyloid membrane and a broad band of vitreous gel adhering to the mac-

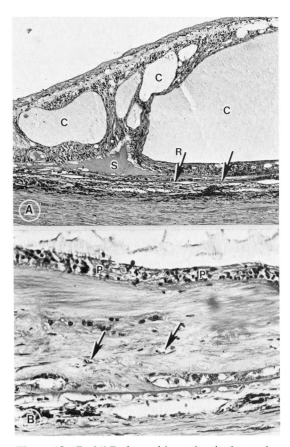

Figure 13-17. *(A)* Patient with a subretinal vascular net *(arrows)* demonstrating shallow serous retinal detachment and marked cystoid degeneration (C). Note that cystoid spaces (C) in the outer plexiform layer extend to the inner layers of the retina. There is a marked loss of photoreceptor cells. *(B)* Subretinal neovascular net *(arrows)* in the same case shown in *A* demonstrates degeneration of the photoreceptor cells (P).

not show inflammatory infiltrate in the retina, although Martin and associates did observe vasculitis in eyes with CME.[37] Combining the observations of vitreous prolapse and Müller cell edema in CME, Tessler hypothesizes that vitreous traction on Müller cells may cause malfunction of ionic exchange in Müller cells leading to CME.* It is an interesting hypothesis that needs more supporting evidence.

CME ASSOCIATED WITH UVEITIS

CME occurs in patients suffering from anterior or posterior uveitis and pars planitis. Beçhet's disease, acute nongranulomatous iridocyclitis, and nematode enophthalmitis have been associated with CME. A mild anterior uveitis is frequently seen in patients with aphakic CME. While the causes of some of these ocular inflammatory conditions have yet to be determined, patients who exhibit marked perivasculitis, extensive fluorescein leakage into the vitreous, and severe CME tend to suffer from severe visual loss (Fig. 13-20). Interestingly, while retinal edema in pars planitis tends to be generalized, it is most pronounced in the macula. This may be a form of vasogenic edema.

It has been suggested that CME hinges on endogenous mediators such as prostaglandins, especially in patients with anterior uveitis.[26–28,51] Corticosteroid has been used with variable success for the treatment of CME that frequently recurs after termination of therapy. Therapeutic trials of CME with 1% fenoprofen, a prostaglandin synthesis inhibitor, were inconclusive.[3] The observation that indomethacin administered before cataract surgery may ameliorate fluorescein leakage in CME suggests that it may be related to endogenous mediators.[32,39–44] However, in spite of the fluorescein angiographic improvement with this treatment, patients do not show significant recovery in visual acuity when compared with controls.[76,77]

* Personal communication

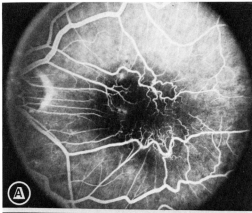

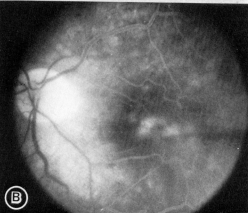

Figure 13-18. Patient with cellophane retinopathy shows a preretinal membrane tugging on the retina and causing irregular tortuosity of the retinal vessels *(A)*. Perimacular leakage is noted in the late venous phase of the fluorescein angiogram *(B)*.

CME ASSOCIATED WITH DRUGS AND PHARMACOLOGIC AGENTS

The administration of epinephrine, particularly to an aphakic patient, may produce CME.[33] Discontinuation of the treatment frequently leads to improvement of the edema and to the recovery of visual acuity. Nicotinic acid administration for treatment of hypercholesterolemia has caused CME that showed no leakage on fluorescein angiography. The edema quickly subsided with the discontinuation of nicotinic acid.[15]

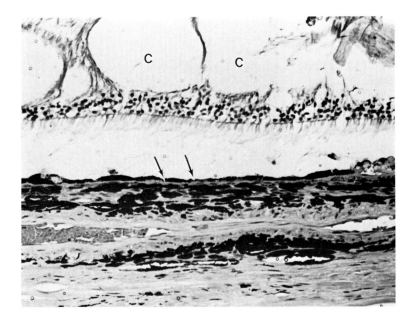

Figure 13-19. CME (C) in a case of traumatic retinopathy. The RPE *(arrows)* is atrophic and thinned. The choriocapillaris is largely absent. (Hematoxylin and eosin, original magnification × 220) (Tso MOM: Pathology of cystoid macular edema. Ophthalmology 89(8): 902–915, 1982)

PATHOGENESIS OF CME

I believe that CME is a mulifactorial syndrome comprising at least four sets of primary pathogenetic factors:[65] (1) disruption of the blood–retina barrier at the retinal vasculature and at the RPE; (2) vascular disturbances resulting in retinal ischemia and formation of cysts; (3) intraocular events, such as inflammatory diseases, vitreous traction, and ocular hypotony that may be mediated through mechanical, physiologic, or biochemical pathways; and (4) systemic disease such as diabetes mellitus, hypertension, and others that affect the dynamics of retinal and choroidal circulation and retinal tissue compliance.

Blood–Retina Barrier

Clinical and laboratory evidence points to the prominent role that the disruption of the blood–retina barrier plays in CME.[5,49,61] Its daily fluctuating clinical course and the spontaneous resolution of CME in some cases suggests that the disease process intermittently interferes with a physiologic process. Leakage of fluorescein into the swollen retina and vitreous, observed by fluorescein angiography and vitreous

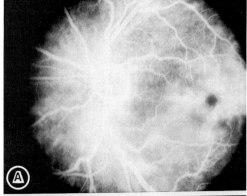
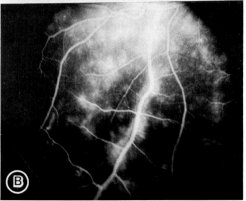

Figure 13-20. *(A)* Patient has pars planitis and marked CME. *(B)* Perivascular leakage is prominent.

fluorophotometry, implicates disturbances of the blood–retina barrier in the disease process. Disruption of the barrier function of the retinal capillary is indicated in some cases of CME by fluorescein leakage in the perimacular retinal capillaries. Whether disruption of the outer blood–retina barrier at the RPE is an important pathogenetic factor still is not known. Fluorescein angiography does not effectively detect generalized seepage of tracer through the RPE. Disruption of the RPE, such as that seen with the subretinal pigment epithelial neovascular net in age-related disciform macular degeneration undoubtedly would lead to cystoid degeneration of the macula.

To study both inner and outer blood–retina barrier disruptions in cataract extraction, we performed lens extraction on rhesus monkeys.[72] Fluorescein angiography failed to show in the monkeys the classic petalloid leakage pattern seen in cases of human CME (Fig. 13-21). However, light and electron microscopic studies with horseradish peroxidase tracer demonstrated leakage from both the retinal vasculature and the RPE (Fig. 13-22–13-25). The RPE was focally decompensated, and the cytoplasm of some cells was infiltrated by the tracer (see Fig. 13-24). This type of intracellular infiltration of tracer probably represents fluorescent staining seen clinically by fluorescein angiography. The bright choroidal fluorescent background could have masked subtle fluorescein staining of the

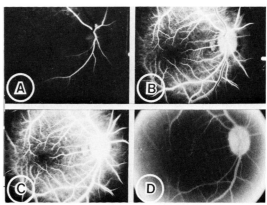

Figure 13-21. Fluorescein angiograms of the retina of a rhesus monkey 14 days after intracapsular lens extraction with vitreous loss. No perimacular capillary abnormalities or petalloid leakage pattern is noted. However, horseradish peroxidase tracer study of this eye, which was enucleated 24 hours after the angiogram, showed diffuse leakage from the retinal vessels and the RPE. (Tso MOM, Shih CY: Experimental macular edema after lens extraction. Invest Ophthalmol 16:381–392, 1977)

RPE in the angiogram. Some horseradish peroxidase tracer passed through the RPE to the subretinal space. However, the tracer did not diffuse throughout the interphotoreceptor matrix of the entire subretinal space; it remained localized in the macular area. The photorecep-

Figure 13-22. Unstained section of the macula of a rhesus monkey two days after extracapsular lens extraction with vitreous. Horseradish peroxidase tracer leaks profusely from the retinal vessel, particularly the veins (V). Extravasated tracer *(arrows)* was noted around the blood vessels. Leakage through the RPE *(arrowhead)* extends into the subretinal space. (Unstained Epon section, original magnification × 165) (Tso MOM, Shih CY: Experimental macular edema after lens extraction. Invest Ophthalmol 16:381–392, 1977)

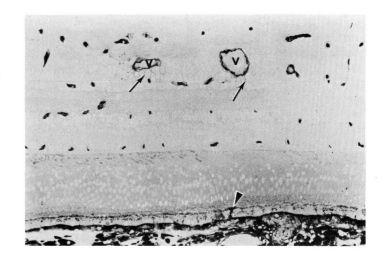

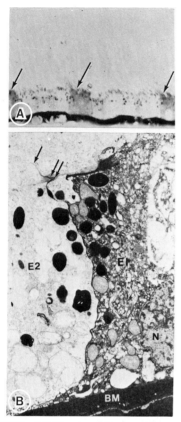

Figure 13-23. *(A)* Horseradish peroxidase perme-
ates the cytoplasm of three retinal pigment
epithelial cells *(arrows).* (Unstained Epon section;
original magnification × 350). *(B)* Tracer material
diffusely infiltrates the cytoplasm of the pigment
epithelial cells (E1) but the cytoplasm (E2) is free of
tracer material. The cell junction *(double arrows)*
remains competent, and no tracer material is
present inferior to the cell junction; N, nucleus;
BM, Bruch's membrane. (Original magnification × 7200) (Tso MOM, Shih CY: Experimental
macular edema after lens extraction. Invest
Ophthalmol 16:381–392, 1977)

tor cells exhibited mild disruption of the outer
segments (see Fig. 13-25).

Leakage of tracer was also observed from the
retinal vessels, particularly the large retinal
veins (see Fig. 13-22, 13-23). Tracer seeped into
the cytoplasm of the endothelial cells and extended along the basement membrane of the
endothelial cells and pericytes into the extracellular space between neuronal and glial cells of
the retina. In other areas, many pinocytotic vesicles filled with tracer were seen at the ablumenal
side of the endothelial cells. Monkeys with vitreous loss during lens extraction tended to exhibit
increased retinal vascular leakage. No cystoid
spaces were noted histopathologically, but the
Müller cells of some of the animals showed
moderate swelling (Fig. 13-26). One month after
surgery, retinal leakage gradually decreased and
cystoid degeneration did not occur. This type of
leakage was most likely comparable to angiographic CME seen in routine cataract extractions, in which staining of the macula was frequently noted and healed spontaneously
postoperatively.

In a recent study performed in our laboratory,
five rhesus monkeys underwent subtotal vitrectomy through a pars plana approach.[47] One of
the animals developed diffuse fluorescein leakage in the macular region, but it did not show the
classic petalloid pattern. Injected horseradish
peroxidase tracer leaked through the RPE and
retinal vasculature, but no cystoid spaces were
observed in the retina histologically. No edema
was noted in the Müller cells in these monkeys
(Fig. 13-27). Vitrectomy disrupted the blood–
retina barrier at the RPE and retinal capillaries.

Photic injury inflicted by the operating microscope during lens extraction has been postulated to cause CME. Photic injury damages the
RPE, as evidenced by diffuse fluorescein leakage into the subretinal space.[48,65,68,70,74] However, leakage from retinal capillaries has not
been noted, and the discrete petalloid leakage
pattern has not been seen. Even so, photic injury
inflicted by the operating microscope has not
been ruled out as one of many contributory factors to CME.

Experimentally, we produced small, mild foveal burns in monkeys. The retinal pigment epithelial lesion quickly healed.[67] However, three
to four years later, abnormal basement membrane was produced by the RPE, and mild cystoid degeneration was observed in Henle's fiber
layer.

To examine further the importance of
chronic retinal pigment epithelial insufficiency
and leakage in the pathogenesis of CME, the

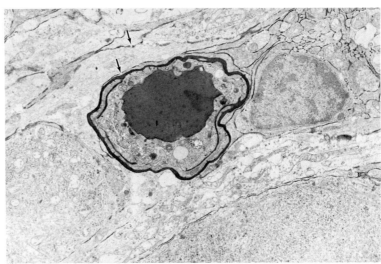

Figure 13-24. Disruption of the blood–retina barrier at the retinal capillary of a monkey after lens extraction. Tracer *(arrows)* infiltrates the basement membrane of the retinal capillaries as well as the surrounding interstitial space. (Original magnification, ×11,400) (Tso MOM: Pathology of cystoid macular edema. Ophthalmology 89(8): 902–915, 1982)

eyes from rhesus monkeys were exposed to the light of an indirect ophthalmoscope (American Optical) set at 7.5 volts, directed at the macular area.[60,68,74] The retina was exposed for 1 to 2 hours. The eyes were studied by ophthalmoscopy, fundus photography, and fluorescein angiography, and the eyes were enucleated at 18 months to five years and 10 months after light exposure. Clinically, focal raised yellowish lesions were seen in the posterior pole by ophthalmoscopy and fluorescein angiography (Fig. 13-28). Histopathologically, the regenerated RPE proliferated to form a placoid lesion, but the horseradish peroxidase tracer study showed persistent leakage from the choroid through the damaged RPE to the subretinal space (Fig. 13-29) for as long as 5 years following photic injury. However, CME was not seen in any of the monkey eyes. The experiment clearly demonstrates that while chronic disruption of the blood–retina barrier may be an important factor in CME, it is not necessarily the primary pathogenetic mechanism.

Ischemic Damage With Cyst Formation

One of the main features of CME is cyst formation. Cystic spaces develop in Henle's fiber layer, the outer and inner nuclear layers, and occasionally in the ganglion cell layer of the

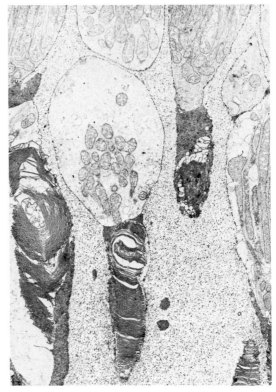

Figure 13-25. Disruption of the photoreceptor lamellae in a monkey that had lens extraction and diffuse leakage of RPE. (Original magnification × 11,780) (Tso MOM: Pathology of cystoid macular edema. Ophthalmology 89(8): 902–915, 1982)

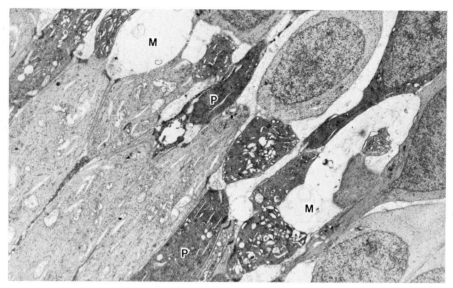

Figure 13-26. Edema of Müller cell around the external limiting membrane in a monkey after lens extraction. Horseradish peroxidase tracer infiltrated into the cytoplasm of the photoreceptor cells (P). The Müller cells (M) have vacuolated watery cytoplasm. (Original magnification × 6840) (Tso MOM: Pathology of cystoid macular edema. Ophthalmology 89(8): 902–915, 1982)

macula. In some cases, cystoid degeneration involves the entire posterior pole of the retina.

When eyes with CME are studied pathologically, the cysts are almost always so large in the late stage of the disease that they are undoubtedly extracellular. In the early stages of the disease, however, edema may occur intracellularly. The contents of most of the cysts are usually watery and transudative in nature and fail to stain in paraffin sections. Although fluorescein angiography cannot detect whether edematous fluid is extracellular or intracellular, the gross

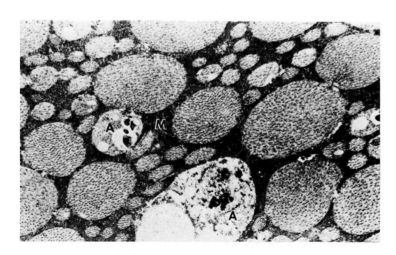

Figure 13-27. Retina of a rhesus monkey with total vitrectomy and angiographic CME. There is no Müller cell (M) swelling, but the axons (A) show vacuolation and degenerative changes (Original magnification × 6000) (Tso MOM: Animal modeling of cystoid macular edema. Surv Ophthalmol 28:512–519, 1984)

petalloid pattern seen by fluorescein angiography strongly suggests the presence of extracellular fluid in cystoid cavities. Fluid in these spaces appears to turn over slowly, as fluorescein staining of the cyst persists for many minutes. While staining of the retinal cysts may suggest leakage from the retinal or choroidal vasculature, prolonged hyperfluorescence may result from delayed reabsorption of dye that leaks into the retinal spaces. Recent studies by Cunha-Vaz[5] have suggested that extracellular fluid around normal retinal vessels is rapidly absorbed by active transport into the vascular lumen.*

The reabsorption probably involves the perivascular glial cells as well as the retinal pericytes and endothelial cells. Müller cells are believed to transport fluid from the vitreous cavity to the subretinal space or vice versa. Dysfunction of these cells may cause the transport of extracellular fluid to fail and may be one of the factors accounting for the persistence of extravasated fluid in the cystoid spaces. Indeed, Fine and Brucker observed Müller cell swelling as an early sign of CME in patients with peripheral malignant melanomas.[8]

Histologic sections of eyes from patients with CME show loss of outer and inner nuclear layers of the retina, suggesting definitive cell necrosis. Loss of vision in patients with CME is consistent with neuronal damage observed histologically. Many of these patients have retinal vascular abnormalities. However, generalized ischemic changes such as central retinal artery occlusion lead to extensive retinal infarction, but not cyst formation. Only multifocal ischemia with localized loss of retinal tissue may produce cystoid degeneration.

To study the clinical features and histopathologic changes in multifocal ischemic retinopathy, talc retinopathy was induced in rhesus monkeys with repeated intravenous injections of talc twice weekly for 3 1/2 to 10 months.[29–31] Initially, small emboli lodged in the pulmonary capillaries. Collaterals subsequently developed, and small talc particles passed into the systemic circulation and were deposited in the retinal and

* Personal communication

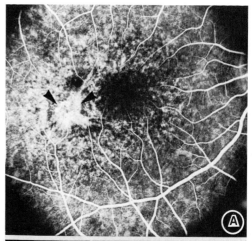
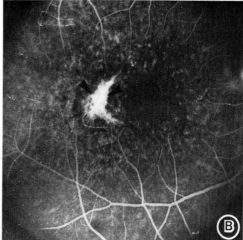

Figure 13-28. Macula of a rhesus monkey after exposure to the light of an indirect ophthalmoscope for 90 minutes, showing a hyperfluorescent scar *(arrowhead)* in the arteriovenous phase *(A).* The retinal lesion *(arrowhead)* stains with fluorescein in the late venous phase *(B).* The angiographic pattern is distinctively different from CME. (Tso MOM: Animal modeling of cystoid macular edema. Surv Ophthalmol 28:512–519, 1984)

choroidal vasculature, particularly in the posterior pole. Fluorescein angiography disclosed distinctive precapillary arteriolar occlusion, capillary nonperfusion, and abnormal foveal avascular zones with retinal vascular leakage. Histologically, microinfarction produced small cystoid spaces in the outer plexiform layer, the

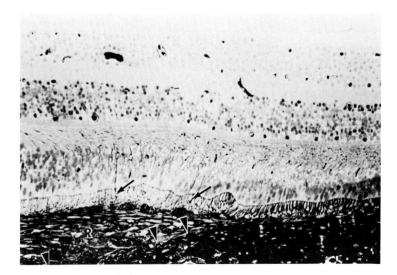

Figure 13-29. The macula of a rhesus monkey exposed to the light of an indirect ophthalmoscope. A placoid proliferation of retinal pigment epithelium (R) has developed. Horseradish peroxidase tracer *(arrow)* passes into the subretinal space and outlines the photoreceptor elements. Note the absence of cystoid macular degeneration. Bruch's membrane is indicated by the arrowheads. (Toluidine blue, original magnification × 260)

outer and inner nuclear layers, and the ganglion cell layer of the macula (Fig. 13-30, 13-31). Cystoid bodies scattered in the retina. This experiment confirmed that multifocal infarction causes multiple cysts to form in the retina.

Experiments in branch retinal vein occlusion induced by retinal photocoagulation in monkeys also demonstrate that focal ischemia will lead to the formation of mutliple cysts in the outer plexiform layer and in the inner and outer nuclear and ganglion cell layers.[60] The cystoid spaces are filled with exudate and are surrounded by swollen glial and neuronal cells (Fig. 13-32). Surprisingly, glial elements that normally expand and proliferate in retinal infarction do not proliferate to fill the cystoid spaces. Few macrophages, if any, are seen. When the ischemic process is chronic, dissolution and removal of necrotic retinal tissues proceed slowly and fail to provide sufficient stimuli to provoke retinal gliosis.

If CME is caused by multifocal ischemia with

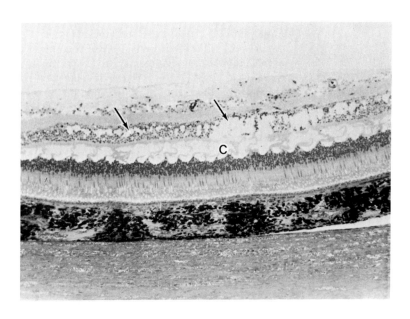

Figure 13-30. Macula of a rhesus monkey with talc retinopathy exhibits cystoid degeneration (C) in the outer plexiform layer. Some of the cysts extend into the inner nuclear layer *(arrows).* (Toluidine blue, original magnification × 82) (Tso MOM: Pathology of cystoid macular edema. Ophthalmology 89(8): 902–915, 1982)

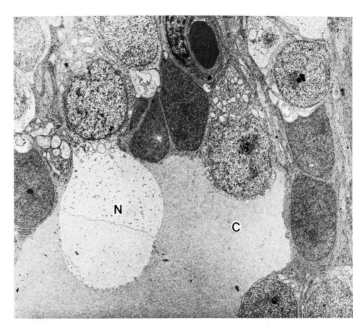

Figure 13-31. Cyst (C) in a monkey with talc retinopathy. Note the swelling of the neuronal cells (N) in the inner nuclear layer, surrounding the cystoid space. (Original magnification × 4400) (Tso MOM, Pathology of cystoid macular edema. Ophthalmology 89(8):902–915, 1982)

tissue loss, an explanation is needed for the recovery of 20/20 vision by many patients after remission of the disease. Frisen believes that only 44% of the neuronal channels in the retina are required for 20/20 vision.[9,10] Thus, even when half of the retina has been infarcted, the patient could still retain 20/20 vision after the active disease process subsides.

INTRAOCULAR EVENTS ASSOCIATED WITH CME

Intraocular events, such as inflammation, vitreous traction, anterior or posterior uveitis, ocular hypotony, and others are commonly associated with CME. The pathogenetic relationship between macular edema and pathologic processes elsewhere in the eye is not known. A biochemically mediated pathway or a still undefined pathophysiologic mechanism may be involved. It has been proposed that CME may be related to prostaglandin production. Patients with CME had a response rate of 70% with topical and systemic steroids, which is comparable to the spontaneous remission rate.[19] Prophylactic administration of systemic indomethacin after

cataract surgery appears to decrease the fluorescein angiographic incidence of CME significantly.[32] Topical indomethacin before and shortly after cataract extraction also reduces the incidence of fluorescein angiographic CME prophylactically, but has no direct effect on the visual outcome.[35,76,77] Topical fenoprofen, a nonsteroidal anti-inflammatory drug, did not produce a significant effect in a small series of patients with chronic CME, although topical fenoprofen improved CME in four patients whose symptoms were exacerbated when the drug was withdrawn.[3]

In a further attempt to produce CME experimentally in rhesus monkeys, cryotherapy was applied to the ciliary body to produce anterior uveitis with prolonged ocular hypotony.[71] These animals demonstrated diffuse fluorescein leakage and edema in the macula and optic disc, even though a petalloid pattern of leakage was not seen. Histopathologic studies showed extensive disruption of the blood–retina barrier of the RPE and retinal vasculature (Fig.13-33–13-35). Horseradish peroxidase leaked through the RPE into the subretinal space. Leakage from the retinal vasculature was traced into perivascular neural and glial tissues, but no cystoid de-

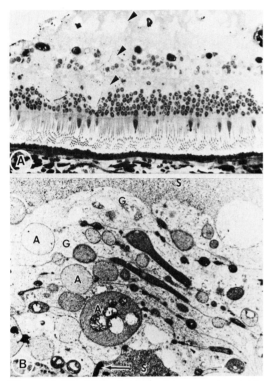

Figure 13-32. *(A)* Retina of a rhesus monkey with experimental retinal vein occlusion showing cystoid edema *(arrowheads)* in the outer plexiform layer, inner nuclear layer, and nerve fiber layers. (Toluidine blue, original magnification × 260). *(B)* Electron micrograph of the wall of the cystoid spaces (S) shown in *A*. The glial cells (G) and the axons (A) in the vicinity of the cystoid spaces are swollen. Fibrin *(arrow)* is deposited in the extracellular space. (Original magnification × 5000) (Tso MOM: Animal modeling of cystoid macular edema. Surv Ophthalmol 28:512–519, 1984)

generation was observed in the macular area. This experiment showed that ocular inflammation and hypotony disrupted the blood–retina barrier, but no cystoid degeneration developed.

Tessler, in his 1986 O'Connor lecture, suggested that some intraocular events result in vitreous traction, producing a mechanical pull on the retina with subsequent dysfunction of the Müller cells. Edema of these cells may be the early stage of development of CME. An inflammatory mediator may superimpose on this cascade of events, resulting in CME.

Jampol proposes that chronic exposure to ultraviolet (UV) light of low intensity in the aphakic patient may be partially responsible for CME.[27] In a prospective randomized study of 297 patients, the effects of a UV-blocking filter on the operating microscope were evaluated to determine the incidence of CME in patients undergoing extracapsular cataract extraction with implantation of a posterior lens chamber. Kraff and coworkers showed that the presence of the UV-blocking filter made no difference in the angiographic incidence of CME or on the visual outcome in these patients.[34] However, patients who received a UV-blocking intraocular lens showed statistically significant lower rates of CME.

SYSTEMIC DISEASES ASSOCIATED WITH CME

Elderly patients with diabetes mellitus and hypertension often are predisposed to CME. The effect of systemic circulatory changes on retinal vasculature in the pathogenesis of CME has not been conclusively defined, although diabetes and hypertension may decrease retinal and choroidal blood flow and inflict retinal ischemic changes. However, monkeys with diabetes experimentally induced for 10 years (from intravenous streptozotocin injections) and increased glucose levels (350 to 500 mg/dl) have shown no incidence of CME.

THERAPEUTIC APPROACHES TO CME

Since CME is a final common pathway of many different disease processes, treatment of any given case of this syndrome depends on the basic pathologic processes involved. Since the primary pathogenetic mechanisms of CME have not been definitively determined, many of the therapeutic approaches are relatively empirical, and most are not very effective. However, since a number of predisposing factors of CME have been defined, prophylactic therapy ap-

Figure 13-33. Disruption of the blood–retina barrier in the macula of a rhesus monkey that had cryotherapy and ocular hypotony. Horseradish peroxidase tracer infiltrates through the RPE into the retina, appears in the subretinal space and in the cytoplasm of the photoreceptor cells, and passes along the axons *(arrow)* into the cone pedicles and rod spherules. Tracer is also observed in the cytoplasm of the Müller cells *(arrowheads)*, extending from the external limiting membrane to the internal limiting membrane of the retina. (Unstained Epon section, original magnification × 260) (Tso MOM: Animal modeling of cystoid macular edema. Surv Ophthalmol 28:512–519, 1984)

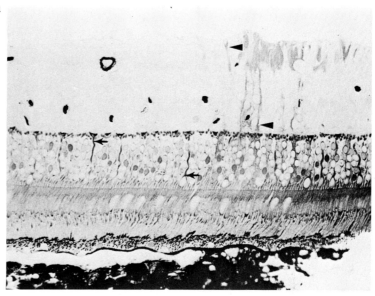

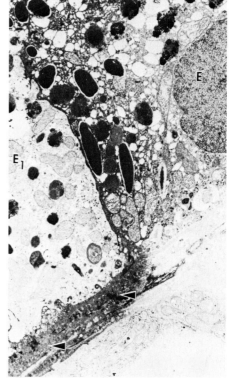

Figure 13-34. Disruption of the blood–retina barrier in the RPE of a monkey that had cryotherapy and ocular hypotony. Tracer material passed into the cytoplasm of a decompensated pigment epithelial cell (E). The adjacent pigment epithelial cell (E1) is free of tracer material. Tracer material *(arrowheads)* accumulates in Bruch's membrane beneath the pigment epithelial cells. (Original magnification × 12,000) (Tso MOM: Animal modeling of cystoid macular edema. Surv Ophthalmol 28:512–519, 1984)

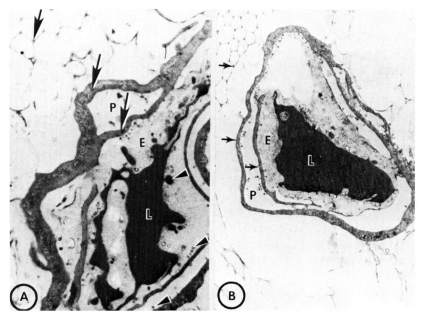

Figure 13-35. Disruption of the blood–retina barrier in the RPE of a monkey that had cryotherapy and ocular hypotony *(arrowheads).* *(A)* Tracer material *(arrows)* passes along the basement membrane of the endothelial cells (E) and pericytes (P) into the interstitial space. (Original magnification ✕ 5000). *(B)* Tracer material is seen within the cytoplasm of the endothelial cell (E) and freely infiltrates into the interstitial space. (L, lumen of blood vessels, P, pericyte; unstained section, original magnification ✕ 25,000) (Tso MOM: Animal modeling of cystoid macular edema. Surv Ophthalmol 28:512–519, 1984)

pears to produce more promising results than does the treatment of established CME.

Prophylactic Therapy for CME

Prophylactic treatment for CME in patients who are predisposed to this disease should be begun when a surgical procedure is planned and performed. Cataract extraction with an intact posterior capsule is associated with a lower incidence of CME. A high incidence of CME is associated with iris-supported intraocular lenses, which should not be used. Loose and improperly placed anterior chamber lenses frequently cause CME and should be avoided in patients who have a history of CME in the contralateral eye. Unexpected complications, such as vitreous loss during a surgical procedure, should be judiciously handled by automated vitrectomy or cellulose sponge vitrectomy so that vitreous incarceration in the wound is prevented.

Systemic hypertension and diabetes mellitus are known to predispose patients to CME. Control of these systemic diseases would be beneficial before the planned procedures. However, the beneficial effects have not been unequivocally proved. In patients with ocular diseases such as uveitis, pars planitis, iridocyclitis, and other intraocular inflammations, the inflammatory process should be controlled as much as possible before the surgical procedure. Medical prophylactic therapy using anti-inflammatory drugs such as topical indomethacin is reported to be associated with a lower incidence of angiographic CME. However, none of these studies have demonstrated that eventual visual acuity was significantly improved or that the effect was sustained for more than a year.[26,27] Other pharmacologic agents known to induce CME, such as epinephrine, should be avoided by patients at risk for this syndrome.

Therapy for Established CME

Most patients with CME initially show some evidence of inflammatory reactions in the anterior chamber. Perilimbic injection and cells or flares in the anterior chamber or in the vitreous are frequently noted. Patients with these anterior chamber reactions may be given topical steroids, but no random clinical trials regarding their efficacy have been performed. The use of topical steroids may induce rising intraocular pressure, and McEntyre suggests that CME clears because of the increased intraocular pressure.[36] While this is also my clinical impression, studies with appropriate controls have not been reported. We performed a small double-masked randomized trial of topical 1% fenoprofen, a nonsteroidal anti-inflammatory agent for the treatment of established CME.[3] No statistically significant effect was demonstrated because there were too few cases in the study. However, four patients whose conditions improved with topical fenoprofen suffered repeated recurrence of the condition when treatment was discontinued.

Surgical intervention, such as vitrectomy or YAG laser treatment, in patients with vitreous incarceration in wounds, may have been beneficial. Fung has reported a prospective randomized study to demonstrate the efficacy of vitrectomy in CME patients with vitreous incarceration.[11-13] Preliminary results suggest a beneficial effect.

In a recent study, photocoagulation using a grid pattern of laser burns has been beneficial for some patients with diabetic macular edema, particularly those with microaneurysms and focal ischemia and leakage.

While some therapeutic approaches discussed have a favorable effect on CME, the ultimate solutions depend on the future determination of the primary pathogenetic mechanisms of CME.

REFERENCES

1. Boniuk M: Cystic macular edema secondary to vitreoretinal traction. Surv Ophthalmol 13:118–121, 1968
2. Brownstein S, Orton R, Jackson WB: Cystoid macular edema with equatorial choroidal melanoma. Arch Ophthalmol 96:2105–2107, 1978
3. Burnett J, Tessler H, Isenberg S, et al: Double-masked trial of fenoprofen sodium: Treatment of chronic aphakic cystoid macular edema. Ophthalmic Surg 14:150–152, 1983
4. Cogan D: Pseudoretinitis pigmentosa. Arch Ophthalmol 81:45–53, 1969
5. Cunha-Vaz JG, Travassos A: Breakdown of the blood-retinal barriers and cystoid macular edema. Surv Ophthalmol (Suppl) 28:485–492, 1984
6. Early Treatment Diabetic Retinopathy Study Research Group: Photocoagulation for diabetic macular edema. Arch Ophthalmol 103:1796–1806, 1985
7. Ferris FL, Patz A: Macular edema, a complication of diabetic retinopathy. Surv Ophthalmol (Suppl) 28:452–461, 1984
8. Fine BS, Brucker AJ: Macular edema and cystoid macular edema. Am J Ophthalmol 92:466–481, 1981
9. Frisen L, Frisen M: A simple relationship between the probability distribution of visual acuity and the density of retinal output channels. Acta Ophthalmol 54:437–444, 1976
10. Frisen L, Frisen M: Micropsia and visual acuity in macular edema: A study of the neuro-retinal basis of visual acuity. Albrecht von Graefes Arch Klin Exp Ophthalmol 210:69–77, 1979
11. Fung WE: Anterior vitrectomy for chronic aphakic cystoid macular edema. Ophthalmology 87:189–193, 1980
12. Fung WE: Surgical therapy for chronic aphakic cystoid macular edema. Ophthalmology 89:898–901, 1982
13. Fung WE: The national, prospective randomized vitrectomy study for chronic aphakic cystoid macular edema: Progress report and comparison between control and nonrandomized groups. Surv Ophthalmol (Suppl) 28:569–575, 1984
14. Gass JDM: Nicotinic acid maculopathy. Am J Ophthalmol 76:500–510, 1973
15. Gass JDM: Lamellar macular holes: A complication of cystoid macular edema after cataract extraction. Arch Ophthalmol 94:793, 1976
16. Gass JDM: Stereoscopic Atlas of Macular Diseases: Diagnosis and Treatment, 3rd ed. St Louis, CV Mosby, 1977
17. Gass JDM, Anderson DR, Davis EB: A clinical, fluorescein angiographic and electron microscopic correlation of cystoid macular edema. Am J Ophthalmol 100:82–86, 1985
18. Gass JDM, Norton EWD: Cystoid macular edema and papilledema following cataract extraction: A fluorescein funduscopic angiographic study. Arch Ophthalmol 76:646–661, 1966
19. Gass JDM, Norton EWD: Follow-up study of cystoid macular edema following cataract extraction. Trans Am Acad Ophthalmol Otolaryngol 73:665–682, 1969

20. Gutman FA: Macular edema in branch retinal vein occlusion: Prognosis and management. Trans Am Acad Ophthalmol Otolaryngol 83:488–495, 1977

21. Gutman FA, Zegarra H: Macular edema secondary to occlusion of the retinal veins. Surv Ophthalmol (Suppl) 28:462–470, 1984

22. Henkind P: First International Cystoid Macular Edema Symposium. Surv Ophthalmol (Suppl) 28:431–577, 1984

23. Hidayat AA, Fine BS: Diabetic choroidopathy: Light and electron microscopic observations of seven cases. Ophthalmology 92:512–522, 1985

24. Irvine AR: Cystoid maculopathy. Surv Ophthalmol 21:1–17, 1976

25. Jaffe NS, Clayman HM, Jaffe MS: Cystoid macular edema after intracapsular and extracapsular cataract extraction with and without an introcular lens. Ophthalmology 89:25–29, 1982

26. Jampol LM: Pharmacologic therapy of aphakic cystoid macular edema: A review. Ophthalmology 89:891–897, 1982

27. Jampol LM: Aphakic cystoid macular edema. Arch Ophthalmol 80:1134–1135, 1985

28. Jampol LM, Sanders DR, Kraff MC: Prophylaxis and therapy of aphakic cystoid macular edema. Surv Ophthalmol (Suppl) 28:535–539, 1984

29. Jampol LM, Setogawa T, Rednam KRV, et al: Talc retinopathy in primates: A model of ischemic retinopathy: I. Clinical studies. Arch Ophthalmol 99:1273–1280, 1981

30. Kaga N, Tso MOM, Jampol LM, et al: Talc retinopathy in primates: A model of ischemic retinopathy: II. A histopathologic study. Arch Ophthalmol 100:1644–1648, 1982

31. Kaga N, Tso MOM, Jampol LM: Talc retinopathy in primates: A model of ischemic retinopathy: III. An electron microscopic study. Arch Ophthalmol 100:1649–1657, 1982

32. Klein RM, Katzin HM, Yannuzzi LA: The effect of indomethacin pretreatment on aphakic cystoid macular edema. Am J Ophthalmol 87:487–489, 1979

33. Kolker AE, Becker B: Epinephrine maculopathy. Arch Ophthalmol 79:552–562, 1968

34. Kraff MC, Sanders DR, Jampol LM, et al: Effect of an ultraviolet-filtering intraocular lens on cystoid macular edema. Ophthalmology 92:366–369, 1985

35. Kraff MC, Sanders DR, Jampol LM, et al: Prophylaxis of pseudophakic cystoid macular edema with topical indomethacin. Ophthalmology 89:885–890, 1982

36. McEntyre JM: A successful treatment of aphakic cystoid macular edema. Ann Ophthalmol 10:1219–1224, 1978

37. Martin NF, Green WR, Martin LW: Retinal phlebitis in the Irvine–Gass syndrome. Am J Ophthalmol 83:377–386, 1977

38. Michels RG, Green WR, Maumenee AE: Cystoid macular edema following cataract extraction (the Irvine–Gass syndrome): A study clinically and histopathologically. Ophthalmic Surg 2:217–221, 1971

39. Miyake K: Prevention of cystoid macular edema after lens extraction by topical indomethacin. (I) A preliminary report. Albrecht Graefes Arch Klin Ophthalmol 203:81–88, 1977

40. Miyake K: Prostaglandins as a causative factor of the cystoid macular edema after the lens extraction (II). Acta Soc Ophthal Jpn 81:1449–1464, 1977

41. Miyake K: Prophylaxis of aphakic cystoid macular edema using topical indomethacin. Am Intraocular Implant Soc J 4:17, 1978

42. Miyake K: Indomethacin in the treatment of postoperative cystoid macular edema. Surv Ophthalmol (Suppl) 28:554–568, 1984

43. Miyake K, Miyake Y, Maekubo K, et al: Incidence of cystoid macular edema after retinal detachment surgery and the use of topical indomethacin. Am J Ophthalmol 95:451–456, 1983

44. Miyake K, Sakamura S, Miura H: Long-term follow-up study on prevention of aphakic cystoid macular oedema by topical indomethacin. Br J Ophthalmol 64:324–328, 1980

45. Newsom WA, Hood CI, Horwitz JA, et al: Cystoid macular edema: Histopathologic and angiographic correlations. A clinicopathologic case report. Trans Am Acad Ophthalmol Otolaryngol 76:1005–1009, 1972

46. Norton AL, Brown WJ, Carlson M, et al: Pathogenesis of aphakic macular edema. Am J Ophthalmol 80: 96–101, 1975

47. Puck A, Tso MOM, Peyman G, et al: Pathology of cystoid degenerations of the macula. Invest Ophthalmol Vis Sci 24 (ARVO Supplement):170, 1983

48. Robertson DM, Feldman RB: Photic retinopathy from the operating room microscope. Am J Ophthalmol 101:561–569, 1986

49. Sanders DR, Kraff MC, Lieberman HL, et al: Breakdown and reestablishment of blood–aqueous barrier with implant surgery. Arch Ophthalmol 100:588–590, 1982

50. Schepens CL, Avila MP, Jalkh AE, et al: Role of the vitreous in cystoid macular edema. Surv Ophthalmol (Suppl) 28:499–504, 1984

51. Sears ML: Aphakic cystoid macular edema. The pharmacology of ocular trauma. Surv Ophthalmol (Suppl) 28:525, 1984

52. Sebag J, Balazs BA: Pathogenesis of cystoid macular edema: An anatomic consideration of vitreoretinal adhesion. Surv Ophthalmol (Suppl) 28:493–498, 1984

53. Sipperly JO, Quigley HA, Gass JDM: Traumatic retinopathy in primates. Arch Ophthalmol 96:2267–2273, 1978

54. Stark JW, Maumenee AE, Fagadau W, et al:

Macular edema in pseudophakia. Surv Ophthalmol (Suppl) 28:442–451, 1984

55. Stark WF, Worthen DM, Holladay, et al: The FDA report in intraocular lenses. Ophthalmology 90:311–317, 1983

56. Taylor DM, Sacho SW, Stern AL: Aphakic cystoid macular edema: Long term clinical observations. Surv Ophthalmol Supplement 28:437–441, 1982

57. Tolentino FI, Schepens CL: Edema of posterior pole after cataract extraction: A biomicroscopic study. Arch Ophthalmol 74:781–786, 1965

58. Tolentino FI, Schepens CL, Freeman HM: Vitreoretinal Disorders: Diagnosis and Management. Philadelphia, WB Saunders, 1976

59. Tolentino FI, Schepens CL, Pomerantzeff O: Advances in the technique of vitreous cavity examination. In Purett CDJ (ed): Retina Congress, pp 215–227. New York, Appleton-Century-Crofts, 1974

60. Tso MOM: Photic maculopathy in rhesus monkey: A light and electron microscopic study. Invest Ophthalmol 12:17–34, 1973

61. Tso MOM: Pathology of the blood–retinal barrier. In Cunha-Vaz J (ed): The Blood–Retinal Barrier, pp 235–250. New York, Plenum Press, 1980

62. Tso MOM: Pathological study of cystoid macular edema. Trans Ophthalmol Soc UK 100:408–413, 1980

63. Tso MOM: Pathology and pathogenesis of cystoid macular edema. Ophthalmologica 183:46–54, 1981

64. Tso MOM: Pathology of cystoid macular edema. Ophthalmology 89:902–914, 1982

65. Tso MOM: Animal modeling of cystoid macular edema. Surv Ophthalmol (Suppl) 28:512–519, 1984

66. Tso MOM, Cunha-Vaz J, Blair N, et al: Disruption of blood–retinal barrier in diabetic primate. Invest Ophthalmol Vis Sci 22(ARVO Suppl) 110, 1982

67. Tso MOM, Fine BS: Repair and late degeneration of the primate fovea after injury by argon laser. Invest Ophthalmol Vis Sci 18:447–461, 1979

68. Tso MOM, Fine BS, Zimmerman LE: Photic maculopathy produced by the indirect ophthalmoscope: I. Clinical and histopathologic study. Am J Ophthalmol 73:686–699, 1972

69. Tso MOM, Jampol LM: Pathophysiology of hypertensive retinopathy. Ophthalmology 89:1132–1145, 1982

70. Tso MOM, Robbins DO, Zimmerman LE: Photic maculopathy: A study of functional and pathologic correlation. Mod Probl Ophthalmol 12:220, 1974

71. Tso MOM, Shih CY: Disruption of the blood–brain barrier in ocular hypotony: A preliminary report. Exp Eye Res 23:209–216, 1976

72. Tso MOM, Shih CY: Experimental macular edema after lens extraction. Invest Ophthalmol 16:381–392, 1977

73. Tso MOM, Torczynski E: Architecture of the choriocapillaris and macular edema. In Shimizu K, Oosterhuis JA (eds): XXIII Concilium Ophthalmologicum, p 239. Amsterdam-Oxford, Excerpta Medica, 1978

74. Tso MOM, Woodford BJ: Effect of photic injury on the retinal tissues. Ophthalmology 90:952–963, 1983

75. Wilkinson CP: A long-term follow-up study of cystoid macular edema in aphakic and pseudophakic eyes. Trans Am Ophthalmol Soc 79:810–839, 1981

76. Yannuzzi LA, Klein RM, Wallyn RH: Ineffectiveness of indomethacin in the treatment of chronic macular edema. Am J Ophthalmol 84:517–519, 1977

77. Yannuzzi LA, Landau AN, Turtz AI: Incidence of aphakic cystoid macular edema with the use of topical indomethacin. Ophthalmology 88:947–954, 1981

14

Myopic Chorioretinal Degenerations

Liang-yen Wen

INCREASING INCIDENCE OF MYOPIA

The incidence of myopia has increased dramatically in Taiwan during the past 30 years.[2] A survey in 1954 reported that 13.75% of the students in the Taipei area had visual defects, and 94.27% of the defects were myopia.[8] Ten years later, the incidence of myopia was up to 51% for primary school children, 60% among high school teenagers, and a dreadful 85% among college students.[8,9,16] Deep concern prompted further investigation.

Forty years ago, a group of Japanese researchers selected populations of Taiwanese offshore islanders and aborigines for a study of the incidence of myopia, because of their geographical and tribal isolation.[20] Minimal visual disturbance was noted in school pupils and adults. Thirty years later, investigators examined the same tribes, which had since become "modernized." One third exhibited abnormal vision. The pathogenesis of the rising incidence of myopia is still obscure and probably multifactorial.[1,4,9] Only 5% to 8% of myopia is hereditary, so environmental factors must play a role in the development of myopia in young children. Various factors such as close work, reading, television viewing, reading Chinese characters, and even the modernization of society have been blamed for the increased occurrence of myopia.[4,21,22]

MYOPIA AND AXIAL LENGTH OF THE EYEBALL

In Tron's figure the mean value of axial length of the eyeball is 23 mm for the population in this study.[17] However in the young Chinese population, there is a 2-mm shift in the axial length of the eyeball to a mean value of 25 mm.[13]

We have observed that mild myopia in some children appears to advance as they acquire higher education. We also have noted more frequently severe myopia among teenagers in our clinical practice today than two or three decades ago. In the early stage, it is difficult to differentiate simple (or "school") myopia from progressive or pathologic myopia.

A simple way to differentiate simple myopia from progressive myopia is to observe changes of axial length with ultrasonography. However, one of our studies showed that patients with simple myopia may also show increased axial length. Others speculate that abnormal changes of the posterior pole provide clues for pathologic myopia.

PATHOLOGIC CHANGES IN MYOPIA

The five clinical signs of myopia are (1) a crescent around the optic disc (Fig. 14-1, 14-2), (2)

242

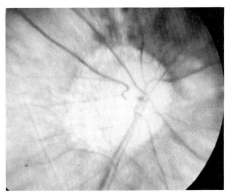

Figure 14-1. Myopic crescent in the temporal aspect of the optic nerve head. Note protrusion of the optic nerve head and abnormal position of the major retinal arteries.

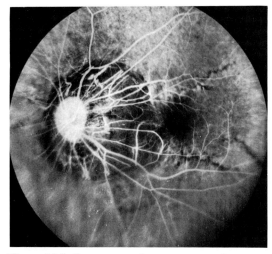

Figure 14-3. Lacquer cracks are rupture of RPE/Bruch's membrane.

lacquer cracks (Fig. 14-3), (3) tessellation of the fundus, (4) chorioretinal degeneration (Fig. 14-4 – 14-6), and (5) macular degeneration (Fig. 14-6). As myopia progresses, these fundus changes worsen (see Fig. 14-2). Severity of the pathologic changes also correlates with advancing age. As a myopic person grows older, retinal chorioretinal changes may advance. Patients with monocular myopia (a congenital anomaly) show retinal degeneration similar to that of patients with bilateral myopia.

Myopic crescent of the RPE – Bruch's membrane – choriocapillaris complex at the peripapillary area is commonly seen in many middle-aged and elderly myopic patients and is occasionally seen in normal and hyperopic individuals.[19] We do not believe that it is a specific sign for myopia. The myopic crescent may increase in size with age. In eyes with advancing myopia, the edge of the crescent may be the site of initial progressive chorioretinal degeneration, which gradually extends to involve the whole posterior pole.

Lacquer cracks are fine yellow-white lines at

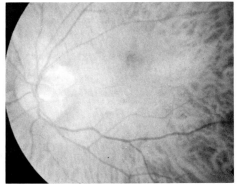

Figure 14-2. Myopic crescent in the superior temporal aspect of the optic nerve head. Note that the optic nerve head is tilted.

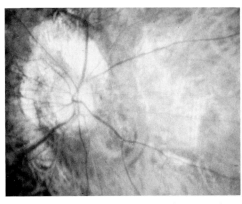

Figure 14-4. Chorioretinal atrophy in the peripapillary region, extending to involve the posterior pole.

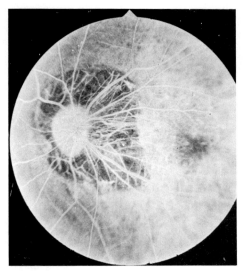

Figure 14-5. Fluorescein angiogram of a patient with myopic degeneration, initially in the peripapillary region and extended toward the entire posterior pole.

the posterior pole and are ruptures of the RPE – Bruch's membrane – choriocapillaris complex, mostly found in patients aged 30 to 50 years.[6,14,15,19] As these patients advance in age (50 – 70 years), lacquer cracks may coalesce and appear as patches of chorioretinal atrophy or

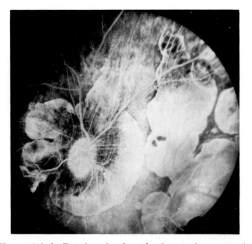

Figure 14-6. Patchy chorioretinal atrophy around the optic disc and the posterior pole. The atrophic area has a discrete border and scalloping edge reminiscent of gyrate atrophy.

develop into focal areas of subretinal neovascularization. In our previous study, 8% of our myopic patients had lacquer cracks when compared to 4.3% of the patients in Curtin's study.[3] Some lacquer cracks may resemble angioid streaks.

Chorioretinal atrophy is seen mostly around the optic disc area and posterior pole. It may be focal or diffuse, usually starting at the border of the myopic crescent and extending gradually to involve the entire posterior pole. Initially there is focal disappearance of the pigment epithelium and choriocapillaris associated with pigmentary clumping. Subsequently, these areas coalesce. Fluorescein angiography may demonstrate loss of the choriocapillaris, occlusion of the large choroidal vessels, and pigment epithelial atrophy. With atrophy of choroidal tissues, the sensory retina degenerates. Many investigators believe that these changes are due to the elongation of the eyeball. Our study showed the degree of diffuse chorioretinal degeneration correlates with the aging process.[5] Furthermore, the focal form of chorioretinal atrophy is seldom seen in the aged because the disease process tends to become diffused with age.[19]

Subretinal neovascularization is caused by the rupture of Bruch's membrane followed by an ingrowth of new vessels similar to those seen in senile macular degeneration. However, myopic subretinal neovascularization is frequently limited and lacks aggressive growth when compared with the neovascularization seen in age-related macular degeneration. In high myopia, subretinal neovascularization is frequently seen at the macular region accompanied by pigment deposits and hemorrhage, giving rise to the Forster-Fuchs spot. This clinical manifestation is exhibited by 18.3% of the aged group, whereas the incidence is less than 1% in the younger group.[19]

OTHER DEGENERATIONS OF THE VITREOUS AND RETINA

A recent investigation revealed that in a total of 204 high myopes of different ages, one third had some peripheral retinal degeneration, including lattice degeneration, "snowball" deposits, and atrophic retinal holes. One fourth had nonspecific changes, such as white-without pressure lesions, shagreen, and irregular pigmentation. The remaining 44.6% appeared normal.[19]

Little or no vitreous traction is found in most myopic patients with macular holes.[12] However, it is well documented that the incidence of peripheral retinal detachment in myopia is many times higher than that of the average population. Schepens postulates that deficiency of the retinal attachment plays an important role in precipitating retinal detachment.[12]

MYOPIA AND GLAUCOMA

No apparent increase in the prevalence of glaucoma has been observed in our myopic populations, as reported by other investigators.[7] This is probably due to the relatively low incidence of chronic open-angle glaucoma in the Chinese (0.6%–0.7%).[7,10]

BIOCHEMICAL STUDIES ON HIGH MYOPIA

In 1973 Takki found elevated blood ornithine levels in patients with gyrate atrophy, an inborn deficiency of ornithine amino-transferase (OAT).[15] The ocular findings in these patients included myopia (5–10 D), opacities in the lens and vitreous, and marked characteristic chorioretinal atrophy with scalloped edges. Because of some similarity between the fundus picture of gyrate atrophy and that of high myopia with chorioretinal degeneration, we studied a group of patients to determine if there are similar blood changes in high myopia.

More than 1,000 individuals were selected for the study. A group of more than 50 Chinese medical students and 50 Caucasians residing in Taiwan served as the control group. Five hundred forty-four subjects of all ages with varying degrees of myopia have been evaluated (Table 14-1). The serum ornithine levels of 150.7 μM and 150.6 μM were found in the control groups. The value was 213.5 μM in the myopic group. This difference is considered statistically significant. However, the plasma ornithine

Table 14-1. Serum L-ornithine Level (μM) of Normal Subjects and Myopic Patients

	Mean +/− SD (sample size)
Chinese subjects	150.7 +/− 41.8 (56)
Caucasian subjects	150.6 +/− 63.5 (59)*
Myopic patients	213.5 +/− 98.9 (544)†

Significantly different based on Chinese subject t-test
Levels of significance: * not significant; † $p \ll 0.005$

level in patients with gyrate atrophy was usually 10 times higher than in those with myopia.[18] This study is still in progress, and final results will be reported later.

REFERENCES

1. Angle J, Wissmann DA: The epidemiology of myopia. Am J Epidemiol 111:220–227, 1980
2. Chang JM, Hou PK: Ophthalmological observation on "human dock" (health examination) cases. Trans Soc Ophthal Sinicae 5:26–37, 1966
3. Curtin BJ, Karlinn DB: Axial length measurements and fundus changes of the myopic eye. Am J Ophthalmol 71:42–53, 1971
4. Duke-Elder S: System of Ophthalmology, Vol V: Ophthalmic Optics and Refraction, p. 340. St. Louis, Henry Kimpton, 1970
5. Kao KD, Wen LY: The age difference in degenerative high myopias. Trans Soc Ophthal Sinicae 21:24, 1982
6. Klein RM, Curtin BJ: Lacquer crack lesions in pathologic myopia. Am J Ophthalmol 79:386–392, 1975
7. Lee PF: Mass screening for glaucoma among Chinese. Trans Soc Ophthal Sinicae 1:19–25, 1962
8. Lin HM: Statistics on ocular diseases and defects among the students in Taipei. Chinese Med 1:27, 1954
9. Lin LK, Hung PT, Ko LS: Survey of the refraction status among the primary school children in Taipei. Tran Soc Ophthal Sinicae 19:8–62, 1980
10. Liu CH: Tonometric survey in Chinese over forty. Selected papers, pp 53–58, Selected papers of National Defense Medical Center, Taipei, Republic of China, 1963
11. Na Y, Huang SY: Visual acuity survey among the pupils of junior middle schools in Taipei. Trans Soc Ophthal Sinicae 13:47–51, 1974
12. Schepens CL: Retinal detachment and allied diseases. p 51. Philadelphia. WB Saunders, 1983
13. Sheu MM: Studies on ocular refraction and its

components. Master of Science Thesis, Kaoshiung Medical College, Republic of China, 1982

14. Shimizu M: Study on myopic fundus. Acta Soc Ophthal Jpn 63:375–393, 1959

15. Takki K: Gyrate atrophy of the choroid and retina associated with hyperornithinaemia. Br J Ophthalmol 58:3–23, 1974

16. Tang KY: Studies on myopia of Ku-ting Primary School, Taipei, Master of Science Thesis, National Defense Medical Center, Republic of China, 1967

17. Tron E: Ueber die optischen Grundlagen der Ametropie. Graefe Arch Ophthal 132:182, 1934

18. Wen LY, Juang TY, Wuu JA, et al: Serum ornithine levels in some ocular disorders. Biomed Metab Biol 35:83–87, 1986

19. Wu QC, Wen LY, Chou TH: Fluorescein angiography in assessing the choroidal and retinal changes in high progressive myopia. Trans Soc Ophthal Sinicae 21:33, 1982

20. Yamaji R, Yoshida S, Uchida H, et al: Study of the visual acuity and refraction of the Yami on Botel Tobago island (Lan-yu). Doc Ophthal Proc 28:13–18, 1981

21. Young FA: Intraocular pressure dynamic associated with accommodation. Doc Ophthal Proc Series 28:171–176, 1981

22. Young FA: The development and control of myopia in human and subhuman primates. Contacto 19:16–31, 1975

15

Retinal Photocoagulation Therapy: Clinical Application and Biological Basis of Therapeutic Effects

Mark O. M. Tso

Retinal photocoagulation therapy has been applied with beneficial effects on a wide spectrum of diseases of the retina and choroid.[7,26] In principle, it is a destructive method of treatment by which normal or diseased tissues of the retina and choroid are destroyed and removed. However, this therapeutic measure is dependent on several important pathophysiologic characteristics of retinal and choroidal diseases. Because many retinal and choroidal diseases are discretely localized, the removal of diseased tissues may improve the function of the remaining healthy tissues. Graded photocoagulation treatment may achieve controlled destruction of the retinal tissues resulting in various healing patterns and the production of different therapeutic effects. Regeneration of glial cells, retinal pigment epithelial cells, and vascular elements after the destructive photocoagulation process may provide a new baseline from which the remaining healthy retinal tissues can function. Leakage from the diseased retinal pigment epithelium (RPE) or retinal vasculature may be eliminated by the healthy regenerated tissues.

Supported in part by Research Grant EY 1903, EY 06761 (Dr. Tso); Core Grant EY 1792 and Training Grant EY 7038 from the National Eye Institute.
Dr. Tso is the recipient of the Research to Prevent Blindness, Inc., Senior Scientific Investigator's Award, 1987.

Finally, diffuse destruction of the retina by panretinal photocoagulation in diseases such as proliferative diabetic retinopathy appears to reduce the metabolic activity of the entire retina and minimizes excessive reactive proliferation in the pathologic healing process.

VARIATIONS OF PHYSICAL PARAMETERS ON BIOLOGICAL EFFECTS OF PHOTOCOAGULATION THERAPY

The manipulation of various physical parameters used in photocoagulation treatment modalities may achieve a desired therapeutic effect. The physical parameters include exposure time, spot size, wave length, and level of energy.

Exposure Time

In general, the shorter the exposure time, the more localized the retinal lesions. The resulting retinal burn will have a sharp margin, as is required in the treatment of macular lesions. However, a short exposure time of less than 0.1 second tends to produce a microexplosion at the level of the retinal pigment epithelium (RPE), resulting in choroidal hemorrhage. With a longer exposure time of 1.0 to 2.0 seconds, the

247

retinal burns tend to spread laterally, producing pyramidal lesions, with widest destruction at the RPE and choroid. The longer the exposure time, the greater the energy delivered to the retina and the more severe the retinal burn. These severe burns extend posteriorly deep into the choroid, spread laterally along the RPE and involve the retinal vasculature anteriorly. To produce heavy photocoagulation burns for therapeutic purposes, the exposure time may be prolonged to 1.0 or more seconds, provided that the patient's eye is immobilized.

Spot Size

Retinal burns created with a large spot size of 500 to 1000 nm are likely to have an indiscrete margin and to spread laterally along the RPE. For diseases such as diabetic retinopathy, in which the purpose of therapy is to decrease the general metabolic demand, large spots will be more effective. After a retinal burn is inflicted, the reactive proliferation of the retinal glial cells and pigment epithelial cells takes place mostly at the periphery of the burn spot, where the burned tissues meet the normal retina. In very large spots, the healing process may fail to reach the center of the burn, which becomes atrophic but does not form a strong chorioretinal scar.

Wave Length

The various wave lengths of laser light produce retinal burns of different intensities and ophthalmoscopic appearances. The absorption spectra of melanin granules, retinal vessels, and xanthophyll in the macular area vary, resulting in theoretically different quantities of energy being absorbed by different structures with various wave lengths.

In general, blue-green argon laser energy produces a whitish retinal burn and is well absorbed by the retinal vasculature. The red krypton laser light tends to penetrate deep into the choroid and be absorbed by the melanin granules of the RPE and uveal melanocytes to produce a somewhat gray retinal burn seen by ophthalmoscopy. The red laser wave length will not be effectively absorbed by retinal vessels or vitreous hemor-

rhage. Therefore, it is not used in the treatment of retinal vascular disorders, but it can minimize unnecessary energy absorption in patients with vitreoretinal hemorrhage. The green laser and krypton laser lights are absorbed poorly by xanthophyll pigment of the macula, suggesting that these wave lengths are more effective for macular photocoagulation therapy.

However, we have compared chorioretinal lesions produced by photocoagulation with green (514 nm), yellow (577 nm), orange (600 nm), and red (630 nm) dye laser wave lengths in the macula and retina of normal cynomolgus monkeys.[1] Acute retinal burns inflicted by all wave lengths studied 24 hours after photocoagulation showed severe necrosis of the RPE and outer retina, indicating that melanin is the primary site for the absorption of energy in the retina and choroid regardless of the laser wave lengths. When compared with green, yellow, and orange laser lights, the red laser wave length produced more severe thrombosis and destruction in the choroid, more damage in the Müller cells, and pyknosis of the inner layers of the retina (Fig. 15-1). However, histologic study of the chronic retinal lesions inflicted by these four wave lengths one month after photocoagulation showed identical degrees of damage and healing. Furthermore, acute and chronic juxtafoveal nonconfluent lesions of 100 microns in diameter, inflicted with 0.1 second of exposure, produced by 4 wave lengths of the orange laser light (590, 595, 600, and 605 nm) were comparable clinically and histopathologically.

In contrast, Smiddy and coworkers reported that orange laser wave lengths of 595 nm and 600 nm produced more severe inner retinal damage than did other wave lengths from 560 nm to 630 nm.[13] However, in their study, the retinal lesions were produced by multiple confluent and overlapping burns, making a comparison between lesions created in their investigation and in our study very difficult. Orange laser energy is absorbed well by the retinal vasculature and may be used to treat retinal vascular lesions. The experience and skill of the surgeon, however, are more important in producing the desirable therapeutic effect than variations in the wave length of the laser light.

Figure 15-1. *(A)* Acute retinal lesion produced by green argon laser light (514 nm) at the posterior pole of a rhesus monkey eye shows necrosis of the outer layers of the retina, including the RPE and photoreceptor cells. The choriocapillaris is mildly involved in the burn. (Original magnification × 200). *(B)* Acute retinal lesion produced by a krypton laser light (630 nm) at the posterior pole of a rhesus monkey eye. The parameters employed are identical to those used to produce the burn shown in *A* (spot, 100 *μ*; duration, 0.1 second; power, 100 milliwatts). Note that the laser burn produces necrosis of the photoreceptor cells, pigment epithelium, and choriocapillaris and involves the larger choroidal vessels *(large arrows)*. Pigment-laden macrophages *(arrowheads)* infiltrate the choroidal stroma, and Müller cell fibers in the inner layers of the retina *(small arrows)* exhibit densification of the cytoplasm. The internal limiting membrane is wrinkled. The krypton laser energy penetrates deeper into the choroidal tissue than the green argon wave length and more extensively involves the inner layers of the retina. (Original magnification × 200) (Wallow IHL, Tso MOM: Retinal repair after xenon arc photocoagulation. II. The evolution of retinal lesions in the rhesus monkey. A clinical and light microscopic study. Am J Ophthalmol 75:610, 1973; published with permission from The American Journal of Ophthalmology)

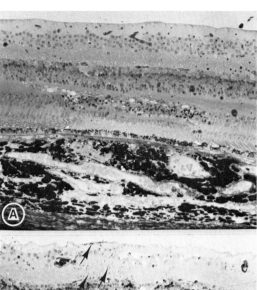

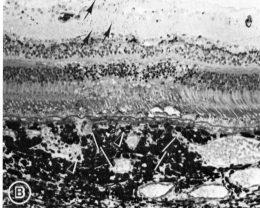

Energy Dose

By varying the power of the inflicting laser or xenon arc light, graded retinal damage may be produced for a variety of retinal diseases induced by different pathogenetic mechanisms.[11,16-23] Photocoagulation lesions may be categorized into 4 grades by severity. This graded damage is best observed ophthalmoscopically if the exposure time is prolonged to 0.5 or 1.0 second, but it may also be seen in burns inflicted by shorter exposure times. The amount of energy required to produce different grades of lesions varies with the individual because of the pigmentation, location of the fundus, and focusing of the laser beam. The clinical appearance of the lesion remains one of the principal guides to the operating surgeon.

A grade I lesion is characterized by a faint grayish spot that becomes more apparent ophthalmoscopically 10 to 30 seconds after application (Fig. 15-2). The lesion increases in prominence 1 to 2 days after treatment. When these lesions were studied histopathologically in human patients whose eyes were enucleated 24 hours after treatment, the burn appeared confined to the RPE, which had become vacuolated and edematous (Fig 15-2A).[16,22] The photoreceptor outer segments were minimally affected, and the photoreceptor nuclei were spared. The endothelial cells of the choriocapillaris were mildly edematous. Similar retinal lesions were studied histopathologically in the rhesus monkey 1 to 3 months after treatment.[17,21] The necrotic RPE was removed, Bruch's membrane was relined by depigmented pigment epithe-

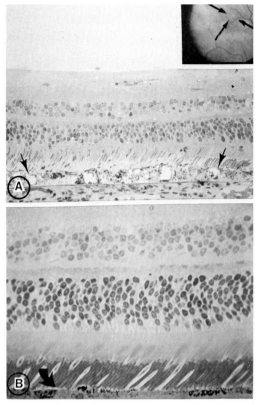

Figure 15-2. *(A)* A grade I retinal burn in a human eye. The lesion *(arrows)* is confined to the RPE and choriocapillaris. The photoreceptor elements are mildly involved, but the photoreceptor nuclei are spared. Clinically, a grade I burn appears as a grayish spot *(arrows)* on the inset. *(B)* The histologic appearance of a similar grade I retinal burn inflicted on a rhesus monkey retina. The eye was enucleated 4 weeks after exposure. The RPE *(arrow)* has been repopulated to line Bruch's membrane, but the cells remain depigmented. The photoreceptor elements have regenerated over the pigment epithelium. The photoreceptor nuclei remain unchanged. (Tso MOM, Wallow IHL, Elgin S: Experimental photocoagulation of the human retina. I. Corelationship of physical, clinical, and pathological data. Arch Ophthalmol 95:1035–1040, 1977; copyright 1977, American Medical Association)

lium, and photoreceptor elements had regenerated over the RPE (Fig. 15-2B). The photoreceptor nuclei remained unremarkable. The main therapeutic value of a grade I lesion is debridement of RPE, which provides a stimulus

to the surrounding pigment epithelial cells to proliferate and form a new layer of cells overlying Bruch's membrane. This type of photocoagulation burn may be used for the treatment of RPE diseases.

In the grade II lesion, the retinal burn appears ophthalmoscopically as a whitish spot surrounded by a grayish ring (Fig. 15-3). The white center is caused by necrosis of the photoreceptor nuclei, while the RPE involvement extends beyond the photoreceptor cell necrosis as a grayish ring (Fig. 15-3A). When these lesions were studied histopathologically in enucleated experimental human eyes, the RPE, photoreceptor elements, and outer nuclear layer were necrosed, but the cells in the inner nuclear layer were spared.[15] The choriocapillaris in these lesions was thrombosed.

Similar lesions were studied histopathologically in rhesus monkeys 1 to 3 months after photocoagulation.[17,21] The necrotic RPE and photoreceptor cells were removed, Bruch's membrane was relined by depigmented retinal epithelium, and pigment-laden macrophages were still in the subretinal space. Müller cell processes extended into the subretinal space to form a new external limiting membrane, but the photoreceptor nuclei were removed. In this reparative process, no chorioretinal scar was formed (Fig. 15-3B). Thus, the grade II burn removed pigment epithelium and photoreceptor cells without producing a chorioretinal scar or involving the inner layers of the retina and the retinal vasculature. The grade II lesion is usually of little therapeutic value since it does not produce chorioretinal adhesive scars or occlude leaking retinal vessels.

A grade III lesion is ophthalmoscopically characterized by a dense white spot with two surrounding grayish rings (Fig. 15-4). When studied histologically, these lesions showed necrosis of the RPE and outer and inner nuclear layers. The whitish center of the retinal lesions correlated with necrosis of the inner nuclear layers. The surrounding two rings corresponded to widespread necrosis of the outer nuclear layer and RPE that extended beyond the inner nuclear layer. In the healing phase (Fig. 15-5), these burns induced a moderate proliferation of RPE cells that extended into the retina. The astrocytes and Müller cells from the retina reached down into the subretinal space to intertwine with the proliferated RPE to form a chorioretinal scar. In these lesions, the retinal capillaries were occluded in the inner nuclear layer and in the choriocapillaris.

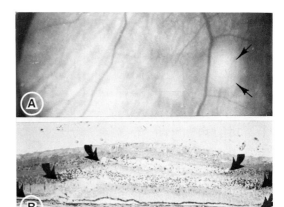

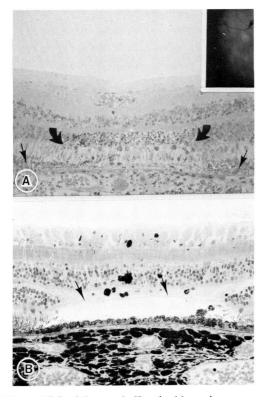

Figure 15-3. *(A)* A grade II retinal burn in a human eye. The RPE, photoreceptor elements, and outer nuclear layer are necrosed, but the cells in the inner nuclear layer are spared. The RPE damage *(small arrows)* extends beyond photoreceptor cell necrosis *(curved arrows)*. Inset: The clinical appearance of a grade II burn showing a whitish central spot and a surrounding grayish ring *(arrow)*. *(B)* A similar lesion inflicted on the retina of a rhesus monkey. The eye was enucleated 3 months after exposure. The necrotic RPE and photoreceptor cells have been removed, and Bruch's membrane has been relined with the pigment epithelium. Müller cells extend into the subretinal space to form a new external limiting membrane *(arrows)* despite the absence of photoreceptor nuclei. Pigment-laden macrophages are still present in the outer layers of the retina; however, no chorioretinal adhesion has developed.

Figure 15-4. *(A)* A grade III retinal burn *(arrows)* is characterized by a dense whitish spot and two surrounding grayish rings. *(B)* Histopathologically, there is necrosis at the RPE and at the outer and inner nuclear layers *(arrows)*. The whitish center of the retinal lesion shown in *A* corresponds to the necrosis of the inner nuclear layer. The surrounding two rings correlate with the widespread necrosis of the outer nuclear layer and pigment epithelium beyond the inner nuclear layer. (Original magnification × 80) *(A,* Tso MOM, Wallow IHL, Elgin S: Experimental photocoagulation of the human retina. I. Corelationship of physical, clinical, and pathological data. Arch Ophthalmol 95:1035–1040, 1977; copyright 1977, American Medical Association)

Grade III lesions may be subdivided into three degrees—mild, moderate, and severe. The whitish center varies in intensity ophthalmoscopically across each level and differs by the extent of necrosis observed histopathologically in the inner retinal layers. In a mild lesion, the inner nuclear layer is slightly involved, and proliferation of the glial cells in the retina is mild, so that a weak chorioretinal scar forms (Fig. 15-5A). A moderate lesion stimulates the retinal glial cells and retinal pigment epithelial cells to produce a strong chorioretinal adhesion (Fig. 15-5B). In severe lesions, the retinal burn may be so marked that the retinal pigment epithelium may fail to grow across Bruch's membrane. Grade III lesions are most useful in the treatment of a number of retinal diseases.

Grade IV lesions are retinal burns with a very intense whitish center surrounded by sloping white rings. When examined histologically, the

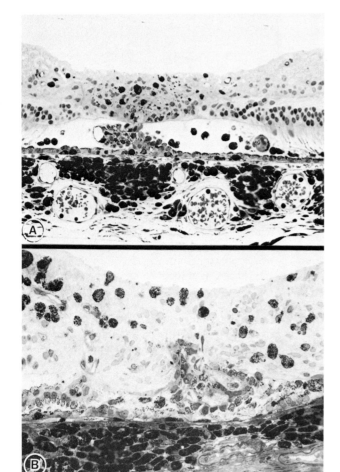

Figure 15-5. *(A)* A mild grade III retinal burn was inflicted on the retina of a rhesus monkey. Three months later, proliferation of the RPE extends across the subretinal space to form a moderate chorioretinal scar. (Original magnification × 150) *(B)* A moderate grade III retinal burn produced a strong chorioretinal scar composed of proliferated retinal pigment epithelial cells interdigitating with retinal glial cells. (Original magnification × 300) *(A,* Wallow IHL, Tso MOM: Retinal repair after xenon arc photocoagulation. II. The evolution of retinal lesions in the rhesus monkey. A clinical and light microscopic study. Am J Ophthalmol 75:610, 1973; published with permission from The American Journal of Ophthalmology)

lesion shows a full-thickness necrosis of the retina involving all layers including the internal limiting membrane (Fig. 15-6A). The high temperature generated by photocoagulation "mummifies" the plasma membrane of the retinal cells, and the cellular outline is temporarily preserved (Fig. 15-6B). The whitish center corresponds to full-thickness necrosis of the retina, and the rings represent the widening necrosis of the photoreceptor cells and RPE into the adjacent retina. The retinal vessels in the nerve fiber and inner nuclear layers show coagulation necrosis and occlusion.

A histologic study of similar lesions in monkeys 1 and 3 months after photocoagulation showed atrophy of the entire retina, resulting in a thin glial membrane bridging across the lesion (Fig. 15-6C). The pigment epithelium frequently failed to proliferate, and chorioretinal adhesions did not form. At times, internal limiting membrane would rupture, allowing a preretinal glial membrane to grow over the atrophic retina. Grade IV lesions are used to destroy retinal and choroidal tumors.

THERAPEUTIC APPLICATION OF PHOTOCOAGULATION TREATMENT FOR RETINAL DISEASES

Debridement of the RPE

In certain diseases of the RPE such as central serous choroidopathy, the cells are decompen-

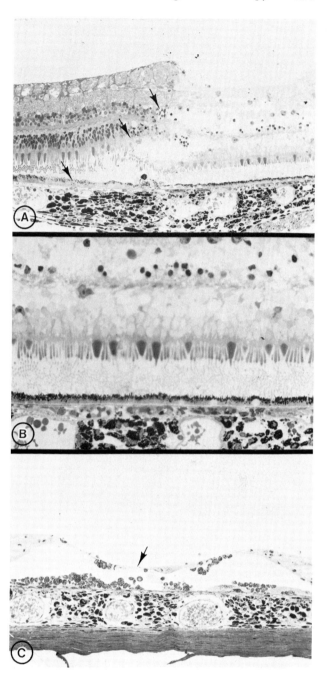

Figure 15-6. *(A)* A grade IV retinal burn shows intense necrosis of all retinal layers *(arrows)* including the internal limiting membrane *(arrowhead)*. (Original magnification × 300) *(B)* The intense heat of the retinal burn has mummified the photoreceptor elements so that the outline of the cell is relatively preserved, even though the cells are necrosed. *(C)* In the healing phase, all the necrotic tissues have been removed, resulting in a thin, bare, glial membrane *(arrow)* reaching across the scar. The RPE cells have barely proliferated to cover Bruch's membrane. (Original magnification × 130)

sated and functionally incompetent. This results in the disruption of the blood–retina barrier and the failure of the transport of fluid to or from the subretinal space. The cells, however, are not necrotic and do not excite a macrophagic or reparative response.[14] Fluorescein angiography discloses leakage of dye from the choroid through these decompensated RPE cells into the subretinal space, revealing an associated serous detachment of the retina (Fig. 15-7). Frequently, the decompensated RPE may heal spontaneously, and the blood–retina barrier is re-formed and the serous retinal detachment improves. In patients with recurrent central serous retinal detachment, photocoagulation may be indicated. In such cases, retinal burns of grade I intensity may be applied at the site of the leakage to cause necrosis of the RPE while inflicting only minimal damage on the photoreceptor cells (Fig. 15-8). The resulting reactive proliferation of RPE around the lesion will reform the blood–retina barrier and re-establish an effective pump for the subretinal fluid so that the serous retinal detachment will settle.

Occlusion of Retinal Vascular Leakage

Photocoagulation is used to obliterate leaking retinal vessels. Leaking microaneurysms are lo-

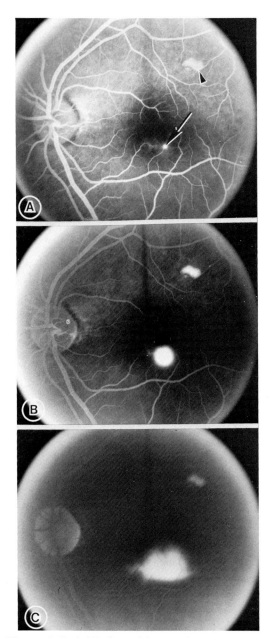

Figure 15-7. *(A)* Patient with central serous choroidopathy demonstrates focal leakage of the RPE in the paramacular area *(arrow)*. Note the small focal retinal pigment epithelial detachment *(arrowhead)*. *(B, C)* Leakage from the RPE increases in size and spreads in the subretinal space beneath the serously detached retina, while the pigment epithelial detachment remains the same size.

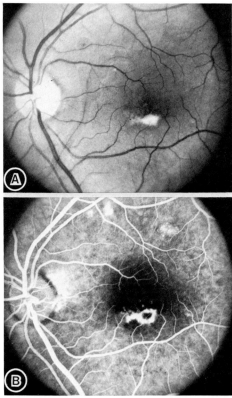

Figure 15-8. After repeated attacks of central serous choroidopathy, the patient in Figure 15-7 received mild photocoagulation treatment to necrose the RPE. The blood–retina barrier is reformed by the proliferated RPE, and the serous retinal detachment settles. *(A)* fundus photograph; *B,* fluorescein angiogram.

cated in the inner nuclear layer, while leaking macroaneurysms usually develop from the larger retinal vessels in the nerve fiber layer (Fig. 15-9). Thus, to treat leaking microaneurysms, a grade III mild to moderate retinal burn will effectively occlude the lesion in the inner nuclear layer. However, grade III severe to grade IV photocoagulation burns may be required to occlude macroaneurysms in the nerve fiber layers of the retina.

A recent report by the Early Treatment Diabetic Retinopathy Study Research Group (ETDRS) recommends focal photocoagulation of clinically significant diabetic macular edema.[5] The microaneurysms are photocoagulated to achieve "definite whitening" around the microaneurysm or "darkening of the microaneurysm itself." These burns correspond to

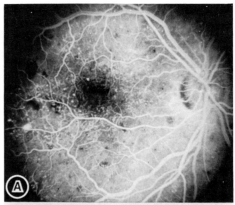

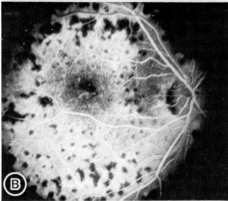

Figure 15-10. *(A)* A patient with diabetes has moderate macular edema and background retinopathy. *(B)* The microaneurysms and focal leakage in *A* are treated with grade III mild to moderate photocoagulation burns.

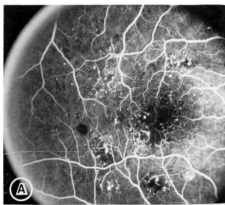

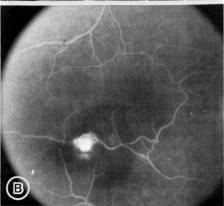

Figure 15-9. *(A)* Microaneurysms in an eye with diabetic retinopathy are located mostly in the inner nuclear layer of the retina. *(B)* A macroaneurysm is found in the nerve fiber layer of the retina.

a grade III mild to moderate photocoagulation lesion (Fig. 15-10). This report also describes a treatment regimen in which light to moderate intensity burns are placed in a grid pattern to treat diffuse leakage or nonperfused areas within two disc diameters of the center of the macula. These mild burns appear to be grade I to II burns, which would bring about RPE cell necrosis. The effectiveness of this mode of treatment suggests that RPE malfunction may be one of the pathogenetic factors of diabetic macular edema. Indeed, we have observed decompensation of the RPE in rats with streptozotocin-induced diabetes and have postulated that photocoagulation treatment of diabetic retinopathy may act as a form of debridement of the RPE followed by healing and the re-establishment of the blood–retina barrier.[14]

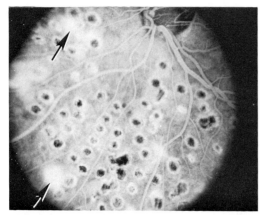

Figure 15-11. A patient with proliferative diabetic retinopathy is treated with panretinal photocoagulation consisting of grade III mild to moderate burns. The arrows denote leakage from vitreous neovascularization.

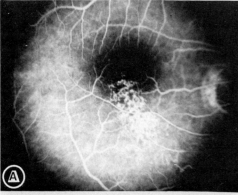

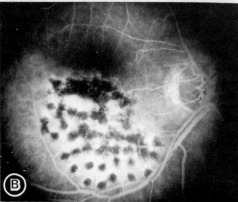

Figure 15-12. *(A)* Patient with branch retinal vein occlusion and retinal telangiectasia and edema. *(B)* The affected area was treated with quadrantal scattered photocoagulation burns.

Therapy for Proliferative Retinopathy

Panretinal photocoagulation is the standard treatment for diabetic proliferative retinopathy (Fig. 15-11). It is also recommended for certain cases of branch retinal vein occlusion (Fig. 15-12) resulting in macular edema or retinal, vitreous, or iridic neovascularization.[2,3] The exact therapeutic mechanism has yet to be determined. It has been proposed that the destruction of retinal tissue by photocoagulation will reduce the metabolic demand of the retina.[23] Increased diffusion of oxygen from the choroidal circulation into the atrophic retina after treatment has been another proposed mechanism.[4] To reduce retinal metabolic demand, grade III mild to moderate burns are probably required, as the outer layers of the retina will be destroyed and a chorioretinal scar will be formed to give added beneficial effect to prevent possible subsequent vitreoretinal traction and retinal detachment.

Occlusion of the Subretinal Pigment Epithelial Neovascularization

One of the important uses of photocoagulation is to occlude subretinal pigment epithelial neovascularization in age-related macular degeneration.[8–10] Human and monkey experimental studies have shown that grade II to grade III burns occlude the choriocapillaris in the normal retina. It is important to note, however, that in the subretinal pigment epithelial neovascular net, the feeding choroidal arterioles are deep in the midchoroidal stroma and may have to be occluded to prevent recurrence in some cases (Figs. 15-13–15-17). To achieve this, grade III moderate to severe burns are needed. On the other hand, we have observed the recurrence of subretinal pigment epithelial neovascular nets that appeared to have been completely ablated previously (Fig. 15-17). There is a strong possibility that vasoproliferative factors from the diseased retina may stimulate recurrence, but the pathogenetic mechanisms have not been definitively determined. The krypton laser may have value in this therapeutic measure, as the laser light appears to penetrate deeper into the cho-

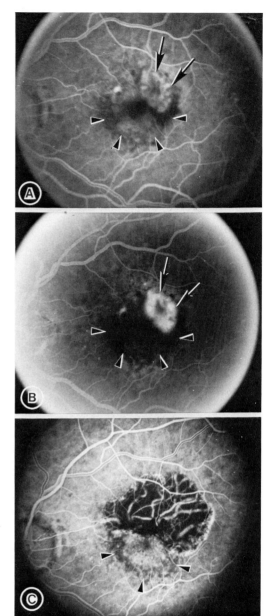

Figure 15-13. *(A)* A patient with subretinal pigment epithelial neovascularization *(arrows)* in the paramacular area. Hemorrhage *(arrowheads)* in the subretinal pigment epithelial space spreads around the entire macular area. *(B)* The late venous phase of the fluorescein angiogram reveals hyperfluorescence of the subretinal pigment epithelial neovascular net *(arrows)* and hypofluorescence of the spreading subretinal pigment epithelial hemorrhage *(arrowheads)*. *(C)* After photocoagulation and ablation of the subretinal pigment epithelial net, visual acuity improved from 20/80 to 20/25. Irregular mottling *(arrowheads)* of the inferior macula persists as the blood is absorbed.

roid than the argon blue-green laser wave length.[1] A subpigment epithelial neovascular net overlying the maculopapillary bundle may be occluded by grade III moderate retinal burns, which will spare the nerve fiber layer of the inner retina and avoid complicating scotomas (Fig. 15-16).

Production of Chorioretinal Adhesions

Photocoagulation is used to produce chorioretinal adhesions to seal off a retinal hole in the prevention of retinal detachment (Fig. 15-18). Grade III mild to moderate lesions are best suited for this purpose. A grade II lesion does not

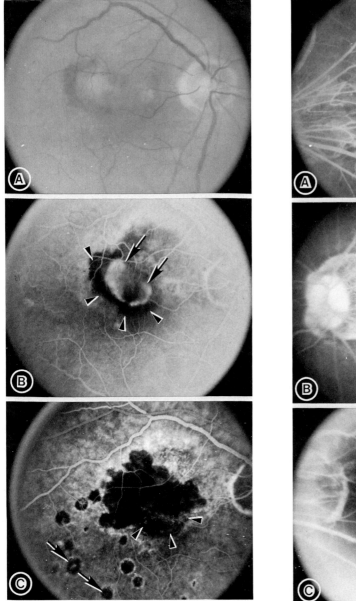

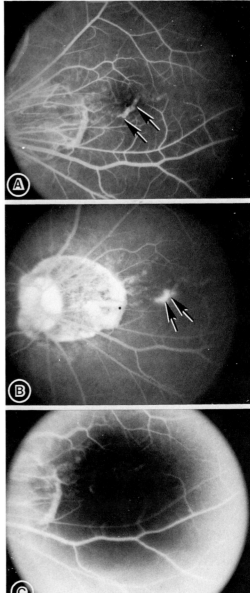

Figure 15-14. *(A)* Patient with age-related macular degeneration has a subretinal pigment epithelial neovascular net involving the superior half of the fovea. *(B)* Fluorescein angiogram demonstrates diffuse leakage of the pigment epithelium overlying the neovascular net *(arrows)* and the hypofluorescent hemorrhage *(arrowheads)* that extends over the entire macular area. *(C)* After photocoagulation, the neovascular net was ablated. Irregular mottling secondary to subretinal pigment epithelial hemorrhage *(arrowheads)* was observed in the inferior half of the fovea. Visual acuity improved from 20/100 to 20/40 after treatment. Arrows indicate laser test spots.

Figure 15-15. *(A)* Subretinal pigment epithelial neovascular net *(arrows)* in patient with myopic macular degeneration. Visual acuity decreased to 20/100. *(B)* The RPE exhibits diffuse leakage *(arrows)* overlying the neovascular net. *(C)* After ablation of the neovascular net, visual acuity increased to 20/40.

produce chorioretinal adhesion. It further weakens the chorioretinal attachment due to the re-formation of the external limiting membrane with the loss of photoreceptor cells. Grade IV lesions produce such an atrophic scar that no firm chorioretinal adhesion of considerable strength will form. Thus, it is most important in this therapeutic procedure to inflict the correct amount of retinal damage to induce proper chorioretinal adhesion.

Treatment of Retinal or Choroidal Neoplasms

Photocoagulation therapy has been used to destroy various tumors, such as retinoblastoma

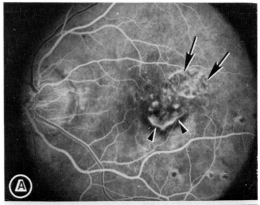

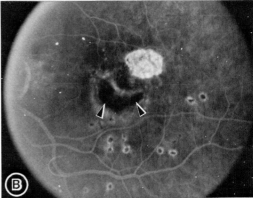

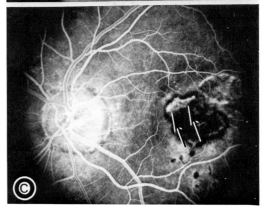

Figure 15-17. A patient with age-related macular degeneration. *(A)* Photocoagulation was applied superotemporally to the fovea to occlude a neovascular net *(arrows)*. One year later, a second neovascular net developed in the inferior macular region *(arrowheads)*. *(B)* The inferior neovascular net was completely ablated *(arrowheads)*. Around the lesion, secondary staining of the necrotic pigment epithelium is seen. *(C)* One month later, the neovascular net *(arrows)* recurred.

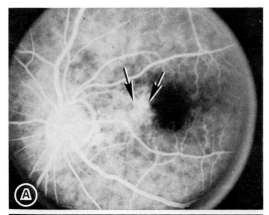

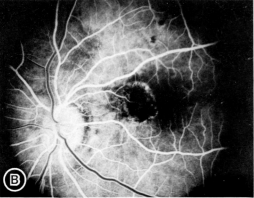

Figure 15-16. *(A)* Subretinal pigment epithelial neovascular net *(arrows)* occurs beneath the maculopapillary bundle. *(B)* The neovascular net was treated with grade III moderate photocoagulation burns, and the patient retained a visual acuity of 20/25 after treatment.

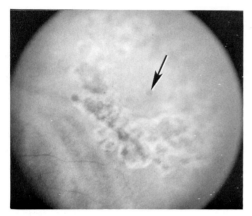

Figure 15-18. A peripheral retinal hole *(arrow)* is sealed off by grade III moderate to severe burns.

heavy photocoagulation treatment to lesions at the equatorial or peripheral retina, where the choroidal arterioles lie in the same plane as the choriocapillaris, may occlude one of the choroidal arterioles, resulting in triangular retinal whitening secondary to choroidal ischemia.[6,25]

Excessive destruction of retinal tissues and rupture of the internal limiting membrane may lead to preretinal membrane formation (Fig. 15-19). Alternatively, rupture of the internal limiting membrane may produce a retinal hole, which will be detrimental in the treatment of macular lesions (Fig. 15-20). In addition, the failure to occlude abnormal vessels completely, particularly in the subretinal pigment epithelial

and malignant melanoma of the choroid, and tumor-like congenital or developmental abnormalities such as *angiomatosis retinae* and retinal telangiectasia of Coats' disease. To occlude the blood supply to these retinal or choroidal lesions, grade III severe to grade IV retinal burns are needed. It is doubtful that photocoagulation burns can reach into the deep choroid to produce necrosis of a malignant melanoma of considerable thickness.

Complications of Photocoagulation Therapy

In patients with opaque ocular media such as corneal opacity, cataract, and vitreous or retinal hemorrhages, the radiant energy of the photocoagulation treatment is absorbed by these ocular media, resulting in damage to the tissues. It is interesting to note, however, that lens opacity produced by the argon laser does not progress, but remains stationary for months.[12]

Excessive energy may cause a microexplosion in the retinal or choroidal vasculature, causing retinal or choroidal hemorrhage. Thus, when heavy photocoagulation burns are needed, it is better to prolong the exposure time, increasing the total dose of energy delivered, rather than to raise the level of energy, risking complicating hemorrhage. Accidental burns to the macular tissue will result in loss of central vision. Also,

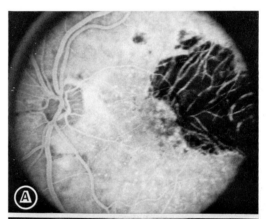

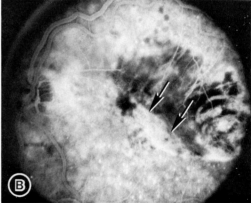

Figure 15-19. *(A)* Patient with subretinal pigment epithelial neovascular net was treated with severe grade IV burns. *(B)* Three months later, a preretinal membrane *(arrows)* developed and leaked fluorescein diffusely.

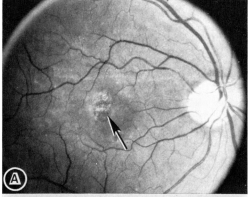

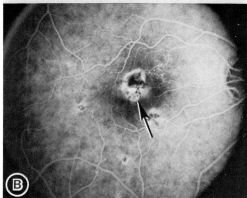

Figure 15-20. The fundus photograph *(A)* and fluorescein angiogram *(B)* of a patient with a perifoveal subretinal pigment epithelial neovascular net which was treated by heavy photocoagulation burns. The internal limiting membranes ruptured, causing a foveal hole *(arrows in A and B).*

neovascular net, may induce these new vessels to recur in damaged retinal tissues and exacerbate the neovascularization process. Occlusion of large retinal arteries and veins may lead to retinal ischemic infarction.

Occasionally, after panretinal photocoagulation, there is a rise in intraocular pressure. The pathogenetic mechanism is not yet known. Patients with extensive panretinal photocoagulation may develop mild anterior and posterior uveitis, or they may complain of mild photophobia with cells and flare in the anterior chamber. These complications should, therefore, be carefully observed and treated accordingly.

REFERENCES

1. Borges JM, Charles HC, Lee CM, et al: A clinicopathologic study of dye-laser photocoagulation in primate retina. Retina 7: 46–57, 1987
2. Branch Vein Occlusion Study Group: Argon laser photocoagulation for macular edema in branch vein occlusion. Am J Ophthalmol 98:271, 1984
3. Branch Vein Occlusion Study Group: Argon laser scatter photocoagulation for prevention of neovascularization and vitreous hemorrhage in branch vein occlusion. Arch Ophthalmol 104:34–41, 1986
4. Diddie KR, Ernest JT: The effect of photocoagulation on the choroidal vasculature and retinal oxygen tension. Am J Ophthalmol 84:62–66, 1977
5. Early Treatment Diabetic Retinopathy Study Research Group: Photocoagulation for diabetic macular edema. Early Treatment Diabetic Retinopathy Study Report Number 1. Arch Ophthalmol 103:1796–1806, 1985
6. Goldbaum M, Galinos SO, Apple D, et al: Acute choroidal ischemia as a complication of photocoagulation. Arch Ophthalmol 94:1025–1035, 1979
7. L'Esperance FA: Ophthalmic Lasers: Photocoagulation, Photoradiation and Surgery, 2nd ed. St Louis, CV Mosby, 1983
8. Macular Photocoagulation Study Group: Argon laser photocoagulation for senile macular degeneration: Results of a randomized clinical trial. Arch Ophthalmol 100:912–918, 1982
9. Macular Photocoagulation Study Group: Argon laser photocoagulation for ocular histoplasmosis: Results of a randomized clinical trial. Arch Ophthalmol 101:1347–1357, 1983
10. Macular Photocoagulation Study Group: Argon laser photocoagulation for idiopathic neovascularization: Results of a randomized clinical trial. Arch Ophthalmol 101:1358–1361, 1983
11. Powell JO, Tso MOM, Wallow IHL: Recovery of the retina from argon laser radiation. Ann Ophthalmol 6:1003, 1974
12. Shapiro A, Tso MOM, Goldberg MF: A clinicopathologic study of an argon-laser induced cataract. Arch Ophthalmol 102:579–583, 1984
13. Smiddy WE, Patz A, Quigley H, et al: Histopathology of the tunable dye laser in primate retina. Invest Ophthalmol Vis Sci (Suppl) 27:219, 1986
14. Tso MOM: Pathology of the blood-retinal barrier. In Cunha-Vaz JG (ed): The Blood–Retinal Barrier, pp 235-250, New York, Plenum Press 1980
15. Tso MOM, Cunha-Vaz JG, Shih CY, et al: Clinicopathologic study of blood–retinal barrier in experimental diabetes mellitus. Arch Ophthalmol 98:2032–2040, 1980

16. Tso MOM, Wallow IHL, Elgin S: Experimental photocoagulation of the human retina. I. Correlations of physical, clinical, and pathological data. Arch Ophthalmol 95:1035–1040, 1977

17. Tso MOM, Wallow IHL, Powell JO, et al: Recovery of the rod and cone after photic injury. Trans Am Acad Ophthalmol Otolaryngol 76:1247, 1972

18. Wallow IHL, Davis MD: Clinicopathologic correlation of xenon arc and argon laser photocoagulation. Arch Ophthalmol 97:2308–2315, 1979

19. Wallow IHL, Lund OE, Gabel VP, et al: A comparison of retinal argon laser lesions in man and in cynomolgus monkey. Albrecht von Graefes Arch Klin Exp Ophthalmol 189:159–164, 1974

20. Wallow IHL, Tso MOM: Failure of formation of chorioretinal adhesions following xenon arc photocoagulation. Mod Probl Ophthalmol 12:189, 1974

21. Wallow IHL, Tso MOM: Retinal repair after xenon arc photocoagulation. II. The evolution of retinal lesions in the rhesus monkey: A clinical and light microscopic study. Am J Ophthalmol 75:610, 1973

22. Wallow IHL, Tso MOM, Elgin S: Experimental photocoagulation of the human retina. II. Electron microscopic study. Arch Ophthalmol 95:1041–1050, 1977

23. Wolbarsht ML, Landers MD III, Rand L: Modifications of retinal vascularization by interaction between retinal and choroidal circulation. Invest Ophthalmol Vis Sci (Suppl) 17:224, 1978

24. Yannuzzi LA, Gitter KA, Schatz H: The Macula. Baltimore, Williams & Wilkins, 1979

25. Yoneya S, Tso MOM: Angioarchitecture of the human choroid. Arch Ophthalmol 105:681–687, 1987

26. Zweng HC (ed): Recent Advances in Photocoagulation. International Ophthalmology Clinics, vol. 16, no 4. Boston, Little, Brown, 1976

16

Fundus Flavimaculatus and Retinitis Pigmentosa

David A. Newsome
Paul Blacharski

Retinal dystrophies and degenerations cause severe visual loss in populations around the world. This group of diseases provides many challenges for the clinician, ranging from difficulties in diagnosis to frustrations of having little other than genetic counseling and routine follow-up examinations to offer the patient.

Fluorescein angiography provides the clinician with valuable information to diagnose and manage a variety of retinal dystrophies and degenerations. The purposes of this chapter are to provide an overview of two of the most frequently seen retinal dystrophies, fundus flavimaculatus and retinitis pigmentosa, and to highlight the use of fluorescein angiography in the evaluation of the management of patients affected by these diseases.

FUNDUS FLAVIMACULATUS

Definition

Fundus flavimaculatus is a bilateral, progressive, familial degeneration inherited as an autosomal-recessive trait that is characterized by subretinal yellow flecks and macular atrophy. Although it is relatively common, precise rates of occurrence for the disease are not available; we estimate its prevalence at 1:10,000 to 1:15,000. This disease has markedly varied forms of presentation and can be confused with

several other conditions (Table 16-1). The term *fundus flavimaculatus* was introduced by Franceschetti in 1962.[58] The condition, however, was comprehensively described by Stargardt in 1909.[133] We have found that Stargardt's disease and fundus flavimaculatus are one and the same, based on the ophthalmoscopic, functional, angiographic, and evolutionary characteristics of our cases; a review of the comprehensive clinical description by Stargardt; and the functional characteristics defined in recent work. Irvine has pointed out that "Stargardt's original papers show that the macular degeneration he described is identical to what has recently been called fundus flavimaculatus with atrophic macular degeneration."[77] Francois has shown that Stargardt's disease and fundus flavimaculatus have identical clinical, electrophysiologic, and genetic characteristics.[60] Anmarkrud[9] has remarked that the "similar angiographic picture with abolished visibility of the choroid circulation . . . may be further evidence that fundus flavimaculatus and Stargardt's disease is [sic] the same disease with a different expression."

Patients with fundus flavimaculatus show a variable electroretinographic finding, ranging from completely normal to some loss of cone amplitudes to a reduction of both cones and rods. The electro-oculogram also varies. Goldmann perimetry may disclose some mild constriction of peripheral field. Also, a central sco-

Table 16-1. Differential Diagnosis of Fundus Flavimaculatus

Drusen
Adult vitelliform foveal dystrophy
Macular pigment epithelial dystrophies
Cone dystrophy
Vitelliform macular degeneration (Bests' disease)
Fundus albipunctatus (with comet-shaped dots)
X-linked juvenile retinoschisis
X-linked retinitis pigmentosa carrier
Olivopontocerebellar degeneration retinopathy
Myotonic dystrophy maculopathy
Flecked retina of Kandori and other rare flecked retinal syndromes

toma is evident when macular atrophy is present.

Fluorescein angiography has aided in the diagnosis of fundus flavimaculatus. Since its development by Flocks and coworkers in 1959 and its modification for human use by Novotny and Alvis in 1960, fluorescein angiography has provided a wealth of information for the diagnosis and management of myriad retinal diseases.[55,112,113] Ernest and Krill first reported on fluorescein studies in fundus flavimaculatus in a comparison with drusen.[46] Several other investigators have offered early accounts of the angiographic features of the disease.[2,4,12,34,59,81] The most characteristic finding is a "silent" or "absent" choroid, described initially by Bonnin in 1971 (Fig. 16-1).[27] Other features include peripapillary sparing from flecks, transmission defects of the macula, peripheral reticular pigment

patterns, multifocal choroidal atrophy, choroidal neovascularization, and retinal neovascularization.[38,40,51,82,89] The angiographically silent choroid has been noted in as few as 50% to as many as 88% of patients.[26,60,129] We have examined angiographic negatives of 71 patients with fundus flavimaculatus and have confirmed the high frequency and diagnostic importance of this feature. We have also observed less common findings not previously emphasized or noted in the literature, such as peripheral histoplasmosis-like spots, reticular pigmentary changes, and multifocal choroidal atrophy of the macula (Table 16-2). Of our 71 patients, 62 had adequate pictures to evaluate choroidal fluorescence. Fifty-five (89%) had blocked choroidal fluorescence. Seven did not show the absence of choroidal fluorescence. The angiograms of the remaining nine were not diagnostic because of limited field, poor quality, or diffuse macular atrophy without peripheral views. We noted that 15 (21%) patients had central choroidal atrophy, 4 (5%) of whom showed a multifocal pattern. One patient (1%) had a monocular choroidal neovascular membrane, and 6 (8%) had peripheral pigmentary reticular changes. These last findings appeared similar to those associated with age-related macular degeneration but were more extensive (extending to the posterior pole) and generated a different angiographic appearance. (See Periphery in Fundus Flavimaculatus.)

Fluorescein angiography must include views of the periphery, either by use of a wide-angle camera (60°) or by "sweeping" the periphery

Table 16-2. Choroidal Fluorescence

	Number of Patients	Percentage
Males	26	36
Females	45	64
Mean age (yr)	22	
Absent choroidal fluorescence (*n* = 62 with angiograms)	55	89
Macular/choroidal atrophy	15	24
Peripheral reticular degeneration	6	10
Multifocal atrophy	4	5
Choroidal neovascularization	1	1

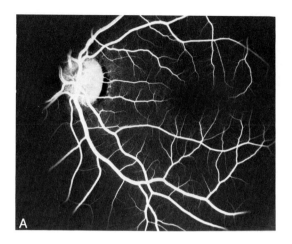

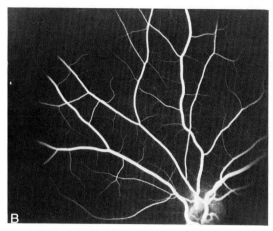

Figure 16-1. Fluorescein angiogram of a 20-year-old woman with 20/40 visual acuity. *(A)* Choroidal fluorescence and other transmission defects are totally absent during the arteriovenous phase. *(B)* The mid-periphery demonstrates the diffuse nature of the absent choroidal fluorescence. *(C)* After 8 years, mottled hyperfluorescence is seen with diffuse atrophy of the pigment epithelium of the macula and hypofluorescence in the fovea corresponding to pigmentary hyperplasia. This later feature confirms the presence of an intact choroidal circulation not visualized in the earlier angiogram.

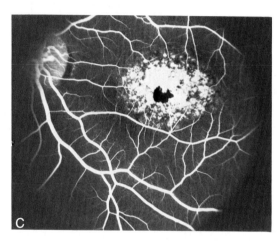

with a 30° or 45° camera. Diffuse macular and posterior pole atrophy, with corresponding transmitted fluorescence, often masks the silent choroid (Fig. 16-2, 16-3).

A review of the negatives helps to minimize variability that occurs in reproduction, including under- and overexposure, which makes analysis difficult and inconclusive. It is also important to remember that angiographic findings may vary, depending upon the portion of the chorioretinal complex studied.

Choroid in Fundus Flavimaculatus

The absence of choroidal fluorescence can be present throughout the entire fundus, and is generally a diffuse, uniform, bilateral phenomenon that is not segmental or focal. Rarely, we have seen slight asymmetry between the two eyes or variability within one eye in which the medial retina has increased absence of choroidal fluorescence. Thus, the peripheral retina will exhibit reduced or absent choroidal fluorescence in association with extensive macular degeneration or atrophy. Fish reported 37 cases of posterior retinal dystrophy with a dark choroid.[51] Of those, 34 demonstrated flecks, while the remaining 3 had a bull's-eye pattern not inconsistent with early fundus flavimaculatus. Their cases included patients with Stargardt's disease, bull's-eye maculopathy, cone dystrophy, butterfly dystrophy, and cone-rod dystrophy. Many reported cases include fluorescein angiograms that show the silent choroid, although the authors did not specifically comment upon this feature.[5,100,101,138,140]

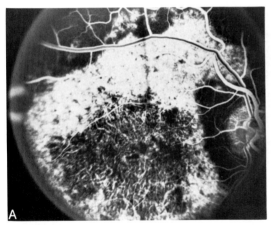
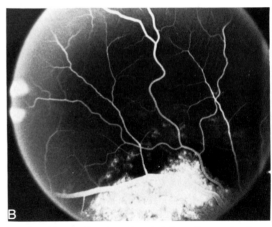

Figure 16-2. Fluorescein angiogram of a 38-year-old man with 20/40 visual acuity. *(A)* Prominent chorioretinal atrophy is surrounded by diffuse pigment epithelial atrophy. Note peripapillary sparing of defects. *(B)* A peripheral view shows blocked choroidal fluorescence and more typical adjacent patchy transmission defects.

We believe that the diffuse absence of choroidal fluorescence is unique to fundus flavimaculatus, although Bonnin noted it in 3% of patients with acute posterior multifocal placoid pigment epitheliopathy (APMPPE).[27] These findings have not been confirmed. Certainly, the active lesions of APMPPE block choroidal fluorescence locally, but it is not the diffuse blockage typical of fundus flavimaculatus.[64] We have examined two sisters with the multicentric form of choroidal atrophy which could have been confused with APMPPE, except that it was familial, bilateral, progressive, and had peripheral findings including flecks and absent choroidal fluorescence (Fig. 16-4). Other diseases showing local (macular) absence of choroidal fluorescence associated with abnormal pigment material include Best's disease and adult vitelliform dystrophy.[65,96]

Etiology of the Absent Choroid

The silent choroid was initially thought to result from a choroidal circulation problem.[27] Other

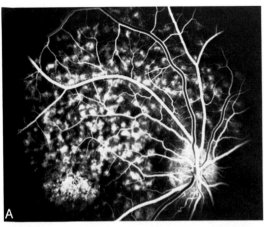
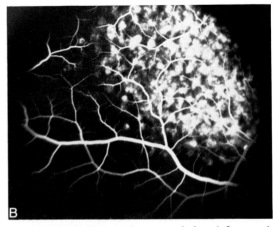

Figure 16-3. *(A)* The macula demonstrates mottled atrophy surrounded by patchy transmission defects and peripapillary sparing. *(B)* The inferotemporal field shows the absent choroidal fluorescence, which was less evident in *A*, demonstrating the importance of the "sweep" to display this feature.

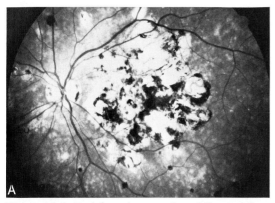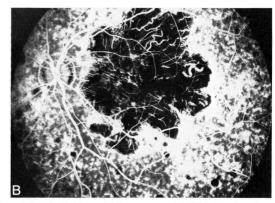

Figure 16-4. Red-free photograph and fluorescein angiograph of a 36-year-old woman with 20/400 visual acuity. *(A)* Demonstrated are multifocal chorioretinal atrophy, peripapillary atrophy, and smaller round peripheral lesions similar to those of the ocular histoplasmosis syndrome. Also present are irregular subretinal defects and marked pigmentary hyperplasia. The patient has a documented 10-year history of progressive disease and a sibling 8 years older with a similar-looking fundus. *(B)* Fluorescein angiogram demonstrates chorioretinal atrophy and the more typical patchy hyperfluorescent defects.

authors have proposed different causes for this feature, including (1) blockage of fluorescence by the sensory retina; (2) a masking effect between the choroid and the retinal vessels from a substance absorbing, emitting, or exciting light; (3) an abnormal absorbing layer at the level of the pigment epithelium; and (4) an abnormal lipofuscin-like material in the pigment epithelial cells blocking the excitatory blue wave length of the fluorescein angiography.[3,9,45,51] If choroidal nonperfusion produced the dark choroid, there would be a marked electroretinographic reduction, which is not found in fundus flavimaculatus. Buettner and colleagues showed that experimental deprivation of the choroidal blood flow caused a marked electroretinographic reduction in a matter of hours.[35] Moreover, in most areas of RPE atrophy, the choroidal fluorescence is usually present.

In 1979, Anmarkrud reviewed the histopathologic work by Klein and Krill and stated that it is likely that a diffuse deposit at the level of the pigment epithelium, Bruch's membrane, or the outer segment of the retina blocks the transmission of light.[9,81] A clinicopathologic study by Eagle and coworkers refined this observation.[45] The authors noted a marked accumulation of an abnormal lipofuscin-like material throughout the entire pigment epithelium. They concluded,

"the generalized choroidal hypofluorescence seen in early cases . . . is readily explained by the well-known ability of lipofuscin to absorb the blue excitatory wave lengths during fluorescein angiography." The accumulation of this abnormal material in the pigment epithelium was confirmed by Frangieh and colleagues.[62] Thus, where a window defect (due to atrophy or hypopigmentation, for example) occurs in the pigment epithelium, we see choroidal fluorescence.

In contrast to previous histopathologic work, a recent clinicopathologic study by McDonnell and associates in a case of fundus flavimaculatus found no evidence of the accumulation of lipofuscin-like material.[90] Only some cells with distended apices contained tubulovesicular material. Fluorescein angiography had not been performed. The authors stated that this may have represented a different pigment epithelial disorder that shares a similar ophthalmoscopic picture.

We have chosen the word *absent* to describe this phenomenon of the choroid rather than *silent, blocked,* or *dark,* used by others. The blue excitatory wave length of the fluorescein camera flash is absorbed by the abnormal pigment contained within the pigment epithelium, thus obscuring fluorescence of the choroid. *Blocked flu-*

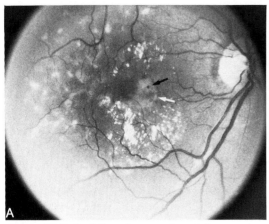 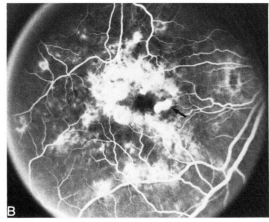

Figure 16-5. Red-free photograph and fluorescein angiogram of a 66-year-old woman with 20/60 visual acuity. *(A)* Red-free photograph shows an area of choroidal obscuration *(white arrow)* associated with a spot of hemorrhage *(black arrow)* medial to the fovea and surrounding lipid, all of which suggest a choroidal neovascular membrane. Throughout the remaining macula are subretinal flecks characteristic of fundus flavimaculatus. The fellow eye has a symmetric appearance except for the area of leakage. *(B)* Corresponding angiogram exhibits the choroidal neovascular membrane and its associated leakage *(arrow)*. Other areas are hyperfluorescent and without leaks. Flecks are distributed in a reticular configuration more typical of those seen in the periphery.

orescence implies that fluorescence exists but cannot be seen. In reality, it has not occurred, so *absent* is a more accurate characterization.

The pattern of flecks has been postulated by Hayreh to "resemble the choriocapillaris pat-

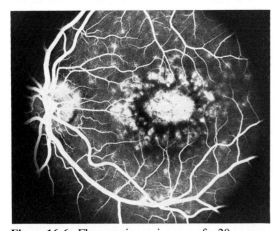

Figure 16-6. Fluorescein angiogram of a 20-year-old woman with 20/120 visual acuity. The macula shows mottled hyperfluorescence surrounded by a ring of irregular and densely spaced transmission defects and a more peripheral zone of more widely spaced defects. The absent choroidal fluorescence is mildly obscured by the overlying flush of the retinal capillaries.

tern."[69] The flecks in fundus flavimaculatus, Hayreh believes, "resemble venous segments of choriocapillaris units" both in morphology and distribution. The relationship between the choriocapillaris and flecks, which are comprised of distended abnormal lipofuscin-laden pigment epithelial cells, is not completely understood.

Subretinal Neovascularization in Fundus Flavimaculatus

Choroidal neovascularization is a rare complication of fundus flavimaculatus (Fig. 16-5). Paufique and Hervouet noted this finding in a histopathologic study.[116] In case No. 18 of a series of patients described by Klein and Krill, it was reported: "the left macula [has] a coarser lesion consisting of a choroidal atrophy involving the macula with characteristic peripheral flecks. The retinal neovascularization occurred in the inferior and superior arcades at the margin of atrophy."[81]

Macula in Fundus Flavimaculatus

The macula may be entirely devoid of pigment epithelial transmission (window) defects other

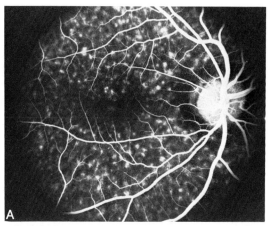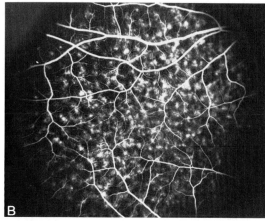

Figure 16-7. *(A)* Fluorescein angiogram represents the relatively even distribution of transmission defects with peripapillary sparing. Between the defects is absent choroidal fluorescence. *(B)* The temporal retina discloses continued widespread distribution of defects.

than absent choroidal fluorescence (see Fig. 16-1). However, there may be a spectrum of pigment epithelial defects (Fig. 16-6, 16-7) including frank atrophy of the choriocapillaris and pigment epithelium (see Fig. 16-2). More commonly, there are patchy transmission defects. During the arterial phase, many macular flecks or other atrophic lesions fluoresce early and become more intense late in the angiogram. There is no leakage unless there is choroidal neovascularization. Frequently, there are multiple, uniformly spaced, irregular patches that do not transmit fluorescence uniformly. In contrast, some flecks may not fluoresce early in their course of evolution. It has been postulated that intact, enlarged pigment epithelial cells that correspond to clinically visible flecks do not transmit fluorescein unless they have been fragmented, which disperses their contents and exposes the underlying choroid. This explanation is supported by histologic and chemical analyses.[3,50,81,96] Other times, more transmission defects are noted than those that correspond to clinical flecks.[12]

Early macular lesions include hypofluorescence of the fovea surrounded by a ring of transmission defects (see Fig. 16-1*C*); a bull's-eye lesion, centered on the fovea and confined to the area of the normal oval macular reflect (Fig.16-8), and the mottled transmission defect of the macula without isolated lesions (Fig. 16-9). All of these examples demonstrate the

surrounding dark choroid. Hypofluorescence of the fovea may represent increased pigmentation secondary to RPE hyperplasia.[59]

The late stages may include total atrophy of the pigment epithelium and choriocapillaris resulting in visualization of the larger choroidal vessels. This pattern of atrophy can range from a solitary area of atrophy to multicentric and irregular lesions (Fig. 16-10), similar to that seen in APMPPE or presumed ocular histoplasmosis syndrome. With progression, the patchy trans-

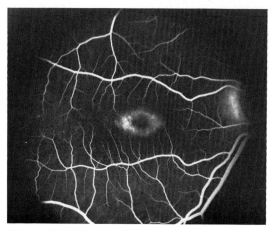

Figure 16-8. Fluorescein angiogram of a 12-year-old girl with 20/50 visual acuity. The macula has a bull's-eye transmission defect with relative foveal sparing. Temporal to the defect are very faint patchy transmission defects. Surrounding the retina is the absent choroidal fluorescence.

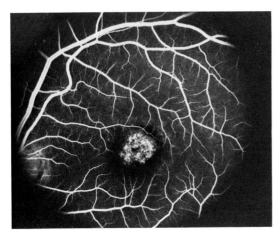

Figure 16-9. Fluorescein angiogram of a 17-year-old boy with 20/120 visual acuity. The macula reveals mottled transmission defects with a zone of early patchy hyperfluorescent defects. In the unaffected portion is diffuse absence of choroidal fluorescence.

mission defects corresponding to flecks can extend beyond the arcades and include the medial retina as well. We also noted in several patients that areas of hyperfluorescence take on a reticular or netlike appearance (Fig. 16-11). This configuration, however, is more commonly noted in the periphery (see Periphery in Fundus Flavimaculatus).

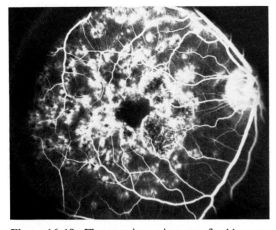

Figure 16-10. Fluorescein angiogram of a 44-year-old man with 20/20 visual acuity. The foveal sparing of defects has an adjacent zone of contiguous defects. Medial to the fovea are multifocal patches of chorioretinal atrophy. The absent choroidal fluorescence is peripheral.

Peripapillary Changes

We and another group have noted an absence of transmission defects in the peripapillary area (see Fig. 16-3).[51] The peripapillary choroid has a different vascular configuration in that there are anastomoses between the recurrent pial vessels and the posterior ciliary vessels, whereas the remaining choroid has a lobular configuration, each lobule supplied by a separate arteriole.[35] Whether this anatomic difference is related to the peripapillary sparing is not fully understood. This finding, however, is not unique to fundus flavimaculatus. We have observed similar sparing in several cases with widespread drusen, particularly the fine cuticular type that is dominantly inherited. Although they are not specifically commented on, those drusen can be seen in published photographs.[11,12,60,67,68,77,81,82,85,95,111,115,126,136]

Periphery in Fundus Flavimaculatus

As the disease progresses, flecks often extend beyond the macula to the midperiphery and medial retina (see Fig. 16-7). In the far periphery, these flecks form a reticular or netlike pattern. Angiographically, they appear like irregular hypofluorescent lines bordered by hyperfluorescence. The surrounding retina and choroid remain relatively hypofluorescent. This reticular pattern often extends into the posterior pole and is frequently associated with chorioretinal atrophy of the macula (see Fig. 16-10, 16-11).

Straatsma and coworkers found a similar angiographic pattern in the reticular degeneration of the pigment epithelium most commonly associated with age-related macular degeneration.[135] Their findings were confined to the equatorial and midperipheral regions, often associated with drusen. In patients with fundus flavimaculatus, we often saw this pattern extending into the macula without drusen. On fluorescein angiography, the polygonal pattern was similar in both cases, with the exception of hyperfluorescent centers in macular degeneration. Based on these differences, fundus flavimaculatus appeared to have a unique reticulation not found in age-related macular degeneration.

We observed one patient with chorioretinal

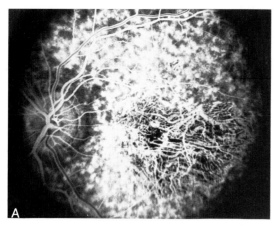 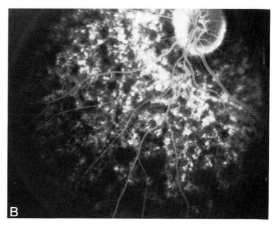

Figure 16-11. Fluorescein angiogram of a 45-year-old woman with 20/400 visual acuity. *(A)* The macula has marked chorioretinal atrophy showing the remaining larger choroidal vessels. There are contiguous transmission defects extending into the far periphery and relative peripapillary sparing. *(B)* The mid-periphery demonstrates the reticular pattern of transmission defects.

atrophy that extended beyond the arcades. With time, the patchy fluorescence corresponding to the flecks stopped spreading, but became more confluent. Several others have reported cases that show choroidal atrophy beyond the arcades.[6,52,60,85]

Other findings in fundus flavimaculatus include round, isolated "punched-out" areas of chorioretinal atrophy that become smaller toward the periphery. These can appear very similar to those found in the ocular histoplasmosis syndrome (see Fig. 16-4). It is conceivable that some of these patients may have had histoplasmosis. In our cases, two sisters, born 9 years apart, had very similarly progressive conditions, making the diagnosis of histoplamosis unlikely.

Summary

Fundus flavimaculatus, a bilateral progressive retinal degeneration characterized by yellowish flecks and continual atrophy of the macula, can be difficult to diagnose in the early and late stages. Besides the clinical, electrophysiologic, and psychophysical testing, fluorescein angiography is very helpful in the diagnosis of this phenotypically variable condition.

The pattern and distribution of flecks, peripapillary sparing, and patterns of progression may be explained on the basis of the choroidal circulation pattern. Each lobular configuration is supplied by an end arteriole except for the peripapillary region, which includes anastomotic vessels.[90] The macular area is often affected first with flecks, which appear later in the periphery. Atrophy also occurs in the macula, varying from a solitary lesion to a multifocal pattern. Rarely is atrophy found in the periphery; however, when present, it is similar to a punched-out spot due to histoplasmosis.

An abnormal lipofuscin-like substance accumulates throughout the pigment epithelium, absorbing the exciting blue wave length and preventing choroidal fluorescence during fluorescein angiography. The reason for this localized accumulation is not known, and no systemic diseases are associated.

The appearance of flecks and the reticular pattern may be influenced in some manner by the choroidal circulation. It is known that the blood flow and metabolism are higher in the macula than elsewhere in the retina. Individual physiologic variations could explain the variable degree of macular degeneration. Those cases not demonstrating a dark choroid may represent some other flecked retinal or pigment epithelial dystrophy. Choroidal and retinal neovascularization are infrequently reported complications of fundus flavimaculatus. The flecks can appear in the fovea rapidly, with loss of vision.

We advise that patients be given a somewhat

guarded prognosis, although their visual acuity is usually 20/200 or better. Yearly follow-up is recommended. There is currently no known treatment for fundus flavimaculatus.

RETINITIS PIGMENTOSA

Definition

The clinical syndrome diagnosed as retinitis pigmentosa is almost certainly caused by many different pathogenetic mechanisms. These mechanisms produce retinal and other ocular changes that appear to be the final common pathway of various disease processes. Through the years, much confusion has surrounded the nature and diagnosis of retinitis pigmentosa. Donders perhaps contributed initially to this confusion by using the name *retinitis pigmentosa,* which inaccurately implies an inflammatory condition.[42,43] Leber introduced the term *tapetoretinal degeneration,* which is confusing since bilaterally inherited diseases should be classified as dystrophies.[87] Although not all cases diagnosed as retinitis pigmentosa have an apparent genetic basis, as far as we know, at least one third to one half do.[29,30,92] Because the name *retinitis pigmentosa* is so widely known and used, it is unlikely to be changed. It is important, however, that those who use it understand its history and relationship to our contemporary understanding of the disease process. It is likely that the definitive understanding of the pathophysiologic mechanisms operative in retinitis pigmentosa will evolve from molecular biological studies.

The retinitis pigmentosa disease process is found worldwide at an estimated prevalence of about 1:4000 to 1:7500.[7,36,74,109] The prescribed anatomic and functional findings necessary to make the diagnosis of retinitis pigmentosa are given in Table 16-3. Most of these classical findings have been noted by ophthalmologists in the last century.[88,98] Bell and Nettleship have since reviewed these hallmarks.[15,103]

Optic nerve pallor is not a criterion for retinitis pigmentosa. In fact, optic nerve color may be relatively normal until extremely late in the course of the disease. Similarly, intraretinal pigment migration, the pathophysiologic basis for the clinically appreciated pigmentary characteristics of "bone spicules," need never be present to make the diagnosis. In our experience, patients who have no visible intraretinal pigmentation initially will develop some bone spiculation and perivascular pigment-bearing cell migration after approximately 3 to 5 years. Since the major clinically appreciable feature in the pigment epithelium is widespread hypopigmentation, the use of the term *retinitis pigmentosa sine pigmento* is unnecessary. We suggest that this term be abandoned.

The essential findings of the syndrome outlined in Table 16-3 can be associated with other changes, such as prominent pigmentary alter-

---

Table 16-3. Essential Criteria to Diagnose Typical Retinitis Pigmentosa

Functional
  Slowly progressive clinical course
  Nightblindness or elevated dark adaptation thresholds
  Peripheral visual field loss
  Visual acuity 20/50 or better until late in the course of the disease
Anatomic
  Vitreous changes (cells, condensations, and posterior separation) present to some extent
  Retinal pigment epithelial hypopigmentation and mottling
  Intraretinal pigment migration present in most but not all advanced cases (not necessary for diagnosis)
  Retinal vessel narrowing present except in very early stages
  Macular changes (loss or broadening of foveal reflex, epiretinal membrane) present in very earliest stages

---

ations in the macula early in the course of the disease. Such patients can be classified as having atypical retinitis pigmentosa, a useful designation implying that the patient will have progressive vision loss as well as an early disability of central acuity.

In a recent study, we detected an apparently progressive sensorineural hearing loss in about 22% of individuals with retinitis pigmentosa. The finding gives credence to frequent patient complaints about the onset of progressive hearing loss in their mid-thirties to early forties. Because this loss is not always present, it is not a hallmark of typical retinitis pigmentosa. This finding suggests that Usher's syndrome, a profound congenital sensorineural hearing loss with a later (5 to 15 years of age) onset of pigmentary retinopathy indistinguishable from retinitis pigmentosa, may be a part of the entire disease spectrum. The recent finding of common defects in ciliated cells further strengthens this notion.[10,75]

Since the etiology of retinitis pigmentosa is not known, any antecedent cause, such as trauma, retinal detachment, ocular surgery, or drug exposure, should be referred to as secondary pigmentary retinopathies. Similarly, when the pigmentary retinopathy is associated with a systemic metabolic disease, for example, in Kearns–Sayre syndrome of Refsum's disease, the term *secondary pigmentary retinopathy* rather than retinitis pigmentosa is preferred.[107]

Clinical Characteristics

Assessment of the functional and anatomical hallmarks of retinitis pigmentosa in evaluation of known or suspected patients with retinitis pigmentosa (see Table 16-3) begins with the history. Many patients with retinitis pigmentosa do not complain of night blindness, even on direct questioning. A simple test of visual acuity in dim illumination can be performed by placing two or three silvery coins or other objects of interest on the floor of the examining room after the lights have been lowered to a rather dim level. This is particularly effective with children and often can show difficulty with night vision in an objective situation that may have been denied subjectively.

The family history should be recorded in detail, including the ages of the parents, ages and sexes of siblings, and the ocular status of all family members. About half or more of large groups of patients with retinitis pigmentosa from around the world do not have identifiable family histories.[29,74,79] Thus, simplex or isolated cases predominate. Of the classifiable conditions, autosomal-dominant and -recessive modes are more common than X-linked.[107] Information obtained from the family history and, whenever possible, the examination of immediate family members, is vitally important. These data are critical to classify the patient and to offer counseling, both to the individual patient and for family planning purposes.

A careful refraction is also important in the evaluation of the patient with retinitis pigmentosa. Myopia is more common in persons with retinitis pigmentosa than in the general population. Some observers have also thought that some genetic types of retinitis pigmentosa display astigmatism, along with the myopia, with unusual frequency.[20,128] If a suspected patient or a person at high risk (such as a sibling of an affected patient) has over 2 or 3 diopters of myopia and more than 1 diopter of astigmatism, that person is at risk for the disease and should be evaluated further.

A complete ophthalmic examination is required. In time, well over 50% of patients with retinitis pigmentosa develop posterior subcapsular type cataracts.[41,53,70,73] Serial documentation of the worsening cataractous changes and its progressive effects on vision can be important in deciding whether and when the patient should undergo cataract surgery.

Some patients with retinitis pigmentosa may have unilateral or bilateral optic nerve head drusen, some of which may be prominent. Although originally described by some authors as astrocytic hamartomas of the optic nerve head, it has been definitively shown by Puck and colleagues that they are drusen.[14,39,117,118] The possible effects of such drusen on visual fields and on the evaluation of glaucoma should be kept in mind. There appears to be no definitive association between retinitis pigmentosa and glaucoma or keratoconus, in contrast to reports in the older literature.

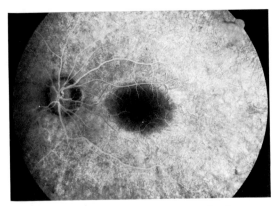

Figure 16-12. The late venous phase of a fluorescein angiogram of the left eye in a 23-year-old woman. The family has a well-documented history of dominantly inherited retinitis pigmentosa. The mottled choroidal pattern shows preserved macular pigment epithelium. Note few peripheral bone spicules in this wide-angle view.

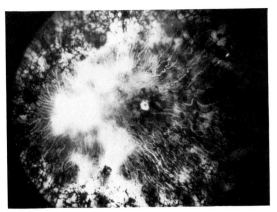

Figure 16-14. The late phase angiogram of the left eye of a 53-year-old man with a well-documented dominantly inherited retinitis pigmentosa. Symptoms of night blindness appeared at age nine. Dye leaks from the optic nerve and areas where the choriocapillaris is present. The foveal pigment epithelium is remarkably preserved. Visual fields showed 5-degree central islands with the V 4E Goldmann stimulus; best corrected visual acuity is 20/40 bilaterally.

Role of Fluorescein Angiography in Retinitis Pigmentosa

Retinitis pigmentosa is a progressive condition and early investigators often performed fluorescein angiography on persons who had moderately advanced or advanced disease. Advanced cases demonstrate atrophy of the choriocapillaris and changes in choroidal pigment cells.

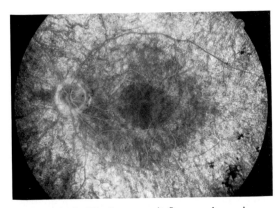

Figure 16-13. The late transit fluorescein angiogram of the left eye of a 27-year-old man, a dizygotic twin. Both twins have retinitis pigmentosa with relatively preserved macular pigment epithelium and a faint bull's-eye pattern. Visual acuity in this eye is 20/30. A small amount of cloudy hyperfluorescence appears in the macular region 65 seconds after injection. Central retinal thickening was noted biomicroscopically, along with mild to moderate changes in an epiretinal membrane.

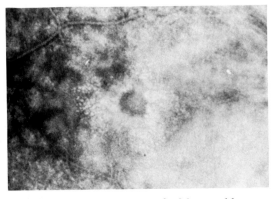

Figure 16-15. The right eye of a 26-year-old man with isolated retinitis pigmentosa reveals a cystoid pattern of dye accumulation immediately surrounding the fovea 6 minutes after injection. Note the microcystic pattern temporal to the fovea and the large amount of fluffy dye accumulations throughout the posterior pole. Some dye also leaked from the optic nerve head, and a patch was noted in the nasal periphery. Both eyes appeared similar: best corrected visual acuity was 20/50 bilaterally.

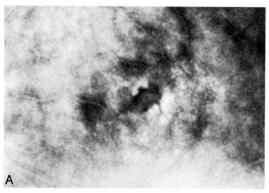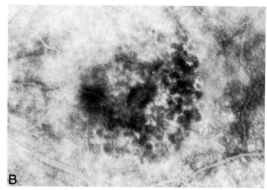

Figure 16-16. *(A)* The left macula of the patient shown in Figure 16-15 discloses cystoid and microcystic edema and diffuse dye accumulation 6 minutes after the intravenous injection of 5 ml sodium fluorescein. Treatment included the placement of a grid of 100-μ argon green laser spots (power set to produce a light burn), 500 μ from the center of the fovea. *(B)* At the 9-month follow-up, the amount of dye accumulation is obviously reduced. The pretreatment best corrected visual acuity was 20/50; after treatment it was 20/30. Visual acuity was stable by 2 years after treatment.

Other choroidal tissues can appear similar to those observed in choroideremia. Earlier in the course of retinitis pigmentosa, a generalized mottling of the RPE may be apparent, with a prominent choroidal pattern due to the widespread hypopigmentation of the RPE. Bonespicule pigmentation blocks choroidal fluorescence (Fig. 16-12). In the macula, fluorescein angiography can reveal a biomicroscopically subtle bull's-eye pattern (Fig. 16-13). Such patterns can be seen in 15% to 20% of patients with retinitis pigmentosa and are frequently compatible with good vision.[70]

It has been recognized for over a decade that fluorescein leakage accompanies retinitis pigmentosa.[76,86] Recently, different anatomic sites associated with fluorescein leakage have been emphasized.[105,106,131,132] Fluorescein leakage is common, and has been found in at least 75% of eyes in one large series (Fig. 16-14).[106] Fluorescein leakage in the macula can be associated with retinal thickening or cystoid edema (Fig. 16-15) and untimely reduction in central acuity. The recognition of clinically significant macular edema in retinitis pigmentosa is important because a light grid of laser photocoagulation can reduce edema and improve visual acuity in at least some patients (Fig. 16-16).[108]

Frequently, retinitis pigmentosa is associated with Coats' types of retinal vascular abnormalities.[56,99,127] Fluorescein angiography can help evaluate the extent of vascular abnormalities and assess the response of the eye to any laser treatment that might be performed.

Retinal neovascularization is a rare complication of retinitis pigmentosa.[32,107] Considering our current understanding of the pathogenesis of retinal neovascularization in such conditions as diabetes mellitus, it is somewhat surprising that we do not see isolated retinal neovascularization more often.[134] It is likely that relatively intact ischemic retinas exist for long periods, at least in the posterior pole in retinitis pigmentosa. Cases of neovascularization in nondiabetic patients have been reported, however, and scatter argon laser photocoagulation has helped reduce new vessel growth.[107]

In cases of unilateral or highly asymmetric retinitis pigmentosa, fluorescein angiography of the affected eye can aid in assessing whether the contralateral eye is lagging in the evolution of the disease process or is indeed normal.[61,72,83,130,139] Occasionally, we have examined persons diagnosed with unilateral retinitis pigmentosa who have some mottling of the RPE on fluorescein angiography as the only abnormal anatomic or functional finding in the unaffected fellow eye. All of the individuals whom we have followed up with unilateral and highly asymmetric retinitis pigmentosa have had at least some degree of fluorescein dye accumulation in the macula of the affected eye, usually in a cystoid pattern.

The presence of true full-thickness macular

holes in retinitis pigmentosa has probably been overstated in the older literature.[54,93] The presence of an epiretinal membrane can produce a pseudo-hole type of appearance.[1] Furthermore, because the mechanical effect of the vitreous may be important in producing a full-thickness central macular hole, the early posterior vitreous separation so common in retinitis pigmentosa may provide some protection. Some investigators have thought that the absence of dye accumulation in the central fovea with the presence of a cystic type appearance represents a lamellar hole.[54] We believe it is necessary to wait at least 10 minutes before judging whether or not fluorescein dye accumulates in the macula, because the process of dye accumulation can be slower in those with retinitis pigmentosa than in persons with other disease processes.

Perifoveal telangiectasia has been reported with variable frequency in retinitis pigmentosa, most commonly in younger people and in association with the presence of cystoid macular edema.[71,132] In more than 120 patients with retinitis pigmentosa studied by fluorescein angiography, we found perifoveal telangiectasia to be uncommon, even though cystoid macular edema may be prominent. Perifoveal retinal vascular telangiectasia is probably under-recognized in the general population. Telangiectasia could occur with retinitis pigmentosa by chance or as a response to humoral factors involved in producing blood–retina barrier alterations.

Carriers of X-linked retinitis pigmentosa can be identified with the use of fluorescein angiography. The angiogram can highlight subtle disturbances of the RPE that may be difficult to appreciate ophthalmoscopically. Combined with electrophysiologic studies, these observations offer a powerful diagnostic tool in the detection of carriers and of individuals at high risk for the development of the disease.[19,24] Vitreous fluorophotometry may also add to our knowledge of the retinitis pigmentosa process.

Management and Treatment Alternatives in Retinitis Pigmentosa

Electrophysiologic studies performed over the last 4 decades have enhanced our ability to diagnose, detect, and classify retinitis pigmen-

tosa.[17,18,91] The electroretinogram in the older literature was rather consistently reported as being nonrecordable.[25,120] Contemporary techniques involving brighter stimuli and, more important, computer averaging and improved corneal electrodes have permitted the detection of small amplitude responses in a large percentage of patients.[66,123,124] An electroretinogram should be performed as part of the initial evaluation of a patient with retinitis pigmentosa. In some instances, it can be useful in following the progress of the disease.[21]

Visual field determinations are the bulwark of the initial evaluation and of routine follow-up visits. A calibrated Goldmann perimeter with the I-4E, III-4E, and V-4E stimuli can, in the hands of a trained technician, provide a relatively reliable and repeatable result that will allow the ophthalmologist to counsel the patient about the state of the retinitis pigmentosa process and the degree of progression.[122] For the patient, the two most important measurements are visual acuity and the amount of peripheral vision. Serial visual fields are recommended. The eventual importance of automated perimetry in the evaluation and follow-up of patients with retinitis pigmentosa is not yet clear.[78]

Color vision testing, using a color-matching, 15-cap test such as the Farnsworth D-15, is quick and practical. The result can help to evaluate changes in the macula in typical retinitis pigmentosa and to differentiate the disease from other conditions.

Numerous psychophysical and quantitative reflectometry studies have been performed in laboratories worldwide. These results have been used to subclassify patients with retinitis pigmentosa, although no general agreement has been reached.[107] Once an accurate diagnosis of the retinitis pigmentosa process has been made, the ophthalmologist should be prepared to counsel the patient about the future course of visual deterioration and the possibility that other family members may be affected. It has been thought that it may be possible to predict the course of an individual patient from the biological activity of the retinitis pigmentosa process in other family members. This has not been corroborated. In fact, variations of the phenotypic as well as the biologic expression of the retinitis pigmentosa process within a single family are striking. We recently examined four of eight siblings from a family with dominantly inherited retinitis pigmentosa. One male sibling complained of poor night vision and difficulties with central vision in his twenties. Although central visual acuity was good (20/30), he had a bull's-eye pattern in the macula, and the electrophysiologic findings showed cone responses were somewhat more affected than rod responses. His visual fields exhibited peripheral loss. The exact diagnosis was unclear until two sisters were examined. They had the typical anatomic and functional findings of retinitis pigmentosa. An additional male sibling demonstrated the findings of early typical retinitis pigmentosa. This pedigree illustrated variability, even within a sibship, and the difficulty of distinguishing moderately advanced, cone/rod dystrophy from retinitis pigmentosa. The term *cone/rod dystrophy* describes an electrophysiologic diagnosis that has been applied most often to early cases of retinitis pigmentosa. It appears to be more useful as a laboratory diagnosis than a clinical diagnosis, except in very rare cases.

Management of Patients With Retinitis Pigmentosa

In an initial evaluation, the absence of a heredity history should prompt a serologic test and FTA for syphilis. Clinical evidence of extra digits, ataxia, hearing problems, or other systemic signs or symptoms should suggest appropriate laboratory tests or referrals. Once an accurate diagnosis has been made, the ophthalmologist should inform the patient about the need for continued follow-up, including a yearly eye examination and visual field testing.

Fluorescein angiography plays an important role in the precataract surgical assessment of a patient with retinitis pigmentosa. The disruption of the macular pigment epithelium and presence of macular edema greatly influence the visual outcome and therefore, patient satisfaction with daily function. In our experience, patients with realistic expectations from cataract extraction and intraocular lens implantation have usually been satisfied.[13,47,110] The use of posterior chamber intraocular lenses for patients with retinitis pigmentosa offers the advantage of minimal optical distortion. Moreover, no associated adverse effects have developed or have shown acceleration or other untoward influences on the disease process.[110]

Fluorescein angiography has also been useful to assess macular edema. We recently reported positive benefits in some patients with retinitis pigmentosa and macular edema after grid laser photocoagulation.[108] A very light pigmented epithelial burn of 100-μm size, using either an 0.05- or 0.1-second exposure time has effected a permanent reduction in angiographically visible edema (see Fig. 16-16) and at least a stabilization of visual acuity after more than 3 years of follow-up in some cases. The number of persons treated in the pilot study was small, and the study was not randomized. A larger prospective randomized trial is currently under way.

An important element in the management of patients with retinitis pigmentosa is to provide adequate genetic counselling for the individual and family members. Examination of close blood relatives and ancestors is helpful. X-linked retinitis pigmentosa is probably underdiagnosed because the patient's mother often is not examined.[24] Although many families with typical dominant- or recessive-type inheritance patterns have affected and unaffected members in proportions conforming (in general) to Mendelian laws, it is important to avoid giving extremely precise numbers. For example, estimates show that gene frequency for retinitis pigmentosa in the general population of the United States is about 1 : 100.[28,31] Thus, an individual with isolated or recessive disease has approximately the same chance of marrying a spouse carrying a retinitis pigmentosa gene. It is reasonable to advise such a person that the chance of having affected children is less than 1 : 100.

Aids for poor vision and night mobility can be helpful to patients with retinitis pigmentosa.[57] In general, low vision and mobility training is best undertaken before visual acuity falls below the 20/80 level. Mobility training can benefit persons who have only tunnel vision with central fields less than 20° in each eye.

The ophthalmologist should also arrange for examination of family members at high risk for the development of the disease. The positive side should be emphasized. We have seen no individuals older than 5 years of age with normal evaluation findings and electrophysiologic responses who have developed the retinitis pigmentosa process.

Update on Pathogenetic Mechanics and Recent Laboratory Advances in Retinitis Pigmentosa

The cause of the retinitis pigmentosa process is unknown, and it is unclear whether the photoreceptors or the RPE cells are primarily affected.[44,104,107] The chorioretinal complex consists of highly interdependent cell layers. To date, it has not been possible to differentiate between a primary defect in one layer and a secondary deterioration of the other layers. Recent ultrastructural studies have confirmed the early loss of rod photoreceptor outer segments and the relative preservation of cone outer segments.[63,84,94,121,125,137] However, in several cases, the remaining cone outer segments have been abnormally shortened and vacuolated. These changes have also occurred in some remnant rod outer segments in eyes from individuals with less-advanced disease. The possible causes of such a photoreceptor abnormality include a defect in a structural gene or in the synthetic enzymes or their products involved in the elaboration of photoreceptor outer segments.

Several investigations correlating biochemical studies of one eye and histologic studies of the fellow eye from persons with retinitis pigmentosa have focused on cyclic nucleotide molecular species and concentrations.[49] These studies have been inspired in part by the finding of a rise in cyclic CMP that coincides with the degeneration of photoreceptors in a mouse mutant with an inherited retinal dystrophy.[48] Other studies have assessed the concentration of retinoid-binding protein in the interphotoreceptor matrix, a molecular species important to the vitamin A economy in the chorioretinal complex.[33] Since the photoreceptors are a major source for the synthesis of this material, it is not surprising that concentrations have been low or absent in the interphotoreceptor space in eyes with advanced disease.[119]

Exciting molecular biological observations have recently been reported in X-linked retinitis pigmentosa. The use of recombinant DNA probes (L1.28) has shown a polymorphic locus on the short arm of the X-chromosome close to the Duchenne muscular dystrophy gene locus that is associated with X-linked retinitis pigmentosa.[22,23,102,114] The calculated closeness of the actual linkage of the L1.28 probe to the X-linked retinitis pigmentosa gene is not thought to be sufficient to allow the use of this probe for antenatal diagnosis at present. The success in discovering probes that lie on either side of the genetic locus for other X-linked eye diseases such as choroideremia provides hope for future successes in retinitis pigmentosa. Work is also under way to clone the gene of X-linked retinitis pigmentosa and to seek the genetic locus in autosomal forms of the disease. Recent studies revealing serum lipid abnormalities in at least some subtypes of retinitis pigmentosa are exciting.[8,37] Further results are expected from ongoing studies in this area.

As with many diseases of serious consequence and unknown etiology, a wide variety of ineffective treatments have been tried, ranging from trephination, placental extract injections, and light deprivation, to dietary supplementation.[107] Two treatment trials of dietary vitamin and mineral supplementation are currently under way in the United States.[16,80] An additional treatment trial is being initiated by Newsome, Bazan, and Dorsey involving the administration of mixed gangliosides by a therapeutic strategy that has been applied with varying success to some central nervous system degenerative disorders.*

REFERENCES

1. Allen AW Jr, Gass JDM: Contraction of a perifoveal epiretinal membrane simulating a macular hole. Am J Ophthalmol 82:684–691, 1976
2. Amalric P: Interet du test a la fluoresceine dans l'etude de certaines degenerescences tapeto-retiniennes et en particulier dans le fundus flavimaculatus. Ophthalmologica 154:367–372, 1967
3. Amalric P: Dystrophie maculaire de type Stargardt avec absence totale de visualisation ango-

* Personal communication

graphique. Bull Soc Ophtalmol Fr 77:913–918, 1977

4. Amalric P, Bessou P, Pitet L, et al: Interet de l'angiographie fluoresceinique au cours du fundus flavimaculatus. Bull Mem Soc Fr Ophtalmol 81:537–550, 1969

5. Amalric P, Kment H, Remky H: Fundus flavimaculatus. Klin Monastbl Augenheilkd 150:625–636, 1967

6. Amalric P, Teulieres J, Stanbuk M: Fundus flavimaculatus modifie de facon brutale par une arteriographie carotidienne. Bull Soc Ophtalmol Fr 76:125–128, 1976

7. Ammann F, Klein D, Franceschetti A: Genetic and epidemiological investigation on pigmentary degeneration of the retina and allied disorders in Switzerland. J Neurol Sci 2:183–196, 1965

8. Anderson RE, Maude MB, Lewis RA, et al: Abnormal plasma levels of polyunsaturated fatty acid in autosomal dominant retinitis pigmentosa. Exper Eye Res (In press)

9. Anmarkrud N: Fundus fluorescein angiography in fundus flavimaculatus and Stargardt's disease. Acta Ophthalmol 57:172–182, 1979

10. Arden GB, Fox B: Increased incidence of abnormal nasal cilia in patients with retinitis pigmentosa. Nature 279:534–536, 1979

11. Babel J: Le fundus flavimaculatus: Etude clinique, functionnelle et genetique. Arch Ophthalmol 32:111–121, 1972

12. Babel J, Farpour H: Les lesions de la choroide dans les heredo-degenerescences a la lumiere del la fluor-retinographie. Ophthalmologica 156:305–312, 1968

13. Bastek JV, Heckenlively JR, Straatsma BR: Cataract surgery in retinitis pigmentosa patients. Ophthalmology 89:880–884, 1982

14. Bec P, Mathis A, Adam P, et al: Retinitis pigmentosa associated with astrocytic hamartomas of the optic disc. Ophthalmologica 189:135–138, 1984

15. Bell J: Retinitis pigmentosa and allied diseases. In Bell J (ed): The Treasury of Human Inheritance vol. 2, pp 1–28. Cambridge, Cambridge University Press, 1922

16. Berson EL: Nutrition and retinal degenerations: Vitamin A, taurine, ornithine and phytanic acid. Retina 2:236–254, 1982

17. Berson EL, Gouras P, Gunkel RD: Rod responses in retinitis pigmentosa, dominantly inherited. Arch Ophthalmol 80:58–67, 1968

18. Berson EL, Kanters L: Cone and rod responses in a family with recessively inherited retinitis pigmentosa. Arch Ophthalmol 84:288–297, 1970

19. Berson EL, Rosen JB, Simonoff EA: Electroretinographic testing as an aid in detection of carriers of X-chromosome-linked retinitis pigmentosa. Am J Ophthalmol 87:460–468, 1979

20. Berson EL, Rosner B, Simonoff BA: Risk factors for genetic typing and detection in retinitis pigmentosa. Am J Ophthalmol 89:763–775, 1980

21. Berson EL, Sandberg MA, Rosner B, et al: Natural course of retinitis pigmentosa over a 3-year interval. Am J Ophthalmol 99:240–251, 1985

22. Bhattacharya SS, Clayton JF, Harper PS, et al: A genetic linkage study of a kindred with X-linked retinitis pigmentosa. Br J Ophthalmol 69:340–347, 1985

23. Bhattacharya SS, Wright AF, Clayton JF, et al: Close genetic linkages between X-linked retinitis pigmentosa and a restriction fragment length polymorphism identified by recombinant DNA probe L1.28. Nature 309:253–255, 1984

24. Bird AC: X-linked retinitis pigmentosa. Br J Ophthalmol 59:177, 1975

25. Bjork A, Karpe G: The electroretinogram in retinitis pigmentosa. Acta Ophthalmol 29:361–376, 1951

26. Bonnin P, Passot M, Triolaire-Cotten M-T: Le signe du silence choroidien dans les degenerescences tapeto-retiniennes posterieures. In De-Laey JJ (ed): International Symposium of Fluorescein Angiography, pp 461–463. The Hague, Dr W Junk Publishing, 1976

27. Bonnin P: Le signe du silence choroidien dans les degenerescences tapeto-retiniennes centrales examinees sous fluoresceine. Bull Soc Ophtalmol Fr 71:348–351, 1971

28. Boughman JA: Population genetic studies of retinitis pigmentosa. PhD Thesis, Indiana University, 1978

29. Boughman J: Genetic analysis of heterogeneity and variation in retinitis pigmentosa. Birth Defects, 18:151–160, 1982

30. Boughman JA, Conneally PM, Nance WE: Population genetic studies of retinitis pigmentosa. Am J Hum Genet 32:223–235, 1980

31. Boughman JA, Schwartz MF: Genetics, counselling and antenatal diagnosis. In Newsome DA (ed): Retinal Dystrophies and Degenerations. New York, Raven Press (in press)

32. Bressler NM, Gragoudas ES: Neovascularization of the optic disc associated with atypical retinitis pigmentosa. Am J Ophthalmol 100:431–433, 1985

33. Bridges DG, O'Gorman S, Alverez RA, et al: Vitamin A store and interstitial retinol-binding protein in an eye with recessive retinitis pigmentosa. Invest Ophthalmol Vis Sci 26:684–691, 1985

34. Brown N, Hill DW: Fundus flavimaculatus. Br J Ophthalmol 52:849–852, 1968

35. Buettner H, Machemer R, Charles S, et al: Experimental deprivation of choroidal blood flow. Am J Ophthalmol 75:943–952, 1973

36. Bunker CH, Berson EL, Bromley WC, et al:

Prevalence of retinitis pigmentosa in Maine. Am J Ophthalmol 97:357–365, 1984

37. Converse CA, Hammer HM, Packard CJ, et al: Plasma lipid abnormalities in retinitis pigmentosa and related conditions. Trans Ophthalmol Soc UK 105: 508–512, 1983

38. Coscas G, Gaudric A, Barthelemy F: Un cas de fundus flavimaculatus avec neovaisseaux preretiniens. J Fr Ophtalmol 3:27–32, 1980

39. DeBustros S, Miller NR, Finkelstein D: Bilateral astrocytic hamartomas of the optic nerve heads in retinitis pigmentosa. Retina 3:21–23, 1983

40. Deutman AF: Stargardt's disease. In Deutman AF (ed): The Hereditary Dystrophies of the Posterior Pole of the Eye, pp 100–171. The Netherlands: Van Gorcum Comp NV Assen, 1971

41. Dilley KJ, Bron AJ, Habgood JO: Anterior polar and posterior subcapsular cataract in a patient with retinitis pigmentosa: A light microscopic and ultrastructural study. Exp Eye Res 22:155–167, 1976

42. Donders FC: Torpeur de la retine congenitale hereditaire. Ann Oculist 34:270–273, 1855

43. Donders FC: Beiträge zur pathologischen Anatomie des Auges: Pigmentbildung in der Netzhaut. Arch Ophthalmol 3:139–150, 1857

44. Duke-Elder S, Dobree JH: The tapetoretinal degenerations. In Duke-Elder S (ed): Diseases of the Retina: System of Ophthalmology, vol 5, pp 574–666. London, Kimpton, 1967

45. Eagle RC, Lucier AC, Bernardino VB, et al: Retinal pigment epithelial abnormalities in fundus flavimaculatus. Ophthalmology 87:1189–1200, 1980

46. Ernest JT, Krill AE: Fluorescein studies in fundus flavimaculatus and drusen. Am J Ophthalmol 62:1–6, 1966

47. Fagerhold PP, Phillipson BT: Cataract in retinitis pigmentosa: An analysis of cataract surgery results and pathologic lens changes. Acta Ophthalmol 63:50–58, 1985

48. Farber DB, Flannery DB, Bird AC: Abnormal distribution pattern of cyclic nucleotides in retina affected with retinitis pigmentosa. Invest Ophthalmol Vis Sci 27 (Suppl):56, 1986

49. Farber DB, Lolley RN: Enzymatic basis for cyclic GMP accumulation in degenerative photoreceptor cells of mouse retina. J Cyclic Nuc Res 2:139–148, 1976

50. Feeney L: Lipofuscin and melanin of human retinal pigment epithelium. Invest Ophthalmol Vis Sci 17:583–600, 1978

51. Fish G, Grey R, Sehmi IKS, et al: The dark choroid in posterior retinal dystrophies. Br J Ophthalmol 65:359–363, 1981

52. Fishman GA: Fundus flavimaculatus: A clinical classification. Arch Ophthalmol 94:2061–2067, 1976

53. Fishman GA, Anderson RJ, Lourenco P: Prevalence of posterior subcapsular lens opacities in patients with retinitis pigmentosa. Br J Ophthalmol 69:263–266, 1985

54. Fishman GA, Fishman M, Maggiano J: Macular lesions associated with retinitis pigmentosa. Arch Ophthalmol 95:798–803, 1977

55. Flocks M, Miller J, Chao P: Retinal circulation time with the aid of fundus cinephotography. Am J Ophthalmol 48:3–6, 1959

56. Fogle JA, Welch RB, Green WR: Retinitis pigmentosa and exudative vasculopathy. Arch Ophthalmol 96:696–702, 1978

57. Fonda G: Low vision correction in retinitis pigmentosa and associated diseases. Int J Rehabil Res 3:39–43, 1980

58. Franceschetti A: Über tapeto-retinale Degeneration im Kindesalter. In Sautter H (ed): Entwicklung und Fortschritt in der Augenheilkunde, pp 107–120. Stuttgart, Ferdinand Enke Verlag, 1963

59. Francois J, DeLaey JJ: L'angiographie fluoresceinique dans les degenerescences maculaires juveniles. Arch Ophthalmol 29:497–508, 1969

60. Francois P, Turut P, Peuch B, et al: Maladie de Stargardt et fundus flavimaculatus. Arch Ophthalmol 35:817–846, 1975

61. Francois J, Verriest G: Retinopathie pigmentaire unilaterale. Ophthalmology 124:65–88, 1952

62. Frangieh GT, Green WR, Maumenee IH: Fundus flavimaculatus: Clinical observations of two brothers during 38 years, and histopathologic studies in one brother. Presented before the XXIV International Congress of Ophthalmology, San Francisco, October–November 1982

63. Gartner S, Henkind P: Pathology of retinitis pigmentosa. Ophthalmology 89:1425–1432, 1982

64. Gass JDM: Acute posterior multifocal placoid pigment epitheliopathy. Arch Ophthalmol 80:117–185, 1968

65. Gass JDM: A clinicopathologic study of a peculiar foveomacular dystrophy. Trans Am Ophthalmol Soc 72:139–156, 1974

66. Goodman G, Gunkel R: Familial electroretinographic and adaptometric studies in retinitis pigmentosa. Am J Ophthalmol 46:142–178, 1958

67. Hadden OB, Gass JDM: Fundus flavimaculatus and Stargardt's disease. Am J Ophthalmol 82:527–539, 1976

68. Hammerstein W, Leide E: Die Bedeutung der Fluoreszangiographie für die Diagnosis der Stargardtschen Makuladegeneration. Klin Monastbl Augenheilkd 178:20–23, 1981

69. Hayreh SS: Segmental nature of the choroidal vasculature. Br J Ophthalmol 59:631–648, 1975

70. Heckenlively J: The frequency of posterior subcapsular cataract in the hereditary retinal degenerations. Am J Ophthalmol 93:733–738, 1982

71. Heckenlively JR, Martin DA, Rosalies TO: Telangiectasia and optic atrophy in cone-rod degenerations. Arch Ophthalmol 99:1983–1991, 1981

72. Henkes HE: Does unilateral retinitis pigmentosa really exist? An ERG and EOG study of the fellow eye. In Burian HM, Jacobson JH (eds): Clinical Electroretinography. Proceedings of the Third ISCERG Symposium, pp 327–350, London, Pergamon Press, 1966

73. Horwitz J, Neuhaus R, Dockstader J: Analysis of microdissected cataractous human lenses. Invest Ophthalmol Vis Sci 21:616–619, 1981

74. Hu DN: Genetic aspects of retinitis pigmentosa in China. Am J Med Genet 12:51–56, 1982

75. Hunter DG, Fishman GA, Mehta RS, et al: Abnormal sperm and photoreceptor axonemes in Usher's syndrome. Am J Ophthalmol 104:385–389, 1986

76. Hyvarinen L, Maumenee AE, Kelley J, et al: Flourescein angiographic findings in retinitis pigmentosa. Am J Ophthalmol 71:17–26, 1971

77. Irvine RA, Wergeland FL: Stargardt's hereditary progressive macular degeneration. Br J Ophthalmol 56:817–826, 1972

78. Jacobson SG, Voigt WJ, Parel J-M: Automated light- and dark-adapted perimetry for evaluating retinitis pigmentosa. Ophthalmology 93:1604–1611, 1986

79. Jay B, Bird A, Jay M: The incidence of the different genetic forms of retinitis pigmentosa. Doc Ophthalmol 17:313–318, 1978

80. Karcioglu ZA: Zinc in the eye. Surv Ophthalmol 27:114–122, 1982

81. Klein BA, Krill AE: Fundus flavimaculatus, clinical, functional and histopathologic observations. Am J Ophthalmol 64:3–23, 1967

82. Klein R, Lewis RA, Meyers SM, et al: Subretinal neovascularization associated with fundus flavimaculatus. Arch Ophthalmol 96:2054–2057, 1978

83. Kolb H, Galloway NR: Three cases of unilateral pigmentary degeneration. Br J Ophthalmol 48:471, 1964

84. Kolb H, Gouras P: Electron microscopic observations of human retinitis pigmentosa, dominantly inherited. Invest Ophthalmol Vis Sci 13:487–498, 1974

85. Krill AE: Fundus flavimaculatus. In Krill AE (ed): Krill's Hereditary Retinal and Choroidal Disease. Vol II: Clinical Characteristics, pp 749–787. Hagerstown, Harper & Row, 1977

86. Krill AE, Archer D, Newell FW: Flourescein angiography in retinitis pigmentosa. Am J Ophthalmol 69:683–690, 1970

87. Leber T: Die *pigment Degeneration* der Netz-

haut und die mit ihr verwandten Erkrankungen. In Graefe-Saemich: Handbuch der gesamten Augenheilkunde, 2nd ed, vol 7, No 1–2:1125–1176, 1916

88. Liebreich R: Abkunft aus Ehen unter Blutsverwandten als Grund von *Retinitis Pigmentosa.* Deutsche Klinik Bd 13:53–55, 1861

89. Leveille S, Morse PH, Burch JV: Fundus flavimaculatus and subretinal neovascularization. Ann Ophthalmol 14:331–334, 1982

90. McDonnell PJ, Kivlin JD, Maumenee IH, et al: Fundus flavimaculatus without maculopathy. Ophthalmology 93:116–119, 1986

91. Marmor, MF: The electroretinogram in retinitis pigmentosa. Arch Ophthalmol 97:1300–1304, 1979

92. Massof RW, Finkelstein D, Boughman JA: Genetic analysis of subgroups within simplex and multiplex retinitis pigmentosa. Birth Defects 18:161–166, 1982

93. Merin S: Macular cysts as an early sign of taperetinal degeneration. J Paediatr Ophthalmol 7:225–228, 1970

94. Meyer KT, Heckenlively JR, Spitznas M, et al: Dominant retinitis pigmentosa: A clinicopathologic correlation. Ophthalmology 89:1414–1424, 1982

95. Michels RG: Flecked retinal syndrome. Int Ophthalmol Clin 17:35–62, 1977

96. Miller SA: Fluorescence in Bests' vitelliform dystrophy, lipofuscin, and fundus flavimaculatus. Br J Ophthalmol 62:256–260, 1978

97. Moloney JBM, Mooney DJ, O'Conner MA: Retinal function in Stargardt's disease and fundus flavimaculatus. Am J Ophthalmol 96:57–65, 1983

98. Mooren A: De la retinite pigmenteuse. Ann Oculist 41:21–31, 1859

99. Morgan WE III, Crawford JB: Retinitis pigmentosa and Coats' disease. Arch Ophthalmol 79:146–149, 1968

100. Morse P, Smith V, Pokorny J, et al: Fundus flavimaculatus with cystoid macular changes and abnormal Stiles-Crawford effect. Am J Ophthalmol 91:190–196, 1981

101. Motolese E, Caporossi A, Sansone M: Forme miste di fundus flavimaculatus e malattia di Stargardt. Bull Oculist 60:513–518, 1981

102. Mukai S, Dryja TP, Bruns CAP, et al: Linkage between the X-linked retinitis pigmentosa locus and the L1.28 locus. Am J Ophthalmol 100:225–229, 1985

103. Nettleship E: Some hereditary diseases of the eye. Ophthalmoscope 4:493–506, 550–556, 1906

104. Newsome DA: The immune system in retinitis pigmentosa. In Lavail M, Anderson R, Hollyfield J (eds): Retinal Degeneration: Experimental and Clinical Studies, pp 75–90. New York, Alan R Liss, 1985

105. Newsome DA: Letter to editor. Am J Ophthalmol 102:409, 1985

106. Newsome DA: Retinal fluorescein leakage in retinitis pigmentosa. Am J Ophthalmol 101:354–360, 1986

107. Newsome DA: Retinitis pigmentosa, Usher's syndrome and other pigmentary retinopathies. In Newsome DA (ed): Retinal Dystrophies and Degenerations. New York, Raven Press (In press)

108. Newsome DA, Blacharski PA: Grid photocoagulation for macular edema in patients with retinitis pigmentosa. Am J Ophthalmol 103:161–166, 1987

109. Newsome DA, Milton RC, Frederique G: High Prevalence of eye disease in a Haitian locale. J Trop Med Hyg 86:37–46, 1983

110. Newsome DA, Stark WF Jr, Maumenee IH: Cataract extraction and intraocular lens implantation in patients with retinitis pigmentosa or Usher's syndrome. Arch Ophthalmol 104:852–854, 1986

111. Noble K, Carr R: Stargardt's disease and fundus flavimaculatus. Arch Ophthalmol 97:1281–1285, 1979

112. Novotny HR, Alvis DL: A method of photographing fluorescence in circulating blood of the human eye (abstr). Am J Ophthalmol 50:176, 1960

113. Novotny HR, Alvis DL: A method of photographing fluorescence in circulating blood in the human retina. Circulation 24:82–86, 1961

114. Nussbaum RL, Lewis RA, Lesko JG, et al: Linkage relationship of X-linked retinitis pigmentosa to X-chromosomal short arm markers. Hum Genet 70:45–50, 1985

115. Passmore JA, Robertson DM: Ring scotoma in fundus flavimaculatus. Am J Ophthalmol 80:907–912, 1975

116. Paufique L, Hervouet F: Anatomie pathologique d'un cas de maladie de Stargardt. Bull Mem Soc Fr Ophthalmol 76:108–114, 1963

117. Pillai S, Limaye SR, Saimoruch LB: Optic disc hamartoma associated with retinitis pigmentosa. Retina 3:24–26, 1983

118. Puck A, Tso MOM, Fishman GA: Drusen of the optic nerve associated with retinitis pigmentosa. Arch Ophthalmol 103:231–234, 1985

119. Rayborn ME, Frederick JM, Ulshafer RJ, et al: Histopathology and *in vitro* metabolic studies on tissues from a family with an autosomal dominant form of retinitis pigmentosa. In La Vail MM, Hollyfield JG, Anderson RE (eds): Retinal Degeneration: Experimental and Clinical Studies, pp 37–49. New York, Alan R Liss, 1985

120. Riggs LA: Electroretinography in cases of night blindness. Am J Ophthalmol 38:70, 1954

121. Rodrigues MM, Newsome DA: Retinitis pigmentosa: Electron microscopy and cell culture studies. Birth Defects 18:81–94, 1982

122. Ross DF, Fishman GA, Gilbert LD, et al: Variability of visual field measurements in normal subjects and patients with retinitis pigmentosa. Arch Ophthalmol 102:1004–1010, 1984

123. Rothberg DS, Weinstein GW, Hobson RR, et al: Electroretinography and retinitis pigmentosa: No discrimination between genetic subtypes. Arch Ophthalmol 100:1422–1426, 1982

124. Sandberg MA, Sullivan PL, Berson EL: Temporal aspects of the dark-adapted cone a-wave in retinitis pigmentosa. Invest Ophthalmol Vis Sci 21:765–773, 1981

125. Santos-Anderson RM, Tso MOM, Fishman GA: A histopathologic study of retinitis pigmentosa. Ophthalmic Paediatr Genet 1:151–168, 1982

126. Schiffer HP, Busse H: Beitrag zum Krankheitsbild des Fundus flavimaculatus mit Makuladegeneration. Klin Monastbl Augenheilkd 166:365–368, 1975

127. Schmidt D, Faulborn J: Retinopathia pigmentosa mit Coats-Syndrom. Klin Monastbl Augenheilkd 157:643–652, 1970

128. Seiving PA, Fishman GA: Refractive errors of retinitis pigmentosa patients. Br J Ophthalmol 62:163–167, 1978

129. Senikowich DJ, Gass JDM, Nicholson DH: "Dark choroid" in Stargardt's disease. Presented at the annual meeting of the Association for Research in Vision and Ophthalmology, May 1–6, 1983, Sarasota, Florida

130. Skalka W: Asymmetric retinitis pigmentosa, leuetic retinopathy and the question of unilateral retinitis pigmentosa. Acta Ophthalmol 57:351–357, 1979

131. Spallone A: Retinal fluorescein leakage in retinitis pigmentosa. Am J Ophthalmol 102:408, 1985

132. Spalton JD, Bird AC, Cleary PE: Retinitis pigmentosa and retinal edema. Br J Ophthalmol 62:174–182, 1978

133. Stargardt K: Über familiare, *progressive degeneration* in der Maculagegend des Auges. Graefes Arch Ophthalmol 71:534–550, 1909

134. Sternberg P Jr, Landers MB III, Wolbarscht M: The negative coincidence of retinitis pigmentosa and proliferative diabetic retinopathy. Am J Ophthalmol 97:788–789, 1984

135. Straatsma BR, Lewis H, Foos RY, et al: Flourescein angiography in reticular degeneration of the pigment epithelium. Am J Ophthalmol 100:202–208, 1985

136. Streicher T, Kremery K: Stargardtova choroba a fundus flavimaculatus. Cs Oftalmol 33:141–146, 1977

137. Szamier RB, Berson EL, Klein R, et al: Sex-linked retinitis pigmentosa: Ultrastructure of

photoreceptors and pigment epithelium. Invest Ophthalmol Vis Sci 18:145–160, 1979

138. Weise EE, Yannuzzi LA: Ring maculopathies mimicking chloroquine retinopathy. Am J Ophthalmol 78:204–208, 1974

139. Weiss JF, Nicholl RJ: Nonsyphilitic unilateral retinitis pigmentosa. Am J Ophthalmol 65:82–87, 1968

140. Zotti A: Fundus flavimaculatus mit sichtbaren Veränderungen nur im Bereich der Macula. Ber Dtsch Ophthalmol Ges 73:215–216, 1975

17

Nutritional Retinopathies

David A. Newsome

Clinical and scientific understanding of the influences of nutrition on the eye has increased remarkably in the past several years. Ever larger numbers of nutrition-related diseases have been observed to be accompanied by prominent ocular manifestations.[30] Certain metabolic disorders that affect the eye adversely can be ameliorated, at least to some extent, by nutritional management.

The eye shares the basic nutritional requirements of other body parts. In addition, certain highly specialized ocular tissues such as the retina have special metabolic requirements. Cells of the sensory retina and pigment epithelium have an avidity for certain nutritional factors (for example, zinc) that results in these tissues exhibiting some of the very highest concentrations of this analyte of any tissue in the body.[10]

It is the purpose of this review to highlight nutrition-related diseases that involve the retina, either primarily or in association with pathologic involvement of other ocular tissues. Acute changes, such as those transitory functional deficits seen after acute excessive alcohol use, will not be considered.[1] Current concepts of the typical ocular symptomatology, clinicopathologic correlations, and nutritional management will be summarized. The nutritional retinopathies can be divided into five categories depending on whether they are related to vitamins, minerals, amino acids, carbohydrate metabolism, or lipoproteins and fat metabolism. It must be remembered that a primary deficiency in one category of nutrient can also have significant secondary effects on uptake, utilization, or other aspects of other nutrients.

VITAMIN-RELATED RETINOPATHIES

Vitamin A

Vitamin A plays a key role in the maintenance of the normal integrity of nearly every tissue in the body. Epithelial tissues are particularly dependent upon an adequate supply of vitamin A.[36] The retina has a unique requirement for vitamin A. Rhodopsin contains the 11-*cis*-retinol form of vitamin A, the form that undergoes biochemical transformation when a photon of light is captured, initiating the visual process. It is this sensitivity to photon capture that allows us to see in dim illumination. Night blindness is one of the earliest symptoms of generalized vitamin A deficiency.[13] The status of a person's dark adaptation can thus be a valuable indicator of the tissue vitamin A concentrations (Table 17-1).[13]

Hypovitaminosis A in children, in its severe forms, can be accompanied by corneal scarring and even melting. Perforation and eventual loss of the eye are common. In a child with hypovitaminosis A, night blindness is frequently the earliest sign. Field workers who are attempting to detect the presence of hypovitaminosis A frequently attempt to elicit a history of night blindness as a tool for determining the prevalence of hypovitaminosis A in a particular area.[38] In many countries where malnutrition is not a problem, hypovitaminosis A can still be seen in patients with certain diseases that produce intestinal malabsorption or chronic pancreatitis, or in patients who have had surgery involving partial bowel resection.[23,40]

Table 17-1. Retinopathies Associated With Vitamin Deficiencies

Disorder	Associated Systemic Diseases	Retinal Manifestations			Associated Ocular Findings	Management
		Clinical	Anatomical	Psychophysical		
Hypovitaminosis A of childhood	Protein-energy malnutrition, usually in 1- to 6-yr-olds	Night blindness; widespread white punctate lesions	Uncertain	Reduced ERG responses; rod responses can be absent, with cone responses near normal; poor dark adaptation	Xerophthalmia and keratomalacia (retinal exam usually impossible with advanced corneal changes)	Replete vitamin A, along with vitamins B, E, and protein calories
Adult hypovitaminosis A	Chronic alcoholism; small bowel disease/resection; chronic liver disease; chronic pancreatitis	Night blindness; widespread white punctate lesions	Uncertain	Reduced rod ERG; poor dark adaptation	Corneal xerosis	Replete vitamin A; vitamin E and zinc may be useful in unresponsive persons
B-complex vitamin deficiency	Malnutrition; some cases with pernicious anemia; alcoholism; multiple neuropathies; organic mental changes	Blurred vision, photobia; loss of macular and nerve fiber layer details; pigmentary disturbance in advanced stages	Loss of outer segments; pigmentary migration	Constricted peripheral visual fields; paracentral/central scotomata; reduced VEP	Angular blepharoconjunctivitis; optic disc pallor	Replete appropriate B-complex vitamins

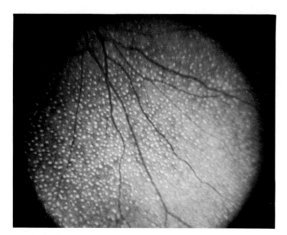

Figure 17-1. This night-blind 10-year-old Haitian female upon presentation showed bilateral retinal white dots with a discrete elevated appearance scattered 360 degrees, with relative foveal sparing. These dots appear to be at the level of the RPE. Dietary history revealed very low intake of vitamin A sources and physical findings compatible with moderately severe protein-energy malnutrition. Ten days after oral vitamin A and protein-calorie repletion, the dots were no longer visible.

Parents of children with night blindness generally notice the profound difficulty the child may have in negotiating after dark, when unaffected children have little or no difficulty. In the case of adult night blindness depending upon the mental status and the life-style of the affected individual, there may be a spontaneous complaint about difficulty seeing in dimly illuminated areas. In the clinical evaluation of persons with chronic alcoholism, chronic liver disease, malabsorption syndromes, or surgical removal of portions of the small bowel, a complete history should include a query about any difficulty in seeing at night.[31]

In childhood hypovitaminosis A retinopathy a striking collection of white dots that are fine, fairly regular, and scattered throughout the fundus has been reported.[37] Psychophysical testing, including electroretinography and dark adaptometry, shows abnormally depressed responsiveness. In the adult, the presence of numerous white dots has also been reported.[23] The rod electroretinographic responses are generally much more affected than are the cone responses. Visual acuity is usually normal.

A 14th-century Dutch poet may have been referring to his observations of the successful treatment of adult night blindness when he wrote: "He who cannot see at night must eat the liver of the goat. Then he can see all right."[6] Replacement of vitamin A generally leads to improvement in the subjective functional, but not always in the objective retinal changes associated with hypovitaminosis A in adults and children (see Table 17-1). The "massive dose" program recommends 100,000 IU retinol palmitate for infants less than 2 years old, and 200,000 IU for older children. The dose is repeated every 6 months.[31] In children, hypovitaminosis A is almost always accompanied by protein energy malnutrition (Fig. 17-1). Thus, appropriate therapy includes the administration of adequate protein calorie intake.[37] The response of adults to vitamin A administration has been known for many years but may be slower and less complete than that of children.

Unfortunately, the isolated administration of vitamin A has had no documented effect on the progressive night blindness of retinitis pigmentosa. Vitamin A administration is a part of the therapeutic attack in individuals with the autosomal-recessive disorders, abetalipoproteinemia, and hypobetalipoproteinemia.[5,8,16]

Vitamin B

As with vitamin A, vitamin B has widespread effects throughout the body and on ocular tissues. In contrast to vitamin A, which is stored in the liver and is fat soluble, the B vitamins are water soluble and are not stored to any significant extent in tissues.

Clinical observations over the past few centuries have underscored the importance of the B vitamins in maintaining normal retinal integrity and function, as well as the integrity and function of the optic nerve. The vitamin B deficiency states pellagra and beriberi have been known for many centuries to cause visual impairment in eyes that otherwise appeared sound. Nutritional amblyopia, as this deficiency state is termed, produces a gradual decrease in central visual acuity with relative sparing of peripheral vision. Some contraction of the peripheral visual field in B deficiency state has been reported, but not confirmed by all observers.[8] Visual acuity can be reduced to the 20/200 level, color vision can be moderately to severely impaired, and retinal hemorrhages may be present. If the optic nerve is also affected, temporal pallor can be seen with the ophthalmoscope. Temporal pallor is almost always present in very longstanding cases.

Alcohol and tobacco as causative factors in nutritional amblyopia have been described in the literature for well over 100 years.[16] However, current evidence indicates that the name *tobacco–alcohol amblyopia* is, indeed, a misnomer for what really is a B vitamin–group deficiency state.[6] Because pernicious anemia or an isolated vitamin B_{12} deficiency can cause, in rare instances, an optic neuropathy, if visible optic nerve changes are present, the appropriate blood studies to test for pernicious anemia should be performed.

The clinical evaluation of persons suspected of having a vitamin B complex deficiency state and who complain of diminution of central vision acuity and color vision should include, besides refraction and formal color vision evaluation, stereoscopic color fundus photography and fluorescein angiography, since the only visible retinal change may be a loss of macular details.[3] It is important to rule out other types of macular pathology. The administration of relatively high and frequent doses of vitamin B_{12} along with other vitamins of the B complex generally provides prompt and relatively complete remission of visual defects. Some individuals may require chronic maintenance on a dietary supplementation with B-complex vitamins (see Table 17-1).

Vitamin E

Since the requirements for vitamin E in humans appear to be generally lower than for the other major fat-soluble vitamin, vitamin A, and because there are many dietary sources of vitamin E, the presence of a vitamin E-deficient state in man has not been well documented. Because vitamin E has a synergistic interaction with vitamin A, as well as an epithelial-supportive spectrum of effects plus antioxidant effects, an inadequate supply of vitamin E in the body has been associated by some with a greater retinal sensitivity to light damage and more rapid progression of such degenerative diseases simulating retinitis pigmentosa.[14,15] Data firmly linking these associations are sparse. In one very demanding study, primates were maintained for over 24 months on a vitamin E–deficient diet.[12] They developed a striking degeneration of the macula along with dissolution and vacuolation of the outer segments of the rods and cones. These changes were interpreted as being consistent with lipid peroxidation, as well as, perhaps, with loss of normal anabolic functions at the level of the outer retina. It must be remembered that additional antioxidant factors such as vitamin C may also play a key role, both independently and synergistically.[43]

Available evidence suggests that the administration of a nontoxic dose of vitamin E any time a hypovitaminosis A condition is being treated may be a helpful adjunct. There is no convincing published evidence that vitamin E administration affects the course of macular degeneration or the occurrence of aphakic cystoid macular edema. There is, likewise, no indication that ingestion of 200 IU of vitamin E daily exacerbates these conditions.

Mineral-Related Retinopathies

The retina and the RPE have some of the highest trace mineral concentrations of any body tissues.[4,10] The precise explanation for the very high concentration of copper in the retina and the RPE is unknown. It may be related to the necessity for trace minerals such as zinc and copper as cofactors for many of the important metabolic enzymes in these tissues, and the very high metabolic demand of these tissues. Zinc also has retinally important actions distant from the eye; it has a key role in the release of retinol binding protein from the liver.[35]

Two trace-element deficiencies have been associated with retinal changes (Table 17-2). In Menke's syndrome, which involves a copper deficiency, degeneration of the pigmented epithelium and the inner retina has been described.[22,45] If the syndrome is treated in infancy with intravenous copper, an amelioration of the

Table 17-2. Retinopathies Associated With Disorders of Mineral Metabolism

Disorder	Associated Clinical Features	Retinal Features	Other Ocular Findings	Management
Copper deficiency (Menke's kinky hair syndrome)	X-linked recessive; mental retardation, failure to thrive; hair and bone abnormalities	Pigmentary changes; loss of nerve fiber layer and macular details; vessel tortuosity	No significant changes	IV copper administration early in infancy may reverse disease; serial serum level determinations
Iron deficiency anemia (severe)	Generalized weakness, fatigue, weight loss, blurred vision	Retinal edema, hemorrhages, exudates; papilledema	Conjunctival pallor	Ferrous iron administration; follow hemoglobin, hematocrit, erythrocyte indices; treat associated problems
Zinc deficiency	Failure to thrive (in children); night blindness; chronic alcoholism; liver disease; pancreatitis; acrodermatitis enteropathica	Whitish punctate accumulations, in some cases	Corneal deposits; optic disc pallor	Oral or IV zinc administration (up to 150 mg daily for acrodermatitis enteropathica); serial serum level determination; quantitate dark adaptation; treat associated problems

retinal dysfunction can be achieved.[26] In severe iron deficiency, retinal edema and hemorrhages have been frequently reported in association with papilledema when the anemia is of great enough severity. Repletion of iron stores results in a complete resolution of these changes.[19]

Zinc deficiency, which is perhaps most frequently seen in individuals with chronic alcoholism or chronic pancreatitis, is commonly associated with complaints of difficulty in adapting to the dark.[40] The night blindness may be unresponsive to vitamin A but alleviated by zinc administration in some cases.[28] In the relatively rare condition, *acrodermatitis enteropathica,* the subjective night blindness can be alleviated by oral zinc administration.[27] One case of zinc deficiency associated with Crohn's disease and parenteral nutrition resulted in a moderately severe deterioration of macular function with the appearance of a maculopathy. The maculopathy was ameliorated by zinc administration. There was a concomitant slight serum copper deficit that was also supplemented.[46]

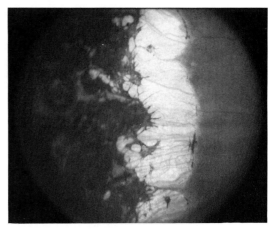

Figure 17-2. The temporal fundus of the right eye of this 35-year-old woman with undetectable fibroblast ornithine amino transferase activity and elevated serum ornithine shows the typical scalloped appearance of gyrate atrophy of the choroid. The eyes had asymmetric involvement. Corrected acuity was 20/80 OD and 20/160 OS. There was a small central posterior subcapsular cataract OS. The heavy hyperpigmentation shown here is typical of the retinal periphery. More posteriorly, intraretinal pigment migration can resemble that seen in the eyes of some persons with retinitis pigmentosa.

AMINO ACID–RELATED RETINOPATHIES

The retina and the RPE, like all other tissues, require a group of eight essential amino acids. Dietary protein is the major source of amino acids in man. The association of retinopathy with pure protein deficiency is extremely uncertain. An isolated severe protein deficiency is quite rare. As mentioned above, the treatment of hypovitaminosis A in children generally involves treating the concurrent protein energy malnutrition. However, protein-calorie malnutrition in an individual with an adequate liver supply of vitamin A does not generally result in even subjective complaints of night blindness.

Three rare disorders of amino acid metabolism have been associated with pigmentary retinopathies. Cystinosis and homocystinuria, both recessively inherited disorders, are associated with a variety of ocular changes, including a peripheral pigmentary retinopathy (see Table 17-2).[32,44] Because the systemic findings in these disorders can be overwhelming, the oc-

ular manifestations may be overlooked. Conversely, the ophthalmologist may be called upon, in a case of a child with various systemic problems and no definite family history, to search for ocular findings that may give a clue to the underlying illness. Thus, in a child with the mild form of cystinosis and visible deposits in the anterior segment that can be identified in biopsy specimens, the careful examination for the presence of retinal changes and documentation of retinal function should be a part of the complete evaluation. Nutritional management of these two disorders can ameliorate the effects of these diseases. They require the supervision of an experienced pediatric nutritionist.

The rare disease known as gyrate atrophy of the choroid is the major manifestation of the recessively inherited disease hyperornithinemia (Fig. 17-2). This disease is related to a deficiency of the enzyme ornithine aminotransferase.[34] The greatest concentration of persons with this disease is found in northern Europe. Because the enzyme deficiency can be detected in skin fibroblasts and peripheral blood mononuclear cells, studies of these cells may be helpful in diagnosing suspected cases where the serum amino acid and urinary amino acid changes are borderline.[42] It is not completely understood why this generalized enzyme deficiency seems to cause only severe disease of the chorioretinal complex.[2]

Because gyrate atrophy of the choroid can lead to blindness, much emphasis has been placed on dietary management. Two principal tactics have been tried. These include the administration of pyridoxine, which is helpful in some cases, or the restriction of arginine intake.[18,25] In some instances, combined therapy has also been tried. Dietary restriction of arginine places many restrictions on the patient and requires careful monitoring to avoid hyperammonemia.

RETINOPATHIES RELATED TO DISORDERS OF CARBOHYDRATE METABOLISM

Diabetes mellitus of sufficient duration is almost always associated with a characteristic microvascular retinopathy.[7] A detailed discussion on the pathogenesis and the relationship between the abnormalities of carbohydrate metabolism in diabetes mellitus and the development of diabetic retinopathy is discussed elsewhere in this volume and in an enormous literature. For the purposes of the present discussion, we can focus on one key issue apropriate to our discussion of nutritional retinopathies: What is the relationship between the development and progression of diabetic retinopathy and blood sugar control? Published studies, nearly all of which have been questioned by one or another group of investigators in the field, have shown either a small but definite beneficial effect of good control or no detectable effect. In a recently reported study of individuals on the continuous subcutaneous infusion pump or on twice-daily insulin by injection regimens, after an average follow-up of about 1 year, there was a favorable treatment effect among those individuals on the pump.[21,24] This is in contrast to results of earlier studies with a shorter follow-up that showed that there may even be a deleterious effect on diabetic retinopathy when patients were switched from insulin administration to the continuous subcutaneous infusion modality.[21]

Regardless of the outcome of future studies, since there are efficacious treatments available for various stages of diabetic retinopathy, it will continue to be advisable that every patient with diabetes mellitus have periodic retinal evaluations by an ophthalmologist with special interest and experience in that area.

RETINOPATHIES RELATED TO DISORDERS OF LIPOPROTEIN AND FAT METABOLISM

The sensory retina, like other nervous tissue, has a high lipid content. Very low dietary fat intake has not been shown to have retinal effects in man. In experimental animals made deficient in fatty acids, the administration of linoleic and arachidonic acids have improved electroretinographic responses. These same animals also exhibited clinical signs of decreased visual acuity. In contrast, in humans with elevated lipoproteins, there can be exudation of fatty material into the retina, with attendant retinal edema and visual reduction, if the macula is involved.[20] With certain types of hyperlipoproteinemia, the occurrence of cholesterol embolization to the retina with effects ranging from no visual symptoms to central retinal artery occlusion can be seen.[17] Dietary management of these disorders must be tailored to the particular abnormality, and has been shown to be successful in a number of well-designed and -executed clinical trials.[9] In fact, some of the hyperlipoidemias, especially type IV, will respond to weight loss alone. Because of reported side-effects, the pharmacologic management of these entities is less safe.

Three rare hereditary diseases that involve disorders of fat metabolism can produce severe retinal degenerative changes. Each of these can be ameliorated, at least to a certain extent, by dietary management. Abetalipoproteinemia, the Bassen–Kornzweig syndrome, a recessive condition manifested by malabsorption and steatorrhea, ataxia, acanthocytosis, and premature cardiovascular disease, is usually accompanied by a pigmentary retinopathy resembling retinitis pigmentosa (Fig. 17-3). The ocular manifestations include difficulties with dark adaptation, reduced peripheral vision, reduced electroretinogram responses, pigment clumping and migration into the sensory retina, retinal vessel attenuation, and optic nerve pallor.[39] The optic nerve pallor may not represent true optic atrophy. Histopathologic examination, in a limited number of cases, has shown that abetalipoproteinemia is associated with early loss of both rods and cones as well as more widespread outer nuclear changes than are seen in comparably advanced cases of typical retinitis pigmentosa.

In contrast to typical retinitis pigmentosa, the disease manifestations in abetalipoproteinemia appear to be linked to the failure of vitamin A transport. In some instances, parenteral vitamin A administration has resulted in improved electroretinographic functioning.[11] The concomitant oral administration of vitamins A and E, along with the restriction of dietary fats, has, in other cases with long-term follow-up, resulted in slowing of the progressive retinal and neurologic changes.[29]

Familial hypobetalipoproteinemia, which is dominantly inherited, can also be associated

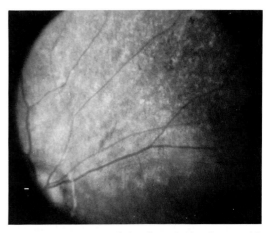

Figure 17-4. The medial retina of this 13-year-old boy with phytanic aciduria and multisystem neurologic disease shows loss of pigment and a "salt-and-pepper" mottling typical of Refsum's disease. This picture of pigment disturbance is similar to that seen in a variety of metabolic diseases with associated retinopathy.

with a pigmentary retinopathy that resembles typical retinitis pigmentosa.[47] This entity also seems to be linked to abnormalities of vitamin A transport. Nutritional management, including vitamin administration and dietary restrictions, have not proved as successful in these patients as in those with abetalipoproteinemia.

Refsum's disease is associated with an absence of the enzyme phytanic acid alpha-hydroxylase. This absent enzyme appears responsible for allowing phytanic and other fatty acids to accumulate in nervous tissues, including the sensory retina. The pigmentary retinopathy that accompanies this disease is a variable phenocopy of typical retinitis pigmentosa. (Fig. 17-4). Histopathologic examination of ocular tissues from individuals with Refsum's disease has shown marked lipid deposition throughout the sensory retina and in other ocular tissues.[41]

Refsum's disease can be ameliorated by strict dietary management. Rich sources of phytanic acid, such as fatty meats, seafood, nuts, and dairy products, must be avoided. Although such dietary restriction has produced a definite improvement in the neurologic manifestations of Refsum's disease, a similar improvement in retinal function in afflicted persons has been documented only occasionally.[33]

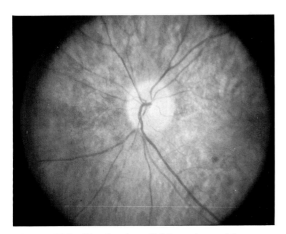

Figure 17-3. The fundus of this patient with electrophoretically demonstrated abetalipoproteinemia (Bassen–Kornzweig) shows widespread but mild pigment mottling. Both retinas have similar appearance.

REFERENCES

1. Adams AJ, Brown B: Alcohol prolongs time course of glare recovery. Nature 257:481–483, 1975
2. Arshinoff SA, McCulloch JC, Phillips MJ, et al: Amino acid metabolism and liver ultrastructure in hyperornithinemia with gyrate atrophy of the choroid and retina. Metabolism 28:979–88, 1979
3. Bietti A: Ueber Augensveränderungen bei Pellagra. Klin Mbl Augenheilk 39:337–350, 1901
4. Bowness JM, Morton RA, Shakir MH, et al: Distribution of copper and zinc in mammalian eyes: Occurrence of metals in melanin fractions from eye tissues. Biochem J 51:521–530, 1952
5. Calhoun FP: Alterations in the visual fields associated with pellagra. Am J Ophthalmol 13:834–837, 1918
6. Carroll FD: Nutritional amblyopia. Arch Ophthalmol 76:406–411, 1966
7. Engerman R: Pathophysiology of diabetic retinopathy. Report of the National Commission on Diabetes #3, DHEW #NIH 76-1023, pp 194–95. Washington, DC, US Government Printing Office, 1976
8. Fine M, Lachman GS: Retrobulbar neuritis in pellagra. Am J Ophthalmol 20:708–714, 1937
9. Frederickson DA, Goldstein JL, Brown MS: The familial hyperlipoproteinemias. In Stanbury JS, Wyngaarden JB, Frederickson DS (eds): The Metabolic Basis of Inherited Disease, 4th ed, pp 604–655. New York, McGraw-Hill, 1978
10. Galin MA, Nano HD, Hall T: Ocular zinc concentration. Invest Ophthalmol 1:142–148, 1962
11. Gouras P, Carr RE, Gunkel RD: Retinitis pigmentosa in abetalipoproteinemia: Effects of vitamin A. Invest Ophthalmol 10:784–793, 1971
12. Hayes KC: Retinal degeneration in monkeys induced by deficiency of vitamin E or A. Invest Ophthalmol 13:499–510, 1974
13. Hecht S, Mandelbaum J: The relation between vitamin A and dark adaptation. JAMA 112:1910–1916, 1937
14. Herrmann RK, Robison WG Jr, Bieri JG: Deficiencies of vitamins E and A in the rat: Lipofuscin accumulation in the choroid. Invest Ophthalmol Vis Sci 25:429–433, 1984
15. Hess HH, Newsome DA, Knapka JJ, et al: Effects of sunflower seed supplements on reproduction and growth of RCS rats with hereditary retinal dystrophy. Lab Animal Sci 31:482–88, 1981
16. Hirschberg J: Tobacco and alcohol amblyopia. Br Med J 2:810–811, 1879
17. Hollenhorst RW: Significance of bright plaques in the retinal arterioles. JAMA 178:23–29, 1961
18. Kennaway NG, Weleber RG, Buist NRM: Gyrate atrophy of the choroid and retina with hyperornithinemia: Biochemical and histologic studies and response to vitamin B. Am J Hum Genet 32:529–41, 1980
19. Kolker AE: Ocular manifestations of hematologic disease. In Brown EB, Moore CV (eds): Progress in Hematology, vol 5, pp 354–389. London, Heinemann, 1966
20. Kurz GH, Shakib M, Sohmer KK, et al: The retina in type 5 hyperlipoproteinemia. Am J Ophthalmol 82:32–43, 1976
21. Lauritzen T, Frost-Larsen K, Larsen H-W, et al: Effect of 1 year of near-normal blood glucose levels on retinopathy in insulin-dependent diabetics. Lancet 1:200–208, 1983
22. Levy NS, Dawson WW, Rhodes BJ, et al: Ocular abnormality in Menke's kinky-hair syndrome. Am J Ophthalmol 77:319–325, 1974
23. Levy NS, Toskes PP: Fundus albipunctatus and vitamin A deficiency. Am J Ophthalmol 78:926–929, 1974
24. Lindsey PS, Plotnik LP, Georgopoulos A: Insulin pump: Effect on diabetic retinopathy. Invest Ophthalmol Vis Sci (suppl) 22:69, 1982
25. McInnes RR, Arshinoff SA, Bell L, et al: Hyperornithinemia and gyrate atrophy of the retina: Improvement of vision during treatment with a low-arginine diet. Lancet 1:513–517, 1981
26. McLaren DL: Nutritional Ophthalmology, p 214. London, Academic Press, 1980
27. Matta CS, Felker GV, Ide CH: Eye manifestations in acrodermatitis enteropathica. Arch Ophthalmol 93:140–142, 1975
28. Morrison SA, Russell RM, Carney EA, et al: Zinc deficiency: A cause of abnormal dark adaptation in cirrhotics. Am J Clin Nutr 31:276–381, 1978
29. Muller DPR, Lloyd JK, Bird AC: Long term management of abetalipoproteinemia. Arch Dis Childhood 52:209–214, 1977
30. Newsome DA: The eye. In Paige DM (ed): Manual of Clinical Nutrition. Pleasantville NJ, Nutrition Publications, 1983
31. Patek AJ, Haig C: The occurrence of abnormal dark adaptation and its relation to vitamin A metabolism in patients with cirrhosis of the liver. J Clin Invest 18:609–616, 1939
32. Presley GD, Stinton IN, Sidbury JB: Ocular defects associated with homocystinuria. South Med J 62:944–946, 1969
33. Refsum S: Heredopathia atactica polyneuritiformis phytanic acid storage disease (Refsum's disease) with particular reference to ophthalmological disturbances. Metabol Ophthalmol 1:73–81, 1977
34. Simell O, Takki K: Raised plasma ornithine and gyrate atrophy of the choroid and retina. Lancet i:1031–33, 1973

35. Smith JE, Brown ED, Smith JC Jr: The effect of zinc deficiency on the metabolism of retinol-binding protein in the rat. J Lab Clin Med 84:692–697, 1974

36. Smolin G, Okumoto M, Friedlaender M, et al: Herpes simplex keratitis treatment with vitamin A. Arch Ophthalmol 97:2181–83, 1979

37. Sommer A: Field guide to the detection and control of xerophthalmia. Geneva, World Health Organization, 1978

38. Sommer A, Hussaini G, Muhilal, et al: History of night blindness: A simple tool for xerophthalmia screening. Am J Clin Nutr 33:887–91, 1980

39. Sugar A, Podos SM: Ophthalmic aspects of inborn errors of metabolism. In Mausolf FA (ed): The Eye and Systemic Disease, pp 48–87. St Louis, CV Mosby, 1980

40. Toskes PP, Dawson W, Curington C: Non-diabetic retinal abnormalities in chronic pancreatitis. N Engl J Med 300:942–946, 1979

41. Toussaint D, Danis P: An ocular pathologic study of Refsum's syndrome. Am J Ophthalmol 72:342–347, 1971

42. Vallee D, Kaiser-Kupfer MI, Del Valle LA: Gyrate atrophy of the choroid and retina: Deficiency of ornithine aminotransferase in transformed lymphocytes. Proc Natl Acad Sci USA 74:5159–61, 1977

43. Woodford BJ, Tso MOM, Lam K-W: Reduced and oxidized ascorbates in guinea pig retina under normal and light-exposed conditions. Invest Ophthalmol Vis Sci 24:862–867, 1983

44. Wong VG, Leitman PS, Seegmiller JE: Alterations of pigmentary epithelium in cystinosis. Arch Ophthalmol 82:267–268, 1967

45. Wray SH, Kuwabara T, Sanderson P: Menke's kinky hair disease: A light and electron microscopic study of the eye. Invest Ophthalmol Vis Sci 15:128–138, 1976

46. Yassur Y, Snir M, Melamed S, et al: Bilateral maculopathy simulating "cherry-red spot" in a patient with Crohn's disease. Br J Ophthalmol 65:184–188, 1981

47. Yee RD, Herbert PN, Bergsma DR, et al: Atypical retinitis pigmentosa in familial hypobetalipoproteinemia. Am J Ophthalmol 82:64–71, 1976

5

Retinal Inflammatory Diseases

18

AIDS and Opportunistic Retinitis

Lee M. Jampol

In the early 1980s an apparently new disease syndrome was first recognized in the United States. Acquired immunodeficiency syndrome (AIDS) is characterized by the occurrence of multiple opportunistic infections and in some cases, Kaposi's sarcoma, in previously healthy patients.[5] These patients have impaired T cell function with a decreased number of T helper cells (OKT4 cells) and reversal of the normal T cell helper/suppressor cell ratio in the peripheral blood. Over 40,000 cases of AIDS have now been confirmed, and the mortality rate in patients approaches 100% with long-term follow-up. The disease was first noted in New York City, Miami, Los Angeles, and San Francisco, although cases have now been reported from all parts of this country, the European continent, the Caribbean, and Central Africa. A larger group of patients with fever, lymphadenopathy, and similarly reduced T cell function (called pre-AIDS, AIDS–related syndrome, or AIDS prodrome) has been identified. Some but not all of these patients will show progression to full-blown AIDS. The population at risk for pre-AIDS is the same as that for AIDS. AIDS shows a predilection for the following groups:

- Homosexual males, especially those with multiple sexual partners
- Intravenous drug users without homosexual experience
- Haitian immigrants living in the United States
- Hemophiliacs, especially those receiving Factor VIII concentrate

- Patients receiving blood transfusions from patients with AIDS or pre-AIDS
- Heterosexual partners of patients with AIDS, pre-AIDS, or at risk for AIDS
- Children born to mothers with AIDS or pre-AIDS, or in a high-risk group for these abnormalities
- Some patients with AIDS or pre-AIDS do not fit into any of the above high risk groups.

Kaposi's sarcoma is an unusual condition characterized by red or purple nontender, non-ulcerating macules, papules, plaques, and nodules scattered on the skin or mucous membranes. The conjunctivae or the eyelids can be involved. Histopathologically spindle-shaped cells with vascular slits and endothelium-lined channels are seen. Kaposi's sarcoma occurs frequently in equatorial Africa but was seen rarely in the United States, and then usually in elderly Italian or Jewish men. Recently this tumor has been appearing in young patients with AIDS. Kaposi's sarcoma in these patients is aggressive, with widespread skin involvement, early lymph node infiltration, and often visceral involvement. The tumor may involve the bone marrow, spleen, liver, lung, gastrointestinal tract, and other areas. Some patients with AIDS have also developed other tumors, especially non-Hodgkin's lymphomas. The most prominent feature of AIDS is the occurrence of the multiple opportunistic infections. *Pneumocystis carinii* infections often cause pneumonitis. The patients frequently show evidence of herpesviruses including herpes simplex, cytomegalovirus, and Epstein–Barr virus. Other opportunistic organisms that are described in these patients include *Candida, Toxoplasma,* and *Cryptococcus.*

Because of the reduced T helper cells, AIDS patients show markedly abnormal cell-mediated immunity. They demonstrate cutaneous anergy and impaired lymphocyte transformation. In general, humoral immunity is normal, and the patients often show hypergammaglobulinemia.

With the sudden appearance of AIDS, various theories came forward as to its origin including its possible relation to cytomegalovirus infection, the recreational use of amyl nitrite and other nitrites by the populations at risk, hepatitis B virus infection, chronic antigenic stimulation secondary to multiple infections, immunosuppression related to semen, and other causes. The most promising theory, however, was that AIDS represented spread of a new virus, most likely a virus transmitted horizontally through intimate contact or by blood products. Thus, its epidemiology was similar to that of hepatitis B virus. Vertical transmission (mother to fetus) also seemed possible occasionally. A retrovirus, human T cell, lymphotropic virus, subgroup III (HTLV III), now called human immunodeficiency virus (HIV), has been widely isolated from tissues and peripheral blood of patients with AIDS or pre-AIDS and has now been established as the cause of AIDS.[2,3,11] Serologic evidence of past or present infection with this virus has been found almost universally in patients with AIDS or pre-AIDS. A very closely related virus, the lymphadenopathy-associated virus (LAV) has been identified by a group in France at the Pasteur Institute in patients with AIDS or pre-AIDS.[1,7,13] Similar retroviruses have been isolated from AIDS patients in San Francisco.[8] These retroviruses contain a magnesium-dependent reverse transcriptase that is capable of directing the synthesis of DNA from viral RNA in the affected cells. This DNA then can cause malignant transformation of the cells (which is seen with HTLV subgroups I and II), or it may cause death or a loss of function of the infected cells (for example, HIV). These viruses replicate preferentially in the helper T cell population and may be cytopathogenic. This explains the loss of these T cells in patients with AIDS or pre-AIDS.

Serologic evidence of infection with HIV is found in patients with AIDS and pre-AIDS using the specific Western Blot technique or the less specific ELISA test. This is true for all subgroups with AIDS including homosexual males, patients receiving transfusions, and drug addicts. Viral isolation has been possible in many of these patients. Some studies have suggested that HIV may have originated in Central Africa where, interestingly, Kaposi's sarcoma is endemic.[12] It has been suggested that this virus either changed its behavior or was then transmitted to the populations that are presently at risk. Concern has been expressed that the virus may continue to spread to the remainder of the population including normal heterosexuals. The potential for this widespread transmission is uncertain.

One of the benefits of the isolation of the retrovirus causing AIDS is the ability to screen blood and blood products to prevent horizontal transmission of the virus by blood. A cheap, easily performed test for screening donated blood for antibodies to HIV has been developed. This advance has eliminated almost all transfusion-associated AIDS. Screening of large populations will then also allow the detection of asymptomatic people with evidence of previous viral exposure. Longitudinal follow-up on these patients can determine their future risk for development of pre-AIDS or AIDS. Serologic testing also assists in the earlier diagnosis of AIDS. Hopefully, the isolation of the virus will allow the development of effective antiviral agents or a vaccine. Several antiviral agents and vaccines are presently being tested.

Treatment of AIDS has been inadequate. The mortality rate with long-term follow-up is very high. Kaposi's sarcoma can be treated by local excision or radiotherapy, but it is extremely difficult to cure in these patients. Individual opportunistic infections can be managed with appropriate antimicrobial drugs although the long-term results are poor. Repeated infections with other organisms frequently occur. Antiviral agents (e.g., acyclovir for herpes simplex infections), antifungal agents (e.g., amphotericin B for many fungal infections), and antibiotics should be used as necessary.

OCULAR MANIFESTATIONS OF AIDS

Ocular manifestations of AIDS are common.[4,9,10] Because patients with AIDS may initially present with ocular symptomatology, the ophthalmologist should be aware of these manifestations. Most patients with AIDS, however, are known to be ill systemically, and often the diagnosis of AIDS has been made before the patient first develops ocular symptoms.

The commonest ocular manifestation of AIDS is the appearance of multiple cotton wool spots in the fundus. Small hemorrhages may also be seen. Cotton wool spots are not pathognomonic of AIDS or of any opportunistic infection; they are nonspecific. It was initially suggested that these cotton wool spots might represent retinal infection with *Pneumocystis.*[6] This, however, has been disputed, and no confirmation has been forthcoming.

Kaposi's sarcoma may involve the conjunctiva or the lids. Such tumors may be asymptomatic and may be one of the first manifestations of AIDS. Local excision or radiotherapy can be used.

Other malignancies including lymphomas may involve the eye, orbit, and adnexae. In addition, central nervous system involvement by lymphomas or by opportunistic infections may produce ocular motility abnormalities including cranial nerve palsies and nystagmus.

The most common serious ocular manifestation of AIDS is the occurrence of opportunistic retinitis. Patients so affected may have no complaints or may complain of blurred vision. The commonest cause of retinitis is the cytomegalovirus. Involvement may be unilateral or bilateral. Anterior segment inflammation (flare, cells, fine keratic precipitates) is usually present, but often is low grade. Examination of the retina reveals scattered yellow-white areas of necrotizing retinitis with multiple vascular occlusions and retinal hemorrhages (Fig. 18-1); it has been called "cottage cheese with catsup" or "pizza

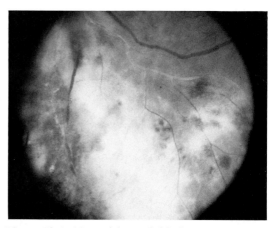

Figure 18-1. Necrotizing retinitis from cytomegalovirus. Characteristic signs include vascular sheathing and occlusion, hemorrhages, and whitening of retina.

pie" retinopathy. Less commonly, optic disc edema and exudative or rhegmatogenous retinal detachment may occur. Areas of previous retinitis may heal with pigment stippling and scarring, or the retinitis may progress to retinal necrosis with retinal tear formation and vitreous organization. The appearance of the retinitis in patients with AIDS is similar to that in patients otherwise immunosuppressed (organ transplants, malignancies). Histopathologically, patients with AIDS may more frequently show a polymorphonuclear leukocytic infiltration in the eye,[12] probably owing to the fact that they have normal polymorphonuclear leukocytes as compared to other severely immunosuppressed or otherwise immunodebilitated patients. Herpes simplex can cause a similar necrotizing retinitis in patients with AIDS although this is much rarer.

Central nervous system toxoplasmosis is commonly seen in patients with AIDS, and occasional cases of ocular toxoplasmosis have been reported. Other fungal infections may also involve the retina including *Cryptococcus* and *Candida. Mycobacterium avium* has also been reported to affect the retina and choroid. It is to be expected that other opportunists, such as *Nocardia,* will also be reported in the eyes of these patients.

Therapy of the retinitis depends upon the individual organism involved. Cytomegalovirus retinitis is a very poor prognostic sign, and many of these patients do not survive long after the diagnosis is made. DHPG (ganciclovir), a new antiviral derivative related to acyclovir has shown some efficacy against CMV retinitis, but relapses are seen when the drug is discontinued. Herpes simplex retinitis may be treated with acyclovir. Toxoplasmosis can be treated with sulfonamides and clindamycin, but the use of corticosteroids and Daraprim does not seem wise in these patients. Fungal infections such as *Cryptococcus* can be treated with systemic amphotericin B. As mentioned above, the appearance or even the occurrence of *Pneumocystis* retinitis has not been confirmed, although recently *Pneumocystis choroiditis* has been documented.

REFERENCES

1. Barré-Sinoussi F, Cherman JC, Rey F, et al: Isolation of T-lymphotropic retrovirus from a patient at risk for acquired immune deficiency syndrome (AIDS). Science 200:868–871, 1983
2. Broder S, Gallo RC: A pathogenic retrovirus (HTLV-III) linked to AIDS. N Engl J Med 311:1292–1297, 1984
3. Gallo RC, Salahuddin SZ, Popovic M, et al: Frequent detection and isolation of cytopathic retroviruses (HTLV-III) from patients with AIDS and at risk for AIDS. Science 224:500–503, 1984
4. Jampol LM, Tessler HH: The acquired immunodeficiency syndrome (AIDS) II. Ocular findings. In Ernest JT (ed): 1983 Year Book of Ophthalmology pp. 305–307. Chicago, Year Book Medical Publishers, 1983
5. Jampol LM, Tessler HH: The acquired immunodeficiency syndrome (AIDS) I. Systemic findings. In Ernest JT (ed): 1983 Year Book of Ophthalmology, pp 201–204. Chicago, Year Book Medical Publishers, 1983
6. Kwok S, O'Donnell JJ, Wood IS: Retinal cotton-wool spots in a patient with *Pneumocystis carinii* infection. N Engl J Med 307:184–185, 1982
7. Laurence J, Brun-Vezinet F, Schutzer SE, et al: Lymphadenopathy-associated viral antibody in AIDS: Immune correlations and definition of a carrier state. N Engl J Med 311:1269–1273, 1984
8. Levy JA, Hoffman AD, Kramer SM, et al: Isolation of lymphocytopathic retroviruses from San Francisco patients with AIDS. Science 225:840–842, 1984
9. Palestine AG, Rodriques MM, Macher AB, et al: Ophthalmic involvement in the acquired immunodeficiency syndrome. Ophthalmology 91:1092–1099, 1984
10. Pepose JS, Hilbourne LH, Cancilla PA, et al: Concurrent herpes simplex and cytomegalovirus retinitis and encephalitis in the acquired immune deficiency syndrome (AIDS). Ophthalmology 91:1669–1677, 1984
11. Popovic M, Sarngadhavan MG, Read E, et al: Detection, isolation, and continuous production of cytopathic retroviruses (HTLV-III) from patients with AIDS and pre-AIDS. Science 224:497–500, 1984
12. Saxinger WC, Levine PH, Dean AG, et al: Evidence of exposure to HTLV-III in Uganda before 1973. Science 227:1036–1038, 1985
13. Vilmer E, Barré-Sinoussi F, Rouzioux C, et al: Isolation of a new lymphotropic retrovirus in two hemophilia B siblings, one presenting with acquired immunodeficiency syndrome. Lancet 1:753–757, 1984

19

Immunology of Retinal and Choroidal Disease

Henry J. Kaplan

For many years, ophthalmologists have identified various clinical inflammatory disorders of the posterior segment of the eye without understanding their etiologies or pathogeneses. Even where the putative pathogenic agent has been identified, as in toxoplasma retinochoroiditis, the reason for recurrent disease is unknown. With the application of modern concepts of immunology to inflammatory disorders of the eye, there is renewed hope that insights into the etiology and pathogenesis of many of these disease entities will be forthcoming.

This chapter will present a review of certain basic features of the immune response and apply these concepts to two common clinical inflammatory disorders of the posterior segment, toxoplasma retinochoroiditis and the presumed ocular histoplasmosis syndrome. Although some experimental data exist to support these concepts in ocular disease, many are still hypothetical and await verification. Nevertheless, their existence should stimulate fruitful clinical research in the near future.

This work is supported in part by NIH grant #EY03723 and in part by an unrestricted grant to the Department of Ophthalmology from Research to Prevent Blindness, Inc., New York. Dr. Kaplan is a Research to Prevent Blindness Olga Keith Weiss Scholar.

THE IMMUNE RESPONSE TO ANTIGEN

When a host encounters a protein or other immunogen that it recognizes as nonself, a complex cellular response designed to protect it from the possible harmful effects of the protein ensues. For example, if the protein is associated with a pathogenic organism, the immune response is designed to contain and destroy that pathogen; if it is on the cell surface of a neoplastic cell, that cell is killed. Although the immune response may occasionally go awry and cause iatrogenic (autoimmune) disease, it usually functions very effectively.

As our knowledge of the immune response increases, the complexity of the latter becomes more apparent. Nevertheless, it can be conceptualized as having two basic components: generation of the immune response to antigen and regulation of that response.

Generation of the Immune Response

When the immune system responds to an antigen, a complex series of events is initiated.[20] However, the ultimate result is either the production and secretion of antibody (immunoglobulin) into the blood and other body fluids

Lymphoid Differentiation

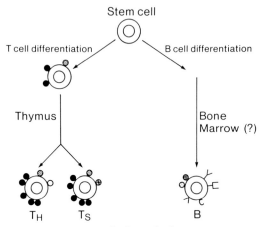

Figure 19-1. Stem cells from the bone marrow migrate to the thymus, where hormonal factors stimulate differentiation into helper T cells (T_h) or suppressor/cytotoxic T cells (T_s). They can be identified by the presence of common (T-11, ◒) and unique (T-4 = helper, ○; T-8 = suppressor/cytotoxic, ⊕) differentiation antigens on their cell membrane surfaces. B lymphocytes are also derived from stem cells and may differentiate in the bone marrow. Their cell membrane surfaces also possess distinctive markers (⊕ = B-1, ☉ = Ia, Y = surface immunoglobulin).

(humoral immunity) or the generation of sensitized lymphocytes (cellular immunity).

The agent of cellular immunity is the lymphocyte. Although lymphocytes are morphologically identical, they are functionally heterogeneous. They express an array of cell-surface molecules (markers) that define two major populations, T and B cells, and their subsets (Fig. 19-1).[39]

Lymphocytes interact with each other as well as with macrophages to allow selective expansion or suppression of specific populations (clones) of lymphocytes. Each lymphocyte clone has a unique receptor on its cell surface, which allows it to recognize and combine optimally with one antigen. Combination of this protein receptor (which on B cells has been identified as an immunoglobulin molecule and on T cells as a heterodimer, composed of two polypeptide chains) with antigen results in the transmission of a signal across the cell membrane, which "activates" the lymphocyte and can result in selective proliferation and expansion of that lymphocyte clone.

Although numerous cellular interactions are involved in the generation of an immune response to antigen, there are essentially three distinct types: antigen recognition by macrophages and presentation to T cells (macrophage–T cell interaction); antibody production in response to antigen (T–B cell interaction); and augmentation or inhibition of T cell activity (T–T cell interaction).

Macrophage–T Cell Interactions

The induction and antigen-responsiveness of T cells is often macrophage dependent (Fig. 19-2). A substantial part of antigen phagocytosed by macrophages is catabolized within phagolysosomes. However, a small amount of highly immunogenic antigen can be found associated with the macrophage surface. Although the deg-

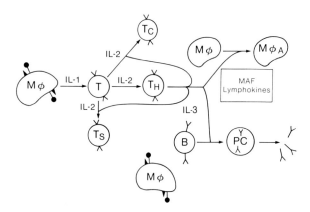

Figure 19-2. The immune response is generated by the interaction of many different cell types, with the assistance of soluble factors. Cells: M𝜙 = macrophage, T = T cell precursor, T_h = helper T cell, T_s = suppressor T cell, T_c = cytotoxic T cell, B = B cell, PC = plasma cell, Y = immunoglobulin, M𝜙A = activated macrophage. Soluble factors: IL-1 = interleukin 1, IL-2 = interleukin 2, IL-3 = interleukin 3, MAF = macrophage activation factor.

radation state of antigen on the macrophage surface is unknown, it may exist solely as its primary amino acid sequence. Surface antigen is intimately associated with the products of a specific region of the major histocompatability complex (MHC), called the *I region* (which codes for Ia molecules).

The MHC is a genetic segment that codes for the classic transplantation antigens (HLA-A, -B, and -C) and I region–associated antigens (HLA-D/DR). The I region, first identified in mice, codes for both protein molecules (called Ia antigens) expressed on the cell membrane of monocytes, B cells, and activated T cells; and immunologic responsiveness (through Ir genes) of T cells to protein antigens.[33]

The manner in which Ia molecules interact with antigen or T cells is not clear. Two explanations have been proposed to explain the requirement for Ia homology. In the first hypothesis, Ia molecules facilitate cell interaction. An immune T cell with two membrane receptors is envisioned, one interacting with Ia and the other with antigen. In the second hypothesis, Ia is involved in the binding of antigen by the phagocyte, and the immune T cell has an Ia–antigen complex receptor.[52]

Following antigen recognition, there is clonal proliferation and expansion of those precursor T lymphocytes which are directed at the involved antigen. Among the subsets of expanded T cells will be helper T cells.

T–B Cell Interactions

Helper T cells provide both antigen-specific and nonspecific help for B cells, as well as for subsets of T cells involved in cytotoxic or suppressor reactions. It is likely that several distinct categories of helper T cells will eventually be recognized.

The production of antibody to most antigens requires the synergistic cooperation of helper T cells and B cells. The omission of either population will result in limited antibody production or none. This is true in both the primary (on initial antigen exposure) and secondary (after subsequent antigen exposure) antibody responses.

The precise mechanism of T–B cell coopera- tion is variable and probably dependent upon the antigen involved. There is evidence to suggest that in most instances, interaction between helper T cells and B cells is a localized phenomenon involving direct cell contact. However, help can also be mediated, at least in some experimental systems, by soluble factors released by T cells. These T cell factors, collectively known as interleukins (e.g., IL-2, IL-4), are released on T cell stimulation by antigen (see Fig. 19-2). They serve as growth factors for activated T helper and cytotoxic cells (IL-2), and enhance B cell differentiation into plasma cells (IL-4). The importance of these factors in T–B cooperation is still being studied.

T–T Cell Interactions

The immune response to antigen can result in the generation of cytotoxic T cells with the ability to kill allogeneic cells (foreign transplanted cells) or virus-infected syngeneic (host) cells. Optimal generation of cytotoxic cells requires interaction between helper T cells and cytotoxic T cell precursors. The exact nature of the interaction between these cells is unclear, but it may involve direct cell contact or soluble factors.

Multiple cell–cell interactions occur during the generation of an immune response. It is necessary to regulate these interactions so that the net effect of the immune response is appropriate and to prevent the inadvertent destruction of host bystander cells. Although multiple homeostatic controls exist, we will focus solely on the role of T cell suppression in immunoregulation.

Regulatory Mechanisms of the Immune Response

Since the antigen receptor on lymphocyte cell membranes is the only clonally distributed structure, it must be involved in cell regulation. This can occur through either cell receptor interaction with antigen or with receptors directed at the antigen receptor itself (idiotype–antiidiotype recognition).

So far, clonal expansion has been considered in the context of selection by antigen. As such, the regulation of clonal expansion can be

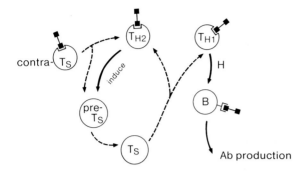

Figure 19-3. The suppressor T cell regulatory circuit influences the production and secretion of antibody as well as the cellular immune response. H represents the help Thy-1 provides for B cell production of antibody. Cells: T_h-1 = helper T cell 1, T_h-2 = helper T cell 2, contra-T_s = contrasuppressor T cell, pre-T_s = suppressor T cell precursor, T_s = suppressor T cell, B = B cell.

achieved by antigen removal with secreted antibody or cytotoxic T cells. The depletion of antigen for lymphocyte receptors serves as a negative feedback for antigen-driven clonal expansion. In addition, another level of control results from the recognition of antigenic determinants on lymphocyte receptors (idiotypes) or other lymphocytes. However, the precise details of the idiotypic–anti-idiotypic network will not be discussed; suffice it to say that multiple mininetworks of regulation exist for each clone expanded.

In addition to the mechanisms mentioned above, there is a prominent level of control mediated by suppressor T cells. Their effect can be either antigen specific or nonspecific. Interaction of antigen with a suppressor T cell results in the generation of a soluble suppressor molecule with I-region specificities which can combine with antigen. Another feature of this factor is that it can be absorbed onto the surfaces of cells that are suppressed, namely, helper T cells. However, the precise mechanism of suppression by this factor is still under investigation.

Experimental studies in mice involving the addition and removal of lymphocyte subsets have shown that there are circuit-like regulatory interactions among suppressor cells.[4] Although the specifics of the regulatory suppressor circuit in man have not yet been identified, it is reasonable to assume that circuits similar to those found in the mouse exist. Thus, a hypothetical regulatory circuit for feedback inhibition of antibody production is presented so that the true complexity of this regulatory mechanism is appreciated (Fig. 19-3).

After interaction with antigen, two different helper cells (T_h-1, T_h-2) are stimulated. Th-1 conveys signals that enhance the production of antibody of B cells. However, Th-2 induces a pre-T suppressor cell (pre-T_s) to become a suppressor cell (T_s), inhibiting the helper function of Th-1. Thus, the system regulates itself by suppressing the signal from the helper T cell to the B cell (feedback inhibition). Recently, a contrasuppressor T cell (contra-T_s) has been discovered which may act to regulate either the signal from Th-2 to the pre-T_s or from the pre-T_s to the T_s. Furthermore, the contrasuppressor cell itself is the product of a mini-network of cellular interactions beginning after antigen stimulation.

It is obvious that the suppressor cell regulatory circuit is complex and that effective modulation of this circuit will require selective enhancement or inhibition of specific subsets. The sophistication of this network is appreciated when one realizes that under physiologic conditions, it must regulate the immune response against one antigen without impairing the response to another. The precise details and interactions of this circuit continue to be refined.

IMMUNOLOGIC INSIGHTS INTO INFLAMMATORY DISEASES OF THE POSTERIOR SEGMENT

Two different posterior segment ocular inflammatory diseases will be discussed. The first, *Toxoplasma* retinochoroiditis, is a disease in which the etiologic agent is known; the second, the presumed ocular histoplasmosis syndrome, is a disease in which doubt exists about the role of histoplasmosis. In each instance, the immunopathologic mechanism of disease will be discussed.

Toxoplasma Retinochoroiditis

Ocular toxoplasmosis is a focal necrotizing inflammation of the retina with involvement of the underlying choroid caused by infection with the protozoa *Toxoplasma gondii* (Fig. 19-4). Although a rare case has been documented following an acquired systemic *Toxoplasma* infection, most cases are thought to be recurrences of congenital infection. *Toxoplasma* lesions are insidious in onset and are usually heralded by floating spots unless they are located in the macula, maculopapular bundle, or optic nerve. Visual acuity can be compromised by dense vitreous opacities or macular edema; rarely, a retinal detachment will follow severe vitritis and vitreous contraction. The diagnosis is made on the basis of the appearance of the lesion, and confirmation is frequently made with a positive antibody titer in either the serum or aqueous humor.

It has been postulated that reactivation of a quiescent toxoplasmosis scar represents a delayed-type hypersensitivity response to *Toxoplasma* sporozoites released from cysts; while, in the cyst, they are antigenically isolated from the host.[42] However, the immune response to toxoplasmosis is much more complex than a simple delayed-type hypersensitivity response. It can be conceptually separated into two stages: the inducer phase, during which antigen interacts with phagocytes, leading to lymphocyte stimulation; and the effector phase, in which cellular cytotoxicity damages the organism.

The Inducer Phase

Initial recognition and processing of *Toxoplasma* antigen involves phagocytosis by macrophages (Fig. 19-5). The ingestion of the antigen by the phagocyte is nonspecific as the cell performs in its primitive capacity as a scavenger. The phagocyte is not activated by contact with *Toxoplasma* antigen and is not cytotoxic. However, it processes the antigen and presents it to T cells in a process regulated by genes of the MHC.[52]

Phagocytes can be divided into two subsets on the basis of the presence or absence of Ia molecules.[43] Although all phagocytes can take up *Toxoplasma* antigen, only those that bear the Ia molecules are capable of cooperating with the T

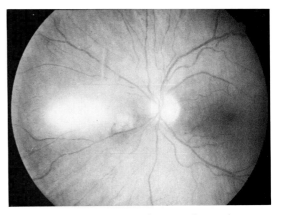

Figure 19-4. Recurrent ocular toxoplasmosis: Acute retinochoroiditis (the white lesion) extends as a satellite from a previously resolved scar of *Toxoplasma* infection. The associated perivasculitis (arterial and venous), as well as vitritis, is a frequent accompaniment of such reactivation.

cell. *Toxoplasma*-specific T cells establish contact and bind only the phagocytes bearing both the *Toxoplasma* antigen and the appropriate Ia antigen. Following this contact, T cell proliferation and differentiation occur, stimulated by macrophage secretion of various growth and differentiation molecules.

The Effector Phase

Once the specific antigen-reactive T cell clone is stimulated, the effector phase of the immune response is entered. Stimulated T cells undergo proliferation and differentiation with the release of soluble mediators (lymphokines) and the expression of cytotoxic, helper and suppressor functions. Primary resistance to *Toxoplasma* infection is mediated by the activated phagocyte, which possesses high cytocidal activity. Phagocytes are not normally capable of killing the *Toxoplasma* organism efficiently; they do so only after interaction with activated T cells.[24] Thus, the antigenic specificity in such reactions resides in the T cell, which, when activated, turns on macrophages to kill in an antigenically nonspecific fashion.[13]

T cells mobilize and activate macrophages through the release of soluble lymphokines. The latter are glycoproteins released by activated T cells and have been characterized by their functional properties, for example, macrophage in-

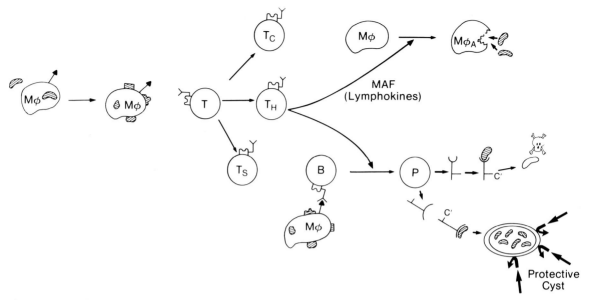

Figure 19-5. Ia⁺ macrophage ingests the toxoplasma organism (◎) and expresses *Toxoplasma* antigens (◎) on its surface. The T cell recognizes the *Toxoplasma* antigen–Ia complex with its receptor (◻) and proliferates and differentiates into various T cell subsets (helper [T$_h$], suppressor [T$_s$] and cytotoxic [T$_c$]). The helper T cell activates the macrophage via MAF; the activated macrophage destroys the *Toxoplasma* organism. Simultaneously, the

helper T cell helps the B cell to differentiate into a plasma cell (P) which secretes either cytotoxic (⊦) or enhancing (⋎) antibody.

hibition factor, macrophage activation factor, and macrophage chemotactic factor.[9,31,53] These lymphocyte mediators are proteins that exert an effect on macrophages regardless of their MHC type and Ia content.

Although the biochemical changes of the activated macrophage have been studied extensively, the mechanism by which cytotoxic activity is mediated is not clear. There is an enhanced synthesis of many enzymes (e.g., plasminogen activator), as well as increased oxidative metabolism and secretion of oxygen-derived products such as superoxide anion and hydrogen peroxide.[11,27] Recent attention has been focused on these latter products as the molecules involved in killing parasites.[37]

Helper T cells also collaborate with *Toxoplasma*-specific B cells to differentiate into plasma cells and secrete anti-*Toxoplasma* antibodies. The spectrum of antibody produced varies significantly with regard to affinity for the organism and functional role. Cytotoxic an-

tibody is secreted which can lyse the free organism in the presence of complement. Alternatively, Shimada and colleagues have demonstrated in vitro that an enhancing antibody is produced which can cause pseudocyst formation in the presence of complement.[44] When encysted, the organism is protected from destruction by either cytotoxic antibody or killer cells. Thus, enhancing antibody is counterproductive to parasite removal and may facilitate re-emergence of the infectious organism and recurrence of disease at a later date.

Thus, the immune response following host contact with *Toxoplasma* is not a simple delayed-type hypersensitivity reaction. There are numerous immunoregulatory factors (both cellular and humoral) that interact with the immune response to terminate or reactivate cytocidal activity which we have not discussed. Analysis of only the inducer and effector phases of the immune response to *Toxoplasma* shows that there are many steps in the sequence at which intervention could either inhibit or enhance immunity. Only with a further understanding of the importance of each of these steps in ocular toxoplasmosis will we be able to select the appropriate time and mode of intervention to eliminate the parasite from the host completely.

The Presumed Ocular Histoplasmosis Syndrome (POHS)

The POHS is a disease complex probably caused by infection with the fungus *Histoplasma capsulatum*. It is confined to individuals who have spent part of their lives in areas where histoplasmosis is endemic. About 88% of affected patients display cutaneous hypersensitivity to histoplasmin; chest and abdominal films show calcified scars in the lungs and spleen.

The disease is first brought to the patient's attention by blurred or distorted vision. Retinal lesions consist of multiple discrete atrophic spots in the choroid and overlying RPE (Fig. 19-6). Histologic examination of these scars reveals multiple lymphocytic foci and occasional breaks in Bruch's membrane associated with ingrowth of abnormal vessels (i.e., a subretinal neovascular membrane). Indeed, the major cause of visual loss is rupture of these blood vessels with a hemorrhagic detachment of the macula. The clinical triad of the POHS consists of multiple atrophic spots with occasional pigment dots, peripapillary atrophy of the RPE and a macular subretinal neovascular membrane.

Immune Response to Histoplasma Capsulatum

The immune response (protection) to *H. capsulatum* appears to be primarily cell mediated, as is the case with other intracellular organisms such as mycobacteria and *Toxoplasma gondii.* Support for this view is provided by (1) the demonstration that lymphocytes from mice injected with a sublethal injection of *H. capsulatum* can inhibit intracellular growth of the fungus in normal mouse macrophages; (2) the demonstration of increased susceptibility to *Histoplasma* infection in congenitally athymic (nude) mice; and (3) evidence for adoptive transfer of immunity against *H. capsulatum* by spleen or perito-

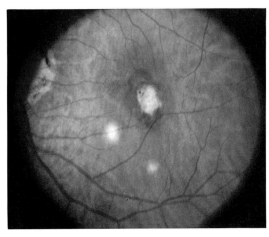

Figure 19-6. The presumed ocular histoplasmosis syndrome: the punched-out, discrete chorioretinal scars typical of this syndrome are observed just beneath the fovea. They are frequently observed only outside the vascular arcades. Together with peripapillary atrophy and the macular subretinal neovascular membrane (the central lesion), they constitute the triad of the presumed ocular histoplasmosis syndrome.

neal cells, specifically T cells, from immunized donors.[21,50,51,57]

The immune response to *Histoplasma* can be conceptually separated into two stages, like that for *Toxoplasma:* the inducer phase, during which antigen is processed by macrophages, leading to lymphocyte stimulation, and the effector phase, during which the organism is killed by activated cells. Since the details of these stages are discussed above for *T. gondii,* they will not be repeated here.

Immunity in the Presumed Ocular Histoplasmosis Syndrome

Most immunologic studies of *Histoplasma* have focused on disseminated disease. However, the overwhelming majority of *Histoplasma* infections are benign and asymptomatic; eye disease is present in only 1 of 666 cases.[41]

Infection is localized to endemic areas where exposure to *H. capsulatum* has been documented by positive skin tests to histoplasmin in 70% to 90% of the population. The peripheral atrophic lesion in the POHS is more common than the macular disciform scar, occurring in

1.6% to 2.5% of people residing in an endemic area. Histoplasmosis is contracted by inhalation of mycelial spores, which undergo transformation to the yeast phase within the lung, followed by dissemination throughout the body via the bloodstream. Most benign infections are thought to occur in adolescence; the presence of eye disease becomes apparent 10 to 30 years later with the development of a disciform macular scar.[17]

The relationship of POHS to *Histoplasma* infection is strongly supported by epidemiologic data. More than 88% of patients with POHS have a positive histoplasmin skin test.[6,18,47] On the other hand, serum antibody to *Histoplasma* is not detected uniformly. Complement-fixing antibody titers are present in 16% to 68% of patients, with only 5% demonstrating antibody to *Histoplasma* on immunodiffusion.[6,25] The low frequency with which antibody is detected is related both to the time lapses between initial infection and eye disease and to the assay method.

Immunologic studies in patients with POHS have shown a difference between those with macular disciform scars and those with peripheral retinal lesions. Weber and Schlaegel first reported that patients with ocular histoplasmosis and macular disease reacted to more skin test antigens than did other uveitis patients.[55] Ganley confirmed this observation when he found increased blast transformation to many different antigens and increased mean induration of the histoplasmin skin test in those patients with macular disease.[14-16]

Human leukocyte antigen (HLA) studies have also indicated a dichotomy between these two groups. HLA-B7 is associated with the disciform macular scar of POHS and not with peripheral lesions.[35,36] However, the DRw2 allele is found with increased frequency in both groups of patients.[36] The significance of these findings will be discussed later.

Recent lymphocyte transformation studies in patients with POHS using various *Histoplasma* antigens, such as products of sonication of yeast-phase *Histoplasma,* commercial histoplasmin, and histoplasmin H-42, have shown increased stimulation ratios compared to matched controls.[6,16] When patients with inactive macular scars were compared to those with peripheral scars, the former were again noted to have significantly increased cellular responsiveness. Unfortunately, there is extensive cross-reactivity between the antigens of *H. capsulatum, Coccidioides immitis,* and *Blastomyces dermatitidis* in lymphocyte transformation assays, so these results must be accepted with caution.[7]

An interesting difference is found when lymphocyte transformation is studied in patients with active histoplasmosis. When compared to healthy patients with positive histoplasmin skin tests, patients with active histoplasmosis demonstrate severe depression of blastogenesis to both mycelial and yeast-phase *Histoplasma* antigens.[8] It appears that suppression of lymphocyte transformation is mediated by *Histoplasma* antibody alone or in conjunction with antigen.

Artz and Bullock have studied both the cell-mediated and humoral immune response to *Histoplasma* in the C_3H mouse following the intravenous inoculation of yeast-phase *H. capsulatum.*[1,2] The disease produced is self-limited, lasting up to 8 weeks after injection. Complement-fixing antibody to the *yeast*-phase of *Histoplasma,* first detected at week 1, peaks at week 3, and has already declined by week 8. In contrast, complement-fixing antibody to the mycelial phase is not observed until week 3 and does not peak until week 18. The kinetics of this humoral response are similar to those reported in humans by Chandler and colleagues.[5]

At the time of initial antibody production to yeast-phase *Histoplasma,* there is a dramatic enlargement of the spleen to three times its normal size and simultaneous atrophy of the thymus. Similar atrophy of the thymus has been observed after intravenous infection with *T. gondii.*[22] These morphologic changes slowly revert toward normal, with the spleen returning to only twice its normal size and the thymus returning to normal size by week 8. It appears that in the first week following infection, thymocytes migrate to the spleen, where further differentiation and clonal expansion occur. In addition to thymocyte migration, antigen-specific trapping of recirculating lymphocytes occurs within the spleen, and it is likely that lymphoid cells specifically committed to *Histoplasma* are retained and further expand the splenic population.[12]

Of most interest is the observation that the cellular immune responses of these mice were diminished considerably. This was associated with the presence of potent immunosuppressor activity in the spleen. From 1 to 3 weeks following inoculation, there was (1) depression of the delayed-type hypersensitivity response to sheep erythrocytes and histoplasmin; (2) impairment of concanavalin A– and histoplasmin-induced blastogenic transformation by splenocytes *in vitro;* (3) depressed cytotoxic activity of spleen cells from infected mice; and (4) extensive suppression by splenocytes from infected mice of the primary antibody response to sheep erythrocytes by normal spleen cultures. With resolution of the infection by week 8, there was a shift of immunoregulatory function from dominant suppressor activity to expression of helper activity.[2]

Nickerson and colleagues further characterized the suppressor response in infected mice and demonstrated suppressor cells in the spleen and lymph nodes that inhibited both a T-dependent (sheep erythrocyte) and a T-independent (trinitrophenol-lipopolysaccharide) antigen.[38] Two populations of spleen cells express suppressor function in this model, one identified as T cells, the other with macrophage-like properties. If these findings are extrapolated to the human situation, it is likely that the depression of lymphocyte transformation noted in patients with active histoplasmosis is mediated at least in part by the generation of suppressor populations within the spleen and the lymphoid system.

Pathogenesis of the Ocular Lesions

How do these events explain the eye disease noted in the POHS? As previously emphasized, the POHS ony rarely follows disseminated infection or chronic pulmonary histoplasmosis; it occurs most frequently after benign disease. The infection is acquired by inhalation of mycelial spores, with subsequent dissemination of the yeast phase of the organism in the bloodstream.

Despite the mild nature of benign disease, multiple foci of dead or latent *Histoplasma* are demonstrable in numerous organs many years later at autopsy.[41]

It is reasonable to assume that throughout the life span of an infected individual, there are multiple asymptomatic transient episodes of *Histoplasma* fungemia originating from any of the foci. The recurrent intravascular dissemination of *H. capsulatum,* with entrapment in the choroid, could explain the changing pattern of peripheral spots that may occur many years later.[29,30,40,50] Smith and associates have clearly demonstrated in the primate that vascular injection of the yeast phase of *Histoplasma* can produce foci of chorioretinitis, which can evolve into an atrophic scar.[45,46,49] Histopathologic examination of active foci reveals organisms surrounded by many mononuclear cells, with frequent disruption of the adjacent RPE and Bruch's membrane.

We know that in mice, fungemia is associated with the development of suppressor cell activity within the spleen and peripheral lymph nodes. Transient immunosuppression may allow replication of *Histoplasma* organisms randomly deposited in the choroid following intravascular dissemination. Clinically, they would appear as active foci of chorioretinitis. Such lesions would block fluorescence in the early phase of fluorescein angiography but would stain in the later phase. If the focus of inflammation is located in the peripheral retina, it would not be noticed by the patient, and a pattern of changing peripheral spots would occur.

On the other hand, if the focus of chorioretinitis were located in the macula, the patient would be symptomatic. Since Bruch's membrane and the RPE adjacent to this focus are frequently disrupted, the development of a subretinal neovascular membrane is not unexpected. Its presence may not be directly related to either the infecting organism or the subsequent immune response but rather, to the unique anatomical properties of the macula which predispose it to subretinal neovascularization in other entities, such as senile degenerative choroidopathy. This would explain the clinical observation that disciform maculopathy in the second eye of an individual with the POHS is usually in an area contiguous to an old atrophic scar.[18,48]

With the re-emergence of helper (and presumably killer) cell activity, the replicating *H. capsulatum* organisms are destroyed by the immune system. As the focus of inflammation in the peripheral lesion resolves, there is atrophy and proliferation of the surrounding RPE. Fluorescein angiography shows the characteristic window defect in the RPE without staining. As inflammation in the macula resolves, the patient's course becomes that of the natural evolution of a subretinal neovascular membrane, namely a serous or hemorrhagic detachment of the RPE or neurosensory retina.

Any explanation of the pathogenesis of the lesions in the POHS must account for the persistence of lymphocytes in the choroid of eyes many years after active disease.[23,32,34,41] Davidorf suggested that the *Histoplasma* organism is phagocytized within the lung by a macrophage, transformed to the yeast phase, and transported to the choroid, where it stimulates the immune response.[10] He postulates that either a small quantity of antigen that initiated the original response remains in the choroid, stimulating a smoldering inflammation, or sensitized T cells remain in the choroid without continued antigenic stimulus.

It is conceivable that *Histoplasma* organisms infect resident cells within the choroid or retina and serve as a persistent antigenic stimulus. However, the infected cells should eventually be destroyed by the immune response (and the nidus of inflammation quieted) unless the infectious organism can multiply and infect adjacent cells. However, organisms cannot easily be identified histopathologically in the choroid or retina.[28,56] Furthermore, it is unlikely that lymphoid cells will remain in the choroid without an antigenic stimulus. When ocular inflammation resolves following an antigenic stimulus, the lymphocytes involved in the immune response exit from the eye so that none can be observed on microscopic examination.[26]

Alternatively, persistent lymphocytic infiltration may reflect periodic seeding of the eye by recurrent fungemia. Other foci within the body could then serve as sources of antigen, so that a changing pattern of lesions would result. It is apparent that, since the POHS is not usually seen after disseminated or chronic pulmonary disease, there must be something unique about individuals with the POHS that predisposes them to eye involvement. Most clinical evidence suggests that these individuals manifest a different immunologic response when confronted with *H. capsulatum.* The uniqueness of their immune responsiveness appears to be genetically regulated.

HLA in the Presumed Ocular Histoplasmosis Syndrome

Braley and colleagues and Godfrey and coworkers were the first to observe an association between HLA-B7 and the POHS.[3,19] However, on further study, Meredith and colleagues demonstrated that the increased frequency of HLA-B7 (77% vs. 26% in controls) was seen only in patients with disciform scarring, not in those with peripheral atrophic spots.[35]

When HLA analysis was extended to include the HLA-D/DR locus, an even stronger association in both clinical subgroups was uncovered with the DRw2 allele.[36] It was found in 81% of patients with disciform scars, 62% of patients with peripheral atrophic scars, and only 28% of controls.

A study of black patients with the POHS demonstrated no HLA-B7 association, but instead showed a strong correlation with DRw2, although at a slightly lower frequency than that found in white patients.* Additionally, linkage disequilibrium for the DRw2 and MB1 alleles was observed in both races. The MB locus lies within the HLA-D/DR complex and contains independently inherited alleles.

The pathophysiologic importance of such a correlation is speculative. However, it is tempting to propose that a distinctive immunologic responsiveness to *H. capsulatum* is associated with the DRw2–MB1 allelic combination, which predisposes to the development of peripheral atrophic spots in the POHS. Furthermore, HLA-B7 may be antigenically modified by the organism so that the HLA-B7–*Histoplasma* complex serves as a target for the

*T.A. Meredith, personal communication

immune response, possibly associated with an increased frequency for disruption of the RPE and Bruch's membrane and the subsequent development of a subretinal neovascular membrane. These hypotheses can be verified experimentally, and it is hoped that their verification will contribute to our understanding of the POHS.

Ocular toxoplasmosis and the POHS are two of the most common inflammatory disorders of the posterior segment. Since the latter disease has been documented in areas of the world where histoplasma is not endemic, doubt has arisen concerning the role of *H. capsulatum* in this disease. Nevertheless, both diseases are characterized by a changing pattern of lesions thought to be related to the immune response to a specific pathogen. As our understanding of the immune response to these two pathogens increases and we further clarify the unique immunologic characteristics of the eye, the reasons for the distinctive clinical characteristics of each disease should become clear. Only then will effective therapeutic intervention be possible so that the destructive visual effects of recurrent inflammation or new lesions will be eliminated.

REFERENCES

1. Artz RP, Bullock WE: Immunoregulatory responses in experimental disseminated histoplasmosis: Lymphoid organ histopathology and serologic studies. Infect Immunol 23:884, 1979
2. Artz RP, Bullock WE: Immunoregulatory responses in experimental disseminated histoplasmosis: Depression of T cell–dependent and T effector responses by activation of splenic suppressor cells. Infect Immunol 23:893, 1979
3. Braley RE, Meredith TA, Aaberg TM, et al: The prevalence of HLA-B7 in presumed ocular histoplasmosis. Am J Ophthalmol 85:859, 1978
4. Cantor H, Gershon RK: Immunological circuits: Cellular composition. Fed Proc 38:2058, 1979
5. Chandler JW, Smith TK, Newberry WM, et al: Immunology of the mycoses. II. Characterizaton of the immunoglobulin and antibody responses in histoplasmosis. J Infect Dis 119:247, 1969
6. Check IJ, Diddie KR, Jay WM, et al: Lymphocyte stimulation by yeast phase *Histoplasma capsulatum* in presumed ocular histoplasmosis syndrome. Am J Ophthalmol 87:311, 1979
7. Cox RA: Cross-reactivity between antigens of *Coccidioides immitis, Histoplasma capsulatum,* and *Blastomyces dermatitidis* in lymphocyte

transformation assays. Infect Immunol 2:32, 1972
8. Cox RA: Immunologic studies of patients with histoplasmosis. Am Rev Respir Dis 120:143, 1979
9. David JR: Delayed hypersensitivity in vitro: Its mediation by cell-free substances formed by lymphoid cell–antigen interaction. Proc Natl Acad Sci USA 56:72, 1966
10. Davidorf FH: The role of T lymphocytes in the reactivation of presumed ocular histoplasmosis scars. Int Ophthalmol Clin 15:111, 1975
11. Drath DB, Karnovsky ML: Superoxide production by phagocytic leukocytes. J Exp Med 141:257, 1975
12. Ford WI: The recruitment of recirculating lymphocytes in the antigenically stimulated spleen. Clin Exp Immunol 12:243, 1972
13. Fowles RE, Fajardo IM, Liebowitch JL, et al: The enhancement of macrophage bacteriostasis by products of activated lymphocytes. J Exp Med 138:952, 1973
14. Ganley JP: Epidemiologic characteristics of presumed ocular histoplasmosis. ACTA Ophthalmol (Copenh) (Suppl): 119, 1973
15. Ganley JP: The role of the cellular immune system in patients with macular disciform histoplasmosis. Int Ophthalmol Clin 15:83, 1975
16. Ganley JP, Nemo GJ, Comstock GW, et al: Lymphocyte transformation in presumed ocular histoplasmosis. Arch Ophthalmol 99:1424, 1981
17. Ganley JP, Smith RE, Knox DL, et al: Presumed ocular histoplasmosis. III. Epidemiologic characteristics of people with peripheral atrophic scars. Arch Ophthalmol 89:116, 1973
18. Gass JDM, Wilkinson CP: Follow-up study of ocular histoplasmosis. Trans Am Acad Ophthalmol Otolaryngol 76:672, 1972
19. Godfrey WA, Sabates R, Cross DE: Association of presumed ocular histoplasmosis with HLA-B7. Am J Ophthalmol 85:854, 1978
20. Golub ES: The Cellular Basis of the Immune Response, 2nd ed, pp 13–68, 235–275. Sunderland, Massachusetts, Sinauer Associates, 1981
21. Howard DH, Otto V: Experiments on lymphocyte-mediated cellular immunity in murine histoplasmosis. Infect Immunol 16:226, 1977
22. Huldt GS, Gard S, Olouson SG: Effect of *Toxoplasma gondii* on the thymus. Nature 244:301, 1973
23. Irvine AR, Spencer WH, Hogan MJ, et al: Presumed ocular histoplasmosis syndrome. A clinicopathologic case report. Trans Am Ophthalmol Soc 74:91, 1976
24. Jones CT, Len L, Hirsch JG: Assessment in vitro of immunity against *Toxoplasma gondii.* J Exp Med 141:466, 1975
25. Jones DB: Presumed histoplasmic choroiditis. A possible late manifestation of a benign disease. In Aiello L, Chick EW, Furcolow ML (eds): Histo-

plasmosis: Proceedings of the Second National Conference. Springfield, Illinois, Charles C Thomas, 1971

26. Kaplan HJ, Streilein JW: Immune response to immunization via the anterior chamber of the eye: I. F_1 lymphocyte–induced immune deviation. J Immunol 118:809, 1977

27. Karnovsky ML, Lazdins JK: Biochemical criteria for activated macrophages. J Immunol 121:809, 1978

28. Khalil MK: Histopathology of presumed ocular histoplasmosis. Am J Ophthalmol 94:369, 1982

29. Krill AE, Chishti MI, Klien BA, et al: Multifocal inner choroiditis. Trans Am Acad Ophthalmol Otolaryngol 73:222, 1969

30. Lewis ML, Van Newkirk MR, Gass JDM: Follow-up study of presumed ocular histoplasmosis syndrome. Ophthalmology 87:390, 1980

31. Mackaness GB: The influence of immunologically committed lymphoid cells on macrophage activity in vivo. J Exp Med 129:973, 1969

32. Makley TA, Craid EL, Long JW: Histopathology of presumed ocular histoplasmosis. Palestra Oftalmol Pan Am 1:71, 1977

33. McDevitt HO, Chinitz A: Genetic control of the antibody response: Relationship between immune response and histocompatability (H-Z) type. Science 163:1207, 1969

34. Meredith TA, Green WR, Key SN, et al: Ocular histoplasmosis: Clinicopathologic correlation of three cases. Surv Ophthalmol 22:189, 1977

35. Meredith TA, Smith RE, Braley RE, et al: The prevalence of HLA-B7 in presumed ocular histoplasmosis in patients with peripheral atrophic scars. Am J Ophthalmol 86:325, 1978

36. Meredith TA, Smith RE, DuQuesnoy RJ: Association of HLA-DRw2 antigen with presumed ocular histoplasmosis. Am J Ophthalmol 89:70, 1980

37. Nathan CF, Silverstein SC, Brukner LH, et al: Extracellular cytolysis by activated macrophages and granulocytes. II. Hydrogen peroxide as a mediator of cytotoxicity. J Exp Med 149:100, 1979

38. Nickerson DA, Havens RA, Bullock WE: Immunoregulation in disseminated histoplasmosis: Characterization of splenic suppressor cell populations. Cell Immunol 60:287, 1981

39. Reinherz EL, Kung PC, Goldstein G, et al: Discrete stages of human intrathymic differentiation: Analysis of normal thymocytes and leukemic lymphoblasts of T cell lineage. Proc Natl Acad Sci USA 77:1588, 1980

40. Schlaegel TF: The natural history of histo spots in the disc macular area. Int Ophthalmol Clin 15:9, 1975

41. Schlaegel TF: Ocular Histoplasmosis. New York, Grune & Stratton, 1977

42. Schlaegel TF: Toxoplasmosis. In Duane TD, Jaeger EA (eds): Clinical Ophthalmology, Vol 4. Philadelphia, Harper & Row Publishers, 1984

43. Schwartz RH, Yano A, Paul WE: Interaction between antigen-presenting cells and primed T lymphocytes: An assessment of Ir gene expression in the antigen-presenting cell. Immunol Rev 40:153, 1978

44. Shimada K, O'Connor GK, Yoneda C: Cyst formation by *Toxoplasma gondii* (RH strain) in vitro. Arch Ophthalmol 92:496, 1974

45. Smith RE, Dunn S, Jester JV: Natural history of experimental histoplasmic choroiditis in the primate. I. Clinical features. Invest Ophthalmol Vis Sci 25:801, 1984

46. Smith RE, Dunn S, Jester JV: Natural history of experimental histoplasmic choroiditis in the primate. II. Histopathologic features. Invest Ophthalmol Vis Sci 25:810, 1984

47. Smith RE, Ganley JP: An epidemiologic study of presumed ocular histoplasmosis. Trans Am Acad Ophthalmol Otolaryngol 75:994, 1971

48. Smith RE, Knox DL, Jensen AD: Ocular histoplasmosis: Significance of asymptomatic macular scars. Arch Ophthalmol 89:296, 1973

49. Smith RE, Macy JI, Parrett C, et al: Variations in acute multifocal histoplasmic choroiditis in the primate. Invest Ophthalmol Vis Sci 17:1005, 1978

50. Tewari RP, Sharma DK, Mathur A: Significance of thymus-derived lymphocytes in immunity elicited by immunization with ribosomes of live yeast cells of *Histoplasma capsulatum*. J Infect Dis 138:605, 1978

51. Tewari RP, Sharma DK, Solotorovsky M, et al: Adoptive transfer of immunity from mice immunized with ribosomes of live yeast cells of *Histoplasma capsulatum*. Infect Immunol 15:789, 1977

52. Unanue ER: Cooperation between mononuclear phagocytes and lymphocytes in immunity. N Engl J Med 303:977, 1980

53. Ward PA, Remold HG, David JR: Leukotactic factor produced by sensitized lymphocytes. Science 163:1079, 1969

54. Watzke RC, Claussen RW: The long-term course of multifocal choroiditis (presumed ocular histoplasmosis). Am J Ophthalmol 91:750, 1981

55. Weber JC, Schlaegel TF: Delayed skin test reactivity of uveitis patients. Influence of age and diagnosis. Am J Ophthalmol 67:732, 1969

56. Weingeist TA, Watzke RC: Ocular involvement by *Histoplasma capsulatum*. Int Ophthalmol Clin 23:33, 1983

57. Williams DM, Graybill JR, Drutz DJ: *Histoplasma capsulatum* infection in nude mice. Infect Immunol 21:973, 1978

20

The Role of Vitrectomy in Endophthalmitis

Richard L. Abbott

Endophthalmitis is an inflammatory response to injured intraocular tissues and may be either infectious or sterile in nature. Proper management requires rapid determination of an infectious or sterile etiology, followed by institution of appropriate therapy. Infectious etiologies include both acute and long-term postoperative cases, cases that appear after penetrating trauma to the globe, and those cases that are endogenous—originating from an infectious site elsewhere in the body.

Depending on the underlying etiology and route of infection, the clinical presentation of endophthalmitis can be quite varied and may not demonstrate several of the more classic findings that have been described in this condition (i.e., severe pain, chemosis, lid edema).[10] The clinician should have a high degree of suspicion in any case in which the inflammatory response seems out of proportion for what would normally be expected considering the extent of surgery or trauma and should proceed with a diagnostic workup.

The management of infectious endophthalmitis is one of the most challenging and serious ocular problems confronting the ophthalmologist. During the past decade, numerous diagnostic and therapeutic techniques have been studied with renewed interest both in the laboratory and in clinical studies.[18] The need for new therapeutic modalities was based on discouraging clinical results with conventional therapy, including systemic, periocular, and topical

treatments, and on confirmation in the animal model that dosages of antibiotic necessary for treatment success were lacking in the vitreous.[11]

Intravitreal antibiotic administration and vitrectomy in the management of infectious endophthalmitis are now widely used modes of therapy.[14] Laboratory and clinical studies have demonstrated the relative safety, enhanced delivery, and improved results in both animal models and humans with intraocular antibiotics over more conventional routes of therapy.[5,9,11,15,17] In addition, several studies have shown the use of vitrectomy to offer some distinct advantages over intraocular antibiotics alone.[4,7,17,19]

The role of vitreous surgery in the management of infectious endophthalmitis, however, does remain controversial. Present clinical information on its risk:benefit ratio is inconclusive.[14]

This chapter discusses the rationale and basic principles for using vitrectomy in the management of infectious endophthalmitis. The surgical approach and possible complications will also be discussed.

RATIONALE FOR VITRECTOMY

Conventional methods (systemic, periocular, and topical antibiotics) for the treatment of culture-proven endophthalmitis have traditionally been unsuccessful.[2,8] These poor results are best

313

explained by the relative impermeability of the blood–retina barrier to the antibiotics and the subsequent inability of these drugs to reach the infecting organisms.[16] In addition, the presence of organized inflammatory debris in the vitreous cavity enhances the destructive properties of the infectious process by further prohibiting antibiotic penetration and toxic by-product removal.

Forster and Cottingham developed an animal model to study the possibility of using vitrectomy as a means to remove the bulk of infectious organisms and associated inflammatory debris from the vitreous cavity.[4] Their rationale was based on the general surgical principle of incision and drainage of an abscess in other parts of the body. It seemed reasonable that "draining" the vitreous cavity of this purulent debris would allow greater mobility of the instilled intravitreal antibiotics and the eye's own natural defense mechanisms. Further studies by others have substantiated this basic rationale for using vitrectomy in these cases.[5,6,12]

In summary, the rationale for employing vitrectomy in the management of infectious endophthalmitis is

1. It allows bulk removal of organisms and inflammatory debris.
2. It provides better samples for microscopic examination and cultures.
3. It reduces the likelihood of later intravitreal organization.
4. It improves circulation of intravitreal drugs.
5. It may improve penetration of local and systemic drugs into the vitreous.

INDICATIONS FOR VITRECTOMY

The use of vitrectomy in the management of endophthalmitis can be for either diagnostic or therapeutic purposes. Prior to therapeutic intervention, it is necessary to obtain a diagnostic culture from the vitreous cavity.[10] This can be accomplished with a 23- or 25-gauge needle attached to a 1-ml tuberculin syringe, either through the limbus in aphakic patients or through the pars plana in phakic patients. If an inadequate vitreous sample is obtained or if one suspects a fungal etiology, then the limbal or pars plana incision is enlarged and a vitreous

instrument is introduced to remove formed vitreous. Such a sample, diluted by the irrigating solution, is then passed through a disposable membrane filter system. The filter is then removed in a sterile manner and cut into pieces for appropriate inoculation onto media.[11]

The indications for *therapeutic* vitrectomy in the management of infectious endophthalmitis are not clearly defined. All would agree, however, that prompt initiation of a management plan is necessary when a patient presents with a suspected endophthalmitis.

The duration of the inflammatory response and the organism responsible for the infection together probably are the most critical factors in determining the likelihood of salvaging useful vision by any therapeutic technique. The criteria for using vitrectomy in the management protocol are based primarily on these two factors and relate mainly to more advanced cases of endophthalmitis.

As mentioned previously, part of the rationale for using vitrectomy is to remove the bulk of infecting organisms and associated inflammatory debris and to allow greater antibiotic access to the remaining organisms. Combining this rationale with evidence of either prolonged onset or a particularly virulent organism, or both, the following indications for vitrectomy surgery can be recommended:

- Extensive formation of a vitreous abscess that precludes visualization of the retina[5,13,18]
- Ultrasound evidence of vitreous abscess formation if opacities in the anterior chamber limit visualization of the fundus[5]
- Worsening of the clinical course in eyes initially treated with periocular, systemic, and intraocular antibiotics[13]
- Worsening of the clinical course in untreated eyes with suspected bacterial endophthalmitis of more than 48 hours' duration[5,13]
- Suspected cases of fungal endophthalmitis in which vitreous involvement was widespread and there was a delay in obtaining culture results[18]
- Laboratory evidence of intravitreal gramnegative organisms with severe vitreous involvement

SURGICAL APPROACH

The key to successful management of infectious endophthalmitis cases is to provide the maximum effective therapy with the least amount of delay. Table 20-1 outlines suggested diagnostic

Table 20-1. Diagnostic and Management Protocols in the Surgical Approach

I. Diagnosis
  A. Signs and Symptoms
    1. Pain
    2. Upper lid swelling
    3. Inflamed and chemotic conjunctiva
    4. Corneal edema
    5. Turbid aqueous, hypopyon
    6. Absent red reflex
    7. Poor vision
    8. Increasing cells and membranes in vitreous
    9. Often suppuration at wound
  B. Delay of Onset of Infection Suggests
    1. Mycotic infection (weeks)
    2. Infected filtering bleb (weeks, months, or years)
    3. Fistula or "vitreous wick" to wound (weeks or months)
    4. Bacteria of lesser virulence *(Staphylococcus epidermidis, Propionibacterium acnes)*
II. Preoperative Management
  A. Culture Technique
    1. Culture lid margins, conjunctiva, infected bleb, or flap
    2. Anterior chamber and vitreous aspiration
    3. Obtain Gram's and Giemsa stain of aspirate
    4. Perform Grocott's methenamine silver stain if fungus is suspected
    5. Direct inoculation onto culture media
      a. Blood agar (two plates, 37°C and 25°C)
      b. Chocolate agar (in candle jar)
      c. Brain heart infusion (BHI) broth
      d. Thioglycolate broth (anaerobes)
      e. Sabouraud's agar with gentamicin
  B. Medical Management of Early Cases
    1. Onset of symptoms within 12 to 24 hours
    2. Red reflex present
    3. Early vitreous involvement
    4. Diagnostic workup
      a. Culture lid margins, conjunctiva, and flap
      b. Proceed into diagnostic anterior chamber and vitreous aspiration

     c. Inoculate cultures; obtain appropriate stains
    5. Medical therapy
      a. Intraocular
        Gentamicin, 0.1 mg (100 μg), *and*
        Cefazolin (Ancef), 2.25 mg *and*
        Decadron, 400 μg*
          or
        Gentamicin, 0.1 mg (100 μg), *and*
        Vancomycin, 1 mg *and*
        Decadron, 400 μg*
      b. Subconjunctival
        Gentamicin, 40 mg, *and*
        Cefazolin, 100 mg, *or*
        Methicillin, 100 mg
        Aristocort, 40 mg (periocular)
      c. Topical
        Gentamicin, 9 mg/ml *and*
        Cefazolin, 33 mg/ml
      d. Systemic
        Cefazolin, 1 gram stat; 1 gram every 6 hours (intravenously)
    6. Follow-up management
      a. Observe for 24 hours
      b. Change antibiotics depending on isolate and sensitivity
      c. Continue observation if condition is stable or improving
      d. If condition worsens
        (1) Consider repeat intraocular antibiotics
        (2) Consider vitrectomy
      e. If culture is negative
        (1) Do not repeat intraocular antibiotics
        (2) Consider tapering or discontinuing antibiotics
        (3) Consider increasing steroids
  C. Medical Management of More Advanced Cases
    1. Onset of symptoms later than 48 hours
    2. No red reflex
    3. Significant vitreous involvement
    4. Management
      a. Repeat diagnostic workup and medical therapy
      b. Therapeutic vitrectomy; pass material through membrane filter
      c. Follow-up management as for early cases

---

*The use of intraocular steroids is controversial. Their use may retard the eye's response against *Pseudomonas* and fungal organisms. Argument in favor of their use stresses their ability to potentially lessen the effects of toxins on the retina and to prevent the formation of intravitreal bands.

and management protocols in the approach to these extremely difficult cases.[1,11] The following sections describe the surgical technique and complications of vitrectomy.

Surgical Technique

The following checklist describes steps to be taken in preparation for surgery:

1. Operating room alerted and prepared for a "dirty" case
2. Glass slides and culture media brought to operating room for direct inoculation
3. Antibiotics ordered for intraocular and periocular use
4. General anesthesia arranged, if possible

Although the limbal approach can be used in endophthalmitis cases requiring vitrectomy, poor visualization and increased corneal and iris trauma often make the pars plana approach preferable. In most of these cases, visualization is barely adequate and requires extreme care and skill by the surgeon. Prior to insertion of the vitreous instrument into the eye, any prior surgical wound should be closely checked to ensure tight closure and to avoid possible complications later in the management of the case.[3]

The vitrectomy instrument is carefully introduced into the eye, 3 mm to 3.5 mm posterior to the limbus at an angle aimed toward the center of the vitreous cavity, if a lens is present. Low-suction force is used to first remove the anterior hyaloid face. The iris tissue can be quite necrotic, and care should be taken to avoid contact or traction. After the anterior vitreous is removed, the endoilluminator is introduced for improved visualization. Only a "core" vitrectomy should be done, with no effort made to separate the posterior cortical vitreous from the retina if a posterior vitreous separation is not already present.[13] Extreme care should be taken to avoid any traction on the frequently necrotic retina.[3] The dense vitreous debris should be removed for smear, culture, and sensitivity and may be passed through a millipore filter for increased concentration of the specimen. After the "core" vitrectomy has been completed, in-traocular antibiotics are given into the mid-vitreous prior to closing the vitrectomy wound.

Complications of Vitrectomy

Although vitrectomy has become a frequently used therapeutic modality in the management of the more severe cases of endophthalmitis, there are increased risks associated with this procedure. The performance of vitrectomy in a case of endophthalmitis is difficult because of poor visibility, the necrotic and edematous state of the retina, and diffuse ocular inflammation. Retinal breaks and detachment related to retinal necrosis and surgically induced retinal traction occur in at least 10% of the cases.[3] Other complications may include corneal edema, secondary glaucoma, and cataract formation. As stated above, vitreous surgery should be held in reserve and used for the more severe and progressive cases of endophthalmitis.

REFERENCES

1. Abbott RL: Diagnosis and management of infectious endophthalmitis. Ouctome/Fragmatome Newsletter, p 2. Irvine, California, Cooper-Vision Systems, 1982
2. Allen HG, Mangiaracine AB: Bacterial endophthalmitis after cataract extraction: I. A study of 22 infections in 20,000 operations. Arch Ophthalmol 72:454, 1964
3. Charles S: Endophthalmitis. In Vitreous Microsurgery, p 155. Baltimore, Williams & Wilkins, 1981
4. Cottingham AJ, Jr, Forster RK: Vitrectomy in endophthalmitis: Results of study using vitrectomy, intraocular antibiotics, or a combination of both. Arch Ophthalmol 94:2078, 1981
5. Diamond JG: Intraocular management of endophthalmitis: A systematic approach. Arch Ophthalmol 99:96, 1981
6. Eichenbaum DM, Jaffe NS, Clayman HM, Light DS: Pars plana vitrectomy as a primary treatment for acute bacterial endophthalmitis. Am J Ophthalmol 86:167, 1978
7. Fisher JR, Civiletto SE, Forster RK: Toxicity, efficacy, and clearance of intravitreally injected Cefazolin. Arch Ophthalmol 100:650, 1982
8. Forster RK: Endophthalmitis: Diagnostic cultures and visual results. Arch Ophthalmol 92:387, 1972
9. Forster RG, Zachary IG, Cottingham AJ, Jr,

Norton EWD: Further observations on the diagnosis, cause and treatment of endophthalmitis. Am J Ophthalmol 81:52, 1976

10. Forster RK: Endophthalmitis. In Duane TM (ed): Clinical Ophthalmology, vol 4, Chap 24. Hagerstown, Harper & Row, 1978

11. Forster RK, Abbott RL, Gelender H: Management of infectious endophthalmitis. Ophthalmology 87:313, 1980

12. McGetrick JK, Peyman GA: Vitrectomy in experimental endophthalmitis. II. Bacterial endophthalmitis. Ophthalmic Surg 10:87, 1979

13. Michels RG: Vitreous Surgery, p 345. St. Louis, CV Mosby, 1981

14. Olson JC, Flynn HW, Forster RK, Culbertson WW: Results in the treatment of postoperative endophthalmitis. Ophthalmology 90:692, 1983

15. Peyman GA, Vastine DW, Crouch ER, Herbst RW: Clinical use of intravitreal antibiotics to treat bacterial endophthalmitis. Trans Am Acad Ophthalmol Otolaryngol 78:862, 1974

16. Peyman GA, May DR, Homer PI, Kasbeer RT: Penetration of gentamicin into the aphakic eye. Ann Ophthalmol 7:871, 1977

17. Peyman GH, Vastine DW, Raichand M: Symposium: Postoperative endophthalmitis. Experimental aspects and their clinical applications. Ophthalmology 85:374, 1978

18. Peyman GA, Raichand M, Bennett TO: Management of endophthalmitis and pars plana vitrectomy. Br J Ophthalmol 64:472, 1980

19. Zachary IG, Forster RK: Experimental intravitreal gentamicin. Am J Ophthalmol 82:604, 1976

21

Multifocal Chorioretinopathies

Lee M. Jampol

This chapter reviews the chorioretinopathies that exhibit multiple foci of inflammatory retinal and choroidal involvement with loss of visual function. These diseases include serpiginous choroiditis, bird-shot chorioretinopathy, acute retinal necrosis syndrome (ARN), multiple evanescent white dot syndrome, acute posterior multifocal placoid pigment epitheliopathy (APMPPE), acute macular neuroretinopathy, multifocal choroiditis and panuveitis, and acute retinal pigment epitheliitis. For some of the entities, such as serpiginous choroiditis, the etiology remains uncertain, while etiologic agents have been found for others, for example, acute retinal necrosis syndrome.

SERPIGINOUS CHOROIDITIS (GEOGRAPHIC CHOROIDITIS)

Serpiginous choroiditis is a chronic recurring disease in young to middle-aged patients.[6] Affected individuals often present with unilateral visual loss and multiple exacerbations in the same eye; usually both eyes eventually become involved. The clinical findings include vitreous cells and an occasional inflammatory reaction in the anterior chamber. Ophthalmoscopically, white edematous lesions (Fig. 21-1) appear to arise at the level of the retinal pigment epithelium (RPE) and choroid.

The lesions are most common in the peripap-

This research was sponsored in part by an unrestricted grant from Research to Prevent Blindness, Inc., New York, New York.

illary area, although they may occur in the macula or, more rarely, in other areas of the posterior pole. Recurrences usually extend away from the optic disc in a serpentine fashion, accounting for the name *serpiginous choroiditis.* Recurrent lesions are frequently adjacent to areas of previously healed chorioretinitis. The acute phase of the fluorescein angiogram shows blockage of fluorescence (Fig. 21-2) with later staining.

Inflammatory activity of the lesions last for several weeks, but the RPE and underlying choroidal vessels may gradually atrophy, with associated pigmentary clumping. Patients may have recurrences in either eye, although involvement is usually not simultaneous. In later stages, subretinal neovascularization may be seen. When the macula is involved, permanent central visual loss occurs. Amsler-grid testing reveals dense scotomas corresponding to the areas of healed chorioretinitis.

The etiology of this disease is not known. It has been suggested that tuberculosis may be the cause, but there is no evidence of active infection in the vast majority of patients. Systemic evaluation is usually not revealing. The differential diagnosis includes APMPPE. In patients with APMPPE the lesions usually resolve more rapidly with less atrophy of the choroid. The lesions in APMPPE commonly have a simultaneous onset in both eyes and true recurrences are rare. Patients with serpiginous choroiditis, as a rule, have recurrent episodes with activity present at different times and stages in both eyes. Visual recovery is the rule with APMPPE.

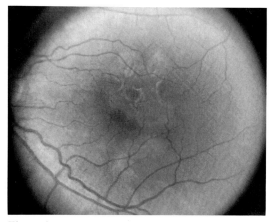

Figure 21-1. Acute white geographic lesions occur in the macula of a patient with serpiginous choroiditis.

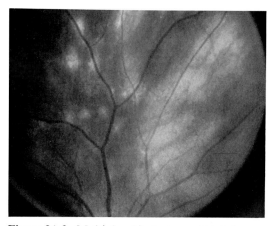

Figure 21-3. Multiple white lesions of bird-shot chorioretinopathy.

No therapy is of proven value in serpiginous choroiditis. Some clinicians believe that systemic or periocular corticosteroids may have an ameliorating effect.

BIRD-SHOT (VITILIGINOUS) CHORIORETINOPATHY

This disease of unknown etiology presents in older persons who suffer from a gradual loss of central vision with or without prominent vitreous floaters.[11] Occasionally, patients have nyc-

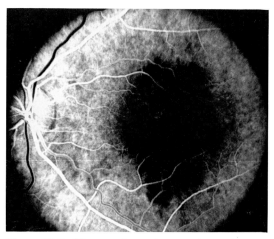

Figure 21-2. Fluorescein angiogram shows dark area corresponding to apparent hypofluorescence of the choroid.

talopia. The visual symptoms may be unilateral or bilateral, and visual acuity may vary from 20/20 to 20/100. Clinical examination shows evidence of chronic intraocular inflammation, characterized by vitreal cells and debris. Patients demonstrate multiple grayish-white or yellowish lesions at the level of the RPE, scattered throughout the posterior pole and midperiphery (Fig. 21-3). Evidence of retinal vascular dilation and leakage, cystoid macular edema, and optic disc edema is often seen. Mild anterior chamber reaction with fine keratic precipitates may be noted. Arteriolar narrowing and vascular sheathing have been described. There are no pars plana exudates, so the disease process may be distinguished from pars planitis. Electroretinographic measurements often show decreased amplitudes. Bird-shot chorioretinopathy follows a chronic course in which the visual function usually relates to the severity of the macular edema rather than the number of vitreal cells. With time, the RPE lesions become more atrophic and multiple depigmented spots may arise. Bird-shot chorioretinopathy is often exhibited in patients who show the HLA-A29 antigen. In addition, studies of lymphocytes in vitro in these patients demonstrate sensitization to retinal S antigen. This evidence suggests that bird-shot chorioretinopathy could be an autoimmune disease.

The differential diagnosis of bird-shot chorioretinopathy includes forms of intermediate uveitis (including pars planitis), the ocular histoplasmosis syndrome, and age-related vitritis. Treatment of bird-shot chorioretinopathy is often unsatisfactory. Systemic or periocular corticosteroids may offer some beneficial effect. The visual outcome, however, is often limited by chronic macular changes. In severe cases, cyclosporin has been tried because of the suggestion that this may be a disorder of the immune process involving T cells. A beneficial effect has been reported with this treatment.

ACUTE RETINAL NECROSIS SYNDROME (ARN)

A recently recognized entity, ARN was probably first reported by Urayama, who named the disease *Kirisawa's uveitis.* Patients present with unilateral or bilateral uveitis. Severe anterior and posterior chamber reactions may be noted, with flare, cells, fibrin, and marked vitritis. Subsequently, a necrotizing retinitis becomes apparent.[4] There is often profound vascular sheathing associated with retinal vascular occlusions, hemorrhage, and retinal infarction. The retinitis is often first seen in the peripheral fundus, although the changes may occasionally be present in the posterior pole. Whitening of the retina (Fig. 21-4) and RPE is seen. Some

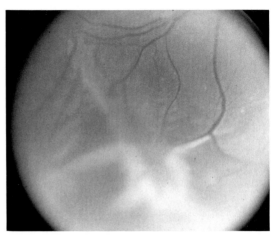

Figure 21-5. Retinal detachment is a complication of acute retinal necrosis syndrome.

patients show choroidal thickening. Serous elevation of the retina may also be exhibited. The retinitis extends posteriorly, with confluence of the lesions. If the macula is involved, central visual acuity is destroyed. Eventually, the lesions heal, and marked pigmentation and scarring develop. A late sequela is the development of vitreoretinal traction with retinal tears and retinal detachment (Fig. 21-5). These detachments are difficult to repair either with standard buckling procedures or aggressive vitrectomy. Loss of vision often occurs despite surgery.

The similarity of the clinical appearance of ARN syndrome to retinitis caused by herpesviruses (e.g., cytomegalovirus) was noted early on. There is now considerable evidence that at least some cases of ARN syndrome are caused by herpes zoster virus.[2] The differential diagnosis of ARN syndrome includes viral retinitis syndromes, disseminated toxoplasmosis of the retina, and necrotizing retinitis such as Bechet's disease. In most cases, the clinical appearance and rapid progression of ARN helps to differentiate the two entities.

No therapy is of proven value. Acyclovir seems to facilitate healing of the retinitis, but does not prevent retinal detachment. Prophylactic vitrectomy, scleral buckling, photocoagulation, and other measures have been advocated to prevent retinal detachment; however, their efficacy is not established.

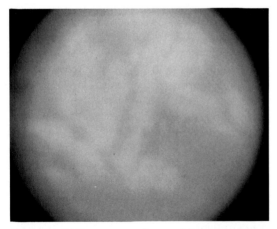

Figure 21-4. Large areas of necrotizing retinitis seen with acute retinal necrosis syndrome.

MULTIPLE EVANESCENT WHITE DOT SYNDROME (MEWDS)

The multiple evanescent white dot syndrome is a recently described syndrome that may lead to unilateral and (occasionally) bilateral loss of vision in young patients, usually females.[7,9] Affected patients present with central visual loss in one eye. Clinical examination reveals granularity in the foveal area (Fig. 21-6) and multiple small (100 to 200 μ) white dots at the level of the RPE (Fig. 21-7). These dots usually appear in the perimacular area and become less prominent at the equator and the fovea. Patients may show signs of intraocular inflammation with vitreous cells and retinal vascular sheathing. Edema of the optic disc may be noted. Fluorescein angiography reveals leakage at the level of the RPE and of the retinal and optic disc vasculature. During the acute phase, electroretinography (ERG) and early receptor potential (ERP) measurements show a markedly diminished amplitude, which may fully recover. Over a period of several weeks the lesions heal, and the white spots disappear. The macular granularity may partially disappear.

The cause of this disease remains uncertain. Systemic evaluations have so far been unrewarding. Occasional reports describe bilateral involvement, rare recurrences, and a delay in onset of the disease between one eye and the

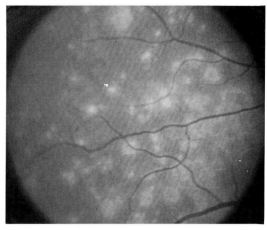

Figure 21-7. Note multiple evanescent white dots. Number of dots may vary from a few to many.

second eye. The excellent visual prognosis, however, militates against medical intervention. Corticosteroids or other therapeutic measures have not been shown to be of value.

ACUTE POSTERIOR MULTIFOCAL PLACOID PIGMENT EPITHELIOPATHY

Acute posterior multifocal placoid pigment epitheliopathy (APMPPE) was first described by Donald Gass in 1968.[5] The onset of the syn-

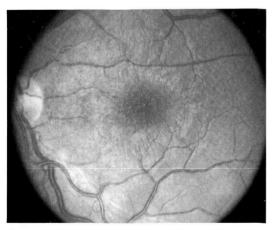

Figure 21-6. Characteristic granular macula with wrinkling of internal limiting membrane in patient with multiple evanescent white dot syndrome.

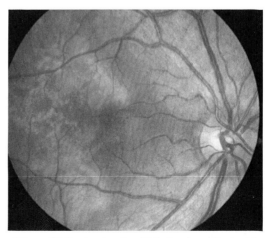

Figure 21-8. Acute placoid lesion in patient with acute posterior multifocal placoid pigment epitheliopathy.

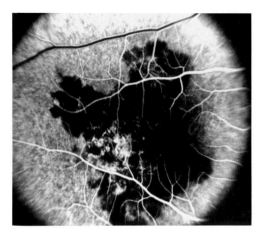

Figure 21-9. Fluorescein angiogram discloses hypoperfusion of choroid or blockage of choroidal fluorescence.

drome is often preceded by an influenza-like illness in young patients, usually adolescents, and is equally distributed among males and females. Both eyes are almost always affected. Patients may show signs of inflammation in the eye, including scleritis, iritis, and vitritis. Disc edema may also be noted. The classic feature of the disease is the presence of multiple, cream-colored, placoid lesions at the level of the RPE (Fig. 21-8). These lesions are geographic in configuration and are scattered around the posterior pole. The fovea may be involved. Initially, fluorescein angiography may show the lesions to be hypofluorescent (Fig. 21-9) with late staining. Controversy in the literature relates to whether the hypofluorescence corresponds to hypoperfusion of the underlying choriocapillaris or to swelling and opacification of the overlying RPE. During the acute phase of the disease, the patient may exhibit central nervous system involvement as manifested by meningeal symptoms and elevated protein levels in the cerebrospinal fluid with pleocytosis. Electroretinographic and electro-oculographic findings are normal. The placoid lesions resolve in 7 to 10 days, with the development of irregular pigmentation. The amount of pigment epithelial and choroidal atrophy is significantly less than that in serpiginous choroiditis. Central visual acuity usually recovers, although this may take months. In a few cases, permanent central visual loss occurs. Rarely, recurrences are observed.

However, serpiginous choroiditis should be considered in the differential diagnosis of these patients.

Whether APMPPE represents a possible viral disease of the RPE or a choroidal ischemic syndrome related to choroidal vasculitis is still unknown. No therapy has proved beneficial.

ACUTE MACULAR NEURORETINOPATHY

Acute macular neuroretinopathy is a rare disease, described in 1975 by Bos and Deutman, which is seen in young adults, mostly women.[1] It may be unilateral or bilateral. Patients complain of impaired vision, although central visual acuity may be normal by the Snellen chart test. Careful examination discloses paracentral scotomas in the involved eye associated with petal-shaped or multiple round lesions in the parafoveal areas, which are a darker red or brown than the surrounding retina (Fig. 21-10). Lesions appear to be present in the deep retina or RPE. The fluorescein angiographic picture is frequently normal, although there may be slight hyperfluorescence in the areas of involvement. Electroretinographic results are normal. Patients have prolonged loss of vision, although there may be a gradual improvement in visual acuity, scotoma size, and ophthalmoscopic appearance. No therapy is of proven benefit. The etiology of the disease remains uncertain.

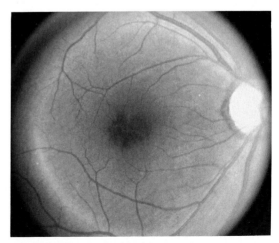

Figure 21-10. Petaloid brown lesions of acute macular neuroretinopathy.

MULTIFOCAL CHOROIDITIS
AND PANUVEITIS

Careful clinical examination in groups of patients with uveitis reveals a subset who present with multifocal areas of choroiditis, often associated with diffuse inflammation or panuveitis.[3] Patients show whitish foci in the peripheral retina, which in time may become confluent and pigmented (Fig. 21-11). There is often marked cellular reaction in the vitreous. Optic disc edema and cystoid macular edema may be present. Involvement may be unilateral or bilateral. Lesions may spare the posterior pole. Retinal vascular sheathing may be present. Peripapillary involvement has also been described. Some of the posterior lesions may develop subretinal neovascularization with destruction of the macula. The cause of this syndrome is unresolved.

A similar clinical appearance may be associated with progressive posterior pole and peripapillary subretinal scarring. This entity has been called *progressive subretinal fibrosis and uveitis* (Fig. 21-12).[10] It is not clear whether it represents a variant of multifocal choroiditis and panuveitis or is a separate disease. Patients often have bilateral progressive scarring in the subretinal space with distortion of the overlying retina. There may be cellular reaction in the vitreous, and there may or may not be discrete focal choroiditis in the periphery.

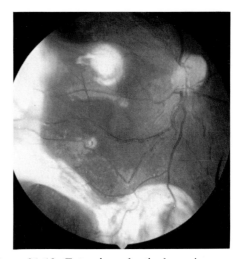

Figure 21-12. Extensive subretinal scarring (subretinal fibrosis).

PUNCTATE INNER
CHOROIDOPATHY (PIC)

Another recently described entity that resembles the two preceding ones is punctate inner choroidopathy.[12] This disease commonly occurs in myopic women who present with blurred vision and paracentral scotomas, unilaterally or bilaterally. Visual acuity may be as poor as finger counting. Examination of the posterior pole in these patients reveals clusters of small yellow-white lesions at the level of the choroid and RPE (Fig. 21-13). During the acute phase of the disease, a small overlying serous

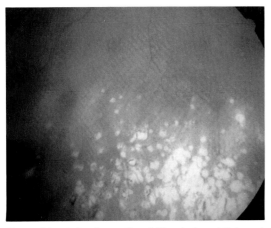

Figure 21-11. Lesions of multifocal choroiditis and panuveitis.

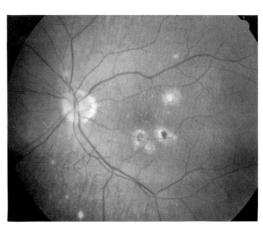

Figure 21-13. Multiple lesions in posterior pole with punctate inner choroidopathy.

detachment of the retina and fluorescein leakage from the lesions may develop. If the peripheral retina is involved, the syndrome may resemble multifocal choroiditis and panuveitis (see above). Subretinal neovascularization may arise as a late sequela in some of these lesions, with destruction of the macula in some patients. The clinical picture may resemble presumed ocular histoplasmosis, myopic chorioretinal degeneration, and multifocal choroiditis and panuveitis. With time, the lesions may enlarge or become pigmented. Recurrences develop and fresh lesions may be seen. Further clinical study is necessary to determine whether multifocal choroiditis and panuveitis, progressive subretinal fibrosis, and PIC represent variants of the same pathologic process. So far, no clues as to the etiology of any of these entities have emerged.

ACUTE RETINAL PIGMENT EPITHELIITIS

This rare disease was first described in 1972 by Alex Krill.[8] Recently, clinicians have questioned whether it is a distinct entity. Krill described young adults who developed an acute visual loss that varied from minimal to the level of 20/100. Some cases were unilateral, others, bilateral. Patients demonstrated normal anterior segments, but small discrete clusters of small brown and grayish spots (usually two to four spots per group) were seen in the involved macula. Sometimes, the spots were surrounded by a small yellow or white halo. Fluorescein angiography during the acute stage showed hypofluorescent areas with a surrounding halo that was sometimes hyperfluorescent. Electroretinography and visual evoked responses were normal. The electro-oculogram was said to be subnormal in amplitude. Lesions evolved over a 6- to 12-week period with a return of central visual acuity in most cases. The lesions darkened and became less prominent. The exact nature of this entity remains uncertain. Further clinical investigations are needed to confirm the existence of this disease as a separate entity.

REFERENCES

1. Bos PJM, Deutman AF: Acute macular neuroretinopathy. Am J Ophthalmol 80:573–584, 1975
2. Culbertson WW, Blumenkranz MS, Pepose JS, et al: Varicella zoster virus is a cause of the acute retinal necrosis syndrome. Ophthalmology 93:559–569, 1986
3. Dreyer RF, Gass JDM: Multifocal choroiditis and panuveitis. Arch Ophthalmol 102:1776–1784, 1984
4. Fisher JP, Lewis ML, Blumenkranz M, et al: The acute retinal necrosis syndrome. Part I: Clinical manifestations. Ophthalmology 89:1309–1316, 1980
5. Gass JDM: Acute posterior multifocal placoid pigment epitheliopathy. Arch Ophthalmol 80:177–185, 1968
6. Jampol LM, Orth D, Daily MJ, et al: Subretinal neovascularization with geographic (serpiginous) choroiditis. Am J Ophthalmol 88:683–689, 1979
7. Jampol LM, Sieving PA, Pugh D, et al: Multiple evanescent white dot syndrome. Arch Ophthalmol 102:671–674, 1984
8. Krill AE, Deutman AF: Acute retinal pigment epitheliitis. Am J Ophthalmol 74:193–205, 1972
9. Meyer RJ, Jampol LM: Recurrences and bilaterality in the multiple evanescent white dot syndrome. Am J Ophthalmol 101:388–389, 1986
10. Palestine AG, Nussenblatt RB, Parver LM, et al: Progressive subretinal fibrosis and uveitis. Br J Ophthalmol 68:667–673, 1984
11. Ryan JT, Maumenee AE: Birdshot retinochoroidopathy. Am J Ophthalmol 89:31–45, 1980
12. Watzke RC, Packer AJ, Folk JC, et al: Punctate inner choroidopathy. Am J Ophthalmol 98:572–584, 1984

6

Retinal Detachment and Vitreal Diseases

22

Management of Complicated Retinal Detachment

Mark S. Blumenkranz

The fundamental principle of retinal reattachment surgery is the same as that laid out by Gonin more than 50 years ago, namely, identification and closure of the retinal break.[14] A variety of surgical techniques have evolved during the ensuing half century. These include, but are not necessarily limited to, the following: the use of scleral imbrication, resection, exoplant, or implant material to produce a buckling effect in the wall of the globe; cryotherapy, diathermy, or photocoagulation to produce an irritative chorioretinal adhesion; and release of accumulated subretinal fluid. A decision on which combination of these techniques to incorporate in the operative procedure represents the balance between the desire to reapproximate the normal retinal position and the wish to avoid unnecessary surgical manipulation and, possibly, complications. Most experienced retina surgeons report long-term surgical reattachment rates of approximately 90%, figures that have remained relatively constant over the past 30 years.[31,35,42] The remaining 10% of cases not amenable to conventional scleral buckling, which are often referred to as *complicated retinal detachments,* are the subject of this chapter.

This investigation was supported in part by the Veterans Administration Hospital, Project #5421-01, Miami, Florida; in part by the Research to Prevent Blindness, Inc., New York, New York; by NIH Research Grants #EY 03934-01A1; #EY 06520 and #EY 05230; and by Core Facility Grant #EY 02180-06.

Rather than rely on retrospective assessment of success or failure to categorize complicated retinal detachment, I find the following mechanistic divisions useful in understanding retinal detachment and in planning surgical therapy.

Classification

TYPE I: Rhegmatogenous Retinal Detachment. The presence of subretinal fluid (usually bullous or convex in appearance) is (solely) pathogenetically related to kinetic interactions between the vitreous body and a visible retinal break (Fig. 22-1).

TYPE II: Tractional Retinal Detachment. The presence of subretinal fluid (flat or concave) is (solely) pathogenetically related to static or kinetic vitreous traction forces in the absence of a detectable retinal break (Fig. 22-2).

TYPE III: Complicated Retinal Detachment. The presence of subretinal fluid is pathogenetically related to the synergistic interaction between a retinal break and vitreous or periretinal tractional forces, either of which alone might not be capable of producing retinal detachment (Fig. 22-3).

TYPE IV: Serous Retinal Detachment. The presence of subretinal fluid is due to an irritative lesion in the choroid, resulting in retinal detachment.

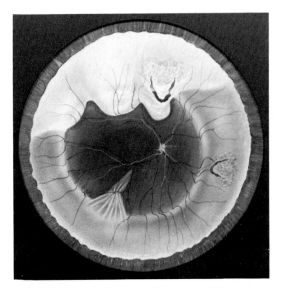

Figure 22-1. Type I retinal detachment (rhegmatogenous). Bullous subretinal fluid is present in association with improperly positioned buckle. Minor proliferative folds inferiorly, indicative of limited PVR, are incidental.

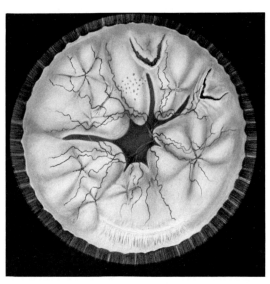

Figure 22-3. Type III retinal detachment (complicated). Mixed mechanism in which retinal breaks, although properly positioned, may leak owing to interaction with contractile membranes. Tight radial folds, often concealing small perioral retinal breaks, are seen inferiorly.

PREOPERATIVE EVALUATION

The Retinal Drawing

Careful preoperative evaluation remains a most critical step in the successful management of complicated retinal detachments. I prefer to use indirect ophthalmoscopy and the newer aspheric 28- and 30-diopter lenses, because they produce a large retinal field in which to evaluate and draw anatomic relationships; permit easy visualization through small pupils (found with iris-plane intraocular lenses, trauma, and surgical miosis); facilitate funduscopy through a gas bubble; and are smaller, lighter, and easier to manipulate. The relative disadvantage of image minification can be overcome by reducing the distance between the lens and the observer. The 20-diopter lens remains preferable for eyes with significant lenticular nuclear sclerosis or intravitreal liquid silicone.

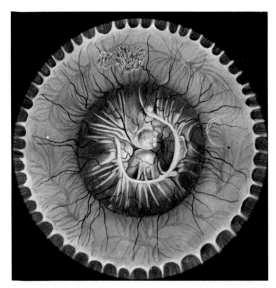

Figure 22-2. Type II retinal detachment (tractional). Shallow, concave retinal elevation with angular configuration of folds and circumferential tractional ridges. (Modified from Schepens C: Retinal Detachment and Allied Diseases. Philadelphia, WB Saunders, 1983)

Meticulous attention should be directed toward identification of all retinal breaks; the distribution, quantity, and appearance of subretinal fluid; the position, extent, and height of any pre-existing buckle; and vitreoretinal and periretinal tractional forces. Particular care should be given to the assessment of epiretinal membranes and their relationship to retinal breaks. The most subtle of these changes are best appreciated by examination with a contact lens.

Subretinal strands may be noted in long-standing retinal detachment. Most will not prohibit satisfactory settling of the retina unless they are intimately associated with a retinal break. The outer retinal opacification that occurs in the presence of preretinal membranes can be misinterpreted as a subretinal membrane, particularly when the preretinal membranes are relatively transparent. The recently proposed classification for proliferative vitreoretinopathy (PVR) standardizes these changes.[43]

In eyes that have undergone vitrectomy, sequential gas–fluid exchange can be performed at the bedside the evening before surgery with topical or local anesthesia after the retinal drawing has been completed. The details of this procedure are explained in a following section. When a 100% exchange has been performed, virtually all the subretinal fluid resulting from unsealed retinal breaks will be reabsorbed within 24 hours, regardless of the duration of the detachment. In this way areas of unresolved traction that might otherwise be obscured can be clearly identified and dealt with intraoperatively. If the exchange has been complete and the bubble has been adequate in size for at least 24 hours, any remaining subretinal fluid can be considered either tractional or exudative, depending on its configuration (type II or type IV). Occasionally, retinal reattachment will be so complete as to require only photocoagulation or intravitreal silicone infusion as a subsequent procedure.[7]

OPERATIVE PROCEDURE

The Role of Vitrectomy and Scleral Buckling

Whether to employ scleral buckling or vitrectomy or a combination of the two depends primarily on the preoperative evaluation. Consideration should be given to the clarity of the ocular media, the number and nature of previous surgeries, and the condition of the sclera. The age and health of the patient and the status of the fellow eye are additional factors in determining whether or not surgery should be performed and in selecting the type of procedure.

Previous reports have adequately demonstrated that scleral buckling alone is not a completely satisfactory solution to the management of PVR in the majority of cases. McMeel and colleagues have reported a 46% 6-month success rate in a large series of retinal detachments complicated by the development of PVR and treated by scleral buckling alone in the era before vitreous surgery.[29] Grizzard and Hilton have described an overall success rate of 34.7% for scleral buckling alone in eyes with varying degrees of PVR. However, eyes with stage C-3 disease or worse had only a 19% success rate.[18] Several guidelines emerge for answering the question: Is scleral buckling alone adequate therapy?

When a retinal break has not been included in or is improperly situated over an existing buckle and is associated with bullous subretinal fluid (type I), *modification of the buckle alone* may be all that is required. This solution is applicable even if significant vitreoretinal proliferative change occurs elsewhere in the fundus, as long as the ability of the break to settle and remain seated on the buckle is not affected. Unfortunately, concomitant adjacent proliferative change does not always allow adequate sealing of the retinal breaks to accomplish resolution of the rhegmatogenous component. In general when prominent star-folds are present in three or more quadrants, the chance for successful repair by buckling alone is considerably reduced.

Similarly, if no open breaks can be identified and the configuration of the detachment (type II) suggests a purely tractional etiology, vitrectomy alone is generally sufficient. This relatively uncommon situation in essence represents the advanced stage of the spectrum of macular pucker. Vitrectomy, membrane segmentation, peeling, and delamination relieve existing tractional forces and allow the retina to settle without the additional procedures of subretinal fluid drainage, tamponade by gas or silicone oil, chorioretinal adhesion production, and buckle modification.

Most often, the situation is not so simple as an unclosed hole or pure tractional detachment, and the choice of surgical procedure is more complex. The decision to modify an existing buckle in conjunction with vitrectomy entails considerable extension of operating time (buckle take-down, scar dissection, suturing, and buckle replacement); risk of perforation in eyes with thin sclera, previous dissection or diathermy, or multiple operations; increased postoperative inflammation (and occasional anterior segment ischemia); risk of postoperative intraocular pressure elevation; increased conjunctival scarring and risk of muscle dysfunction; and increased postoperative pain and disability. For these reasons, the decision to modify or replace an existing buckle in eyes indicated for vitreous surgery should be made with considerable deliberation.

The Scleral Buckle

When an open or leaking break is appropriately positioned over a pre-existing buckle of adequate height and extent, it need not be modified, irrespective of the height of break elevation or volume of subretinal fluid. Similarly, the buckle need not be replaced when no retinal breaks are identified (despite adequate visualization of the fundus) and an encircling buckle of reasonable height and breadth is present. The decision not to modify a pre-existing buckle carries with it significant implications for the surgical management of subretinal fluid and chorioretinal adhesion, as discussed in the following sections.

When retinal breaks can be identified anterior or posterior to a pre-existing buckle, a diligent attempt should be made to seal them with additional buckling material or to replace the buckle with a different element (in most cases). If PVR has developed before the primary scleral buckling procedure, a broad, moderately high, smooth encircling buckle should be placed. This has the advantage of covering seen and unseen breaks and minimizing the effects of pre-equatorial vitreoretinal contracture, which is difficult to remove by vitrectomy. The effect can be

achieved in a number of ways utilizing solid or sponge silicone exoplants. A grooved No. 287 solid silicone tire (MIRA) or oval 5- × 7.5-mm sponge is extremely effective when anchored by stout bites of nonabsorbable 5-0 suture (one or two per quadrant) extending from just behind the rectus insertions to 10 mm posterior. Larger elements such as 281 tires or trimmed 4- × 12-mm sponges can be used, although they are associated with a higher rate of postoperative choroidal detachment, anterior segment inflammation and ischemia, and pain. A surprisingly broad encircling effect can be produced with the use of relatively narrow solid silicone bands (2.5–4.0 mm), in which suture bites of 3.5 to 5.5 mm straddle the equator. In the latter case the height and breadth of the buckle are primarily functions of the horizontal shortening of the band rather than its thickness, width, or suture placement. For example, shortening a 4.0-mm band 15 mm from the normal equatorial circumference of the globe produces a buckle 1.5 mm high and 8.0 mm wide; shortening the same band 30 mm produces a buckle 3.8 mm high and 10 mm wide, comparable to that produced by the larger elements.

Prominently shortened solid silicone bands and larger ovoid elements both produce axial lengthening of the globe.[22] This accentuates the appearance of radial retinal folds (which also occur as the result of circumferential contracture of the nonexcised vitreous base) and promotes leakage of subretinal fluid in an anterior-to-posterior direction through small oral or pre-equatorial breaks (Fig. 22-4). In contrast, round encircling elements and very broad suture placement tend to reduce axial length and, so, counteract retinal shortening and the tendency toward radial-fold formation. The choice of element is influenced by several parameters. Large encircling sponges and tires are advantageous in eyes with posterior breaks (multiple radial elements beneath bands tend to leak) and breaks at widely varying levels, and in eyes with extensive peripheral proliferation producing perioral radial folding. Similarly, shortened bands are preferred in eyes with small or nonvisualized peripheral breaks, primarily posterior proliferation, staphylomatous sclera, or in patients at significant risk for vascular compromise such

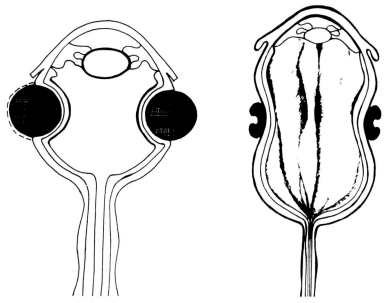

Figure 22-4. Axial elongation is produced by circumferential shortening of solid silicone band. This predisposes to induction of radial folds in retina, which promotes fish-mouthing, particularly in eyes with severe existing peripheral retinal contracture.

as the elderly and those with diabetic microangiopathy, sickle-cell disease, or acute retinal necrosis (all likely to develop type III detachment).

Occasionally, the possible adverse effects of supplemental scleral buckling outweigh the benefits, despite the presence of unsealed retinal breaks. These incude, but are not limited to macular holes, other very posterior breaks, previous extensive scleral dissection and diathermy, severe myopic staphylomatous scleral degeneration, previous scleral rupture, prior necrotizing infectious scleritis necessitating buckle removal, and poor anesthesia risk. While most of these breaks may be flattened intraoperatively, additional measures such as supplemental photocoagulation and vitreous tamponade must be taken to effect long-term closure and to stop leaks.

Chorioretinal Adhesion

Chorioretinal adhesion can be produced in a variety of ways, depending on the initial choice of procedure. If vitrectomy and membrane surgery alone are performed, without modification of a pre-existing buckle, then the approach by necessity must be transvitreal. If a scleral buckle is performed or revised, then the approach may be either transscleral or transvitreal. Both transscleral diathermy and cryotherapy have been advocated as external methods. Transscleral diathermy has the advantage of producing a more localized well-defined lesion with less retinal pigment epithelial fallout than cryotherapy. Additionally, it is claimed that the immediate diathermy lesion may be slightly more adhesive than that produced by cryotherapy, although this is subject to debate.[38] Disadvantages of diathermy are the associated scleral necrosis, which can be partially offset by treatment through partial-thickness scleral flaps, and the need for a large number of applications to cover broad areas. On the other hand, the cryoprobe is relatively easy to manipulate; a smaller number of applications are required to treat a given area with cryotherapy than with diathermy; and there is no need to create scleral flaps.

Additional theoretical issues to be considered in the choice of treatment modality for the production of the chorioretinal adhesion include the duration of internal tamponade required to permit adequate maturation and strengthening of the chorioretinal adhesion; the extent of treatment required to maximize probability of long-term retinal reattachment; and the optimal treatment modality by the transvitreal route.

Experimental cryogenic studies in rabbits indicate that within the first week following moderate treatment, pigment epithelial proliferation is maximal at the periphery of the lesions. Flattened depigmented epithelium slides toward the center of the lesions, where Bruch's membrane is denuded by depolarized injured epithelial cells migrating toward the inner retinal layers. Heavy lesions may result in localized exudative detachments, whereas very light lesions may preserve the outer nuclear layer and prevent the formation of glial pigment epithelial attachments.

Studies of tractional force, however, suggest that all three types of application eventually produce a retinal adhesion. In the months and years following cryotherapy, further remodeling of the adhesion occurs; the pigment epithelium is repolarized and Müller cells form intervillous rather than desmosomal interconnections.[23]

This sequence of events appears quite similar to that of the changes observed following transcorneal argon-laser photocoagulation, although damage to the middle and inner retinal layers in the latter appears to be less severe than in medium and heavy cryo-lesions. Investigations on the adhesive force of the RPE performed on normal and treated rabbits indicate that, besides the cellular proliferative and reparative mechanisms that become active in the second through fourth weeks after treatment, a variety of physiologic mechanisms make an important and immediate contribution to adhesiveness. Intrinsic RPE adhesiveness may be affected by oxygenation, intraocular osmolality, intravascular oncotic pressure, and pharmacologic agents such as Diamox and depolarizing agents.[28] Many of these physiologic mechanisms are deranged in the immediate postoperative period, depending on the choice of surgical procedure, suggesting that retinal adhesiveness may actually be decreased temporarily as a result of treatment. This concept is supported by additional studies in rabbits, in which actual weakening of the RPE adhesion occurred during the first 48 hours and strengthened by 96 hours.[20] Thus, an initial

period of 3 to 4 days appears necessary to re-establish the adhesiveness related to normal physiologic homeostatic mechanisms, and a longer period (approximately 2 weeks) is required to produce newly modeled intercellular complexes.

How extensive treatment should be remains unsettled, although several prudent guidelines are available. Elevated breaks associated with recurrent detachment should be re-treated if the interval between redetachment and primary treatment is greater than 2 weeks. Very heavy or extensive cryotherapy is associated with intravitreal liberation of pigment epithelial cells and marked breakdown of the blood–retina barriers. As this results in the intraocular accumulation of fibrin and other potential growth- and attachment factors contained in serum that are conducive to vitreoretinal proliferation, it should be avoided. In eyes with advanced PVR, I apply argon or krypton laser photocoagulation to the buckle, either intraoperatively or postoperatively when extensive peripheral or equatorial surface proliferation cannot be completely removed surgically. These eyes often hide small perioral breaks within proliferative folds that, although temporarily flattened with gas, leak with resolution of the gas bubble, particularly inferiorly. This complication can be decreased by applying laser spots to the smoothly attached retina on the buckle while there is gas in the eye. This has the added benefit of demarcating or loculating recurrent subretinal fluid to the area of the buckle where extensive proliferative ridges prevent adequate settling of peripheral breaks on even the highest, broadest buckles.

When a very posterior retinal break is encountered or created during vitrectomy and cannot be easily buckled, photocoagulation can be applied in multiple concentric rows posterior to the buckle. The spacing of laser or cryotherapy lesions is of some importance. Kain has shown experimentally that a double row of photocoagulation is more effective than a single row and that heavy lesions are more effective than light lesions in halting the movement of subretinal fluid.[20] Lesions too broadly spaced permit the extravasation of subretinal fluid between individual lesions. However, the proliferation of RPE required to produce chorioretinal adhe-

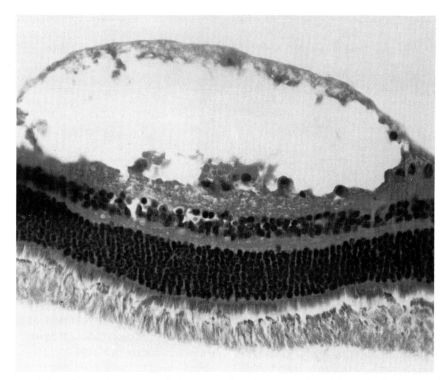

Figure 22-5. Severe inner retinal damage induced by transvitreal (endo-) diathermy with relative sparing of the retina one day following treatment. (H&E, original magnification ×250)

sion takes place at the periphery of the lesion, which also appears to have the strongest attachment in the first days. Thus, lesions should be closely spaced but not directly contiguous or overlapping.[11]

If vitrectomy without manipulation of the scleral buckle is the preferred course of management for recurrent retinal detachment, the chorioretinal adhesion must be produced by a method other than transscleral cryotherapy or diathermy. Several options exist: transvitreal diathermy, transvitreal cryotherapy, transvitreal xenon photocoagulation, or transvitreal argon–laser photocoagulation.[7,10,13,27] Transvitreal argon-laser photocoagulation clearly appears to be the method of choice. We and others have shown that both endodiathermy and endocryotherapy have major drawbacks including severe and frequent preferential damage to the surrounding retina during the creation of lesions.[11]

In rabbits, even light transvitreal diathermy applications with a unimanual bipolar coaxial microprobe (energies .05–.125 joules/25-msec)

produce severe inner retinal necrosis with fragmentation of the internal limiting lamina and loss of axons, ganglion cells, and inner nuclear layers. Despite this extent of retinal injury, pigment epithelial irritation is variable, and the resulting adhesion is unpredictable and often associated with surface retinal proliferation (Fig. 22-5). Heavy lesions produce severe full-thickness retinal necrosis commonly associated with lysis of Bruch's membrane and resultant ingrowth of fibrovascular tissue from the underlying choroid. Endocryotherapy produces a more reliable pigment epithelial lesion without rupture of Bruch's membrane but also results in severe full-thickness retinal necrosis and prominent choroidal engorgement. This is frequently accompanied by transient localized serous detachment delimited at the margins of the lesion by pigment epithelial proliferation. The margins appear to be the points of greatest adhesion both early and late (when there are frequently marked thinning and loss of nearly all retinal elements centrally).

In contrast, transvitreal photocoagulation of

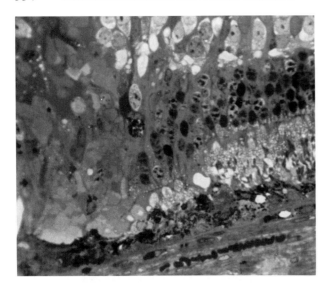

Figure 22-6. Margin of transvitreal argon laser photocoagulation burn in rabbit at 1 week. Note compact pigment epithelial glial adhesion with relative sparing of the inner retina. (Paraphenylenediamine, original magnification ×430)

medium intensity spares the inner retina yet produces a firm predictable chorioretinal adhesion. Xenon arc endophotocoagulation may be applied to eyes filled with fluid. However, argon-laser endophotocoagulation has several additional advantages over xenon-arc including a more favorable wave-length spectrum for producing a pigment epithelial lesion; shorter recycling time between pulses; and the ability to produce a lesion in gas-filled eyes at a safe probe distance from the retina.

Histopathologically, the lesions produced by the argon endolaser in rabbits following vitrectomy through fluid- or air-filled media are essentially identical to those produced by transcorneal argon-laser photocoagulation at similar time intervals. With light to moderate lesions, damage is confined to the pigment epithelium and photoreceptors, but heavy white lesions produce full-thickness necrosis. The lesions appear to have significant strength by 1 week, and epiretinal proliferation and subretinal choroidal fibrovascular ingrowth are extremely uncommon (Fig. 22-6).

Vitrectomy Techniques

The rationale for vitrectomy in the management of complicated retinal detachment includes the following: to alleviate tractional forces either solely responsible for retinal elevation (type II) or contributing to persistent leak-

age through retinal breaks (type III); to provide intraocular space for vitreous substitutes when adequate subretinal fluid cannot be removed; to improve surgical visualization in patients with cloudy or opaque ocular media; and to improve the visual prognosis in eyes with structural abnormalities, such as macular pucker, vitreous incarceration associated with macular edema, translucent vitreous membranes, associated foreign bodies, or dislocated lenses.

In cases of advanced proliferative vitreoretinopathy a three-port system incorporating a separate infusion cannula, light pipe, and cutter is advantageous for the variety of manipulations that may be required.

I routinely remove the lens because it permits more complete removal of the anterior peripheral vitreous; it often becomes cataractous if exposed for extended periods of time to vitreous substitutes such as sulfur hexafluoride (SF_6) or silicone; and postoperative fluid–gas exchange and supplemental photocoagulation are made much simpler in routine or complicated cases, such as a recurrent detachment. For all but the densest cataracts (grade IV nuclear sclerosis), lensectomy is performed with one of several commercially available ultrasonic hand-pieces as an aspirating device. A 20-gauge infusion needle is inserted through the future light pipe site; it is used to inflate the lens, thereby reducing the risk of inadvertent premature capsular rupture, and to cool the emulsified and partially coagulated lens material, which otherwise may clog the aspirating port. With sufficient magnification and attention to detail, it is possible to leave the lens capsule intact to protect the corneal endothelium anteriorly and to prevent accidental loss of lens fragments posteriorly. The intact anterior capsule guards the corneal endothelium until it opacifies intraoperatively or until fluid–gas exchange is performed.

In general, the peripheral vitreous is densely adherent to the pre-equatorial retina and may not be completely removed without substantial risk of producing large or multiple retinal holes. Multiple radial cuts can be made in the condensed vitreous base in valleys between equatorial retinal folds. Areas of persistent contracture can be buckled if they are not located too far posterior to the equator.

Once the formed vitreous gel and easily visible bridging membranes are removed with the vitreous cutter, attention is directed to any closely adherent periretinal membranes to determine whether further dissection is necessary to allow retinal settling. If the retina appears mobile enough at this point to settle with external or internal drainage, no further dissection is performed aside from peeling of macular puckers for the purpose of improving central vision. When retinal settling is uncertain, it can be more accurately assessed by internal fluid gas exchange through a pre-existing or planned retinal break. If gas passes into the subretinal space readily or the retina fails to settle or begins to tear at a distant site, then unresolved tractional forces exist.

Although a great deal has been written about the advantages and disadvantages of sharp dissection using instruments such as hooked needles, forceps, and manual automated right-angle and delaminating scissors, I have found the technique of blunt retinal dissection using the rounded tip of the vitreous cutter (with no suction) counterpoised against the light pipe invaluable in cases of proliferative vitreoretinopathy. The basic premise is that the application of light to moderate tangential force on the retina by two closely apposed blunt instruments which are slowly rotated from one another is much more likely to lyse retina-to-retina adhesions produced by thin surface proliferation

than to produce retinal holes. This technique has the advantage of cleaving tissue along potential or pre-existing anatomic planes in much the same way that blunt dissection with fingers or forceps (rather than scissors or blades) in the subcutaneous tissues of the abdomen reduces the risk of bleeding and inadvertent transection of muscle planes. Transparent surface membranes derived from proliferation along the posterior hyaloid and identifiable only by the abnormal conformation changes in the underlying retina can be lysed in this way. The severed edges can then be grasped and the membrane peeled in large sheets anteriorly with the Sutherland forceps.

One caveat regarding the technique of blunt dissection: Reserve this technique primarily for cases of proliferative vitreoretinopathy in which most of the retina is of normal thickness and tensile strength. In eyes with long-standing or diabetic atrophic detachment, scissor techniques are safer because firm pressure on the retina produces holes. Similarly, other small membranes of glial origin, such as those running along and intimately associated with the vascular arcades or those centered in small star-folds, have firm desmosomal attachment plaques and cannot be easily peeled. These, too, must be segmented or delaminated with the appropriate intraocular scissors or left in place if they can be readily buckled and the risk of major hemorrhage or hole formation appears to be great. Subretinal proliferations including yellow dots composed of macrophages, and connective tissue or glial dendritic strands, plaques, or sheets are a common concomitant of proliferative vitreoretinopathy. As a general rule, the vast majority of subretinal membranes need not be approached surgically in order to bring about retinal reattachment, although in some instances they may result in localized retinal elevation. As long as this does not occur in the macula or in direct communication with a retinal break, the outcome is not compromised. Subretinal strands appear to be particularly common in association with pre-existing choroidal detachment, subretinal hemorrhage, the acute retinal necrosis syndrome, and in areas of prior photocoagulation that soon thereafter became detached.

Drainage of Subretinal Fluid

Because various long-acting gases for intravitreal injection are readily available and because subretinal fluid is reabsorbed in a matter of hours with gas tamponade, essentially irrespective of duration of detachment, drainage should be reserved for the following indications: for eyes undergoing scleral buckling alone without gas injection; as a therapeutic test to determine whether vitreoretinal and retinal–retinal traction forces have been sufficiently relieved to permit complete retinal flattening; for eyes with a large amount of subretinal fluid prohibiting the instillation of an adequately sized gas bubble; for eyes that require intravitreal silicone instillation or endophotocoagulation after scleral buckling, intravitreal gas, and vitrectomy alone have previously failed; for eyes with pre-existing or inadvertent iatrogenic posterior retinal holes easily amenable to internal drainage techniques; and for eyes with so much subretinal fluid that safe insertion and manipulation of vitrectomy instruments are effectively prohibited.

Conversely, drainage need not be done in eyes with limited subretinal fluid, wider funnels that may be easily filled with a large amount of gas, surrounding proliferation or underlying atrophy of the RPE in which planned retinotomy entails considerable risk of later nonclosure, and a pre-existing buckle bed that would be hazardous to open. Drainage may not be necessary even in eyes that may eventually require either laser photocoagulation to the buckle or intravitreal silicone instillation. Photocoagulation can be applied postoperatively with a slit-lamp delivery system. Often the degree of retinal flattening with a gas tamponade is significantly greater after 24 hours than following linear extrusion or passive egress of subretinal fluid.

Several principles generally apply in cases in which conventional or external drainage is indicated. Depending on subretinal fluid distribution, drainage sites, if possible, should be selected anteriorly, immediately adjacent to the rectus muscle insertions, in the bed of the buckle, and beneath pre-existing fixed folds or bullous elevation, to minimize the risks of subretinal hemorrhage and retinal hole formation or incarceration. Light external diathermy to the exposed choroid also reduces the risk of choroidal bleeding into the subretinal space. Closure of the sclerotomy with an absorbable 7-0 suture adds a measure of control, minimizing late accidental incarceration during buckle tightening or subsequent buckle revision.

For internal drainage, it is preferable to utilize any pre-existing breaks than to create additional ones. Retinal breaks have a tendency to enlarge, even when small or tapered internal drainage needles are used. So it is better to enlarge and delineate the break purposely with transvitreal diathermy before drainage than to incarcerate the retinal edge accidentally with the drainage needle, causing jagged enlargement, rips, or retinal vascular bleeding. Delineation with diathermy also highlights the break for subsequent photocoagulation or cryocoagulation when the retina is flat. "Passive egress" occurs when a pressure gradient created by intravitreal gas insufflation drives subretinal fluid into a drainage needle vented to atmospheric pressure by a finger-controlled aperture.[7] The probe tip should be 23-gauge or larger to allow adequate flow for this method. When subretinal fluid evacuation is controlled instead by automated suction transmitted through the needle tip by the surgeon, tips with considerably smaller diameters can be utilized. The advantages over the former method are lower vitreosubretinal pressure gradients and fewer iatrogenic stretch tears in the retina. A peripheral drainage site can be easily buckled, although the evacuation of fluid posteriorly may not be complete. Conversely, posterior drainage sites allow more complete evacuation of subretinal fluid but are difficult to buckle. If posterior sites are elected, they should be placed in the supranasal quadrant to permit the longest internal gas tamponade, resulting in the least visual compromise to the patient. Intraoperative or postoperative photocoagulation is usually sufficient, in conjunction with temporary gas tamponade, to seal the retinotomy permanently unless there are adjacent subretinal strands or epiretinal membranes.

In selected cases of retinal detachment repair, one useful technique is external fluid–gas exchange, in which intravitreal gas is slowly and continuously infused through the cannula as fluid is drained through an external sclerotomy.

It is important to tilt the quadrant of the drain site posteriorly and to avoid forceful gas instillation or sudden bursts of pressure to prevent inadvertent incarceration of the retina by outward pressure of the gas bubble as it rises anteriorly. This complication can be easily recognized by the loss of gas through the sclerotomy; it requires cryopexy or photocoagulation to the drainage bed. Since most retinas will flatten if an adequate gas bubble is placed in a vitrectomized eye, this technique should be reserved for eyes with bullous inferior detachments or eyes in which internal drainage cannot be performed and sufficient release of periretinal tractional forces remains questionable.

Intraocular Gases

The intravitreal instillation of air for the treatment of retinal detachment was first advocated by Rosengren more than 40 years ago.[36] Sterile filtered air remains an excellent method to tamponade retinal breaks internally, although it is rapidly reabsorbed into the vascular compartment and generally vacates the vitreous cavity completely within 5 to 7 days. This fact limits its effectiveness in eyes with inferior retinal breaks or unresolved tractional forces adjacent to the break, which require prolonged internal tamponade while the chorioretinal adhesion becomes established.

Recently, interest has centered on gases that remain in the vitreous cavity for longer periods of time. Sulfur hexafluoride (SF_6), introduced by Norton in the Jackson Lecture of 1972, has been the prototype of long-acting gaseous vitreous substitutes.[32] Although highly lipid-soluble, SF_6 has low solubility in plasma and therefore remains in the vitreous cavity nearly twice as long as air. When pure SF_6 gas is instilled in the vitreous cavity of rabbits, the bubble increases at 24 hours by approximately 150%, with a maximal pressure elevation at 6 hours. This is caused by the rapid influx of venous nitrogen into the intravitreal gas pocket and, because of its reduced solubility, the correspondingly slower efflux of SF_6 into the venous system. Intravitreal SF_6 concentration reduces to 52% at 6 hours and approximately 18% by 24 hours (at which point nitrogen accounts for 71.5% of the volume).

Complete resorption of the bubble occurs within 8 to 10 days in rabbits.[1] While a bubble of 100% SF_6 will expand to approximately 2.5 times its original volume, a mixture of 40% SF_6 and 60% air does not increase the volume of the gas bubble or elevate the intraocular pressure. There appears to be no retinal toxicity of the gas as evaluated by electroretinography or histologic study. Feathery posterior subcapsular cataracts that are partially reversible develop, however, when the gas bubble occupies more than 50% of the vitreous cavity and remains in direct contact with the lens longer than 24 hours.[12] More recently, other potentially useful longacting gases of the perfluorocarbon family have undergone considerable investigation. Perfluoromethane (CF_4), perfluoroethane (C_2F_6), and perfluoropropane (C_3F_8) have intraocular persistence that increases with the length of the carbon chain, as well as more gradual expansion and pressure effects than SF_6. In these gases, the bubble lasts 6, 16, and 28 days, respectively, in the rabbit vitreous.[5] Perfluoro-*n*-butane (C_4F_{10}) expands to five times its original volume slowly over the course of 3 days, begins to shrink at 1 week, and remains in the vitreous cavities of rabbits for up to 3 months.[26,*]

While intravitreal gases are a valuable adjunct to scleral buckling in the treatment of complicated forms of retinal detachment, they are mostly used in conjunction with vitrectomy techniques. The duration of an internal tamponade appears to have significance for longterm success. Clarkson and associates found that when patients with complicated forms of retinal detachment were randomly assigned to treatment with either air or SF_6, patients in the latter group had a statistically significant increased reattachment rate and a slightly higher complication rate.[9] The major complication of intravitreal SF_6 gas use is increased intraocular pressure in the immediate postoperative period. In one study, presumed central retinal artery occlusion and no light perception vision in the immediate postoperative period were encountered in 11% of patients treated with intravitreal SF_6 gas; other investigators have not found the incidence to be as high.[2]

* Robert Machemer, personal communication

In principle, nonexpanding concentrations of gases should be used intraoperatively with large-volume gas fills. Gas should be used with great caution, if at all, in patients with pre-existing glaucoma, rubeosis, or vascular compromise or in those receiving very large buckling elements who have concomitant orbital swelling and vortex vein compromise. Modifications in technique must be employed with automated air injectors for use intraoperatively to achieve reliable gas concentrations. Following total air fill intraoperatively, a minimum of four to five ocular volumes of gas (25–30 cc) of the desired concentration should be flushed through the infusion line manually to achieve this intraocular concentration. Intraocular pressure should remain within the normal range at the end of the procedure but must be remeasured within the first 6 hours postoperatively when expansile gases are used. This is particularly important when nitrous oxide is used for general anesthesia; it should be discontinued before gas insufflation to prevent ocular overfilling.

POSTOPERATIVE MANAGEMENT

Sequential Fluid–Gas Exchange

When air or nonexpansile gases are used, the degree and duration of the internal tamponade may be insufficient to permit the chorioretinal adhesion to mature before rhegmatogenous or tractional forces redetach the retina. Because expansile gas concentrations may cause acute pressure elevation, one solution is to repeat the fluid–gas exchange postoperatively on one or more occasions. In this way, other complicating variables such as acute orbital swelling, severe intraocular inflammation, systemic hypotension, and intravenous anesthetic partial pressures are reduced, and the intraocular pressure can be monitored more conveniently. The technique is applicable to aphakic, phakic, or pseudophakic eyes that have previously undergone vitrectomy for the following indications: rhegmatogenous redetachment caused by breaks elevated over a buckle, unbuckled posterior breaks, or an "invisible" break; nonclearing opacities of the media such as hemorrhage and

early fibrin pupillary membrane; postoperative photocoagulation; prolonged internal tamponade; and before filling the cavity with silicone.

Technique

When no additional procedures such as photocoagulation are anticipated, fluid–gas exchange can be performed in aphakic eyes with use of topical anesthesia in the outpatient clinic or at the bedside, without an assistant. Topical proparacaine and gentamicin drops are instilled with mydriatics to maximize pupillary dilation. A lid speculum is inserted, and the patient is positioned face down on a stretcher or bed with the chin resting on both hands or on a pillow and the forehead and nose extended over the edge. A total of 8 cc of sterile air or gas is drawn in a 10-ml syringe through a 0.22-μ Millipore filter, and a ½-inch, 27-gauge needle is fitted to the syringe. The surgeon sits comfortably on the floor or on a low stool. A cotton-tipped applicator held in the nondominant hand is used to stabilize the globe 180 degrees from the intended entry site at the limbus. For a right-handed surgeon, the entry site is nasal in right eyes and temporal in left eyes in a very shelved direction through the limbus, past Descemet's membrane. The needle is then directed posteriorly into the midpupillary plane, the applicator is dropped, and the left hand is used to stabilize the barrel of the syringe while the right hand works the plunger (Fig. 22-7). Since the needle tip is directed posterosuperiorly in the inverted eye, as fluid is aspirated into the syringe, it flows toward the plunger, while the gas for injection remains superiorly in the syringe and needle. Using only one entry site, fluid can be sequentially aspirated while gas is injected, thus reducing the risk of hemorrhage, infection, and leakage. With this technique the exact volume exchange can be determined, the fluid can be saved for analysis, the intraocular pressure and volume can be precisely normalized during the exchange, and intraocular fluid is not vented on the floor or the surgeon.

In general, a 27-gauge needle is optimal; a 25-gauge needle has slightly better flow but tends to leak, whereas a 30-gauge needle has poor flow and tends to produce "fish eggs." As the exchange nears completion, the needle is directed in a progressively more anterior (corneal) direction to remove the remaining intraocular fluid, gravitating into the anterior chamber and angle recesses. A fresh cotton-tipped applicator is grasped in the left hand and used to judge the intraocular pressure before removing the needle from the eye, again in a very shelved fashion to avoid leakage. Leakage also can be minimized by sliding the applicator over the extraction site at the moment when the needle is withdrawn. If the iris is poorly dilated or the anterior chamber is flattened, the gas bubble will tamponade the site and result in a small focal peripheral synechia. In such cases, the eyes should be left slightly softer than normal, as the expected leakage of gas, which serves as a safety valve, does not occur after the exchange. The intraocular pressure may then rise to very high levels if expansile gases are used. It is important to avoid nicking the iris and effecting extreme variations in the intraocular pressure in either direction, since both complications produce pain and occasional hyphema. If iris bleeding occurs and is not removed or if the eye is left too soft, a fibrin pupillary membrane may occur the following day. This membrane is not to be confused with a hypopyon, and it clears in 5 to 7 days (see Fig. 22-5).

Several modifications of this technique are necessary in phakic or pseudophakic eyes. Entry must be made via the pars plana, necessitating a retrobulbar anesthetic. The patient is positioned on the side of the eye to be treated, and the dependent temporal portion of the globe is always chosen for entry. The physician is seated on the side of the stretcher, entry is made with the dominant hand inferiorly, and the needle's position in the midvitreous cavity is ascertained with the indirect ophthalmoscope and condensing lens held in the nondominant hand. This same hand is then used to stabilize the syringe for sequential exchange. As the eye is filled, the needle is slowly withdrawn inferiorly, where the remaining fluid collects dependently rather than anteriorly. Great care should be taken to avoid accidentally nicking the crystalline lens. In this fashion it is possible and, in fact, rather easy to achieve greater than a 95% gas fill in a previously vitrectomized phakic eye that requires either prolonged tamponade or laser photocoagulation or has a nonclearing vitreous hemorrhage.

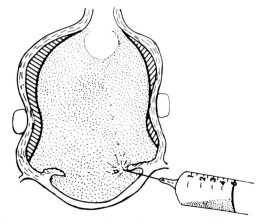

Figure 22-7. Technique of postoperative fluid gas exchange. With the patient and the syringe in the inverted position, the gas bubble is enlarged.

In general, in eyes that have significant subretinal fluid occupying the intraocular volume or in which postoperative photocoagulation will not be performed on the same day, I use a moderately expansile concentration of SF_6 gas (50%–70%) and leave the eye relatively soft. Although the presence of gas in the anterior chamber suggests a total fill, the patient's face-down position allows significant amounts of intraocular fluid to occupy interstices between the individual smaller bubbles or "fish eggs." Thus, as the bubble slightly and slowly expands, it replaces any subretinal fluid and residual intraocular fluid. If photocoagulation is to be performed the same day, if there is no subretinal fluid present, or if a smaller bubble is already present, I use a lower nonexpansile (20%–30%) concentration of SF_6 and leave the eye firm at the end of the procedure (generally less than 30 mm Hg).

If recurrent detachment appears in eyes with a significant rhegmatogenous component and no visible retinal break, I perform fluid–gas exchange using a mixture of either 50% SF_6 gas or air on the evening before surgery with use of topical anesthesia. A slightly expansile concentration of SF_6 gas is preferable, because the effective intravitreal volume increases as the subretinal fluid is evacuated overnight. Thus, the gas bubble is large enough to achieve retinal flattening within 12 to 48 hours. If complete flattening has been achieved by the following morning (common), I place a 19- or 20-gauge needle through the pars plana into the gas-filled eye for infusion. For aphakic eyes, a 30-gauge needle is placed through the limbus. If complete retinal flattening does not occur on the first day following preoperative fluid–gas exchange, the relative components of tractional and exudative detachment can be assessed and the appropriate measures (surgical delay or membrane dissection and retinotomy) can be taken before intravitreal instillation of silicone.

Mild to moderate pain that may occur on the night of the procedure can be treated with analgesics. A topical cycloplegic steroid and an antibiotic are generally applied every 6 hours, and the intraocular pressure and light perception are checked at 2 and 6 hours following exchange, if an expansile concentration of gas is used. If the intraocular pressure is markedly elevated (> 40 torr) or rapidly increasing from a low level, it is relatively easy to aspirate 0.5 cc of gas through the limbus with a tuberculin syringe at the patient's bedside. In eyes with small pupillary apertures, the anterior chamber may occasionally be flattened by an expanding gas bubble the following day. In virtually all instances they will spontaneously re-form in 5 to 7 days. Although many eyes develop small peripheral anterior synechiae and corneal scars at the needle tract sites, neither have caused significant visual morbidity or chronic glaucoma in patients with otherwise successful results.

Results of Fluid–Gas Exchange

As of May 1984 we have performed more than 200 fluid–gas exchanges on 130 patients; follow-up has been complete on 108. The most frequent indication was PVR (43 patients) followed by giant retinal tear (16 patients), recurrent rhegmatogenous detachment (14 patients), and trauma (9 patients). The remainder included recurrent diabetic vitreous hemorrhage and a variety of other indications. None of the 108 patients developed endophthalmitis or lost light perception due to elevated intraocular pressure. In 72% of patients, the ocular media were clear enough within the first 48 hours to permit laser treatment, if indicated. The gases used most frequently were either sterile room air or 50% SF_6, although in some cases up to 100% SF_6 was used. Only 5% of the patients receiving gas had a pressure on the operative or following day exceeding 40 mm Hg; none exceeded 50 mm Hg. More than 90% of the patients who underwent postoperative fluid–gas exchange for a retinal detachment achieved complete reattachment within 48 hours; but only 60% maintained this reattachment through the follow-up period.

These findings indicate that, at least as a temporary measure before the introduction of either silicone or laser photocoagulation, the procedure has significant benefits with no great attendant risks or discomfort to the patient.

Postoperative Photocoagulation

Although sequential fluid exchange results in reabsorption of subretinal fluid in more than 90% of instances, the recurrence of subretinal fluid in the immediate postoperative period as the gas bubble resorbs indicates either insufficient maturation of the chorioretinal adhesion or a missed retinal break. In either event, additional measures are required to effect long-term retinal reattachment. If no break is identified or if one is visualized and appropriately positioned, I prefer treatment with postoperative photocoagulation. With appropriate flattening of the retina, a retrobulbar anesthetic is administered the day following fluid–gas exchange. In aphakic eyes, treatment is technically easier if the globe is completely filled with gas and no fluid meniscus is present. This can be achieved by supplemental exchange immediately before photocoagulation using the technique described. In either phakic or aphakic eyes, the posterior fundus and peripheral buckle can be easily and clearly visualized as a minified inverted image through the Rodenstock panfunduscopic lens at the slit lamp with low magnification.

I prefer to use the krypton laser postoperatively, as it tends to produce less intraocular smoke than the argon blue-green laser and is more effective in creating a pigment epithelial lesion in eyes with shallow neurosensory elevation. In eyes with limited proliferation, I confine treatment to a triple or quadruple row of 500-μ

burns on the buckle for 360 degrees. If breaks are identified posterior to the buckle or if previous treatment has failed, additional concentric rows are placed posterior to the buckle. The objective of this treatment is to seal the retinal breaks and to delimit areas of localized peripheral subretinal fluid and tractional elevation from visually significant posterior retina. There is no evidence to indicate that postoperative scatter photocoagulation either tacks down the retina or destroys proliferating cells. For that reason burns should be nearly confluent for good barrier effect and confined to the vicinity of the buckle.

Early complications of photocoagulation include pain, choroidal detachment, exudative retinal detachment, elevated intraocular pressure, and hole formation. These can be minimized by reducing energy settings. Late complications include tractional tears at photocoagulation sites and subretinal proliferative membranes. With the recently available argon laser endoprobes, these techniques can now be performed intraoperatively through air following evacuation of the subretinal fluid, a technique recently described by Parke and Aaberg.[34]

Other Vitreous Substitutes

Silicone

Liquid silicone may be used for a long-term tamponade of retinal breaks. Cibis initially reported anatomic reattachment in eight of 13 patients with PVR; complications included silicone globules in the anterior chamber in two patients and subretinal silicone in two others.[8] A subsequent report described anatomic retinal reattachment at 6 months in only nine of 33 cases, including eyes with PVR, giant retinal tear, and atrophic retinal detachment. Complications of silicone migration into the anterior chamber occurred in eight cases; glaucoma, in five; and cataract, in three eyes with persistent anatomic detachment.[44] Subsequent reports indicated that success rates varied between 5% and 79%.[16,17,37]

Technique

Previously, silicone oil was used primarily as an alternative or adjunct to conventional techniques of scleral buckling, usually during the external drainage of subretinal fluid. Results were surprisingly good compared with techniques of conventional scleral buckling without the use of vitrectomy.

More recently, silicone oil has been employed as an adjunct to both conventional scleral buckling and vitrectomy techniques in the treatment of PVR (Fig. 22-8 and 22-9).[15,21] Following the removal of cortical vitreous and peeling, segmentation, and delamination of pre- and subretinal membranes, the subretinal fluid is drained internally through a tapered cannula, while silicone oil is infused simultaneously through the preplaced cannula until the retina has completely flattened.

I perform a conventional air–fluid or gas–fluid exchange with either external or internal drainage, depending on the circumstances, until the retina is completely flattened. Following this, silicone oil is injected either through the infusion cannula or through a separate, longer infusion cannula held directly over the optic nerve head, with fiberoptic endoillumination. This technique minimizes the possibility of subretinal silicone infusion by completely flattening the retina and allows an adequate assessment of the preretinal membrane surgery before the introduction of silicone in the eye. If pneumatic exchange under constant pressure through a mechanized air pump does not flatten the retina, further membrane dissection or a retinotomy can be performed; also, trapped subretinal air can be evacuated internally by applying external pressure to the globe or performing additional relaxing retinotomies. Introducing silicone into air-filled eyes with large posterior retinal breaks or relaxing retinotomies requires care to maintain the intraocular pressure at a relatively high level to prevent the rolling of cut retinal edges and inadvertent subretinal silicone infusion. This can be accomplished by maintaining constant pressure on the air infusion pump and introducing silicone through a separate hand-held infusion cannula.

Complications

Major complications of silicone use include cataract (ranging from 49%–65% within 3 years), glaucoma (15%), and band-shaped or vascular-

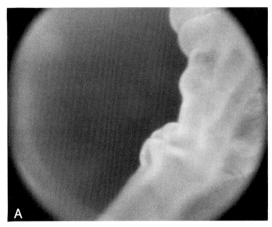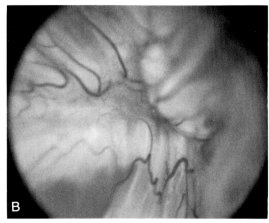

Figure 22-8. Preoperative appearance of 23-year-old one-eyed man with *(A)* giant retinal tear and *(B)* severe PVR (Stage D-3). Visual acuity improved to 20/70.

ized keratopathy (7%).[16,17] For these reasons, it appears prudent to remove silicone between 3 and 6 months following successful reattachment and cessation of the vitreoretinal proliferation or in eyes at the first sign of silicone intolerance. Eyes with total silicone replacement may develop corneal decompensation and opacifying edema following removal of the silicone.

Whether or not silicone is toxic to the retina remains controversial. While initial reports indicated that silicone was toxic to the retina, recent studies in rabbits have not confirmed these findings.[34] Although silicone has been thought

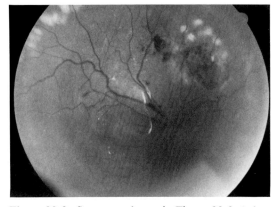

Figure 22-9. Same eye shown in Figure 22-8, 1 day following vitrectomy, lensectomy, membrane dissection, and silicone oil injection. Visual acuity ultimately improved to 20/200. Superonasal retinotomy drainage site is surrounded by endophtocoagulation scars.

to be an electrical insulator (thus rendering ERG criteria unreliable), Ober and associates (1983) obtained ERG recordings in rabbits under topic and phototopic conditions. They found silicone-injected eyes to be comparable to saline-injected control eyes. No appreciable difference between the groups was noted in pathologic changes in the retina such as ganglion-cell degeneration, Müller-cell swelling, and retinal hemorrhages.[35]

Indications

Indications for the use of intravitreal silicone are still evolving. In addition to PVR, intravitreal silicone has been useful in the treatment of giant retinal tears. I reserve use of silicone for the following indications: eyes having previously undergone vitrectomy and membrane surgery that develop retinal redetachment due to a significant rhegmatogenous component (type III); eyes with multiple and large posterior retinal breaks accompanied by residual traction in which demarcating photocoagulation would not appear to be effective; and "only" eyes in which retinal reattachment cannot be achieved but which show partial flattening after intravitreal silicone tamponade.

Other Viscoelastic Surgical Adjuvants

Healon and other synthetic glycosaminoglycans provide internal tamponade by virtue of increased surface tension (compared with aqueous or liquid vitreous) and they facilitate a variety of intraoperative microsurgical maneuvers involving the retina, including unfurling of giant retinal tears and facilitation of membrane dissection. The viscoelastic substance is either insinuated into the potential space between the retina and periretinal membrane, or it is used as a substitute for gas during internal drainage of subretinal fluid. The latter method is employed for the repair of multiple posterior breaks, areas of unresolved vitreoretinal traction, or retinal shortening.

The most commonly available viscoelastic substitute currently available is sodium hyaluronic acid (Healon), which is prepared from purified fraction of rooster comb. It is similar in composition to the hyaluronic acid normally found in human vitreous in conjunction with type II collagen. Healon is a sterile, noninflammatory, nonantigenic preparation of variable molecular weight. Stenkula and Ivert used Healon to treat 103 cases of complicated retinal detachment, including 37 patients with PVR, and achieved a 30% success rate at 6 months. Elevated intraocular pressure greater than 30 torr was noted in nine eyes (9%) and mild vitreous haze was observed in 33%.[39]

I have found Healon extremely helpful in unfolding giant retinal tears greater than 180 degrees before using the inverted gas exchange. Healon achieves a nearly complete flattening of the retina intraoperatively for the placement of full-thickness retinal and pigment epithelial cryopexy lesions and obviates the need for specialized techniques such as retinal incarceration or transvitreal suturing. In my experience, when large quantities of Healon are left in the aphakic vitrectomized eye, significant elevation of the intraocular pressure has without fail been a complication. Healon is particularly useful in eyes with a combined giant retinal tear and severe PVR. Inverted fluid–gas exchange alone does not produce retinal flattening in these eyes, and conventional supine internal fluid–gas exchange results in significant posterior slippage of the giant tear or subretinal gas infusion. By infusing Healon directly over the optic nerve through a hand-held cannula while simultaneously venting vitrectomy infusion fluid

through a preplaced cannula or a separate drainage cannula using coaxial illumination, it is possible to flatten the posterior retina and to unfold and anteriorly reposition curled retinal flaps in the fluid-filled eye. Healon has the advantage of being heavier than aqueous. Unlike silicone, which tends to rise over the fluid meniscus during internal subretinal fluid drainage, Healon remains posterior and flattens the retina in a posterior-to-anterior direction. Retinal slippage is avoided, and optical aberration is minimized in phakic eyes. One potential disadvantage of Healon is related to its high viscosity. The occasional difficulties noted in removing Healon, even with the vitreous cutting instrument, can be minimized by diluting it with vitrectomy-infusion solution and using high vacuum pressures and a large-bore cannula.

Antiproliferative Therapy

Successful long-term retinal reattachment in complicated forms of retinal detachment appears to depend on the prolonged tamponade of all retinal breaks by either internal or external means and the prevention of reproliferation and contractile membrane forces.[27] Cellular membrane proliferation as a cause for failure in retinal detachment has received increasing attention. A number of pharmacologic agents have been tested for their ability to inhibit intraocular proliferation in cell culture in experimental animal models of PVR.

Five-fluorouracil (5-FU) is a synthetic pyrimidine analog in which a fluorine atom is substituted for a hydrogen atom. In other respects it is identical with the native molecule uracil, a necessary component for RNA synthesis. When 5-FU is administered to rapidly dividing cells in therapeutic concentration, growth is almost immediately curtailed without unacceptable toxicity to metabolically active but nondividing cells. Continuous exposure to concentrations as low as 0.3 μg/ml produces significant inhibition of cells in culture.[41] The drug is rapidly transported out of the eye with an apparent half-life of approximately 3.3 hours in phakic nonvitrectomized eyes, and 1.4 hours in aphakic vitrectomized eyes.[19] This can be partially retarded by injecting the drug in a vehicle of Healon in aphakic vitrectomized eyes with intact posterior capsules.[45] While continuous exposure of target cells such as liberated RPE, glia, and fibroblasts to low doses of the drug appear to be optimal, pulsed or short-duration exposure to higher concentrations of the drug may be a reasonable therapeutic alternative. Dosages of 1 mg in an isolated intravitreal injection or daily 0.5-mg injections in the aphakic vitrectomized eye have been safe in studies with rabbits.[5,6,41]

In a previously published series, 22 consecutive patients with advanced stages of PVR (C3–D3) were treated with a combination of vitrectomy, scleral buckling, gas–fluid exchange, and postoperative photocoagulation in addition to fluorouracil therapy. Intravitreal 5-FU was administered to 55%; subconjunctival 5-FU, to 64%; and both, to 18% of the patients. After 6 months or longer, 64% of patients had permanently attached retinas. Of the 22 patients, 13 regained at least ambulatory vision. No retinal toxicity directly attributable to the drug was observed. Late healing of corneal epithelial defects was seen in 18% of patients, and subtle subepithelial and anterior corneal stromal scarring was noted in 32%. There were no severe or visually significant side-effects.[5]

Dosage

Fluorouracil is commercially available at a concentration of 50 mg/ml in a 10-ml glass vial suitable for parenteral administration. For subconjunctival injection, 0.2 ml of sterile undiluted drug is usually administered in the inferior cul-de-sac with a tuberculin syringe and 27-gauge needle, with or without subconjunctival lidocaine (Xylocaine) to produce a small bleb. The drug is relatively nonirritating by subconjunctival injection when compared with agents such as gentamicin and is well tolerated by most patients, with or without the subconjunctival anesthesia. We administer the drug for 5 consecutive days, beginning on the day of surgery, to patients receiving subconjunctival therapy alone. This obviates the need for injecting the drug into the completely gas-filled vitreous cavity in the immediate postoperative period. In eyes with large corneal epithelial defects, administration of the drug is delayed until the defect has resolved.

For intravitreal injection, we dilute the commercially available drug in sterile nonpreserved saline (1 : 5) to obtain an intravitreal injection of 0.1 ml, for a concentration of 10 mg/ml in a final intravitreal dose of 1 mg. In phakic eyes, this can be administered with a tuberculin syringe and 27-gauge needle via the pars plana. In aphakic eyes injection with topical anesthesia is accomplished through the corneal limbus. While injecting the drug into eyes with a large gas bubble may produce a jet stream of fluid within the eye or temporary pooling of relatively large concentrations of drug on the retinal surface, we have not encountered any direct complications to date.

SUMMARY

I have presented a rather personal view of one possible approach to the analysis and treatment of complicated forms of retinal detachment. Areas of critical importance include analysis of the forces responsible for retinal detachment, choice of appropriate operative procedure and hardware, and postoperative management. Careful preoperative examination and analysis of the detachment necessarily dictate the choice of the operative procedure. Some eyes require only a revision of the scleral buckle, while others need only vitrectomy or some combination of both. The operative procedure should ideally be one that resolves the disequilibrium of forces responsible for detachment while minimizing intraoperative surgical trauma, a strong stimulus for recurrent proliferation. Extended internal tamponade appears to be an important prerequisite for successful long-term reattachment. The choice of silicone or various long-acting gases remains a personal one, as does the selection of a buckling element.

Postoperative management is important to the ultimate success of these patients. Supplementation with gas or silicone injection, photocoagulation, and drug therapy appears to have a place although the exact indications for each and their interrelationships are still evolving.

Last, careful consideration of the therapeutic objectives and patient education are extremely important. Because the majority of eyes, even those with a successful anatomic result, do not regain good macular function, various factors need to be carefully considered before therapy is instituted. These include status of the fellow eye, age of the patient, and suitability for multiple potential therapeutic interventions.

REFERENCES

1. Abrams GW, Edelhauser HF, Aaberg TM, et al: Dynamics of intravitreal sulfur hexafluoride gas. Invest Ophthalmol 13:863–868, 1974
2. Abrams GW, Swanson DE, Sabates W, et al: The results of sulfur hexafluoride gas in vitreous surgery. Am J Ophthalmol 94:165–171, 1982
3. Blumenkranz MS, Byrne SF: Standardized echography for the detection and characterization of retinal detachment. Ophthalmology 89:821–831, 1981
4. Blumenkranz M, Claflin A, Hajek A: Selection of therapeutic agents for intraocular proliferative disease. Arch Ophthalmol 102:598–604, 1984
5. Blumenkranz M, Hernandez E, Ophir A, et al: 5-Fluorouracil: New applications in complicated retinal detachment for an established antimetabolite. Ophthalmology 91:122–130, 1984
6. Blumenkranz MS, Ophir A, Claflin A, et al: Fluorouracil for the treatment of massive periretinal proliferation. Am J Ophthalmol 94:458–467, 1982
7. Charles S: Vitreous Microsurgery. Baltimore Williams & Wilkins, 1981
8. Cibis P, Becker B, Okun E, et al: The use of liquid silicone in retinal detachment surgery. Arch Ophthalmol 68:46–55, 1962
9. Clarkson J, Blankenship G: The use of intraocular gas in the management of retinal detachment. Oral Presentation. American Academy of Ophthalmology, October, 1982
10. Delloparta A: A method for sealing macular holes by transbulbar coagulation. Am J Ophthalmol 37:649, 1954
11. Farah M, Blumenkranz M, Hernandez E: Histopathology of argon laser endophotocoagulation in rabbits. Invest Ophthalmol Vis Sci 25:335, 1984
12. Fineberg E, Machemer R, Sullivan P, et al: Sulfur hexafluoride in owl monkey vitreous cavity. Am J Ophthalmol 79:67–76, 1975
13. Fleischman J, Swartz M, Dixon J: Argon laser endophotocoagulation: An intraoperative trans pars plana technique. Arch Ophthalmol 99:1610–1612, 1981
14. Gonin J: The treatment of detached retina by searing the retinal tears. Arch Ophthalmol 4:621–625, 1930
15. Gonvers M: Temporary use of intraocular silicone oil in the treatment of detachment with massive periretinal proliferation. Ophthalmologica 184:210, 1982
16. Grey RHB, Leaver PK: Silicone oil in the treatment of massive periretinal retraction. I: Results in 105 eyes. Br J Ophthalmol 63:355–360, 1979
17. Grey RHB, Leaver PK: Results of silicone oil injection in massive periretinal retraction. Trans Ophthalmol Soc UK 97:238–241, 1977
18. Grizzard WS, Hilton GF: Scleral buckling fo. retinal detachments complicated by periretinal proliferation. Arch Ophthalmol 100:419–422, 1982
19. Jarus G, Blumenkranz MS, Hernandez E et al: Clearance of intravitreal fluorouracil: Normal and aphakic vitrectomized eyes. Ophthalmology 92:91–96, 1985
20. Kain HL: Chorioretinal adhesion after argon laser photocoagulation. Arch Ophthalmol 102:612–615, 1984
21. Lean J, Leaver PK, Cooling RJ, et al: Management of complex retinal detachments by vitrectomy and fluid silicone exchange. Trans Ophthalmol Soc UK 102:203–205, 1982
22. Levada A, Blumenkranz MS: Biometric alterations in the globe following scleral buckling. Invest Ophthalmol Vis Sci 22:53, 1982
23. Lincoff H, Long R, Marquardt, et al: The cryosurgical adhesion. Trans Am Acad Ophthalmol Otolaryngol 72:191, 1968
24. Lincoff A, Lincoff H, Iwamoto T, et al: Perfluoro-N-butane — A gas for maximum duration retinal tamponade. Arch Ophthalmol 101:460–462, 1983
25. Lincoff H, Mardirossian J, Lincoff A, et al: Intravitreal longevity of three perfluorocarbon gases. Arch Ophthalmol 98:1610–1611, 1980
26. Machemer R: Massive periretinal proliferation: A logical approach to therapy. Trans Am Ophthalmol Soc 75:556–585, 1977
27. Mae Y, Matsui M: Ophthalmoscopic model of nerve fiber bundle defects in monkey eyes produced by intraocular retinal coagulation. Jpn J Ophthalmol 26:274–281, 1982
28. Marmor MF, Abdul-Rahim AS, Cohen D: The effect of metabolic inhibitors on retinal adhesion and subretinal fluid reabsorption. Invest Ophthalmol Vis Sci 19:893–903, 1980
29. McMeel W: Oral Presentation. Jules Gonin Club. Cordoba, Argentina, April, 1982
30. Mukai N, Schepens CL: Intravitreous injection of silicone: An experimental study. Ann Ophthalmol 4:273–287, 1982
31. Norton EWD: Retinal detachment in aphakia. Am J Ophthalmol 58:111, 1964
32. Norton EWD: Intraocular gas in the management of selected retinal detachments. Trans Am Acad Ophthalmol Otolaryngol 77: 85–98, 1973
33. Ober RR, Blanks JC, Ogden TE: Experimental retinal tolerance to liquid silicone. Retina 3:77–84, 1983

34. Parke DW, Aaberg T: Intraocular argon laser photocoagulation in the management of severe proliferative vitreoretinopathy. Am J Ophthalmol 97:434–443, 1984

35. Rachal WF, Burton TL: Changing concepts of failures after retinal detachment surgery. Arch Ophthalmol 97:480–483, 1979

36. Rosengren B: The results of treatment of detachment of the retina with diathermy and injection of air into the vitreous. Acta Ophthalmol 16:573–579, 1938

37. Scott JD: Treatment of massive vitreous retraction. Trans Ophthalmol Soc UK 95:429–432, 1975

38. Sipperly J, Machemer R: Histopathologic evaluation of adhesive properties of early lesions in diathermy and cryopexy. Int Ophthalmol 3, 2: 107–110, 1981

39. Stenkula S, Ivert L: Sodium hyaluronate (Healon) as an intravitreal agent in retinal and vitreous surgery. J Ocular Ther Surg 3:110–114, 1984

40. Stern WF, Blumenkranz M: Fluid gas exchange after vitrectomy. Am J Ophthalmol 96:400–402, 1983

41. Stern WH, Guerin CJ, Erickson DA et al: Ocular toxicity of fluorouracil after vitrectomy. Am J Ophthalmol 96:43–51, 1983

42. Tani P, Robertson DM, Langworthy A: Rhegmatogenous retinal detachment without macular involvement treated with scleral buckling. Am J Ophthalmol 90:503–508, 1980

43. The Retina Society Terminology Committee: The classification of retinal detachment with proliferative vitreopathy. Ophthalmology 90:121–125, 1983

44. Watzke RC: Silicone retinopiesis for retinal detachment: A long-term clinical evaluation. Arch Ophthalmol 77:185–196, 1967

45. Woodlief N, Blumenkranz MS, Hernandez E, et al: Extended delivery of therapeutic levels of intravitreal 5-FU. Invest Ophthalmol Vis Sci 25:272, 1984

23

Fluoropyrimidines in the Treatment of Proliferative Vitreoretinopathy and Glaucoma

Michael K. Hartzer
Mark S. Blumenkranz

PHARMACOLOGY OF THE FLUOROPYRIMIDINES

The first fluorinated pyrimidine was synthesized in 1957 as a proposed antimetabolite for the treatment of advanced forms of human cancer.[47] Further development has led to the release of a class of agents that are used clinically in a variety of disease states. 5-Fluorouracil (5-FU) and its deoxyribonucleoside, 5-fluoro-2'-deoxyuridine (5-FUDR), are used in the treatment of solid cancers.[48,55] 5-Fluorocytosine (5-FC) has been shown to be beneficial in the treatment of yeast and fungal infections, and 5-trifluoromethyl-2'-deoxyuridine (trifluorothymidine, Viroptic) has been effective in the treatment of ocular herpes keratitis.[72,106]

The rationale for the synthesis of 5-FU was based on the observed increase in uracil utilization by tumor cells.[87] 5-FU closely resembles uracil, except for the substitution of fluorine for hydrogen at carbon-5 which modifies the reactivity of the molecule but does not significantly alter its size. As a result, 5-FU can replace uracil in all forms of RNA.[45,46]

5-FU also has been effective in controlling the proliferation of nonmalignant cells and in inhibiting the cicatricial response.[31,52,70] In addition to its widespread use in the treatment of ocular neoplasms, it has recently been beneficial in the treatment of ocular proliferative disorders, especially proliferative vitreoretinopathy (PVR), and in preventing the closure of filtering blebs after glaucoma-filtering surgery.[8,11–13,37,51,96]

Metabolism of 5-FU

Experimental evidence indicates that 5-FU is essentially harmless to mammalian cells unless subjected to metabolic activation.[72] For activation to occur, 5-FU must be enzymatically converted into either a ribose or deoxyribose nucleotide form (Fig. 23-1). 5-FU is converted into 5-fluoro-2'deoxyuridine (5-FUDR) by thymidine phosphorylase, which in turn may be phosphorylated by thymidine kinase to form 5-fluorodeoxyuridine monophosphate (5-FUDRP), an active form of 5-FU and a potent inhibitor of the enzyme thymidylate synthetase.

Alternatively, 5-FU may be converted into a ribose sugar by two distinct pathways. It is changed into 5-fluorouridine (5-FUR) via the action of either uridine or deoxyuridine phosphorylase.[59] 5-FUR is then phosphorylated by uridine-cytidine kinase to form 5-fluorouridine monophosphate (5-FURP).[2] 5-FURP can be further phosphorylated to form diphosphate (FURDP) and triphosphate (FURTP), which may be incorporated into RNA (see Fig. 23-1). 5-FU may also be converted directly to 5-FURP by orotic acid phosphoribosyl transferase (OPRTransferase).[84] This enzyme uses 5-phosphoribose-1-pyrophosphate (PRPP), a substrate that is shared with the first step of purine biosynthesis. Competition with purine biosynthesis can affect the rate of conversion of 5-FU to 5-FURP. 5-FURDP may then be converted to its deoxy form, 5-FUDRDP by ribonucleotide reductase, and subsequently converted to 5-FUDRP, the inhibitor of thymidylate synthetase. Thus, 5-FU can be metabolically activated via three pathways. The relative importance of each pathway varies with cell type, and all pathways are not necessarily operative in a single cell.

The incorporation of fluorodeoxyuridine nucleotides into DNA has been under intense investigation. Although 5-FUDRP may be additionally phosphorylated to form the deoxynucleotide triphosphate (FUDRTP), a substrate for alpha DNA polymerase, it was believed that FUDRP was not incorporated in measurable amounts into cellular DNA before enzymes prevented incorporation of uracil into DNA.[18,71] Recently, however, it has been shown that 5-FU can be incorporated into the DNA of murine bone marrow cells and several tumor cell lines.[60,65,88,89]

The catabolism of 5-FU follows the same pathways of uracil and thymidine.[15,16] The rate-limiting step in this pathway is the enzyme dihydrouracil dehydrogenase, which converts 5-FU into 5-F-ureido propionate.

Inhibition of Thymidylate Synthetase and DNA Synthesis

Methylation of deoxyuridylate to form deoxythymidylate is an integral part of the de novo pathway for the synthesis of the latter (see Fig. 23-1). Catalyzed by the enzyme thymidylate synthetase, this reaction requires tetrahydrofolate as a cofactor. Noncompetitive inhibition of this enzyme by 5-FUDRP is the best-understood biological effect of 5-FU and may explain much of the antitumor activity of the drug (see Fig. 23-1).[45,48] This inhibition results in DNA breakage and the so-called thymineless death.[22] Because of the requirement for a reduced folate cofactor, drugs such as methotrexate which inhibit dihydrofolate reductase and thereby decrease the available reduced folate may diminish the inhibitory effects of 5-FUDRP on thymidylate synthetase.[99,101]

Incorporation of FU-modified deoxynucleotides into DNA constitutes another mechanism for toxicity in certain cell lines.[60,65,88,89] This incorporation may be attributable to low activity or saturation of the enzymes designed to exclude uracil from DNA and may result in DNA miscoding or fragmentation.[89] Bone marrow cells in vivo, reportedly have a greater correlation between 5-FU incorporation into DNA and cytotoxicity than between thymidylate-synthetase inhibition and cell death.[89]

Effects of 5-FU on RNA Processing and Synthesis

As described, 5-FU may be converted into ribonucleotides and ultimately incorporated into RNA in most cell types. 5-FURP can replace uridine monophosphate in messenger RNA, which results in miscoding and errors in protein synthesis in *Escherichia coli*.[39,86,108] In HeLa cells, 5-FU is converted into 5-fluorocytosine (5-FC), which is then incorporated into mRNA in place of cytosine and subsequently misread as uracil.[36] Besides coding errors, FU-modified polyadenylic acid RNA was translated 2.5 times faster than unmodified RNA.[20]

Added to its effects on mRNA, 5-FU also affects processing and maturation of ribosomal RNA, but has only minimal effects on the synthesis of preribosomal RNA. Several groups have reported a decrease in both 18s and 28s ribosomal RNA and reduced levels of RNA methylation following exposure to 5-FU, but no change in levels of 45s (preribosomal) RNA.[20,49,108] Others have found an increase in 18s and 28s RNA following exposure to inhibitory doses of 5-FU.[26,27] These authors suggested that the cytotoxic effects of FU incorporation into RNA are due to miscoding, which results in increased rates of protein synthesis and ultimately in metabolic exhaustion of the cell as it attempts to maintain essential enzymatic functions.[26,27]

Exposure to 5-FU also produced changes in the synthesis and metabolism of small nuclear RNA (snRNA) whose functions include mRNA splicing and messenger- and ribosomal RNA

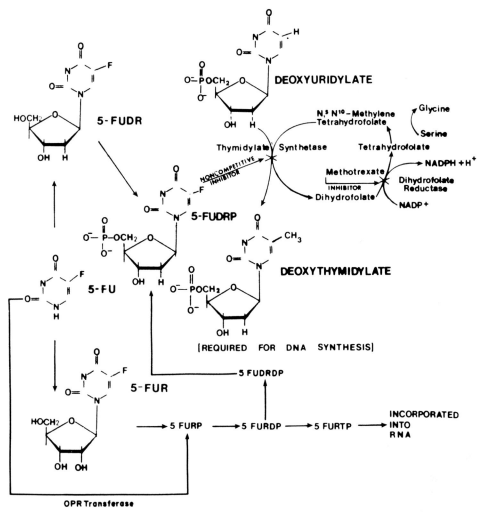

Figure 23-1. Metabolic pathways of 5-fluorouracil (5-FU) and its major metabolites. 5-FU may be converted to 5-FUDRP, which inhibits the enzyme thymidylate synthetase. The resultant lack of intracellular deoxythymidylate for incorporation into DNA leads to "thymidineless death" of cells. 5-FU may also be converted into 5-FURP by two pathways, leading to incorporation into RNA or conversion back to FUDRP and inhibition of thymidylate-synthetase activity.

processing.[3,35] In a human colon-carcinoma cell line, a stronger correlation was shown between cell lethality and incorporation of FU into nuclear RNA than between either DNA or RNA synthesis and cell death.[35]

Effects of DNA and RNA on Cytotoxicity

Heidelberger's early hypothesis suggested that the inhibition of thymidylate synthetase by FUDRP was responsible for most of the ob-served antitumor activity of 5-FU.[45,48] A number of recent reports, however, have indicated that this inhibition failed to account completely for the cytotoxicity of 5-FU in many cell lines.[26,49,67,108] To isolate a single pathway to as-sess the role of 5-FU in cytotoxicity, a number of researchers have attempted to suppress either DNA effects with the addition of thymidine or RNA effects with the addition of uracil. It would be expected that the addition of thymidine would replenish the depleted pool of thymidylate, thereby overcoming the inhibition of thymidylate synthetase and preventing thymineless death. The addition of uracil would be expected to block the RNA effect of 5-FU. In a number of studies in vitro, partial "rescue" of tumor cells by thymidine has been observed.[71,102] Conversely, other studies have demonstrated that increased concentrations of thymidine have led to increased incorporation of 5-FU into RNA and increased antitumor efficacy.[19,30,69,74] These apparently conflicting results can be explained by variations among cell types in the metabolism of 5-FU, the most important of these being the direct conversion of 5-FU to 5-FURP by OPRTransferase (see Fig. 23-1). Cells that can utilize this pathway will convert any available 5-FU into RNA when excess thymidine is present because of competition with 5-FU for the thymidylate synthetase–binding site and the inhibition of conversion of FURDP to FUDRDP. The end result is increased cytotoxicity. If ORPTransferase is absent from the cell or present only in low levels, thymidine will simply reduce the effects of FUDRP on thymidylate synthetase.[72] Thymidine and 5-FU are also catabolized by the same pathway, resulting in a significant decrease in 5-FU clearance following the addition of thymidine.[57]

Concurrent treatment with 5-FU and uridine also produced conflicting findings. Uridine has been used not only as a "rescue agent" to increase the therapeutic index of 5-FU against several mouse tumors, but also to increase the toxicity of 5-FU–treated mouse lymphoma (S-49) cells.[58,59,78] In some mouse tumors, uridine competes with 5-FUR for uridine/cytidine kinase, the rate-limiting enzyme in the pathway, thereby decreasing the incorporation of F-nucleotides into RNA.[58] In other cells, uridine increases the anabolism of 5-FU into RNA, presumably via conversion of 5-FU directly into 5-FURP by ORPTransferase. These authors, however, report that only 50% of the increase in cell lethality following concurrent treatment with 5-FU and uridine could be attributed to an increase in RNA anabolism.[78]

The understanding of 5-FU metabolism is further complicated by the existence of two ribonucleotide pools, one cytoplasmic and the other nuclear.[56,82,90] The rate at which these pools equilibrate with each other varies markedly with cell type.[72] F-RNA may also act as a slow-release depot for FURP, which may then be converted into FUDRP, resulting in long-term inhibition of thymidylate synthetase.[72,93]

OCULAR APPLICATIONS OF FLUOROPYRIMIDINES

Proliferative Vitreoretinopathy

Studies in vitro

Proliferative vitreoretinopathy, progressive traumatic tractional retinal detachment, and intraocular neovascularization represent ocular disease processes characterized by the uncontrolled proliferation of a population of nonneoplastic cells. These cells may be of varied origins, including astroglia, RPE, macrophages, vascular endothelium, myofibroblasts, or fibroblasts.[10,64] From a chemotherapeutic standpoint, any antiproliferating agent capable of selectively inhibiting the growth of these rapidly proliferating cells without producing unacceptable levels of toxicity may prove useful. A number of drugs including antimetabolites, steroids, and nonsteroidal anti-inflammatory agents have been evaluated in vitro, and the fluoropyrimidines have had some of the best therapeutic indices of all drugs tested.[8,9]

The ID_{50} (the concentration of drug required to produce 50% inhibition of cellular proliferation in vitro) of 5-FU and its major metabolites has been determined for a number of ocular cell types; 5-FUR is the most potent, 5-FU has intermediate efficacy, and 5-FUDR is the least effective (Table 23-1).[9,10,61,66,107] 5-FUR was at least 50 times more potent than 5-FU for all cell types tested. The ID_{50} for both 5-FU and 5-FUR were similar for all three cell types, whereas RPE cells and vascular endothelial cells were considerably more resistant to FUDR, indicating either differential rates of uptake or differences in intracellular metabolism.[10] The ID_{50} for both the ribose monophosphate (5-FURP) and deoxyribose monophosphate (5-FUDRP) were similar to 5-FUR and 5-FUDR, respectively (Fig. 23-2). Possibly, these results are due to ex-

Table 23-1. ID$_{50}$ (μg/ml) of 5-FU, 5-FUDR, and 5-FUR

Cell Type	*5-FU*	*5-FUDR*	*5-FUR*
Dermal fibroblasts	0.35	0.19	0.0047
Retinal pigment epithelial cells	0.30	3.08	0.0039
Vascular endothelial cells	0.71	4.08	0.0032

tracellular dephosphorylation of the monophosphates leaving 5-FUR and 5-FUDR as the active compounds.

In contrast, Heath and associates have found 5-FUDR (ID$_{50}$, 0.001 μM) to be 1200 times more effective than 5-FU and seven times more potent than 5-FUR in inhibiting the growth of rabbit fibroblasts.[46] The inhibitory effects of 5-FUDR were completely eliminated by the addition of 20 μM thymidine to the media.[44]

The time dependence of fluoropyrimidine antiproliferative effects on cellular proliferation and their potential reversibility have been investigated. A 24-hour exposure time to 5-FU was nearly as effective as a 72-hour exposure, whereas a 4-hour exposure increased the ID$_{50}$ tenfold (4 μg/ml).[42] Decreasing the exposure time from 72 hours to 1 hour reduced the efficacy of 5-FU 20-fold.[44] The antiproliferative effects of a 24-hour treatment with 1 μg/ml and 5 μg/ml were reversible within 14 days, whereas

proliferation was still inhibited at 14 days following a 10-μg/ml treatment.[42] Similar effects were noted following 24-hour treatment with 5-FUR. Treatment effects with drug concentrations of 10 ng/ml were reversible at 14 days, but those of 50 ng/ml were not reversible within the same period.[42] Using synchronized fibroblastic cultures, it was shown that 4-hour treatments with 10 μg/ml 5-FU during S phase was significantly more effective than during other portions of the cell cycle (Fig. 23-3).[42]

Effects of Fluoropyrimidines on Cell-Mediated Contraction

In addition to pharmacologic modulation of cellular proliferation, control of cellular contractility appears to be of critical importance in preventing the sequels of ocular cicatrization. Using modifications of a procedure developed by van Bockxmeer's group, several investigators have measured the effects of fluoropyrimidines

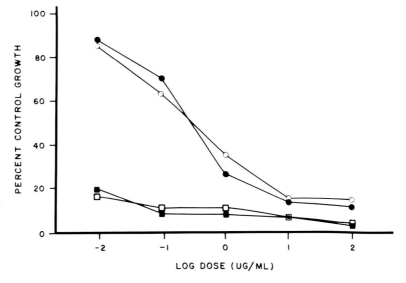

Figure 23-2. Effects of fluoropyrimidine treatment on human fibroblast growth in vitro. 5-Fluorouridine (5-FUR) *(open square)* and 5-fluorouridine monophosphate (5-FURP) *(solid square)* are more than 100 times more effective than 5-fluorodeoxyuridine (5-FUDR) *(open circle)* and 5-fluorodeoxyuridine monophosphate *(solid circle).*

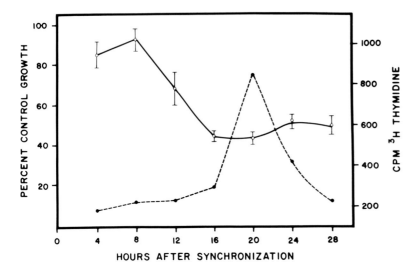

Figure 23-3. Effects of 4-hour treatment of fibroblasts with 10 μg/ml 5-FU during different portions of the cell cycle. Inhibition occurred only when drug was present during the time DNA was being synthesized (S phase). 5-FU inhibition *(solid line)*; labeled thymidine incorporation *(dotted line)*.

and other known and potential anticontractile agents on the cell-mediated contraction of a three-dimensional collagen matrix in vitro.[103] This contractile effect is directly proportional to the number of cells used in the assay, and varies inversely with the collagen concentration in the gel.[41,103,104] The degree of contraction is measured by determining the partitioning of tritiated water between the gel phase and the surrounding media, allowing an estimation of collagen gel volumes.[102-104]

5-FUR was an effective inhibitor of cellular contraction. When present during the assay, 200 μg/ml of 5-FUR reduced contraction by 25%. However, when the cells were exposed to the same drug concentration for 48 hours before the assay, contraction was inhibited by as much as 85% (Fig. 23-4).[41] When fewer cells were used per unit of gel volume, Heath and coworkers reported complete inhibition of contraction with a concentration as small as 300 μM (80 μg/ml) of 5-FUR and, surprisingly, with only 100 μM of 5-FUR in the presence of 20 μM of thymidine.[44] 5-FUDR failed to inhibit contraction at all concentrations tested.[44]

When 5-FU was present at concentrations up to 250 μg/ml during the assay, only limited inhibition of contraction occurs (see Fig. 23-4).[41,44,104] Inclusion of thymidine in the media did not increase inhibition.[44] Preincubation for 48 hours at 250 μg/ml of 5-FU also failed to inhibit contraction using 50,000 cells/

ml of collagen gel.[41] However, exposure to 1 μM (0.13 μg/ml) of 5-FU for 72 hours in the presence of thymidine reportedly inhibited contraction completely.[44] These differences are due to the increased contractility and decreased drug sensitivity of human fibroblasts compared with rabbit fibroblasts.

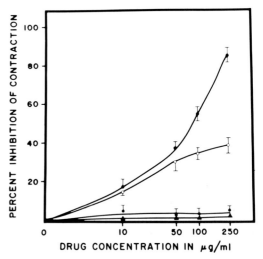

Figure 23-4. Anticontractile effects of 5-FU and 5-FUR on human fibroblasts in a 2-ml collagen lattice. Cells were treated with the drug for 48 hours prior to the contraction assay. Contraction was allowed to occur for 48 hours. 5-FU showed little inhibition even at high concentrations, whereas 5-FUR was almost completely inhibitory at 250 μg/ml.

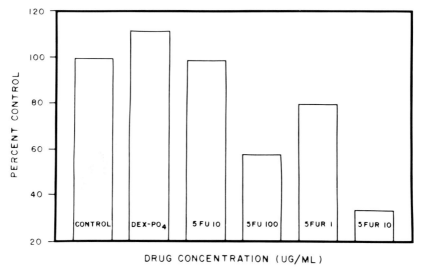

Figure 23-5. Effects of fluoropyrimidines and dexamethasone phosphate on collagen synthesis and secretion by human fibroblasts. Ten μg/ml 5-FUR inhibited collagen to a greater extent than 5-FU or dexamethasone phosphate.

Inhibition of Collagen Synthesis and Extracellular Matrix Production

Preventing the formation of collagenous epiretinal membranes is an important step in the treatment of ocular cicatricial disorders. Colchicine and the vinca alkaloids, although highly retinotoxic, inhibit collagen secretion by interfering with microtubular transport.[14,24] Steroids also effectively inhibit collagen synthesis in many instances, although their mechanisms of action are very complex.[23] In addition, collagen synthesis is inhibited by fluoropyrimidines, especially 5-FUR.[41]

Collagen synthesis was measured by a modification of the method of Peterkofsky and Diegelmann, which utilizes highly purified bacterial collagenase to cleave TCA–precipitable, radiolabelled, proline-containing protein into soluble peptides for scintillation counting.[25,79] Confluent fibroblast cultures were treated with the drug for 48 hours before ^{3}H-proline was added. Treatment with 1 μg/ml and 10 μg/ml of 5-FUR reduced collagen synthesis up to 82% and 33% of the control values, respectively (Fig. 23-5). By comparison, 5-FU was less effective, 100 μg/ml reducing synthesis up to 56% of control. Similar results were obtained when collagen synthesis by human RPE cells was measured. Supraphysi-

ologic concentration (10^{-5}M) of dexamethasone phosphate produced no inhibition and in some cases actually increased collagen synthesis slightly.[41]

Animal Model Studies *in vivo*

Several successful animal models for proliferative vitreoretinopathy (PVR) have been developed. The earliest models relied on the injection of autologous dermal fibroblasts or RPE cells into the vitreous cavity of rabbits.[1,83,100] Later, the injection of 250,000 homologous dermal fibroblasts was demonstrated equally effective in producing tractional detachments, which significantly reduced the technical difficulties associated with the earlier models.[76] This latter model, or variations thereof, has been used to test the ability of a number of antiproliferative drugs, including the fluoropyrimidines, to reduce the incidence of detachment.

Blumenkranz and associates found that a single 1-mg intravitreal injection of 5-FU sufficiently reduced the rate of retinal detachment from 73% in the control group to 31% in the treated group at 4 weeks (Fig. 23-6).[13] Intraocular neovascularization was also significantly reduced in the treated group. Supplementing the intravitreal injection with repeated 10-mg sub-

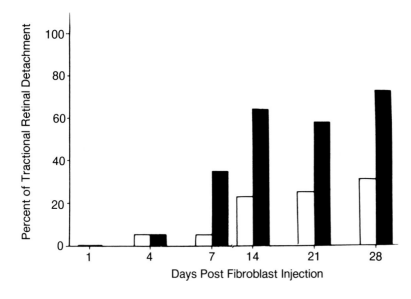

Figure 23-6. Frequency of tractional retinal detachment after injection of heterologous fibroblasts was significantly decreased 1 week after a single 1-mg intravitreal injection of 5-FU. Five-FU–treated eyes *(open bars);* control eyes *(solid bars).*

conjunctival injections of 5-FU further reduced the rate of detachment.[13] These results were confirmed by Binder and associates, who reported a decrease from 75% to 30%.[6] Sunlap and coworkers showed that 1 μM (140 μg) of 5-FU administered intravitreally reduced detachment rates from 63% to 37% when 100,000 fibroblasts were injected, but reported no effect when the number of injected cells was increased to 250,000.[98] A single 1-mg injection of 5-FU lessened intraocular proliferation in 16 of 24 rabbits subjected to double perforation injuries.[4]

Stern and coworkers demonstrated the efficacy of 5-FU in reducing PVR in aphakic vitrectomized eyes after the injection of RPE cells. In eyes receiving 200,000 cells, intraocular injections of 0.5 mg of 5-FU every 24 hours for 7 days reduced rates of detachment from 100% to 66% at 4 weeks. In aphakic vitrectomized eyes receiving 400,000 cells, no difference was reported between control and treated groups at 4 weeks.[96]

Human Clinical Studies
In a pilot study, 22 patients with advanced forms of PVR were treated with a combination of intraocular or periocular 5-FU along with scleral buckling and vitrectomy.[11] Of 22 patients, 12 were given 5 consecutive subconjunctival injections of 10 mg of 5-FU beginning on the day of surgery. Fourteen of 22 received in-

travitreal injections of 1 mg of 5-FU on one or more occasions. Four patients received both subconjunctival and intravitreal injections. After 2 months, 73% of the retinas remained attached and 64% of the patients had ambulatory vision or better. At 6 months, the attachment rate was 60%, and 55% had at least ambulatory vision.[11] Successful attachment rates of 40% and 35% were achieved when only scleral buckling was used.[38,64] No evidence of retinal toxicity was attributed to the administration of the drug. The only complications noted were delayed healing of corneal epithelial defects in 18% of the patients and subtle subepithelial or anterior stromal scarring in 32% of these cases.[11] This study suggested that 5-FU in combination with standard vitrectomy and postoperative fluid–gas exchange may significantly increase the retinal reattachment rates in advanced forms of PVR.[11]

Toxicity Studies
The potential toxicity of 5-FU and 5-FUR following intravitreal injection has been examined by a number of investigators using both histologic and electrophysiologic techniques. Unfortunately, each investigation has been conducted under a different condition, making a comparison of the results difficult. Stern and coworkers determined the toxicity of 5-FU following intravitreal injection into rabbit eyes that had under-

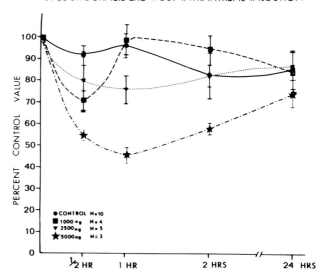

Figure 23-7. Averaged electoretinographic b-wave amplitudes following an intravitreal injection of varying dosages of 5-FU in rabbits as a function of time.

gone a lensectomy-vitrectomy.[95] Eyes that received 1.25 mg every 12 hours for 4 consecutive days followed by 1.25 mg every 24 hours for 3 days showed a decrease of electroretinographic b-waves to 0% of control baseline values and no recovery after 3 weeks. Loss of photoreceptor outer segments and ribosomes, along with corneal opacification, was observed in those eyes as well. A second group, which received 1.25 mg of 5-FU every 24 hours for 7 days, also showed loss of photoreceptors and ribosomes at 9 days, but a return to normal values at 5 weeks. A decrease in b-wave amplitude to 10% of baseline at 2 weeks with a return to 62% at 3 weeks was also reported. A third group of eyes receiving 0.5 mg of 5-FU every 24 hours for 1 week exhibited no signs of toxicity.[95] The effect of lensectomy-vitrectomy on 5-FU toxicity was not determined, but since the rate of clearance of 5-FU from aphakic-vitrectomized eyes is 2.5 times that in normal eyes, one would anticipate that precedent lensectomy-vitrectomy would decrease potential 5-FU toxicity.[53]

Blumenkranz and associates have determined the toxicity of 5-FU following a single intravitreal injection.[11,12] Doses of up to 1.0 mg produced no demonstrable retinal toxicity by electrophysiologic or histologic criteria. A dose of 2.5 mg caused a slight decrease in b-wave amplitude, which returned to normal within 24

hours (Fig. 23-7). In contrast, a single injection of 5 mg of 5-FU effected a significant decrease (52% of normal baseline) in b-wave amplitude, which returned to normal after 2 weeks. This dosage also produced histologic evidence of toxicity, including densification of photoreceptor nuclei, swelling of mitochondria, and disruption of outer-segment plasma membranes. In later stages, retinal atrophy was accompanied by atrophic hole formation. However, no significant damage to retinal inner layers was noted.[11] Other investigators have reported development of a whitish retinal edema, pale optic discs, and multiple atrophic hole formation.[6] Narrowing of retinal vessels and hemorrhages resembling venous thrombosis have also been observed after a single 5-mg injection of 5-FU.[6]

In addition to the studies in vivo, Nao-I and Honda have evaluated the toxic effects of 5-FU on rabbit retinas in vitro.[73] Concentrations up to 10 μg/ml produced no change in b-wave amplitude, while 100 μg/ml and 1 mg/ml significantly reduced b-wave amplitude, and 5 mg/ml resulted in a complete disappearance of the b-wave although recovery occurred within 1 hour after the removal of the drug.[73] Other investigators have found 250 μg/ml to be a nontoxic level for infusion of 5-FU into aphakic eyes, either alone or in combination with other antineoplastic drugs.[5,80,81]

Blumenkranz and coworkers have reported that a single intravitreal injection of 100 μg or less of 5-FUR produced no evidence of retinal toxicity. However, dosages of 500 μg resulted in a significant decrease in b-wave amplitude. Doses of 1 mg produced thrombotic occlusion of medullary ray vessels, preretinal hemorrhage, and retinal neuronal atrophy.[9]

Both 5-FU and 5-FUR caused a decrease in protein synthesis and transport in the neural retina.[63] A single intravitreal injection of 100 μg/ml of 5-FUR decreased axonal protein transport to the superior colliculus by 53%. Injections of 2.5 mg and 1.0 mg of 5-FU reduced transport by 26% and 13%, respectively.[63]

Corneal toxicity has also been described after intravitreal, subconjunctival, and topical application of 5-FU.[37,91,95] When 1.5 mg was administered topically six times per day, corneal epithelial wound healing was decreased by 40%, and the rate of corneal and conjunctival cell mitoses was significantly reduced.[91] In contrast, Jumblatt's group reported that 10 μg/ml of 5-FU had no effect on corneal epithelial wound closure in vitro.[54]

Systemic intravenous treatment with 5-FU has been associated with a number of ocular side-effects including irritative conjunctivitis, epiphora, hyperemia, blurred vision, excessive lacrimation, and severe punctal cannicular stenosis, and oculomotor disturbances, especially weakness of convergence and divergence, have followed treatment with 5-FU.[7,17,21,32,40] Bilateral cicatricial ectropion after the topical application of 5-FU has also been reported.[33] Most of these manifestations of ocular toxicity were reversed within 1 to 2 weeks after the drug was discontinued.[32]

Clearance and Uptake of Fluoropyrimidines

The ocular pharmacokinetics of 5-FU and 5-FUR are well known. Following a single intravitreal injection of 1 mg of 5-FU, peak concentrations of 670 μg/ml were attained in both phakic and aphakic vitrectomized eyes.[53] The drug was cleared approximately 2.5 times more rapidly in aphakic vitrectomized eyes (half-life, 1.4 hrs) than in normal eyes (half-life, 3.4 hrs) during the first 12 hours. After that time, clearance rates were similar in both phakic and apha-

kic eyes. The difference in rates is attributed to loss of barrier functions of the lens and anterior vitreous/hyaloid along with increased outflow through aqueous channels. Clearance from the vitreous is biphasic for both groups of eyes, following first-order kinetics for the first 12 hours and zero-order kinetics thereafter (Fig. 23-8).[53] Thus, potentially therapeutic concentrations remained in the vitreous up to 72 hours after a single intravitreal injection.[8,53] In phakic eyes, 5-FU concentrations in the aqueous humor stayed relatively constant for the first 12 hours (20 μg/ml) and decreased gradually thereafter. Plasma concentrations peaked at 2 hours (0.12–0.15 μg/ml) then declined rapidly.[53]

In aphakic vitrectomized eyes filled with silicone, the amount of 5-FU recovered in the aqueous after a single intravitreal injection was five times greater than that recovered from normal phakic eyes; peak concentrations occurred at 60 minutes.[77] If the aphakic vitrectomized eyes were filled with saline, the amount of drug recovered increased 17-fold.[77]

5-FUR is cleared from the vitreous in a manner similar to 5-FU. Following a 500-μg bolus injection, peak concentrations of 308 μg/ml were achieved. After 2 hours, vitreous concentrations dropped to 198 μg/ml, and to 1.1 μg/ml 48 hours later. Aqueous concentrations reached a maximum of 9.6 μg/ml at 6 hours and dropped to 0.8 μg/ml by 24 hours. Intravitreal concentrations of 5-FUR 48 hours after injection were greater than 20 times the ID_{50} for several ocular cell types in vitro.[11]

The rate of uptake of 5-FU and 5-FUR following subconjunctival injection differs considerably. After an injection of 6.25 mg of 5-FU, peak concentrations of 69.5 μg/ml and 10.5 μg/ml were measured in the aqueous and vitreous, respectively.[85] By 12 hours, concentrations of drug in both chambers had decreased to 0.9 μg/ml, indicating that 5-FU is cleared more rapidly from the aqueous than vitreous under these conditions.[85] Maximum serum levels (558 μg) occurred in the first 30 minutes and decreased to 120 μg by 12 hours.[85]

In contrast, the ocular penetrance of 5-FUR following subconjunctival injection was inferior to that of 5-FU. After a 5-mg injection, peak anterior chamber concentrations (10.7 μg/ml)

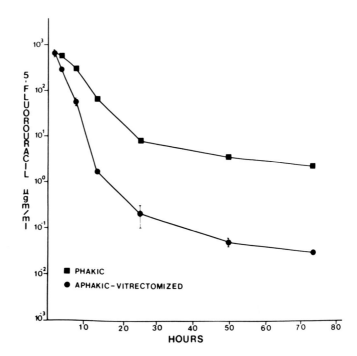

Figure 23-8. Ocular clearance of intravitreal 5-FU from normal or aphakic/vitrectomized eyes following 1-mg injection.

were six times higher than peak vitreous concentrations (1.7 μg/ml), but only about 20% of the concentrations of 5-FU under similar conditions. After 2 hours, concentrations in both eyes were similar to serum concentrations. This suggested that 5-FUR enters the eye primarily through equilibration between the plasma and ocular compartments rather than by moving directly from the subconjunctival space.

When 5-FU was administered topically (7.2 mg, 3 drops), peak aqueous concentrations of 200 μg/ml were measured at 30 minutes. Within 8 hours, aqueous concentrations had decreased to less than 1 μg/ml.[29] Maximum vitreous concentrations (6.8 μg/ml) also occurred at 30 minutes. These concentrations were comparable to those achieved after subconjunctival injection.[29,30]

Sustained-Release Drug Delivery Systems
The rapid clearance of 5-FU and 5-FUR from the eye following subconjunctival or intravitreal injection has provided an impetus for the development of sustained release delivery systems.[53,85] Several investigators have incorporated 5-FU or one of its metabolites into liposomes to increase the therapeutic efficacy of the drug. Fluoro-oratate, a metabolic precursor

of 5-FURP, was reportedly significantly more effective in vitro when encapsulated in liposomes.[43] Its increased efficacy was attributed to the inability of fluoro-oratate to be transported across cell membranes.[43] Liposomes containing 5-FU maintained a relatively constant level of the drug in the anterior chamber for at least 8 hours after subconjunctival injection.[92] 5-FURP, a metabolite found to be very effective in inhibiting cellular proliferation in vitro, was effective in delaying wound healing following glaucoma-filtering surgery when encapsulated into liposomes and injected subconjunctivally.[9,93] The charged phosphate group allowed 5-FURP to be easily incorporated into liposomes at physiological pH. Studies are currently under way to determine the pharmacokinetics of drug release from these liposomes and to determine their ability to decrease the incidence of PVR in an animal model following intravitreal injection.

Fluoropyrimidines have also been embedded into organic copolymers to provide an additional sustained-release system. The most promising of these is ethylene vinyl acetate (EVA), which has a consistency similar to that of silicone rubber and can be molded into "tires" for use as scleral buckles.[34] EVA implants embedded with 5-FU or 5-FUR and placed subconjunctivally were effective in preventing tractional detachments after the injection of 300,000 fibroblasts.[34] 5-FU has also been embedded in bis(*p*-carboxyphenoxy)hexane and sebacic acid, a bioerodable copolymer.[62] Setons of this material were effective in postponing failure following glaucoma-filtering surgery in rabbits.[62]

Other Ocular Applications of Fluoropyrimidines

Glaucoma Filtering Procedures

The goal of glaucoma-filtering surgery is to create a fistula that allows controlled egress of fluid from the eye, thereby lowering intraocular pressure. One of the leading causes of failure is scarring at the surgical site, a process in which fibroblasts play a prominent role. Multiple subconjunctival injections of 3 mg of 5-FU resulted in filtering bleb formation in six of eight treated primates and significantly reduced intraocular pressure when compared with the controls.[37] The only signs of ocular toxicity were corneal epithelial defects and delayed healing of conjunctival incision.[37] Topical application of 5-FU did not promote bleb formation as successfully and was more toxic to the cornea than subconjunctival injections.[50] In a human pilot study, subconjunctival 5-FU was given after filtering surgery in 34 eyes with poor surgical prognosis. Of these, 79% achieved an intraocular pressure of 21 torr or less without serious side-effects.[51] Subconjunctival 5-FU has also been useful in the prevention of posterior capsule opacification following cataract extraction in experimental animals.[105]

In addition, 5-FU has been beneficial in the treatment of Greene's melanoma in an animal model. Following a series of intravitreal injections, all treated animals were free of tumor cells after 2 weeks, whereas all control animals showed viable tumors.[75] All treated animals remained tumor-free 2 weeks after treatment ceased.

REFERENCES

1. Algvere P, Koch E: Experimental fibroplasia in the rabbit vitreous: Retinal detachment induced by autologous fibroblasts. Graefe's Arch Clin Exp Ophthalmol 199:215–222, 1976
2. Anderson E: Nucleoside and nucleoside kinase. In Boyer PD (ed): The Enzymes, pp 49–96. New York, Academic Press, 1973
3. Armstrong R, Takimoto C, Cadman E: Fluoropyrimidine-mediated changes in small nuclear RNA. J Biol Chem 261:21–24, 1986
4. Avni I, Belkin M, Hercberg A, et al: Intravitreal 5-fluorouracil in the prevention of post-traumatic vitreous proliferation. Ophthalmologica 188:5–8, 1984
5. Barrada A, Peyman G, Greenberg D, et al: Toxicity of antineoplastic drugs in vitrectomy infusion fluids. Ophthalmic Surg 14:845–847, 1983
6. Binder S, Riss B, Skorpik C, et al: Inhibition of experimental intraocular proliferation with intravitreal 5-fluorouracil. Graefe's Arch Ophthalmol 221:126–129, 1983
7. Bixenman W, Nicholls J, Warwick O: Oculomotor disturbances associated with 5-fluorouracil chemotherapy. Am J Ophthalmol 83:789–793, 1977
8. Blumenkranz M, Claflin A, Hajek A: Selection of therapeutic agents for intraocular proliferative disease. Arch Ophthalmol 102:598–604, 1984
9. Blumenkranz M, Hajek A, Hernandez E, et al: Fluorouridine: A second generation antimetabolite. Invest Ophthalmol Vis Sci (Suppl) 26:285, 1985
10. Blumenkranz M, Hajek A, Sossi N, et al: Evidence for cell specificity in PVR. Invest Ophthalmol Vis Sci (Suppl) 23:272, 1984
11. Blumenkranz M, Hernandez E, Ophir A, et al: 5-Fluorouracil: New applications in complicated retinal detachment for established antimetabolite. Ophthalmology 91:122–130, 1984
12. Blumenkranz M, Ophir A, Claflin A: A pharmacologic approach to non-neoplastic intraocular proliferation. Invest Ophthalmol Vis Sci (Suppl) 20:200, 1981
13. Blumenkranz M, Ophir A, Claflin A, et al: Fluorouracil for the treatment of massive periretinal proliferation. Am J Ophthalmol 94:458–467, 1982
14. Bunt A: Effects of vinblastine in microtubule structure and transport in ganglion cells of the rabbit retina. Invest Ophthalmol Vis Sci 12:579, 1973
15. Canellakis E: Pyrimidine metabolism. I: Enzymatic pathways of uracil and thymidine degradation. J Biol Chem 221:315–322, 1956
16. Canellakis E: Pyrimidine metabolism. III: The interaction of catabolic and anabolic pathways of uracil metabolism. J Biol Chem 227:701–709, 1957
17. Caravella L, Bruns J, Zangmeister M: Punctal canicular stenosis related to systemic fluoroura-

cil therapy. Arch Ophthalmol 99:284–286, 1981

18. Carradona S, Glazer R: The role of deoxyuridine triphosphate nucleotidohydralase, uracil-DNA glycosylase and DNA polymerase in the metabolism of FUdR in human tumor cells. Mol Pharmacol 18:513–520, 1980

19. Carrico C, Glazer R: Augmentation of thymidine of the incorporation and distribution of 5-fluorouracil in ribosomal RNA. Biochem Biophys Res Commun 87:664–670, 1979

20. Carrico C, Glazer R: Effect of 5-fluorouracil on the synthesis and translation of polyadenylic acid-containing RNA from regenerating rat liver. Cancer Res 39:3694–3701, 1979

21. Christophidis N, Vajda F, Lucas I, et al: Ocular side effects with 5-fluorouracil. Aust NZ J Med 9:143–144, 1979

22. Cohen A: On the nature of thymine-less death. Ann NY Acad Sci 186:292–301, 1972

23. Cutroneo K, Roskowsky R, Counts D: Glucocorticoids and collagen synthesis: Comparison in vivo and cell culture studies. Coll Relat Res 1:557, 1981

24. Davidson C, Green W, Wong V: Retinal atrophy induced by intravitreous colchicine. Invest Ophthalmol Vis Sci 24:301, 1983

25. Diegelmann R, Peterkofsky B: Inhibition of collagen secretion from bone and cultured fibroblasts by microtubular disruptive drugs. Proc Natl Acad Sci USA 69:892–896, 1972

26. Dolnick B, Pink J: 5-Fluorouracil modulation of dihydrofolate reductase RNA levels in methotrexate-resistant KB cells. J Biol Chem 258:13299, 1983

27. Dolnick B, Pink J: Effects of 5-fluorouracil on dihydrofolate reductase and dihydrofolate reductase mRNA from methotrexate-resistant KB cells. J Biol Chem 260:3006–3014, 1985

28. Elford H, Bonner E, Kerr B, et al: The effect of methotrexate and 5-fluorodeoxyuridine on ribonucleotide reductase activity of mammalian cells. Cancer Res 37:4389–4394, 1977

29. Fantes F, Heuer D, Parrish R, et al: Topical fluorouracil: Pharmacokinetics in normal rabbit eyes. Arch Ophthalmol 103:953–955, 1985

30. Fantes F, Parrish R, Heuer D: Subconjunctival fluorouracil: Mechanism of ocular penetration. Invest Ophthalmol Vis Sci (Suppl) 27:322, 1986

31. Ferguson M: The effect of antineoplastic agents on wound healing. Surg Gynecol Obstet 154:421, 1981

32. Fraunfelder F, Meyer S: Ocular toxicity of antineoplastic agents. Ophthalmology 90:1–3, 1983

33. Galentine P, Sloas H, Hargett N, et al: Bilateral cicatricial ectropion following topical administration of 5-fluorouracil. Ann Ophthalmol 13:575–577, 1981

34. Gaynon M, Monroe F, Singh T, et al: Ethylene vinyl acetate delivery system for the sustained delivery of fluorouracil and fluorouridine in a fibroblast model of proliferative vitreoretinopathy. Invest Ophthalmol Vis Sci (Suppl) 27:187, 1986

35. Glazer R, Lloyd L: Association of cell lethality with incorporation of 5-fluorouracil and 5-fluorouridine into nuclear RNA in human colon carcinoma cells in culture. Mol Pharmacol 24:468–473, 1982

36. Gleason M, Fraenkel-Connat H: Biological consequences of incorporation of 5-fluorocytidine in the RNA of 5-fluorouracil-treated eukaryotic cells. Proc Natl Acad Sci USA 73:1528–1531, 1976

37. Gressel M, Parrish R, Folberg R: 5-Fluorouracil and glaucoma filtering surgery. I: An animal model. Ophthalmology 91:378–383, 1984

38. Grizzard W, Hilton G: Scleral buckling for the retinal detachments complicated by periretinal proliferation. Arch Ophthalmol 90:121–125, 1982

39. Gros F, Gilbert W, Hiatt H, et al: Molecular and biologic characteristics of messenger RNA. Cold Spring Harbor Symp Quant Biol 26:111–126, 1961

40. Hammersley J, Luce J, Florentz T, et al: Excessive lacrimation from fluorouracil treatment. JAMA 225:747–748, 1973

41. Hartzer M, Blumenkranz M, Hajek A: The effects of fluoropyrimidines on collagen synthesis and collagen matrix contraction. Invest Ophthalmol Vis Sci (Suppl) 26:26, 1985

42. Hartzer M, Blumenkranz M, Hajek A, et al: Time dependence of fluoropyrimidine effects on cellular proliferation. Invest Ophthalmol Vis Sci (Suppl) 27:187, 1986

43. Heath T, Lopez N, Lewis G, et al: Liposomes as drug carriers in the treatment of PVR. Invest Ophthalmol Vis Sci (Suppl) 26:284, 1985

44. Heath T, Lopez N, Lewis G, et al: Fluoropyrimidine treatment of ocular cicatricial disease. Invest Ophthalmol Vis Sci 27:940–945, 1986

45. Heidelberger C: Fluorinated pyrimidines. Prog Nucleic Acid Res Mol Biol 4:1–50, 1965

46. Heidelberger C: On the rational development of a new drug: The example of fluorinated pyrimidines. Cancer Treat Rep 65:3–9, 1981

47. Heidelberger C, Chaudhuri N, Danenberg P, et al: Fluorinated pyrimidines: A new class of tumor-inhibitory compounds. Nature 179:663–666, 1957

48. Heidelberger C, Danenberg P, Moran R: Fluorinated pyrimidines and their nucleosides. Adv Enzymol 54:58–119, 1983

49. Herrick D, Kufe D: Lethality associated with incorporation of 5-fluorouracil into periribosomal RNA. Mol Pharmacol 26:135–140, 1984

50. Heuer D, Gressel M, Parrish R, et al: Topical

fluorouracil. II: Postoperative administration in an animal model of glaucoma filtering surgery. Arch Ophthalmol 104:132–136, 1986

51. Heuer D, Parrish R, Gressel M, et al: 5-Fluorouracil and glaucoma filtering surgery. II: A pilot study. Ophthalmology 91:384–393, 1984

52. Hughes K: Preliminary report on the effects of a four drug cytotoxic protocol on wound healing in the rat. Clin Oncol 7:235–240, 1981

53. Jarus G, Blumenkranz M, Hernandez E, et al: Clearance of intravitreal fluorourcil: Normal and aphakic vitrectomized eyes. Ophthalmology 92:91–96, 1985

54. Jumblatt M, Neufeld A: A tissue culture assay of corneal epithelial wound closure. Invest Ophthalmol Vis Sci 27:8–13, 1986

55. Kahn S: Tumor biology and its implication for cancer chemotherapy. In Brodsky J, Kahn S, Conroy A (eds): Cancer Therapy III. New York, Grune & Stratton, 1978

56. Khym J, Jones M, Lee W, et al: On the question of compartmentalization of the nucleotide pool. J Biol Chem 253:8741–8746, 1978

57. Kirkwood J, Ensminger W, Roskowsky A, et al: Comparison of pharmacokinetics of 5-fluorouracil and 5-fluorouracil with concurrent thymidine infusions in a phase I trial. Cancer Res 40:107–113, 1980

58. Klubes P, Cerna I: Use of uridine to enhance the antitumor selectivity of 5-fluorouracil. Cancer Res 43:3182–3186, 1983

59. Krenitsky T, Barclay M, Jacquez J: Specificity of mouse uridine phosphorylase: Chromatography, purification, and properties. J Biol Chem 239:805–812, 1964

60. Kufe D, Major P, Egan E, et al: 5-Fluoro-2'-deoxyuridine incorporation in L1210 DNA. J Biol Chem 256:8885–8888, 1981

61. Kwong E, Litin B, Jones M, et al: Effect of antineoplastic drugs in fibroblast proliferation in rabbit aqueous humor. Ophthalmic Surg 15:847–851, 1984

62. Lee D, Flores R, Anderson P, et al: Filtration surgery in rabbits using slow release polymers and 5-FU. Invest Ophthalmol Vis Sci (Suppl) 27:212, 1986

63. Leon J, Hopp R, Mills R, et al: The effect of fluorouracil on protein synthesis in rabbit retina. Invest Ophthalmol Vis Sci (Suppl) 27:304, 1986

64. Machemer R: Massive periretinal proliferation: A logical approach to therapy. Trans Am Ophthalmol Soc 75:556–586, 1977

65. Major P, Egan E, Herrick D, et al: 5-Fluorouracil incorporation in DNA of human breast carcinoma cells. Cancer Res 42:3005–3009, 1982

66. Mallick K, Hajek A, Parrish R: Fluorouracil (5-FU) and cytarabine (Ara-C) inhibition of corneal epithelial cell and conjunctival fibroblast proliferation. Arch Ophthalmol 103:1398–1402, 1985

67. Mandel H: The target cell determinants of the antitumor action of 5-FU: Does FU incorporation in RNA play a role? Cancer Treat Rep 65:63, 1981

68. Martin D, Stolfi R, Sawyer S, et al: High dose 5-fluorouracil with delayed uridine rescue in mice. Cancer Res 42:3964–3970, 1982

69. Martin D, Stolfi R, Spiegelman S: Striking augmentation of the *in vivo* anticancer activity of 5-fluorouracil by combination with pyrimidine nucleosides: An RNA effect. Proc Am Assoc Cancer Res 19:221, 1978

70. Morris T, Lincoln F, Lee A: The effect of 5-fluorouracil on abdominal wound healing in rats. Aust NZ J Surg 48:219–221, 1978

71. Murgo A, Fried J, Burchenal D, Vale K, et al: Effects of thymidine and thymidine plus 5-fluorouracil on the growth kinetics of a human lymphoid cell line. Cancer Res 40:1543–1549, 1980

72. Myers C: The pharmacology of the fluoropyrimidines. Pharmacol Rev 33:1–17, 1981

73. Nao-I N, Honda Y: Toxic effect of fluorouracil on the rabbit retina. Am J Ophthalmol 96:641–643, 1983

74. Nayak R, Martin D, Stolfi K, et al: Pyrimidine nucleosides enhance the anticancer activity of FU and augment its incorporation into nuclear RNA, abstracted. Proc Am Assoc Cancer Res 19:251, 1978

75. Olsen K, Blumenkranz M, Hernandez E, et al: 5-Fluorouracil in the treatment of Greene's melanoma. Invest Ophthalmol Vis Sci (Suppl) 25:84, 1984

76. Ophir A, Blumenkranz M, Claflin A: Experimental intraocular proliferation and neovascularization. Am J Ophthalmol 94:450–457, 1982

77. Orr G, Cohen-Traevert D, Lean J: Aqueous concentrations of fluorouracil after intravitreal injection. Arch Ophthalmol 104:431–434, 1986

78. Parker W, Klubes P: Enhancement by uridine of the anabolism of 5-fluorouracil in mouse t-lymphoma (S-49) cells. Cancer Res 45:4249–4256, 1985

79. Peterkofsky B, Diegelmann R: Use of a mixture of proteinase-free collagenases for the specific assay of radioactive collagen in the presence of other proteins. Biochemistry 10:978–993, 1971

80. Peyman G, Barrada A, Greenberg D, et al: Toxicity of antineoplastic drug combinations on vitrectomy infusion fluid. Ophthalmic Surg 15:844–846, 1984

81. Peyman G, Greenberg D, Fishman G, et al: Evaluation of toxicity of intravitreal antineo-

plastic drugs. Ophthalmic Surg 15:411–413, 1984

82. Plagemann P: Nucleotide pools of Novikoff rat hepatoma cells growing in suspension culture. II: Independent nucleotide pools for nucleic acid synthesis. J Cell Physiol 77:241–258, 1971

83. Radtke N, Tano Y, Chandler D: Simulation of massive periretinal proliferation by autotransplantation of retinal pigment epithelial cells in rabbits. Am J Ophthalmol 91:76–87, 1981

84. Reyes P: The synthesis of 5-fluorouridine-5′-phosphate by pyrimidine phosphoribosyltransferase of mammalian origin. I: Some properties of the enzyme from P-1534J mouse leukemia cells. Biochemistry 8:2057–2063, 1959

85. Rootman J, Tisdall J, Gudauskas G, et al: Intraocular penetration of subconjunctivally administered ¹⁴C-fluorouracil in rabbits. Arch Ophthalmol 97:2375–2378, 1979

86. Rosen R, Rothman F, Weigert M: Miscoding caused by 5-fluorouracil. J Mol Biol 44:363–375, 1969

87. Rutman R, Cantarow A, Paschkis K: Studies in 2-acetylaminofluorine carcinogenesis. III: The utilization of uracil-2-¹⁴C by preneoplastic rat liver and rat hepatoma. Cancer Res 14:119–134, 1954

88. Sawyer R, Stolfi R, Martin D, et al: Incorporation of 5-fluorouracil into murine bone marrow DNA *in vivo*. Cancer Res 44:1847–1851, 1984

89. Scheutz J, Wallace H, Diasio R: 5-fluorouracil incorporation into DNA of CF-1 mouse bone marrow cells as a possible mechanism of toxicity. Cancer Res 44:1358–1363, 1984

90. Shani J, Danenberg P: Evidence that intracellular synthesis of 5-fluorouridine-5′-phosphate from 5-fluorouracil and 5-fluorouridine is compartmentalized. Biochem Biophys Res Commun 122:439–445, 1984

91. Shapiro M, Thoft R, Friend J, et al: 5-Fluorouracil toxicity to the ocular surface epithelium. Invest Ophthalmol Vis Sci 26:580–583, 1985

92. Simmons S, Sherwood M, Nichols D, et al: Pharmacokinetics of a 5-fluorouracil liposomal delivery system. Invest Ophthalmol Vis Sci (Suppl) 27:212, 1986

93. Skuta G, Assil K, Parrish R, et al: 5-FURMP liposomes and filtering surgery in owl monkeys. Invest Ophthalmol Vis Sci (Suppl) 27:212, 1986

94. Spears C, Shani J, Shahinian A, et al: Assay and time course of 5-fluorouracil incorporation into RNA of L1210/0 ascites cells *in vivo*. Mol Pharmacol 27:302–307, 1985

95. Stern W, Guerin C, Erickson P, et al: Ocular toxicity of fluorouracil after vitrectomy. Am J Ophthalmol 96:43–51, 1983

96. Stern W, Lewis G, Erickson P, et al: Fluorouracil therapy for proliferative vitreoretinopathy after vitrectomy. Am J Ophthalmol 96:33–42, 1983

97. Sugita G, Tano Y, Machemer R, et al: Intravitreal autotransplantation of fibroblasts. Am J Ophthalmol 89:121–130, 1980

98. Sunlap M, Wiedemann P, Sorgente N, et al: Effects of cytotoxic drugs on proliferative vitreoretinopathy in the rabbit cell injection model. Curr Eye Res 3:619–623, 1984

99. Tattersall M, Jackson R, Connors T, et al: Combination chemotherapy: The interaction of methotrexate and 5-fluorouracil. Eur J Cancer 9:733–739, 1973

100. Treese M, Spitznas M, Foos R, et al: Experimental tractional retinal detachment in rabbits: Clinical picture and histopathologic features. Graefe's Arch Clin Exp Ophthalmol 214:213, 1980

101. Ullman B, Lee M, Martin D, et al: Cytotoxicity of 5-fluoro-2′-deoxyuridine: Requirements for reduced folate cofactors and antagonism by methotrexate. Proc Natl Acad Sci USA 75:980–983, 1978

102. Umeda M, Heidelberger C: Comparative studies of fluorinated pyrimidines with various cell lines. Cancer Res 28:2529–2538, 1968

103. van Bockxmeer F, Martin C: Measurement of cell proliferation and cell mediated contraction in 3-dimensional hydrated collagen matrices. J Tissue Culture Methods 7:163–167, 1982

104. van Bockxmeer F, Martin C, Constable I: Models for assessing scar tissue inhibitors. Retina 5:47, 1985

105. Walsh P, Stark W, Johnson M, et al: Use of 5-fluorouracil to prevent posterior capsule opacification. Invest Ophthalmol Vis Sci (Suppl) 26:191, 1985

106. Welling P, Awdry P, Bors F, et al: Clinical evaluation of trifluorothymidine in the treatment of herpes simplex corneal ulcers. Am J Ophthalmol 73:932–942, 1972

107. Wiedemann P, Cohen-Travaert D, Sorgente N, et al: *In vitro* evaluation of fluoropyrimidines for proliferative vitreoretinopathy. Invest Ophthalmol Vis Sci (Suppl) 26:284, 1985

108. Wilkinson D, Pitot H: Inhibition of ribosomal ribonucleic acid maturation in Novikoff hepatoma cells by 5-fluorouracil and 5-fluorouridine. J Biol Chem 248:63–68, 1973

24

Surgical Management
of Vitreoretinal Disorders

Wayne E. Fung

Mechanized vitrectomy began in 1972 as the result of the pioneering work of Robert Machemer.[14] For the first time in the entire history of ophthalmology, man invaded the vitreous cavity through the pars plana in a planned, microscopically controlled manner. For those ophthalmologists who were trained to avoid the vitreous whenever possible, this surgical approach bordered on heresy. For those who recognized the heretofore uncontrolled role that the vitreous body exercised upon the retina, this approach represented a quantum leap forward in ophthalmic surgery. Understandably, the comments and predictions about this technique in the early 1970s were based on the fears or promises of what might be forthcoming from this new surgical approach.

Initially, the vitrectomy instruments were rotary-cutting, "full-function" instruments. That is, the cutting action of these instruments was performed by a rotating element revolving within a partially open cylinder, and the outer sleeves of the surgical probe also delivered infusion fluid into the vitreous cavity and illumination for the surgeon's eye. By today's standards, these instruments were fairly crude because of their diameter (3 mm–4.5 mm) and the inefficiency of their cutting action. These disadvantages, however, do not negate the significant ad-

The manuscript was prepared by Peg Brickley, of Pacific Ophthalmic Consultants, San Francisco. All illustrations were drawn by James Brodale, Medical Research Institute, Pacific Medical Center.

vance that was made in ophthalmic surgery by the development of these concepts and instruments.

In the early days of vitrectomy, these multipurpose instruments were expected eventually to reverse all the pathologic processes in the fundus. They were expected to clear vitreous opacities, cut transvitreal membranes, and even attack undesired preretinal membranes. Successes, often dramatic, were achieved in the first two conditions. Even so, complications—retinal dialyses and smaller traction tears—were encountered because of the relatively large size of the intravitreal probe and the relatively poor cutting efficiency of the early rotating mechanisms. Initially, these complications were acceptable because of the nature of the pathology being treated. But it was soon recognized that the pars plana approach and the full-function instrumentation could be improved.

Separating the functions necessary for vitrectomy was first proposed by O'Malley and popularized by Charles.[3,19] Cutting and aspiration, infusion and illumination functions need not be contained in one intravitreal probe, they reasoned. By separating the functions and introducing them into the vitreous cavity by three separate 20-gauge ports, they demonstrated that complications arising solely from instrumentation could be dramatically minimized. "Modern" vitreous surgery was initiated.

This chapter emphasizes the basic principles now used in vitreous surgery, the ocular condi-

362

tions most suitable for this form of invasive therapy, and the major potential complications of these techniques.

BASIC PRINCIPLES

Wound Size. Most pars plana vitrectomies are performed through 20-gauge incisions. These incisions may be made with a disposable 20-gauge needle or with a specialized microvitreoretinal (MVR) blade. The use of smaller incisions dramatically reduced the incidence of retinal dialyses and late postoperative bleeding from the wound sites. With the larger incisions, the potential for neovascular ingrowth in the pars plana region was real; it occurred in approximately 5% of cases. Such ingrowths might then be responsible for intermittent intravitreal hemorrhages.

Wound Location. Initially, incisions were made in the pars plana 4 mm, 5 mm, and sometimes 6 mm posterior to the limbus. Fear of damaging a clear lens was the impetus for placing incisions in these locations. On the other hand, incisions were not placed so far posterior as to threaten the integrity of the peripheral retina.

Over the past several years, most experienced vitreous surgeons began moving their 20-gauge incisions farther foreward. With the proper introduction of the intravitreal instruments, fear of damaging the lens and producing bleeding from the ciliary body progressively subsided. At the present time, this author introduces all instruments and the infusion cannula 3 mm posterior to the surgical limbus, regardless of whether the eye is phakic or not. Incisions at the 3-mm point also allow the introduction of instruments at more of a right-angle approach to the vitreous base. Penetrating the vitreous base at this angle is less likely to transfer traction forces to the peripheral retina than a penetration that runs parallel to the transvitreal fibers of the vitreous base. The latter course travels through a greater portion of this tenacious area of the vitreous and thus has a greater likelihood of transmitting traction forces to the peripheral retina.

Length of the Infusion Cannula. Initially, infusion cannulas were designed to be relatively short (2 mm – 4 mm) for fear of damaging the equatorial portion of the lens. These shorter cannulas run the risk of not penetrating the choroid or the epithelium of the pars plana, especially in recently traumatized or recently operated eyes. Infusion of the fluid into the suprachoroidal space or the subepithelial space immediately introduces a serious complication during surgery. For this reason, this author favors routinely using a 6-mm cannula in both phakic and aphakic eyes. The only exception is in eyes of children under the age of three, when a 4-mm cannula should be used.

In eyes that have recently sustained severe trauma or that are known to have peripheral choroidal detachments, an infusion cannula incorporated with an endoilluminator is least likely to infuse fluid into a space other than the vitreous cavity. In these instances, the infusion line is not activated until the surgeon sees that the endoilluminator light is within the vitreous cavity. The irrigating illuminator is not used on a routine basis, primarily because the amount of illumination is less than that delivered by an illuminator without infusion. This is because the cross-section of the solo illuminator is greater than the cross-section of the fiberoptics combined with the irrigating cannulas.

Limbal Ring and Replaceable Contact Lenses. Pars plana vitrectomy carries with it the need to use a contact lens on the cornea in order to visualize structures beyond the anterior vitreous. Initially, these contact lenses were either free-floating or attached to a handle of some sort. They required constant manipulation by the assistant or the surgeon. In order to obviate this inconvenience, a system of interchangeable contact lenses held in place by a metal ring sutured to the limbus was developed. This system is less traumatic to the corneal epithelium and also affords the opportunity to replace a plano lens with a lens of increasingly stronger prisms for viewing the periphery. Freeing the hands of the assistant is another major advantage.

Intravitreal Scissors. Either manual or automated intravitreal scissors have largely replaced the practice of peeling membranes from the surface of the retina solely by applying traction. When two-handed vitrectomy became established, more preretinal membranes were elevated from the surface of the retina by placing a hook or a bent needle beneath the edge of the membrane and pulling toward the middle of the vitreous cavity. While successful in most cases, this technique carried with it the possibility of creating a retinal tear. Currently, membranes are more commonly segmented or delaminated from the surface of the retina by mechanical scissors. This drastically reduces the probability of transmitting undue traction forces to the retina and reduces the likelihood of ripping blood vessels that course through the connections between the epiretinal membrane and the underlying retina. By using scissors, the incidence of retinal tears and postoperative vitreous hemorrhage has been significantly reduced.

When attempting to peel a preretinal membrane from the surface of the macula, intravitreal scissors may not be useful, owing to the intimate relationship between the membrane and the underlying retina. In these cases, one must still rely on the stripping techniques that employ a bent needle or an intravitreal hook.

Composition of Irrigating Fluids. Experiments have shown that saline solutions fortified with glucose, buffers, and various nutrients are much less damaging to the lens and corneal endothelium than straight saline solutions. Most surgeons now use a balanced salt solution of some sort. In cases where pupillary contraction poses a threat to visualization, 0.5 ml of 1 : 1000 adrenalin is added to 500 ml of irrigating solution. In cases involving prolonged intravitreal dissection in phakic, diabetic eyes, dextrose (3 ml of a 50% dextrose solution in 500 ml of irrigating solution) is frequently used to prevent the formation of lens opacities during the surgery.[10]

Bipolar Coagulation. With the advent of bimanual intravitreal surgery, the opportunity to use bipolar coagulation became apparent. This can be accomplished by activating the metal shafts of each intravitreal probe (endoilluminator and vitrectomy instrument) with various bi-

polar adapters, or by a single probe with bipolar modifications within it. This form of coagulation is particularly useful for any elevated or bridging structure containing blood vessels, and it can also be used on a bleeding structure on the surface of the retina. Liberal employment of these techniques has significantly reduced the incidence and persistence of postoperative intravitreal hemorrhages.

Intravitreal Cryosurgical Probes. Twenty-gauge intravitreal cryoprobes can be used to administer cryosurgery to the edges of flat retinal holes or to stabilize intravitreal objects, such as a totally dislocated lens or a magnetic or nonmagnetic intravitreal foreign body.[2] Intravitreal cryosurgery has not proven to be as useful as intravitreal laser therapy primarily because retina tends to remain adherent to the tips of the cryoprobe, retinal holes may be enlarged by the introduction of the tip of the probe through a retinal hole, and cryosurgically treated choroid becomes engorged with blood. For these reasons, intravitreal laser therapy is gaining in popularity.

Intravitreal Laser Probes. Initially, this advance was made possible by channeling xenon energy through a fiberoptic probe. This technique, however, carries with it the disadvantage of protein coagulating on the tip of the probe during its use because of the heat generated at this point. Therefore, intravitreal laser probes have superseded xenon probes. Laser probes may be used to apply photocoagulation therapy around flat retinal breaks or to administer panretinal photocoagulation to eyes that have chronic intravitreal hemorrhages. Using such probes in combination with internal drainage and fluid – gas exchange has made it possible to treat very posterior retinal breaks with great accuracy, thus avoiding accidental freezing of the optic nerve and macula.

Intravitreal Drainage. In the presence of a retinal detachment secondary to a single retinal break, drainage of subretinal fluid through the vitreous cavity provides the opportunity of flattening the detachment during the pars plana vitrectomy. This drainage can be performed under direct visual control and is aided by suction forces created by linear aspiration consoles. In the presence of a retinal detachment secondary to more than one retinal break, this technique is less satisfactory because subretinal suction is less efficient when a second retinal defect allows fluid to enter the subretinal space.

Fluid–Gas Exchange. Once formed vitreous has been removed from the midportion of the vitreous cavity, the irrigating fluid that occupies the cavity may be replaced with air or an air–gas mixture by simultaneously aspirating the fluid and injecting the gas. The intravitreal gas can be used to tamponade a retinal defect for several days, or the expanding intravitreal bubble can be used to help expand stiffened retina.

Constant Intravitreal Pressure. Air pumps and pressure gauges that allow the constant infusion of air or air–gas mixtures into the vitreous cavity under adjustable pressure now make it possible to perform intravitreal dissection without being concerned about collapse of the globe or damage from undesirably high intravitreal pressures for prolonged periods.

These, then, are the basic principles that constitute modern pars plana vitrectomy. Undoubtedly, with the passage of more time other new and significant surgical techniques will evolve. Any advance that makes epiretinal dissection and visualization of the pathology more efficient will be welcomed.

OCULAR INDICATIONS FOR PARS PLANA VITRECTOMY

Proliferative Diabetic Retinopathy

Without question, this condition is the primary indication for performing pars plana vitrectomy today. The natural course of this condition produces chronic vitreous hemorrhages, detachment of the posterior vitreous face, elevation of preretinal neovascularization, and progressive traction retinal detachments. Each and every one of these conditions lends itself to pars plana vitrectomy. From the surgeon's standpoint, the

critical clinical findings to evaluate are the chronicity of the situation, the relationship between the detaching posterior vitreous face and the retina, and the extent of traction detachments, when present.

Vitrectomy orthodoxy once held that a chronic vitreous hemorrhage should not be removed until it had been present for at least 6 months. In addition, traction retinal detachments should not be operated upon until the detachment "threatens the macula." While these dicta are now generally observed, the relative safety of pars plana vitrectomy using advanced techniques has, in the opinion of this author, modified the timing to some degree. If a diabetic patient has a useful fellow eye, it is reasonable to wait 6 months for a chronic vitreous hemorrhage in the other eye to clear. This is especially true if repeated observation demonstrates gradual clearing of the hemorrhage. On the other hand, if the fellow eye of the patient is blind, a time period of 3 to 4 months might be more reasonable. This is especially true if the eye involved with the chronic hemorrhage shows recurrent bleeding and if the treating surgeon or the primary ophthalmologist knows that the hemorrhages are secondary to bleeding from previously observed, elevated fibrovascular fronds. Under these circumstances, the likelihood of the hemorrhage resolving satisfactorily within 6 months is small, and surgery should not be delayed. When elevated fibrovascular fronds are known to exist, earlier surgery can not only clear the hemorrhage but can also convert the frond into a benign situation, and associated traction detachments can be minimized.

When a traction detachment involves the retina around the disc or along the temporal arcades, especially in the presence of relatively clear media, delaying pars plana vitrectomy until the traction detachment involves the macula is imprudent. With modern techniques, such detachments can be treated much more safely and efficiently before they begin to threaten the macula.

Using intravitreal scissors and intravitreal bipolar cautery, these detachments can be very effectively treated and reversed safely before central vision is threatened. As soon as some space develops between the detaching posterior

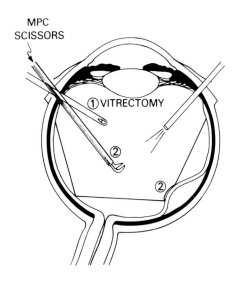

MPC
SCISSORS

① VITRECTOMY

PROLIFERATIVE DIABETIC RETINOPATHY

Figure 24-1. At the present time, the vitrectomy instrument is primarily used to remove formed vitreous between the vitreous base and the site of pathology. (1) Once this goal has been accomplished, the automated scissors are introduced, and the posterior vitreous face and/or preretinal fibrovascular material is lifted off or "circumcised" from its firm attachments to the retina (2).

duced. With these scissors, the detached posterior vitreous face, no matter how limited, is gradually engaged and elevated from the retinal surface. If a point is reached where the detaching posterior vitreous face is firmly adherent to the surface of the retina, the zone is merely "circumcised." That is, the firm attachment is left with the surface of the retina, and this point is cut free from the remainder of the posterior vitreous face. This technique allows the firm attachment to stay with the retina and the remainder of the posterior vitreous face to elevate free of the retina.

Once a posterior vitreous face is completely freed, the intravitreal scissors are extracted and replaced by the vitrectomy instrument, which is then used to remove the entirely detached,

vitreous face and the surface of the retina, vitrectomy is relatively safe. For this reason, the author sees no reason to wait until the macula is threatened.

As recently as 3 years ago, the above statement could not have been made. Separating the posterior vitreous face from the surface of the retina or cutting elevated preretinal bands would have been accomplished through traction provided by bent hooks or needles, or by the cutting action of the vitrectomy instrument itself. Both approaches run the risk of producing retinal tears. The introduction of manual — and especially automated — intravitreal scissors greatly reduced the likelihood not only of retinal tears but also of protracted, postsurgical vitreous hemorrhages. At the present time, the vitrectomy instrument is used only to remove formed vitreous between the vitreous base and the site of pathology (Fig. 24-1). Once this has been accomplished, the vitrectomy instrument is removed, and automated scissors are intro-

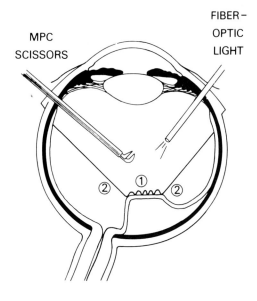

MPC
SCISSORS

FIBER–
OPTIC
LIGHT

② ① ②

TABLE–TOP, DIABETIC DETACHMENT

Figure 24-2. Areas of broad, diabetic traction detachments are best approached by first removing the formed vitreous in the middle of the vitreous cavity *without* removing the detached posterior vitreous face, which extends from the edge of the detachment to the vitreous base. Then, with scissors, the epiretinal membrane over the surface of the detachment is segmented or elevated (1). As this progresses, the lateral traction of the peripheral posterior vitreous face helps to define residual areas on the detachment that require segmenting or elevating. As a last step, the peripheral posterior vitreous face is removed (2).

freely floating posterior vitreous face. Introduction of a bipolar wet-field probe to cauterize the residual "tufts" of fibrovascular tissue on the surface of the retina in various areas is the last step in this procedure. When a diabetic "table-top" traction detachment is present, the situation represents the epitome of diabetic detachments. Experience shows that, following the clearing of central, formed vitreous, one should attack the preretinal membrane on top of the "table," before removing the peripheral detached posterior vitreous face (Fig. 24-2).

In cases involving traction retinal detachments where one is sure the intravitreal dissection has not produced a retinal tear, no further therapy for the traction detachment need be performed. Once the traction forces have been released, absorption of subretinal fluid by the choroid will reattach the retina. On the other

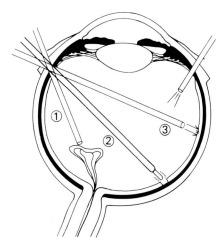

INTERNAL:
① WET-FIELD CAUTERY
② CRYOPEXY
③ LASER THERAPY

Figure 24-4. Once formed vitreous is removed from the central portion of the vitreous cavity, many forms of tranvitreal or *internal* treatment are possible. (1) Bipolar wet-field cautery on a single probe, or bipolar, dual probe, wet-field cautery; (2) cryotherapy; or (3) laser treatment.

hand, if a retinal defect has been created, or if a small defect was present prior to the vitrectomy, this defect must be treated with transvitreal laser or cryosurgery, external cryosurgery, or postoperative laser therapy combined with a buckling procedure or intraoperative fluid–gas exchange.

Special Retinal Detachments

Certain retinal detachments are best approached by pars plana vitrectomy alone or by this approach combined with a standard scleral buckling procedure. Such retinal detachments are those secondary to a macular or a very posterior retinal hole, giant retinal tears, detachments associated with significant proliferative vitreoretinopathy (PVR), or detachments associated with a significant subretinal fibrotic band.

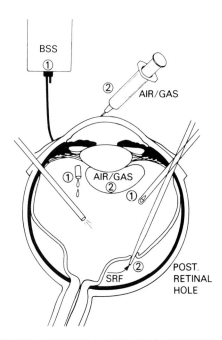

INTERNAL DRAINAGE & FLUID GAS EXCHANGE

Figure 24-3. The pars plana approach to very posterior retinal breaks consists of removing the central vitreous (1) followed by internal drainage of subretinal fluid with simultaneous fluid-and-gas exchange (2). After the break has settled on the choroid, intravitreal laser therapy can be delivered to the edges of the hole (see Fig. 24-4). Less satisfactory is intravitreal or external cryotherapy or postoperative laser therapy.

Macular or Posterior Holes. Repair of macular or very posterior retinal holes is difficult for at least two reasons. First, external cryopexy of

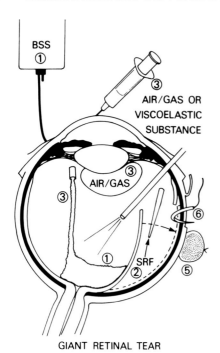

GIANT RETINAL TEAR

Figure 24-5. The posterior flaps of giant retinal tears that are mobile may be stabilized by removing the central vitreous (1), internally draining the subretinal fluid behind the flap (2), and performing a simultaneous fluid-and-gas exchange or injection of a viscoelastic substance (3). After the flap is resting on the choroid (4), it may be stabilized by the buckle alone, by the bubble and a buckle, (5) or by these two plus a transcleral suture (6).

such posterior holes always carries the risk of accidentally delivering cryosurgical energy to the optic nerve. Such an insult to this vital connection to the brain will result in drastically reduced postoperative vision, even though the retina is successfully reattached. Second, placing a buckle in the region of the posterior pole is technically difficult and runs the risk of interrupting important posterior short ciliary vessels. For both of these reasons, such retinal defects are best approached via the pars plana.

These procedures involve (1) pars plana vitrectomy in order to clear a pathway through the vitreous cavity to the posterior defect, (2) transvitreal or "internal" drainage of subretinal fluid through the posterior retinal defect, (3) transvitreal cryosurgery or laser therapy to the edge of the flattened hole, and (4) a fluid–gas exchange

(Fig. 24-3, 24-4). This approach has rendered reparable heretofore inoperable retinal detachments associated with macular holes (like those seen in highly myopic eyes) or very posterior retinal holes.

Giant Retinal Tears. Giant retinal tears present a difficult situation for the standard scleral buckling procedure. Not only is the retinal defect large (at least 90 degrees of arc) but the posterior retinal flap may be extremely mobile or extremely rigid. By employing pars plana vitrectomy techniques, mobile posterior flaps may be stabilized and rigid flaps may be mobilized by stripping the preretinal membranes which are present. When the flap is already mobile, it can be manipulated and partially secured by a fluid–gas exchange or by the layering of viscoelastic substances on its surface (Fig. 24-5). To aid fixation of the mobile posterior flap, transcleral suturing of the posterior flap can be used in conjunction with the intravitreal techniques.[5]

Before embarking on a pars plana vitrectomy, the surgeon should assess whether the situation can be cured with a less hazardous "external" technique. Before the introduction of vitrectomy, many giant retinal tears were cured by one of two techniques: (1) cryosurgery, drainage of subretinal fluid, and injection of air into the vitreous cavity; or (2) cryosurgery, drainage, plus a scleral buckling procedure, with or without intravitreal air. The former technique, cryo-, drainage, air, is often very successful when the retinal flap is mobile and when the giant tear involves the superior, temporal, or nasal quadrant. By positioning the patient properly during the postoperative period, the intravitreal air bubble can unroll and stabilize the retinal flap. This procedure is fast, can be performed under local anesthesia, and is a relatively noninvasive procedure to use in these emergency cases. In a majority of these more "favorable" giant tear cases, the situation can be cured with a simple operation. At the very least, the tear can be reduced in size so that a subsequent scleral buckling procedure is relatively easy and carries a good prognosis. The only disadvantage of this technique is the fact that the patient must be hospitalized for at least 5 to 7 days following surgery in order to carefully monitor the position of the intravitreal bubble in relationship to the edge of the giant tear.[18]

The second technique, cryosurgery, drainage, scleral buckle with or without intravitreal air, is generally successful when the retinal flap does not have a propensity to curl toward the middle of the vitreous cavity. In this type of situation, the scleral buckle can worsen the situation by displacing the retinal flap more posteriorly or by creating a large fish-mouth opening along the tear. It is for this reason that the author favors the nonbuckling approach in amenable cases.

Occasionally, the aforementioned techniques can be assisted by stabilizing the posterior flap of the giant tear if a particular vitreoretinal relationship exists: residual vitreous strands attached to the edge of the flap (Fig. 24-6). In this situation, the free edge of the flap can be tethered to the choroid, making closure of the tear more predictable. This maneuver involves the following indirect ophthalmoscopically controlled steps:

- Recognizing the existence of vitreous strands attached to the far posterior flap by preoperative biomicroscopic examination.
- Surgically attracting the vitreous strand in the tip of a 20- or 23-gauge needle introduced through a sclerotomy placed slightly posterior to the ora.
- Withdrawing the needle with the vitreous attached and purposely incarcerating the vitreous with choroid at the site of the sclerotomy.

By doing this, the free-floating retinal flap now becomes semi-fixed by the vitreous tether, and the orifice of the tear becomes easier to close with either of the aforementioned techniques.[7]

Giant tears associated with a moderate to marked amount of preretinal membrane contraction on the surface of the retinal flap do not have a good prognosis with the two techniques just described. The same can be said for giant retinal tears where the flap is drawn toward the middle of the vitreous cavity by transvitreal membranes or with giant tears in the inferior quadrants. In these situations, the previously

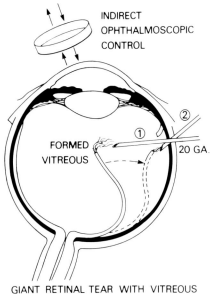

GIANT RETINAL TEAR WITH VITREOUS
ATTACHED TO FLAP

Figure 24-6. When formed vitreous is still attached to the posterior edge of a giant retinal tear, the edge may be tethered to the choroid by introducing a 20-gauge needle attached to a syringe to the vitreous strands (1), aspirating the vitreous into the needle, and (2) incarcerating the vitreous "leash" in the choroid.

described intravitreal approaches constitute the only reasonable modalities to be considered.

Proliferative Vitreoretinopathy. In cases involving significant proliferative vitreoretinopathy (PVR) a pars plana vitrectomy approach is the only technique that has a chance of producing a surgical success. The pathology in these eyes consists of moderate to marked preretinal (and sometimes subretinal) proliferation of fibrotic membranes on one or both surfaces of the retina. This proliferation causes a shortening of the retina in the anteroposterior direction and a contraction of the retina toward the middle of the vitreous cavity.

In its mildest form, PVR is manifested by the presence of "fixed" or star-folds of the retina in one or several locations. In its most advanced form, the retina is drawn to the middle of the vitreous cavity in all quadrants, and the optic nerve cannot be visualized. One other patho-

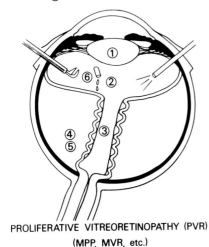

① LENSECTOMY PRN
② VITRECTOMY
③ MEMBRANE PEELING
④ INTERNAL DRAINAGE
⑤ LASER OR CRYOTHERAPY
⑥ FLUID GAS EXCHANGE

PROLIFERATIVE VITREORETINOPATHY (PVR)
(MPP, MVR, etc.)

Figure 24-7. Because PVR is due to the development of epiretinal or subretinal membranes, vitrectomy provides the only direct means of attacking this condition. (*1*) If any cataractous change is present, the lens should be removed before or at the time of surgery. Lens opacities interfere with the surgeon's ability to see details while dissecting membranes off of the surface of the retina, and they increase if gas is left within the vitreous cavity postoperatively. After the vitreous is removed (*2*), the task of membrane segmentation, stripping, or delamination is performed with hooks, picks, forceps, or scissors (*3*). This step must be as complete as possible. An estimation of the success of this membrane removal is then obtained by internal drainage (*4*) and a fluid–gas exchange (*6*). Once the retinal defects are in contact with the pigment epithelium, they are surrounded by internal laser or cryopexy (*5*). External buckling may be required as the last step.

logic condition very frequently exists: an open retinal break or breaks.

In cases with only one or a few peripheral star-folds, the standard scleral buckling approach can be successful in anatomically reattaching the retina, if the breaks can be closed and the star-folds supported by a portion of the buckle. On the other hand, in the more marked cases of PVR, a pars plana approach must be used. The latter cases are treated in a step-wise manner.

The first goal is to mobilize the rigid and contracted retina as much as possible. After the intravitreal structures are removed, one must begin the tedious process of stripping the epiretinal membranes from the surface of the retina in all quadrants without creating new retinal defects. In areas where the preretinal membrane is firmly adherent to the retina, circumcision of the elevated membrane from these points should be performed, rather than forced separation by traction. The stripping and cutting maneuver must be performed in all quadrants, from the pre-equatorial zone to the disc. Once the retina has been mobilized, internal drainage of subretinal fluid through an existing retinal defect will give the surgeon an idea of whether or not the retina will settle back onto the choroid. If it will, intravitreal laser therapy can be applied to the region of the defect(s) and this can be followed by a fluid–gas exchange. After closure of the vitrectomy ports, a scleral buckling procedure can be performed to stabilize the situation (Fig. 24-7).

The prognosis for advanced cases of PVR is in the range of 20% to 50%, even after initial surgical successes, because fibrotic proliferation can return postoperatively, and the retina can be redetached by new forces. One of the main areas of retinal research at this time is the search for a chemical agent that prevents postoperative reproliferation of the preretinal fibrous tissue (See Chap. 22).

In parts of the world where intravitreal liquid silicone can be used, the reported success rate is higher. Liquid silicone is used both as a means of dissecting the preretinal membranes from the surface of the retina and as a tamponade to keep the retina in contact with the choroid. In the United States, liquid silicone is still considered an experimental substance by the Food and Drug Administration, and therefore only a handful of American vitreoretinal surgeons are allowed to use it.

Subretinal Fibrotic Bands and Sheets. Proliferation of fibrotic cells can occur on the undersurface of the retina. Usually, this problem is seen in cases of chronic detachment. The proliferation can produce definitive bands that tent the retina in a "clothesline" fashion, or the fibrosis can produce sheets beneath the retina that behave like a plaque. In general, the bands or sheets are not adherent to the retinal tissue as epiretinal bands and membranes are. The subretinal structures tend to be attached to the retina in isolated spots similar to the supports of a bridge or an elevated highway. The location of these adherent points can be identified by "strumming" the subretinal bands—by stroking the surface of the retina over them and observing the to-and-fro movement of the fibrotic structures between the anchoring points.

When contraction of these subretinal structures causes significant elevation of the retina, closure of more peripheral retinal holes may be made impossible unless the structures are cut. In such instances it is necessary to enter the subretinal space with mechanical scissors through existing or iatrogenically created retinal tears, in order to cut the bands between the anchoring points. Once the bands are cut, they contract toward the fixed points, and the formerly "tented" retina will have a chance to settle toward the choroid (Fig. 24-8).

In detachments where the subretinal bands are peripheral or where they do not elevate the retina for more than 2 mm to 3 mm, this author has allowed them to remain and has proceeded with a standard buckling procedure. If the bands are peripheral, the choroid can be brought to the bands with the buckling element. When the bands are more posterior but thin and not significantly elevated, the buckling procedure can be successful, and the retina may be reattached in the posterior pole. If the bands do not settle, the retina will merely drape itself over the bands, as a sheet does over a clothesline, and remain stationary in this position.

Total Subluxation of the Lenses

This situation usually arises as the result of a lens or the nucleus of a lens being lost in the vitreous cavity at the time of a planned extracapsular cataract extraction. Because this form of cataract surgery is becoming increasingly popular, such cases are occurring more often. Occasionally, the situation is seen following direct trauma to the head or in patients with Marfan's

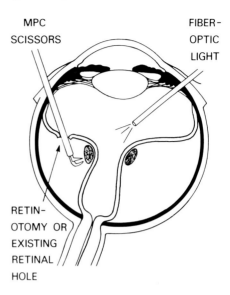

MPC SCISSORS   FIBER-OPTIC LIGHT

RETINOTOMY OR EXISTING RETINAL HOLE

CUTTING SUBRETINAL BAND

Figure 24-8. When subretinal bands prevent settling of the retina, it becomes necessary to cut these structures through an existing retinal defect, if possible, or through an iatrogenically created hole.

syndrome, where the lens can spontaneously slide into the vitreous cavity.

Indications. If the nucleus has moved into the vitreous cavity it must be removed, for its presence will definitely provoke a severe intraocular inflammatory reaction. If the lens capsule of a lens in total subluxation is broken, surgery must be performed for the same reason. Cataract surgeons should understand that these situations do not represent ocular emergencies, for the adverse inflammatory reaction will not develop immediately. When these situations arise, the cataract surgeon should close the cataract wound and inform the patient of the situation. The patient can then be referred to a vitrectomy surgeon in a routine manner.

Occasionally, a lens with its capsule completely intact may sublux into the vitreous cavity. This can occur secondary to direct trauma to the head or in patients with Marfan's syndrome. Surgery is not necessarily mandatory, since the intact capsule will prevent the development of an inflammatory reaction, at least in the near future. This author has seen one patient with Marfan's syndrome go for 20 years before the

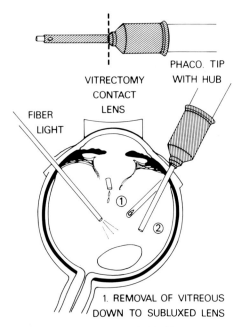

PHACO. TIP WITH HUB

VITRECTOMY CONTACT LENS

FIBER LIGHT

① ②

1. REMOVAL OF VITREOUS DOWN TO SUBLUXED LENS

2. PHACOEMULSIFICATION OF NUCLEUS IN MID VITREOUS

Figure 24-9. To use the Cavitron phacoemulsification tip in the vitreous cavity for the purpose of removing totally dislocated lens material, the three-port vitrectomy system is created. A vitrectomy instrument is initially used to remove the formed vitreous down to the nucleus or lens. Then the "naked" Cavitron tip is exchanged for the vitrectomy instrument after widening the sclerotomy 1 millimeter. If one tries to use the Cavitron handpiece without the silicone hub in place, the first activation of ultrasonic energy will send a fine spray of saline over the surface of the contact lens.

hypermature lens began producing posterior uveitis. With today's advanced vitrectomy techniques, removal of the lens is far safer than it was in the past, and for that reason, this author believes such lenses should be treated rather than observed.

Surgical Technique. There are two basic pars plana approaches: removal with vitrectomy instruments alone and removal with a combination of vitrectomy and phakoemulsification. When employing vitrectomy techniques alone, the three-port approach is preferred over a full-function vitrectomy probe. The convection current generated by the full-function vitrectomy probe makes control of the lens or nucleus difficult.

The vitrectomy-instrument technique consists of clearing the formed vitreous down to the lens, elevating the lens into the midvitreous by suction forces delivered through the cutting port, pressing the lens against the cutting port with the fiberoptic light, then cutting and aspirating. Initially, only a few nibbles will be taken out of the lens before it falls back into the deep portions of the vitreous cavity. By repeating this maneuver, the lens can be crushed or cut into several pieces; each piece is then handled in the same manner until the pieces are small enough to be "ingested" completely through the aspiration port. This technique can be tedious, especially if the nucleus is moderately firm.

A variation of this technique consists of delivering the lens into the anterior chamber with the vitrectomy instrument, constricting the pupil behind the lens, and removing the lens through a limbal incision. When the lens is trapped in the anterior chamber, the corneal endothelium can be traumatized, unless it is protected by a thin layer of viscoelastic substance. This technique is moderately difficult, for placement of the lens in the anterior chamber is not quite as easy as it sounds. The difficulty lies in holding the lens on the tip of the vitrectomy instrument in an attitude that enables delivery through the pupil without having the lens fall back into the vitreous cavity.

The second technique—combined vitrectomy and phakoemulsification—may sound difficult, but it is the most expeditious method this author has found. The basic technique employs the three-port approach. The formed vitreous anterior to the lens or nucleus is removed with standard vitrectomy technique. At this point, the phacoemulsification hand-piece is taken, and the silicone infusion sleeve is cut at the point where the sleeve joins the silicone hub (Fig. 24-9). One now has a naked titanium tip with the sleeveless-silicone hub in its normal position on the phacoemulsification handpiece. The pars plana port used for the vitrectomy instrument is lengthened by approximately 1 mm to admit the naked titanium needle into the vitreous cavity. Under direct visual control the needle is advanced toward the lens or nucleus and brought very close to its surface. Since infusion into the vitreous cavity is being provided through the infusion port, the phakoemulsification hand-piece does not have infusion.

By activating lens suction, the lens or nucleus is drawn to the titanium tip; the lens is elevated into the middle of the vitreous cavity; high suction is activated; the particle is then trapped between the fiberoptic light and the tip; and ultrasound is activated. If the nucleus is soft, the tip will bore into the center of it, and as much of the lens is removed as is possible. If the nucleus is hard, the titanium tip can be driven through the lens nucleus by providing counterpressure with the fiberoptic light. The goal at this stage of the procedure is to bisect the nucleus or lens. Each particle that falls back into the deep portions of the vitreous cavity is then attracted by suction, elevated into the midvitreous and treated in a similar manner. Picking up these particles from the surface of the disc is safer than picking them up from the surface of the macula. This condition can be produced by tilting the globe nasally and rapidly shaking it to and fro.

Phakoemulsification instrumentation expedites the extraction procedure since the aspiration port of the titanium needle is much larger than the cutting port of any vitrectomy instrument and the ultrasonic energy is more efficient at fragmenting the lens than is the cutting action of the vitrectomy instrument. These steps are repeated until all lens fragments are removed. Ultrasonic energy imparted by the shaft on the naked needle does not injure the lips of the sclerotomy.

TRAUMA

Vitrectomy techniques can be applied to a large variety of ocular conditions produced by trauma. This section describes these techniques and goals in four categories: anterior-segment trauma, posterior-segment trauma, perforating injuries of the globe, and intraocular foreign bodies.

Anterior Segment Trauma

Anterior segment trauma consists of one or more of these entities: laceration, hemorrhage, tissue prolapse, traumatic cataract. The first and most important goal is restoring the eye to an intact organ. That is, lacerations or ruptures must be debrided when necessary and closed in a primary fashion. These situations do represent ophthalmic emergencies.

Closure of an anterior-segment wound should be performed with the aid of an operating microscope whenever feasible. The wounds are debrided of foreign or necrotic material; wound edges are prepared for primary closure; and finally, meticulous closure of the defects is accomplished. At the present time, closure is aided by such technical advances as wet-field cautery and viscoelastic substances, the latter being particularly helpful in maintaining an anterior chamber and preventing uveal and lens material from being trapped in the posterior side of corneal lacerations. Once the globe has been closed, the surgeon can decide whether or not to remove a traumatized lens. If removal of a traumatic cataract is elected at the time of a primary closure, a separate limbal or pars plana wound should be used for the approach. Working through the traumatic defect should be avoided because introduction of instruments through such an area only causes swelling of the wound edges and makes primary closure more difficult.

Whether or not to remove a traumatic cataract during the primary procedure depends upon factors such as visualization of the lens through a sutured corneal laceration, the presence or absence of continued bleeding, a general assessment of the amount of traumatic disruption of the globe, and the overall medical status of the patient.

In general, this author favors delaying removal of a traumatic cataract until the primary injury is well healed. This is especially so when the surgeon's view of the anterior segment is compromised by developments that can take place in the cornea or the anterior chamber during the primary repair. When the ocular laceration is associated with a significant lid laceration or a scleral laceration that has produced a vitreous hemorrhage, or when a globe has been severely ruptured, removal of a traumatic cataract would merely protract the surgery and increase the chances of endophthalmitis without adding significantly to the postoperative assessment of the globe's overall status.

In grave situations where the patient's life is endangered, primary closure of the globe should be the only goal during the primary operation. Exceptions to these principles can and do exist, but all factors should be carefully assessed before deciding to remove a traumatic cataract at the time of the initial surgery.

Postoperative evaluation of an eye with a traumatic cataract in place is made less objective because of the inability to view the fundus, but with ultrasonic and computerized tomography and magnetic resonance imaging (MRI) techniques constantly improving, it is becoming less and less of a problem (See Chap. 27).

Performing vitreous surgery as a secondary operation in the presence of a traumatic cataract is not particularly difficult. The first step involves removing the cataract through a limbal or pars plana incision. Vitrectomy should be delayed, if possible, until the cornea has cleared enough to afford an accurate view of the vitreous cavity and retina. In situations where the cornea is markedly scarred from the original surgery, consideration can be given to using an artificial cornea at the time of vitrectomy and combining this procedure with a corneal transplant.[12]

Traumatic Hyphemas

In cases where a total traumatic hyphema ("eight-ball hemorrhage") is present one may have to decide whether or not to remove the anterior chamber clot when uncontrolled secondary glaucoma is present. Assuming that all conservative medical measures have been unsuccessful at controlling the secondary glaucoma and at dissolving the anterior chamber clot, evacuation of the clot using vitrectomy techniques has proven to be very effective.[16]

The technique consists of introducing a small infusion cannula (23-gauge) through the limbus or clear cornea via a "trap" or stab incision with a needle knife. Second, a narrow-diameter vitrectomy instrument is introduced into the anterior chamber through a small limbal incision beneath a conjunctival flap. During the introduction, the surgeon must try to have the cutting port of the instrument facing upward, toward the corneal endothelium. Careful aspira-

tion and cutting are performed in the peripheral portions of the anterior chamber until the tip of the vitrectomy instrument and the cutting port are visualized.

Having reached this goal, the surgeon then gradually advances the vitrectomy instrument toward the center of the anterior chamber. While this is in progress, infusion fluid is introduced to ensure maintenance of a deep anterior chamber, thus protecting the underlying iris and anterior lens capsule. The goal of this operation is reached when the majority of the clot has been removed from the central portion of the chamber.

It is definitely not necessary to aggressively attempt to remove the clot in the chamber angle. Doing so has these disadvantages: bleeding may be renewed and corneal endothelium and iris can be damaged. Postoperatively the clotted blood remaining in the chamber angle will gradually become dislodged and gravitate toward the central and inferior portions of the anterior chamber. If rebleeding should occur at the time of surgery, continued irrigation and aspiration along with raising the intraocular pressure will generally stop it. If these measures fail, the point of bleeding should be localized and penetrating diathermy should be applied through the sclera. If that also fails, the irrigating cannula or needle and the shaft of the vitrectomy instrument can be connected to the bipolar cautery, and coagulating energy can be delivered to the angle, using this two-instrument approach.

Removal of traumatic hyphemas using these surgical approaches should always be performed before blood-staining of the cornea begins. Once the cornea is stained, visualization of anterior-segment structures becomes extremely difficult.

Posterior-Segment Trauma

These situations concern the evaluation of visual acuity, a vitreous hemorrhage, a retinal detachment, or a retained intraocular foreign body. The available diagnostic tools are the direct ophthalmoscope, bright-flash ERG or visual evoked potentials, radiography, computerized tomography, MRI, and vitreous cavity endoscopy.[6,19] The therapeutic tools at our disposal are the vitrectomy instrumentation mentioned previously, intravitreal foreign-body forceps, and scleral buckling techniques where indicated. The controversy at the present time is over the timing of the surgical intervention.

Timing of Surgery. In the presence of a ruptured globe, surgery for the purpose of primary repair of the globe should be performed as soon as is practical, preferably on the day of the injury. If the scleral rupture is anterior to the equator, repair can be made more accurate by the use of microsurgery. However, in situations where the rupture extends posterior to the equator, careful retraction of the surrounding tissues combined with careful intrascleral sutures is the best approach. The goal to be achieved under these circumstances is preservation of the integrity of the globe and avoidance of endophthalmitis.

Perforating Injuries. When a foreign body (usually metallic) perforates both the anterior and posterior wall of the globe, it is the author's opinion that the patient may be observed for 2 to 3 weeks before vitrectomy is contemplated. Assuming that the entrance- and exit wounds are small and self-sealing, as they usually are, immediate emergency steps may not consist of surgical closure of the wound but rather the administration of tetanus toxoid, antibiotics, cycloplegics, and topical steroids.

Because the anterior and posterior wounds are small, the healing mechanisms of the cornea and sclera are capable of closing them permanently. This is true with moderate-sized steel foreign bodies as well as shotgun pellets up to the No. 4 size. If the metallic foreign body is steel (thus possessing sharp edges), missiles as long as 4 mm to 5 mm by 0.3 mm have been known to create wounds that sealed themselves.

In the author's experience, delaying surgery after the accident has yielded extremely good visual results in 9 of 11 patients so treated. The two eyes that did not recover useful vision fell into two unfavorable categories: exit of a shot through the posterior pole of the globe, and a linear tear in the retina caused by the path of the foreign body as it skidded through the retina in a tangential path. In the first instance, a large scar developed in the macula, and in the second instance, an inoperable retinal detachment was present by the time a posterior vitrectomy was performed.

In the other 9 cases, almost complete recovery of central vision was achieved by performing a vitrectomy for removal of the vitreous scaffolding and the intravitreal blood 14 to 21 days after the injury. Provided ultrasonic examination of the globe reveals no retinal detachment, this waiting period between the accident and surgery permits the posterior vitreous face to detach from the surface of the retina and, so, permits complete removal of the posterior vitreous without undue hazard to the retina. The trauma produced by perforation of the retina and the posterior wall of the globe is enough to stimulate a fibroblastic reaction around the exit wound to seal the exit site within the retina. Iatrogenic treatment of the posterior retinal defect is unnecessary. Although contusion of the visual elements in the posterior pole is a theoretical hazard of these missiles, this development appears to be uncommon, provided the missile is traveling at a high velocity or has sharp edges. However, this type of potential injury to the central macula should be mentioned to the patient and the family preoperatively as a possible complication.

In cases where ultrasonic examination of the globe reveals the presence of a concomitant retinal detachment, pars plana vitrectomy should be performed as soon as the situation is diagnosed. Pursuing the retrobulbar foreign body within the orbital tissues does not appear to be necessary in this type of injury. The development of an intraorbital abscess or persistent uveitis has not been a problem.

Retained Intraocular Foreign Bodies. In cases where a magnetic foreign body is present within the vitreous cavity, standard removal with a magnet activated over a sclerotomy in the region of the pars plana or activation over a sclerotomy directly beneath the foreign body is generally successful. If a vitreous hemorrhage obscures the location of the foreign body, a pars plana vitrectomy should be performed to visualize the object, and this maneuver should be combined with removal either by an intravitreal magnet or intravitreal foreign body forceps.

In cases where a nonmagnetic, intraocular foreign body is retained (e.g., shell casing, glass), the performance of a pars plana vitrectomy often reveals the location of the foreign body, which can then be removed with intravitreal foreign-body forceps. (Many are available at this time.) All forceps can be manipulated with one hand and consist of either opposing jaws or three prongs that converge to grasp small objects. The jaws type forceps can further be subdivided according to the type of surfaces on the inner side of the jaws: smooth, cupped, serrated, or diamond-dusted. Diamond-dusted forceps are particularly well suited for grasping smooth objects such as glass or larger bird shot.

Management of Foreign Bodies Incarcerated in the Extraction Sclerotomy. Quite often, the foreign body is larger than the pars plana sclerotomy through which extraction must take place. Even after the sclerotomy is enlarged just before extraction is attempted, the foreign body may become snagged around the edges of the sclerotomy and may remain incarcerated in the wound after the forceps have been removed from the vitreous cavity. This situation poses a dilemma. If one attempts to grasp the foreign body with fine-toothed forceps, there is a definite risk of dislodging the foreign body from the wound and allowing it to fall back into the vitreous cavity. If the surgeon succeeds in grasping the foreign body firmly, a forceful extraction of the object through the lips of the wound may tear adjacent tissues. Both of these complications should be avoided. What, then, is the best way to extract the foreign body?

In the author's experience, the situation is best handled by first removing the intravitreal light source and plugging that sclerotomy with a scleral plug. Second, a command should be given to the operating-room personnel to raise the infusion bottle. This increases the pressure in the vitreous cavity, securing the foreign body in the lips of the extraction site. Now, with both hands free and with the increased intraocular pressure pushing the foreign body outward, the surgeon can carefully dissect the extraction site with fine-toothed forceps and a small sharp

knife. By gradually enlarging the extraction site, the foreign body will present itself, allowing controlled, gradual extraction without risk of its falling back into the vitreous cavity or creating unwanted neuroepithelial tears in the region of the extraction site.

RETROLENTAL FIBROPLASIA

Vitrectomy approach to severe cases of retrolental fibroplasia (RLF) is gradually making inroads in these difficult cases.[3]

Indications. The cases being treated are those with advanced, bilateral disease consisting of severe traction detachments that preclude visualization of the disc (stages IV and V).

Surgical Approach. Because the pars plana in these infants has not developed, the surgical approach is made at a point approximately 1.5 mm posterior to the limbus. The first step involves performing a lensectomy. Next, the retrolental cyclitic membrane is carefully removed. The instrumentation for this step consists of intravitreal scissors to carefully shred the membrane and a vitrectomy instrument to remove the shredded segments. Any blood vessels encountered must be treated with wet-field cautery. Care must be taken to look for retina that might be drawn up into the posterior surface of these cyclitic membranes.

After removal of the cyclitic membrane, intravitreal scissors are used to cut the fibrotic connections between the ciliary body and the peripheral portions of the retina, the so-called anterior loop. Once these connections are cut, the peripheral retina is free of anteroposterior traction forces.

The next step involves releasing the surface of the retina from the centripetal forces that are drawing it in toward the center of the vitreous cavity. This dissection is best performed with intravitreal scissors of some sort. Charles prefers the parallel-cutting Sutherland scissors. All of the above-mentioned dissection attempts to avoid intraocular bleeding and, naturally, iatrogenic retinal defects. After the dissection is com-

pleted, the eye is filled with a viscoelastic substance and the scleral wounds are closed.

Over the 3 years that Charles has been performing this surgery, he has operated upon 375
eyes. The success rate is 45%. Two percent were
found to be inoperable, and 53% failed because
of reproliferation.

CHRONIC APHAKIC CYSTOID MACULAR EDEMA

Incidence. It is well known that the incidence
of angiographically proven cystoid macular
edema (CME) following an intracapsular cataract extraction can be as high as 60% during the
first 2 months following surgery.[11] Fortunately,
if the surgery has been uncomplicated, the overwhelming majority of these eyes recover spontaneously, and central vision is very good. In a
small percentage of these eyes, chronic aphakic
CME develops. These patients' lesions usually
fit all of the criteria encompassed by the term
Irvine-Gass syndrome: an inflamed eye, formed
vitreous adherent to the corneoscleral wound,
generally a peaked pupil, and CME. The CME
in these cases may persist for months or years,
reducing the central acuity of the eye to disap-
pointingly low levels. Steroids or antiprosta-
glandins have been administered by various
routes with favorable results, but lasting cures
with these agents are very rare.

Beginning in the early 1970s a few authors
published their results following the performance of vitrectomy on these chronically irritated
eyes. The success rate in at least two of these
series was in the range of 65%. The series were
relatively small, unrandomized, and uncontrolled.[4,8] Further, the effectiveness of vitrectomy was unproven because the natural history
of aphakic CME is one of sporadic spontaneous
cures. In an effort to subject this surgical approach to scientific testing, this author organized a randomized, controlled, collaborative,
nationwide study sponsored by the Pacific Vision Foundation of San Francisco, California,
in 1979. This study was concluded in January
1984, and the final results can be reported at this
time.[9]

The original cohort consisted of 130 eyes.

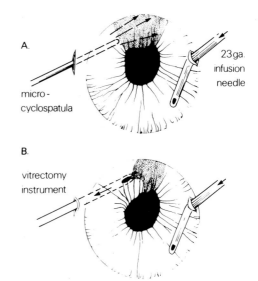

Figure 24-10. The limbal vitrectomy approach for
chronic, aphakic cystoid macular edema has as its
goal restoration of the pupil to as nearly normal a
state as possible. This is easy if the incarcerated
vitreous strand peaking the pupil bridges the iris.
Commonly, however, condensed vitreous is
intimately attached to the iris. To remove these
connections, one must tunnel under the vitreous
sheet *(A)*, and remove it by introducing the
vitrectomy instrument into the tunnel *(B)*. This
maneuver is repeated until all vitreous sheets are
removed from the surface of the iris and the pupil
is round.

One-hundred-fifteen eyes completed the full
9-month protocol. From the visual standpoint,
vitrectomy was proven to be more effective than
control (p = 0.03). The pars plana approach or
a combined limbal and pars plana approach
seemed to have a higher success rate than a strict
limbal approach; this, in spite of the fact that
only 4% of the 130 eyes demonstrated any connection between the detached posterior vitreous
face and the macula. Finally, fluorescein angiography proved to be an unsatisfactory gauge of
the visual success, for vision frequently improved in spite of residual evidence of angiographically positive CME. The profile of the patient most likely to benefit from this procedure
consists of the following criteria: female, nonhy-
pertensive, operated upon by the pars plana approach.

Technique. The goal of surgery was to restore
the pupil and the anterior segment of the eye to

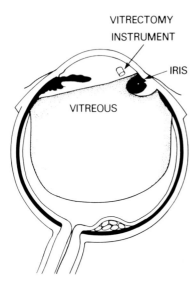

VITRECTOMY
INSTRUMENT

IRIS

VITREOUS

CHRONIC CYSTOID MACULAR
EDEMA IN APHAKIA

Figure 24-11. When the limbal and pars plana vitrectomy approach is used to treat chronic, aphakic cystoid macular edema, the anterior work is pursued as detailed in Figure 24-10. The goal of the pars plana approach is to remove the anterior vitreous and the detached posterior vitreous face. The National Vitrectomy/CME study showed that the pars plana or combined pars plana and limbal approach is more effective than the limbal approach used alone.

as nearly normal a state as possible. This sometimes required approaching the vitreous strands from the inferior quadrants as well as the superior ones. When a pars plana approach was employed, not only was the anterior vitreous removed, but also that in the deeper portions of the cavity. When vitreous plaques are adherent to the surface of the iris, removal is mandatory in order to restore the pupil to its normal state (Figs. 24-10, 24-11).

Complications. A retinal detachment occurred in one of the 47 eyes that received surgery. This detachment developed 2 years after the vitrectomy operation. In the control group (24 eyes), one patient developed a retinal detachment. In addition, a detachment occurred in one eye during the prerandomization period.[9]

COMPLICATIONS OF VITRECTOMY

Besides the usual, rare surgical complications such as endophthalmitis and anesthetic death, vitrectomy carries with it several unique complications (primarily because of the nature of the basic conditions present in those eyes that can benefit most from this surgical approach) —retinal detachment, persistent vitreous hemorrhage, and rubeosis iridis.

Creation of a retinal defect is always possible when one operates in the vitreous cavity. Incomplete cutting of vitreous strands can lead to spaghetti-winding of vitreous strands, producing traction on the retina, which in turn may lead to a retinal defect. This complication was, unfortunately, fairly common in the early days when vitrectomy instrumentation was relatively crude. Today, with better cutting instruments employing either the rotary or the guillotine cutting action, the incidence of traction tears of the retina is greatly reduced. In addition, early vitrectomy techniques attempted to remove attachments to the retina by pulling on those attachments. Today, most preretinal membranes are gently elevated in a progressive fashion until their attachments to the retina are localized. Once these attachments are defined, no attempt is made to pull the attachments free; rather, all membranes connected to the attachment are circumcised. The use of intravitreal scissors for this purpose has greatly reduced the incidence of iatrogenic retinal defects.

In essence, the vitrectomy instrument is now used to clear a path to the pathology, thus allowing the safe introduction of intravitreal scissors. The scissors are now used to perform most of the pre- and epiretinal dissection as well as to cut the bands attached to the retinal surface.

Rubeosis iridis is a complication seen primarily in diabetic eyes. Its incidence rises drastically whenever a detachment develops in a postvitrectomized eye. Treatment of rubeosis iridis consists of reattaching the retina and employing laser therapy in a pan-photocoagulation pattern.

A persistent vitreous hemorrhage may be seen in postoperative diabetic eyes. In order to minimize this complication, any cut preretinal fibrovascular tuft is cauterized intravitreally with bipolar techniques. If such a hemorrhage persists for 6 months, the eye is a candidate for a vitreous wash-out and coagulation of abnormal vessels. When following eyes with a postoperative vitreous hemorrhage, the presence of retinal detachment should be sought with ultrasound. Once a detachment in a vitrectomized eye is discovered, the eye is a candidate for vitreous wash-out combined with a scleral buckling procedure.

REFERENCES

1. Aaberg TM: Pars plana vitrectomy for persistent aphakic cystoid macular edema secondary to vitreous incarceration in the cataract wound. In McPherson A (ed): New and Controversial Aspects of Vitreoretinal Surgery, pp 230–233. St Louis, CV Mosby Co, 1977
2. Bradbury MJ, Fung WE: A new 20-gauge intravitreal cryoprobe. Am J Ophthalmol 90:424, 1980
3. Charles S: Vitreous Microsurgery. Baltimore, Williams & Wilkins, 1981
4. Federman JL, Annesley WH, Sarin LK, et al: Vitrectomy and cystoid macular edema. Ophthalmology 87:622, 1980
5. Federman JL, Shakin JL, Lanning RC: The microsurgery management of giant retinal tears with trans-scleral retinal sutures. Ophthalmology 89:832, 1982
6. Fuller D, Knighton RW, Machemer R: Bright-flash electroretinography for the evaluation of eyes with opaque vitreous. Am J Ophthalmol 80:214, 1975
7. Fung WE, Hall DL, Cleasby GW: Combined technique for a 355° traumatic giant retinal break. Arch Ophthalmol 93:264, 1975
8. Fung WE: Surgical therapy for chronic aphakic cystoid macular edema. Ophthalmology 89:898, 1982
9. Fung WE and the Vitrectomy/ACME Study Group: Victrectomy for chronic aphakic cystoid macular edema, results of a national collaborative, prospective randomized investigation. Ophthalmology 92:1102, 1985
10. Harmann MH, Abrams GW: Prevention of lens opacification during vitrectomy. Ophthalmology 91:116, 1984
11. Irvine AR, Bresky R, Crowder BM, et al: Macular edema after cataract extraction. Ann Ophthalmol 3:1234, 1971
12. Landers MB III, Foulks GN, Landers DM, et al: Temporary keratoprosthesis for use during pars plana vitrectomy. Am J Ophthalmol 91:615, 1981
13. Lightfoot D, Irvine AR: Vitrectomy in infants and children with retinal detachments caused by cicatricial retrolental fibroplasia. Am J Ophthalmol 94:305, 1982
14. Machemer R, Parel JM, Buettner H: A new concept for vitreous surgery. I: Instrumentation. Am J Ophthalmol 73:1, 1972
15. Machemer R: Surgical approaches to subretinal strands. Am J Ophthalmol 90:81, 1980
16. Michels RG, Rice TZ: Bimanual bipolar diathermy for treatment of bleeding from the anterior chamber angle. Am J Ophthalmol 84:873, 1977
17. Michels RG: Vitreous Surgery. St Louis, CV Mosby Co, 1981
18. Norton EWD, Aaberg T, Fung WE, et al: Giant retinal tears. I: Clinical management with intravitreal air. Am J Ophthalmol 68:1011, 1969
19. O'Malley C, Heintz RM: Vitrectomy via the pars plana: A new instrument system. Trans Pac Coast Oto-ophthalmol Soc 53:121, 1972
20. Tso MOM: Pathology of cystoid macular edema. Ophthalmology 89:902, 1982

25

Diagnosis and Management of Intraocular Foreign Bodies

Jorn-Hon Liu

A penetrating injury of the eye with a retained intraocular foreign body (IOFB) is a serious ophthalmic trauma that causes immediate mechanical damage and severe late complications.[11,32,33,35] Retention of a free-floating IOFB in the vitreous cavity may be relatively harmless or it may cause severe vitreoretinal damage and complete disorganization of the globe. In addition, metallic IOFBs such as iron and copper can react chemically with ocular tissues and cause visual impairment.[11] Speedy and accurate diagnosis and effective and appropriate management of these injuries are of utmost importance. This chapter describes methods of diagnostic work-up, approaches to foreign-body extraction, and management of complications.

DIAGNOSTIC WORK-UP

The diagnosis of an IOFB may be made from the clinical history and an ophthalmic examination. Most patients report being struck in the eye by a small chip of material while hammering a piece of metal or working with a spinning machine. Some foreign bodies are neglected for a period of time following the accident until visual symptoms develop. In such cases, diligent inquiry may elicit the history of a minor accident in the past when the patient may have experienced a very sharp pain but no symptom thereafter.

All suspected patients should undergo external examinations, slit-lamp biomicroscopy, and indirect ophthalmoscopy. The slit-lamp examination may show a perforation site in the cornea or a traumatic iridotomy. Pupillary dilation may reveal a foreign body embedded in the lens. Penetrating injury of the lens may be evidenced by a small opacity or a localized grayish patch on the surface of the lens capsule, denoting a sealed penetration site. If the foreign body perforates the conjunctiva and sclera, the site of entry may not be seen, but conjunctival swelling and hemorrhage provide clues to the injury.

Indirect ophthalmoscopy is most useful in the diagnosis of an IOFB in clear ocular media. A relatively small foreign body entering the eye through the pars plana or cornea rarely produces vitreous hemorrhage, provided that the propellant does not penetrate the posterior retina and choroid. In such cases, the IOFB may be seen with an indirect ophthalmoscope. Lenticular injury may result in total lens opacity, which precludes ophthalmoscopic examination. In small penetrating injuries, the lens usually remains relatively clear for the first few days; early ophthalmoscopic examination is therefore very important in the diagnosis of an IOFB. When cloudy media are present and an IOFB is suspected, radiographic examination should be done. Plain films may reveal radio-opaque intraocular or extraocular foreign bodies. Confirmation of an IOFB may need special localization techniques.

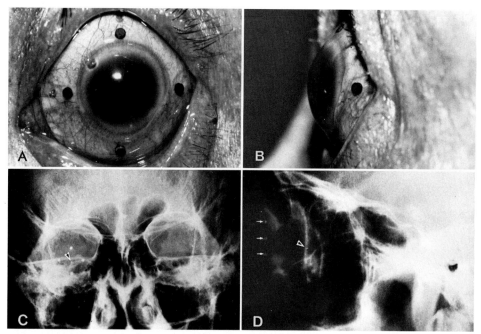

Figure 25-1. Comberg's method for intraocular foreign body (IOFB) localization. Comberg's contact lens with four dots is placed on the eye in the frontal *(A)* and lateral *(B)* views. The radiographs show four dots on posteroanterior *(C)* view and three dots on lateral view *(arrows)* with a small IOFB *(arrowhead, D)*.

Localization of Foreign Bodies

The purpose of localization is to determine whether a foreign body is in the orbit or in some part of the globe. An orbital foreign body may be asymptomatic, but intraocular iron or copper has to be removed early. The location of an IOFB also determines the surgical approach for its removal. The most commonly used localization techniques are Sweet's localization, Comberg's technique, ultrasonography, and computed tomography (CT). Sweet's localization is done by placing a metal indicator at a known distance in front of the cornea and taking two radiographs from the lateral side at a fixed distance and from two separate angles, one horizontally and one slightly tilted. Both radiographs are then placed on Sweet's key plates to obtain the distance of the foreign body from the key lines. These data are then transferred to Sweet's chart to determine the location.[11] This method is popular in the United States.[7,36]

I prefer Comberg's method because it is easier and less complicated to perform than Sweet's method and needs less patient cooperation and attention.[39] A contact lens marked with four lead dots is placed on the surface of the cornea. The contact lens is positioned so that the dots are located at the 12-, 3-, 6-, and 9-o'clock meridians, equidistant from the center of the cornea. Two radiographs are taken, a posteroanterior view and a lateral view.[11] When the side view is taken, the lead dots at the 3- and 9-o'clock meridians coincide on the horizontal plane, so that only three of the four dots appear on the film. The dots indicate the position of the foreign body in relation to the center of the cornea and the limbus (Fig. 25-1). The disadvantage of Comberg's technique is that when a corneal laceration is long and extensive, contact lens placement may be hazardous. Both Sweet's and Comberg's methods have shortcomings. The localization of a foreign body in the globe or orbit is based on the presumption that the eyeball is 24 mm in diameter. It is difficult to localize a foreign body when it is in the vicinity of the posterior scleral coat.

Although ultrasonography has been used in IOFB localization for more than 20 years, it has become popular during the past decade.[1,2,5,30,31]

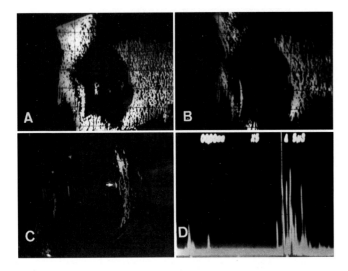

Figure 25-2. Ultrasonographic localization of foreign body. When sensitivity is reduced, the foreign body *(arrow)* stands out at the back of the vitreous cavity on the B-scan *(A, B, C)*. The echo amplitude exceeds sclera and is retained in the A-scan *(D)*.

Some surgeons prefer to use the A-scan (time-amplitude ultrasonogram) over the B-scan.[2,5,31] The two-dimensional B-scan clearly shows the foreign body and the scleral coat simultaneously. The current practice is to use the B-scan to demonstrate the foreign body and the A-scan to observe its echo amplitude for confirmation.[5] Contact- and water-immersion technique are equally effective. It is helpful to obtain a radiograph to show the existence, number, and approximate position of the foreign bodies before performing ultrasonography.

With the B-scan, serial sectioning of the globe is performed initially on the high-sensitivity setting. When a foreign body is suspected, sensitivity is gradually reduced to distinguish the IOFB from vitreal hemorrhages and the scleral coat. The echo of the foreign body persists, while that of the vitreous hemorrhage and global wall disappears (Fig. 25-2). While observing the B-scan, the amplitude of the echo of the foreign body should be watched on the A-scan. Typically, an intravitreal metallic foreign body exhibits a trail of reduplication echoes (or ringing) by ultrasonogram (Fig. 25-3).[3,5] The preretinal and mural foreign bodies sometime show a shadow (anechoic) behind the globe, especially when the IOFB is at the posterior pole.[5] It is difficult to locate an orbital foreign body by ultrasonogram since it provides only indirect evidence such as a trail of reduplication echoes, distortion of the globe, and retrobulbar hemorrhage (Fig. 25-4). Ultrasonography may also be used to measure axial length to augment radiographic localization and to determine magnetic properties using a pulsed magnet.[5]

The CT scan is also beneficial for foreign body localization.[12,17,23] The third and fourth genera-

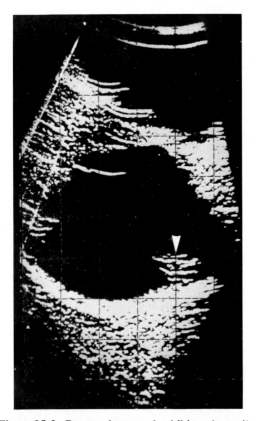

Figure 25-3. B-scan ultrasound exhibits echo trail from the foreign body *(arrow)*.

Table 25-1. Effectiveness of Comberg's Radiographic Technique, Ultrasonography, and Computed Tomography in Locating Foreign Bodies*

Location	No. of Eyes	X-ray	Ultrasonogram	CT Scan
Vitreous	10	9(90%)	10(100%)	10(100%)
Preretina	5	2(40%)	4(80%)	5(100%)
Scleral coat	6	2(33%)	3(50%)	6(100%)
Orbit	5	3(60%)	0	5(100%)

* All eyes had cloudy ocular media (N = 26).

tions of CT scanners have very high resolution, allowing the detection of steel foreign bodies as small as 0.06 mm³ (0.5 mm in diameter).[40] The CT scan has become the most convenient and accurate method of locating foreign bodies. In general, serial cuts 4 mm thick and 4 mm apart are obtained on axial and coronal sections. With adjustments, thinner sections, closer to 2 mm, can be taken. The films are easily read, and the position of the foreign body is readily determined with identification of the global wall and surrounding structures. The CT scan provides a clear visualization of the entire global wall, lens, extraocular muscles, orbital spaces, and periorbital sinuses. It can distinctly demonstrate a foreign body in any of these locations, and will locate multiple small foreign bodies (Fig. 25-5, 25-6).

To compare the accuracy and reliability of Comberg's technique, ultrasonography, and CT scan, we performed all three procedures on 26 consecutive patients with an ocular penetrating injury caused by a missile, resulting in cloudy ocular media.[20] The result of each examination was interpreted and compared with the actual location of the foreign bodies detected by vitrectomy or orbital exploration (Table 25-1). For intravitreal foreign bodies, all three methods performed almost equally well. For orbital foreign bodies with double scleral perforations, a CT scan localized all correctly, Comberg's technique demonstrated three of five, and ultrasonography failed to show any. For preretinal and mural foreign bodies, Comberg's technique failed to detect the exact location of the foreign bodies, ultrasonography pinpointed the location in over half the cases, and a CT scan correctly located all of them (Fig. 25-7 to 25-9).

The ability of CT and ultrasonography to outline the sclera is helpful in locating an IOFB. Ultrasonography alone may be unable to detect the exact location of preretinal, intraretinal, and orbital foreign bodies in double perforations, especially in the presence of thick fibrous tissue

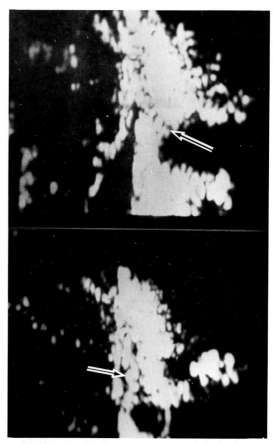

Figure 25-4. Ultrasonograph of double perforating injury demonstrates foreign body track, preretinal organization, and distortion of sclera. Some sonolucent lines *(arrow)* are noted, probably produced by edema or hemorrhage in Tenon's capsule. Location of foreign body could not be pinpointed.

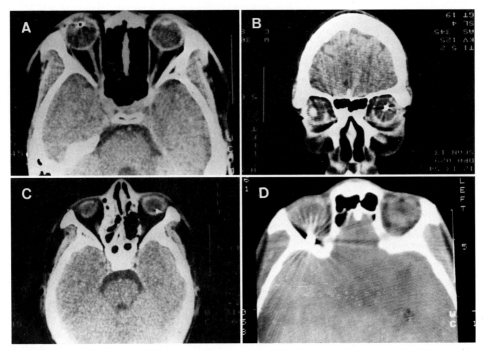

Figure 25-5. CT scan localization of foreign body. *(A)* Foreign body appears in the anterior vitreous cavity. *(B)* Coronal section shows foreign body in the middle of the vitreous cavity. *(C)* Preretinal foreign body is seen. *(D)* Foreign body appears in the upper orbital space.

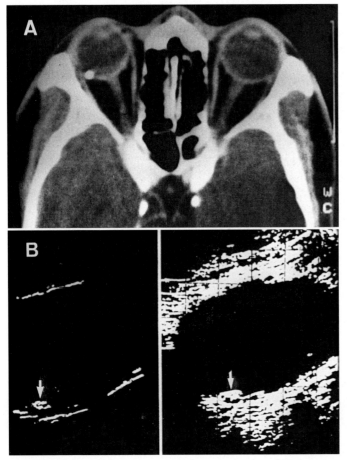

Figure 25-6. *(A)* CT scan shows scleral coat, intraocular and extraocular structures, and a preretinal foreign body. *(B)* Ultrasonograph of the same eye demonstrates a foreign body *(arrow)* on higher-sensitivity *(right)* and lower-sensitivity *(left)* settings.

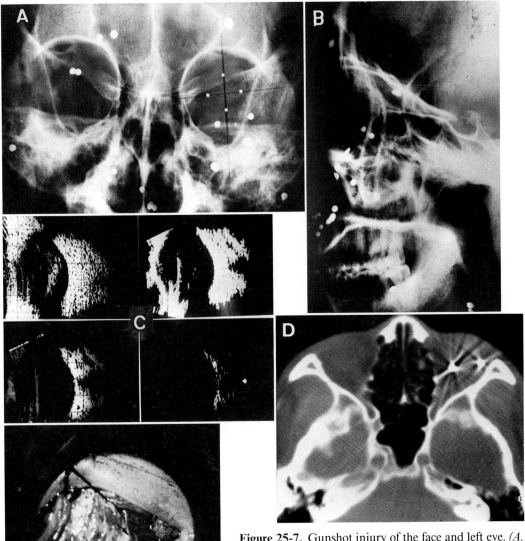

Figure 25-7. Gunshot injury of the face and left eye. *(A, B)* Foreign body on the temporal side was localized in the globe using Comberg's technique. *(C)* Ultrasonograph discloses hemorrhage and hemorrhagic track but no foreign body in the globe. *(D)* CT scan reveals two foreign bodies in the lower portion of the extrascleral orbital region. *(E)* Surgical exploration shows the foreign bodies attached to extrascleral soft tissue *(arrows).*

scar and retinal detachment (Fig. 25-10). However, ultrasonography is very helpful in the management of vitreal and retinal injury.[4] For all cases of suspected IOFB, both CT and ultrasonography should be performed.

GENERAL MANAGEMENT

A penetrating injury with an IOFB should be treated as an emergency. Both perforation of the globe and retention of the foreign body should be considered in the management. A detailed history of the injury and of the patient's medical background should be obtained. Visual acuity should be determined in both eyes and a thorough examination of anterior and posterior segments should be performed. Intraocular pressure is generally not measured with instrumentation if there is an open perforating wound. A metal shield should be placed over the

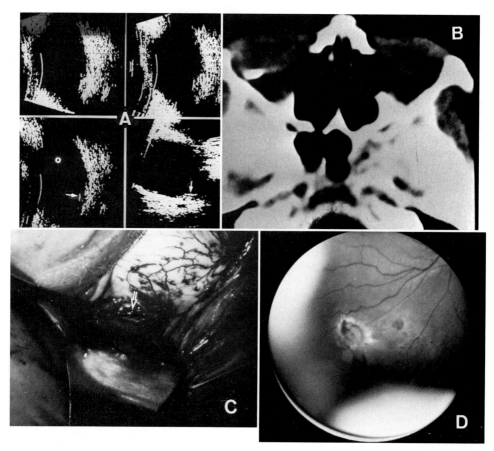

Figure 25-8. Double perforation of the globe by a foreign body. *(A)* Ultrasonograph demonstrates a foreign body that appears to be preretinal *(arrow)*. *(B)* CT scan shows an extrascleral foreign body. *(C)* Exploration of the orbit reveals a foreign body under the inferior oblique stump *(arrow)*. *(D)* Fundus photograph exhibits site of perforation.

injured eye to prevent any additional pressure on the eyeball. A tetanus toxoid injection may be necessary, depending on previous immunization. If available, a sample of the foreign body should be examined. The patient is now ready to undergo foreign body localization.

It must be emphasized that even if the foreign body can be seen by ophthalmoscopy, a plain film or fundus photograph may be necessary for documentation. A treatment approach should be planned based on the findings of the eye examinations and location of the foreign body. If an operation is necessary, a decision must be made to either close the laceration and extract the foreign body at the same time or to perform a primary closure first and extract the foreign body later. If preparation for a complicated procedure is not possible, the second approach will be necessary. If the foreign body is magnetic, removal is usually attempted concomitantly with the primary closure. If removal fails, a later operation may be scheduled.

For a small, sharp-edged laceration, it may not be necessary to repair the wound before removing the foreign body. Surgery is generally preferred with the patient under general anesthesia to avoid undue pressure from the retrobulbar injection of anesthetics. If there is evidence of intraocular infection at the time of foreign body removal, intracameral injections of antibiotics and corticosteroids, such as 200 to 400 μg of gentamicin and 200 to 400 μg of dexamethasone, may be given.[9,13,34,41]

Postoperative care includes prophylactic sys-

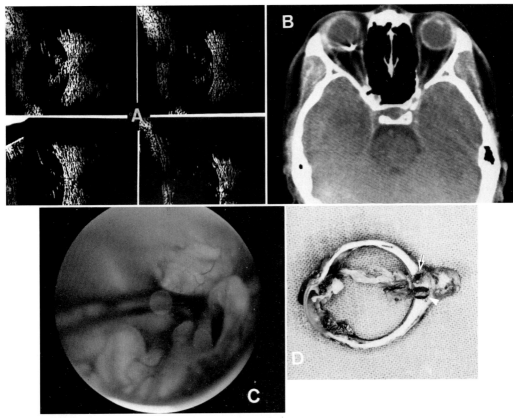

Figure 25-9. Foreign body penetrating the optic nerve. *(A)* Ultrasonograph shows retinal detachment but does not identify the foreign body. *(B)* CT scan demonstrates the foreign body on the outer posterior segment. *(C)* Fundus view reveals a large retinal break. *(D)* Section of enucleated globe discloses foreign body located at the anterior optic nerve *(arrow)*. Foreign body was flipped upward to the side of the original site *(arrowhead)*.

temic antibiotics, and corticosteroids for cases with extensive injury. The eye should be observed for infection, intraocular hemorrhage, and retinal detachment. Ultrasonography may be used to detect retinal detachment if the ocular media are cloudy. Cataract extraction, retinal detachment repair, and vitrectomy may be further indicated in the postoperative period.

EXTRACTION OF FOREIGN BODIES

It is necessary to remove toxic foreign bodies, especially copper and iron, and nontoxic materials that may cause further mechanical damage. An orbital foreign body can be retained or removed at the time that the globe is repaired. In

general, as intraocular foreign bodies may cause vitreoretinal complications later, it is safer to remove them.

The main goal in the extraction of a foreign body is to remove it with minimal damage to the eye. A method should be selected based on this principle. There are five major approaches for the removal of an IOFB: the anterior route, the posterior route, or the pars plana approach with a magnet, the pars plana approach with vitrectomy, and the open sky approach with vitrectomy. Procedures and indications for each are summarized in Figure 25-11.

Anterior Limbal Approach
The anterior approach is chosen when the foreign body is in the anterior chamber, iris, or lens;

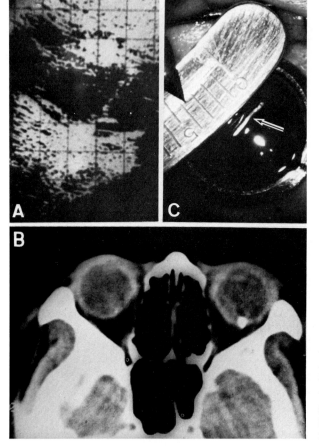

Figure 25-10. *(A)* Ultrasonograph exhibits vitreous hemorrhage and retinal detachment. The foreign body could not be located positively. *(B)* CT scan shows foreign body in the inner layer of the scleral coat. During the vitrectomy, the foreign body was found sticking into the choroid behind the detached retina (not shown). *(C)* Foreign body was identified as a piece of brass *(arrow)*.

in the anterior vitreous cavity and the lens is injured; or when it is too large for other approaches. An incision may be made at the limbus to accommodate the foreign body or the lens. If the foreign body is lodged in the lens, it may be removed with forceps, a magnet, or a cryoprobe. In general, removal of the foreign body through the original corneal perforation wound is not recommended because it is possible to damage the cornea further. If the lens has been injured, it is usually removed during the same operative procedure.

Pars Plana Approach With a Magnet

For a magnetic foreign body floating freely in the vitreous cavity, the pars plana approach is the simplest and least harmful of the five. A 4-mm sclera incision is made 4 mm posterior to and parallel to the limbus. A double-armed suture is placed through both lips of the incision. As both ends of the suture are pulled, the innermost layer of sclera is incised to expose the pars plana uvea. A magnet is placed over the incision, and the foreign body is pulled through the uvea and extracted (Fig. 25-12). The sclerotomy may be widened if it is too small for the foreign body. Occasionally, the foreign body is partially trapped by the vitreous and cannot be attracted to the magnet. When examined by indirect ophthalmoscopy, the foreign body may be seen to move with the magnet but cannot be detached from the surrounding vitreous. To free the IOFB, the surgeon may switch the magnetic action on and off repeatedly, or the extraction of the foreign body may be approached from the opposite direction. Oftentimes, a foreign body bound by the vitreous on one side may be free

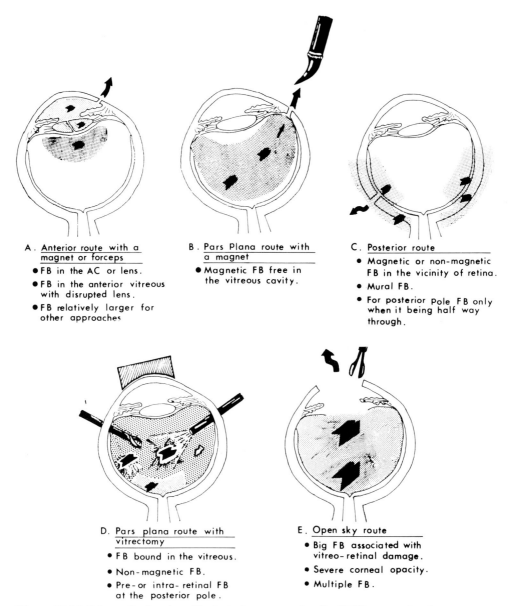

A. <u>Anterior route with a magnet or forceps</u>
- FB in the AC or lens.
- FB in the anterior vitreous with disrupted lens.
- FB relatively larger for other approaches

B. <u>Pars Plana route with a magnet</u>
- Magnetic FB free in the vitreous cavity.

C. <u>Posterior route</u>
- Magnetic or non-magnetic FB in the vicinity of retina.
- Mural FB.
- For posterior pole FB only when it being half way through.

D. <u>Pars plana route with vitrectomy</u>
- FB bound in the vitreous.
- Non-magnetic FB.
- Pre- or intra- retinal FB at the posterior pole.

E. <u>Open sky route</u>
- Big FB associated with vitreo- retinal damage.
- Severe corneal opacity.
- Multiple FB.

Figure 25-11 Schematic drawings illustrate five approaches for IOFB removal and indications for each method: *(A)* anterior limbal approach; *(B)* pars plana approach with a magnet; *(C)* posterior scleral approach; *(D)* pars plana approach with vitrectomy procedure; *(E)* open-sky approach.

on the opposite side, and may be readily removed.

Posterior Scleral Approach

In a posterior approach, a foreign body is removed through the sclera behind the ora serrata. This procedure is indicated when the foreign body is in the vitreous cavity very close to the retina or embedded in the retina or the scleral coat. The standard technique is to localize the foreign body over the sclera with indirect ophthalmoscopy and to mark the site with methylene blue. A 4-mm by 4-mm double-flap trap door is made over the marked area to expose the

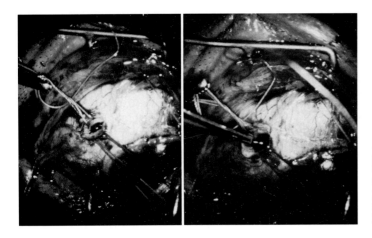

Figure 25-12. Pars plana removal of intraocular foreign body with magnet. *(Left)* The lips of the incision are pulled toward opposite sides to expose the uvea. *(Right)* Foreign body is being extracted by the magnet.

choroid. Light diathermy is applied to the scleral bed, through which extraction of the foreign body is attempted (Fig. 25-13). A magnet should be used for a metallic foreign body. For nonmagnetic objects, an incision is made over the choroid and retina, and the foreign body is expressed by applying gentle pressure on the opposite side of the globe. If the IOFB is small and

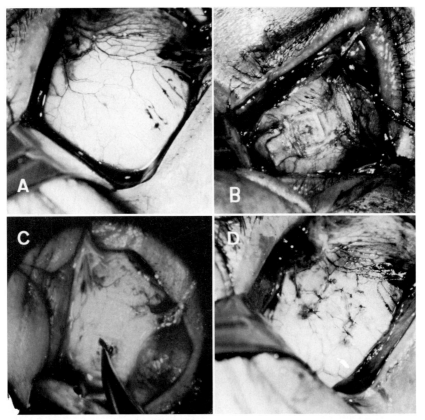

Figure 25-13. Posterior scleral approach of intraocular foreign body removal. Photos: *(A)* The foreign body is localized and marked over the sclera. *(B)* A double-flapped trap door is cut, and diathermy is applied on the scleral bed. *(C)* The foreign body is extracted with a magnet. *(D)* The outer scleral flap is sutured.

(continued)

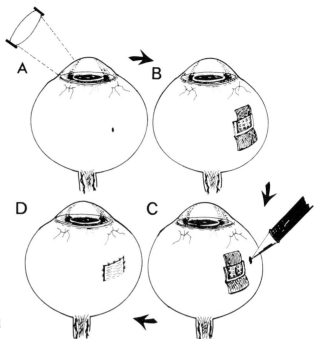

Figure 25-13. *(continued).* Drawing is a schematic rendering of the steps illustrated in Figure 25-13*B*.

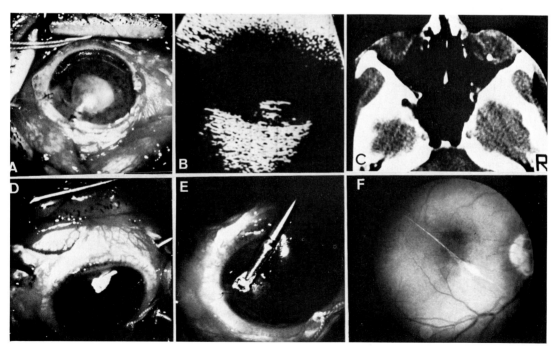

Figure 25-14. Composite picture showing removal of a piece of steel in the vitreous. *(A)* Corneal penetration and lens opacity. *(B)* Ultrasonograph. *(C)* CT scan. *(D, E)* Foreign body is pulled out by forceps. *(F)* Postoperative view of the fundus.

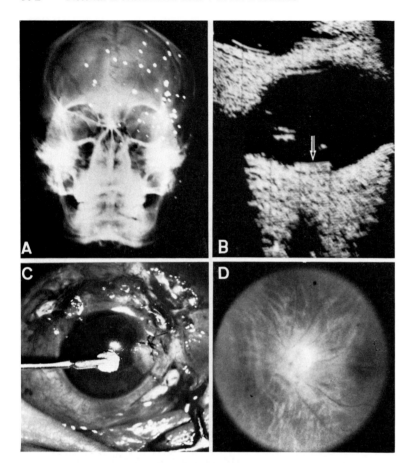

Figure 25-15. Composite picture showing removal of a piece of lead from a patient who sustained a gunshot wound. *(A)* Radiographic view. *(B)* Ultrasonograph exhibits foreign body on the posterior aspect of the globe *(arrow). (C)* Foreign body is removed. *(D)* Postoperative view of the fundus.

located anteriorly, an attempt may be made to grasp the foreign body directly by passing forceps into the vitreous cavity. After the foreign body is removed, the scleral flaps are closed with 8-0 nylon sutures. A local buckle with silicone sponge or silicone plate may be placed as a prophylactic measure against later retinal detachment. If the ocular media are cloudy, it may not be possible to localize the foreign body. In such cases, transillumination is obtained through the pupil, so the shadow cast by the foreign body on the sclera may be observed.[38] Another method is to clear the vitreous opacity with pars plana vitrectomy and then localize the foreign body with indirect ophthalmoscopy. The posterior approach is not recommended for foreign bodies located at or near the macula unless they are at least half-way through the global wall. Otherwise, serious damage may be inflicted on the posterior pole, which is difficult to repair.

Pars Plana Vitrectomy and Foreign Body Removal

A procedure pioneered by Machemer, Hutton, and Michels has become a most important and useful technique in the management of foreign bodies.[16,24-26] This method is indicated when the foreign body is nonmagnetic, when a magnetic foreign body is encapsulated or stuck in organized vitreous or fibrous tissue, or when the foreign body is at the posterior pole and other approaches will endanger the macular area.

It is convenient to use a vitrectomy machine equipped with divided-function probes, such as an ocutome, instead of one with multiple functions. Three sclerotomies are made to accommodate an infusion cannula, an illumination probe, and a cutting-suction probe. The vitreous and blood in the posterior segment are removed until the foreign body is visualized. The foreign body is removed with a pair of Neu-

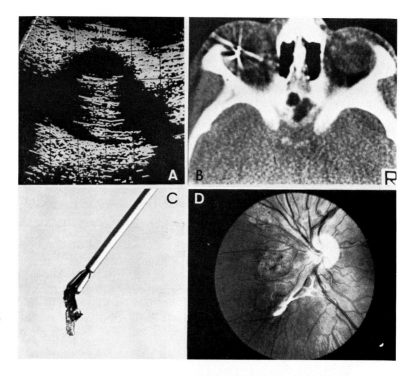

Figure 25-16. Composite picture shows the removal of a piece of brass from an eye injured in a dynamite explosion: *(A)* ultrasonograph; *(B)* CT scan; *(C)* foreign body is removed; *(D)* postoperative view of the fundus.

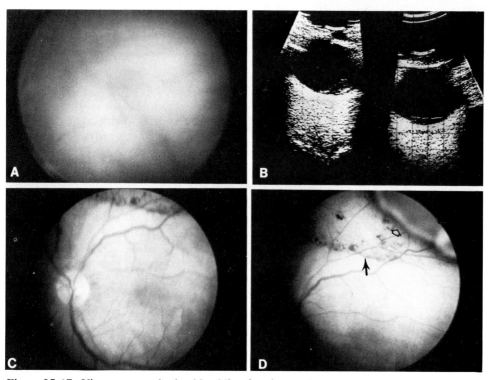

Figure 25-17. Vitrectomy and scleral buckling for vitreous hemorrhage in the eye 4 months after foreign body removal. *(A)* Fundus view is hazy through hemorrhages. *(B)* Ultrasonograph exhibits retinal detachment. *(C, D)* Postoperative fundus view exhibits demarcation line and buckle indentation (arrows).

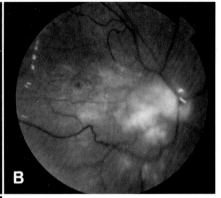

Figure 25-18. Fundus photographs of a patient with a total retinal detachment and proliferative vitreoretinopathy of an uneventful removal of an intraocular foreign body: *(A)* Fundus photograph before operation; and *(B and C)* fundus views after membrane peeling, scleral buckling, and intravitreal silicone oil injection.

bauer's forceps (Figs. 25-14 to 25-16).[28,29] If the IOFB is bound by fibrous tissue, it should be freed and removed. A foreign body adhering to the retina should be gently elevated, freed from one of its margins, and grasped with forceps. An encapsulated foreign body may be incised with a disposable needle before the foreign body is evacuated. This procedure can be difficult and time consuming, especially when the foreign body adheres tightly to the retinal surface. The two-instrument technique is essential for this maneuver. If the ocular media are clear, laser photocoagulation may be applied before removal to prevent accidental damage to the surrounding retina. As the foreign body is extracted, the sclerotomy may need enlarging to avoid additional damage to surrounding structures. After the foreign body is removed, any remaining condensed vitreous and hemorrhage should be entirely removed to prevent subsequent traction on the retina.

Open-Sky Vitrectomy

In this technique, button-shaped pieces of the cornea and lens are excised to remove condensed vitreous and the foreign body under direct visualization. The original corneal button or a donor graft is then sutured back into position. As Hirose and Schepens have reported, this technique is most useful to remove a large foreign body or multiple foreign bodies and to repair extensive vitreoretinal damage caused by the IOFB.[15] It is also indicated when the cornea is very cloudy and a toxic foreign body must be removed quickly. The open-sky technique is rarely used in our daily practice, because most foreign bodies can be removed by other approaches and the damaged vitreous and retina can be managed by simpler techniques, such as a closed pars plana vitrectomy. Furthermore, if a very large foreign body causes severe gross disruption of the globe, there may be no way to salvage the eye. With the recent availabilities of surgical keratoprosthesis, injury associated with corneal opacity may be repaired by the pars plana approach rather than the open-sky approach.[18]

Ancillary Procedures

The most frequently used ancillary procedures are lens extraction, scleral buckling, and pars plana vitrectomy. Lens extraction may be performed by the conventional intra- or extracapsular approach. If the pupil is secluded, if a fibrotic or cyclitic membrane is present, or if the lens is mixed with vitreous or blood, a lensectomy with a vitrectomy instrument is preferred.[10,22] Since most injured patients are young, a sclerotic and hard lens nucleus is rarely a problem.

The conventional scleral buckling procedure may be done in association with IOFB removal for prophylactic purposes or to manage the complication of retinal detachment. Following penetrating injuries with an IOFB, the eye is very susceptible to retinal detachment, which may be caused by a retinal hole inflicted by the foreign body or by traction from vitreous strands. Scleral buckling may be done in combination with a vitrectomy procedure, depending on the condition of the eye. When severe retinal gliosis results in contraction of retina, scleral shortening may be necessary.

Pars plana vitrectomy has been a most useful technique in the management of IOFB injuries, especially when used to treat late complications and sequelae (Fig. 25-17, 25-18).[14,27,37] Vitreous hemorrhage can be removed by vitrectomy to clear the ocular media, restore useful vision, and facilitate visualization of the fundus for retinal repair or removal of an IOFB lodged in the coat of the globe through a posterior approach. To treat a double perforation, it is also necessary to remove vitreous hemorrhage to locate the site of a posterior perforation. Severe tractional retinal detachment and proliferative vitreoretinopathy are common late complications of IOFB injury. They are best treated with vitrectomy, membrane peeling, and the intravitreal injection of silicone oil or gas, such as sulfur hexafluoride or perfluorocarbon. If endophthalmitis has developed, it is possible to salvage the eye with an early vitrectomy together with the intracameral injection of antibiotics and corticosteroids.[6,41]

Table 25-2. Complications of Intraocular Foreign Body Injury of 106 Cases

Complications	No. of Patients
Presented on Admission	
Corneal laceration	40
Scleral laceration	31
Iris prolapse	10
Severe hyphema	12
Lens injury	38
Vitreal hemorrhage	41
Vitreal fibrosis	9
Endophthalmitis	4
Disruption of globe	2
Siderosis	5
Retinal detachment	9
Late	
Retinal detachment	
Repaired	18
Proliferative vitreoretinopathy (final)	8
Inoperable	2
Macular pucker	4
Severe uveitis	11
Bulbar atrophy	14
Recurrent vitreal hemorrhage	3
Partial optic atrophy	1
Macular scar	1

SURGICAL EXPERIENCE IN TAIWAN

Between 1973 and 1982, we treated 106 cases of IOFB injury at the Veterans' General Hospital in Taipei. Patients ranged in age from 6 to 82 years; the majority were between 20 and 40 years. Of these patients, 98 were male and 8 were female. The leading cause of IOFB injury was from a projectile caused by a hammer striking on a metallic object (50 cases). Of these 50 cases, 9 involved the use of a hammer and a chisel; the other 41 resulted from a hammer striking on a

Table 25-3. The Management of 106 Cases of IOFB

Management	No. of Cases
Anterior limbal approach with a magnet or a forceps	10
Pars plana with a magnet	21
Posterior scleral approach with a magnet	10
Forceps under indirect ophthalmoscope	1
Pars plana vitrectomy and forceps	30
Posterior route and pars plana vitrectomy	7
Foreign body not removed:	
Not attempted	9
Failed	16
Eye enucleated as the primary procedure	2
Total	106

Table 25-4. Adjunct Procedures in the Management of Intraocular Foreign Bodies

Management	No. of Cases
Lensectomy (primary and secondary)	41
Secondary vitrectomy	11
Vitrectomy and scleral buckling	9
Scleral buckling	15

variety of metallic objects. The second most frequent cause of injury (24 cases) involved projectiles from the use of a motor-driven machine, including electric drills and electric spinning machines. The 106 foreign bodies included 68 magnetic metallic objects, 34 nonmagnetic metallic objects (13 containing copper and 11 containing lead), and 4 nonmetallic materials (3 glass and 1 plastic chip).

The most frequent site of an IOFB was the vitreous cavity. In 7 cases, the orbital foreign body passed through the globe in transit. The management of these 7 injuries was the same as for those retained in the globe, except that the foreign bodies were not removed. All 7 patients received diagnostic work-up and treatment for complications. Table 25-2 details the early and late complications resulting from 106 penetrating foreign bodies. In some cases, retinal gliosis and siderosis were observed during the first patient visit, indicating long-standing, neglected cases.

Various management approaches are listed in Table 25-3. A total of 30 of the nonmagnetic and magnetic foreign bodies were removed through the pars plana with forceps. Extraction through the pars plana with a magnet accounted for 21 cases. One nonmagnetic foreign body was removed under direct visualization with an indirect ophthalmoscope, a procedure used more frequently in earlier years. Removal was not attempted in 9 cases because the foreign bodies were nontoxic or in the orbit. There were 16 cases in which removal was attempted but failed. Most of these cases were managed before vitrectomy was popularized. Two eyes were enucleated as a primary procedure because the globe suffered gross disruption. Adjunct proce-

Table 25-5. Visual Results After Intraocular Foreign Body Removal (N = 106)

Visual Acuity	No/(%) of Cases		
	1973–77	*1978–82*	*Subtotal*
6/4.5–6/12	10	18	28 (26.4%)
6/15–6/60	6	24	30 (28.3%)
5/60—Finger counting	6	16	22 (20.7%)
Light perception	4	2	6 (5.7%)
No light perception	13	7	20 (18.8%)

Table 25-6. Comparison of Results: 1973–1977 and 1978–1982 (N = 85)*

	1973–1977		1978–1982	
Foreign body	*Success*	*Failure*	*Success*	*Failure*
Magnetic	14	7	35	2
Nonmagnetic	1	6	19	1
Total	15(54%)	13(46%)	54(95%)	3(5%)

* Excludes cases in which removal was not attempted and those of primary enucleation and anterior chamber foreign body.

dures in this series of cases are shown in Table 25-4.

Visual outcome is listed in Table 25-5. There were 26 cases (24.5%) of severe loss of vision to the level of light perception or no light perception. Vision was retained at the level of 6/4.5 to 6/12 in 28 cases (26.4%). Visual results were much better in cases treated in the last 5 years than they were for those treated in the earlier years. Seventeen cases (43%) exhibited vision of light perception or no light perception in the earlier 5 years, compared with nine cases (13%) with such vision who were treated in the recent 5 years. The removal of IOFBs was more successful for cases treated in more recent years (Table 25-6).

DISCUSSION

During the past 10 years, diagnosis and management of IOFBs has changed considerably. As reviewed by Duke-Elder, many techniques were used to locate IOFBs previously, but have been abandoned since the advent of ultrasonography and CT.[11] Radiographic localization, indispensable in the past, has been partially replaced by CT scan. Indeed, the combination of ultrasonography and CT scan alone is frequently adequate for diagnostic work-up. Berman's locator has been useful in the detection of metal during an operation but is rarely used at present.

Methods and routes of IOFB removal have been reviewed extensively by Roper-Hall and Percival.[33,35] Many surgeons prefer an anterior route, while others recommend a pars plana – or direct–posterior approach. I strongly believe the route of removal should depend on the loca-

tion and nature of the foreign body and the associated damage to the globe, as discussed by others.[3,8,27,38] The management of each case should be considered individually. Several British reports maintained that use of a hand-held hammer is the leading cause of IOFB injury in highly industrialized countries.[19,32,35] Findings in our series confirmed these observations.

The prognosis of a patient with an IOFB depends on the size, sharpness, momentum, and nature of the object. Factors leading to permanent visual loss include gross disorganization of the globe, endophthalmitis, retention of a toxic foreign body, persistent inflammation, severe vitreous hemorrhage, and retinal detachment. Each factor can lead to phthisis bulbi.

In reviewing our series of patients, we found the results of the last 5-year period were much better than those of the earlier 5 years. We attribute this to the popularization of vitrectomy, which allows effective and safe removal of traumatic cataracts, condensed vitreous, hemorrhages, and nonmagnetic foreign bodies and enables the repair of complicated cases of retinal detachment.[21,22]

REFERENCES

1. Bronson NR: Techniques of ultrasonic localization and extraction of intraocular and extraocular foreign bodies. Am J Ophthalmol 60:596–603, 1965
2. Bronson NR: Development of a simple B-scan ultrasonoscope. Trans Am Ophthalmol Soc 70:365, 1972
3. Bronson NR: Management of magnetic foreign bodies. In Freeman HM (ed): Ocular Trauma, pp 179–186. New York, Appleton-Century-Crofts, 1979
4. Coleman DJ: Ultrasonic evaluation of the vitre-

ous. In Freeman HM, Hirose T, Schepens CL (eds): Vitreous Surgery and Advances in Fundus Diagnosis and Treatment, pp 63–77. New York, Appleton-Century-Crofts, 1977

5. Coleman DJ, Lizzi FL, Jack RL: Ultrasonography of the Eye and Orbit, pp 258–260. Philadelphia, Lea & Febiger, 1977

6. Cottingham AJ Jr, Forster RK: Vitrectomy in endophthalmitis: Results of study using vitrectomy, intraocular antibiotics, or a combination of both. Arch Ophthalmol 94:2078, 1976

7. Cowden JW, Runyan JE: Localization of intraocular foreign bodies. Further experiences in ultrasonic vs radiologic methods. Arch Ophthalmol 3:299–301, 1969

8. Cridland N: Magnet extraction. In Roper-Hall MJ (ed): International Ophthalmology Clinics, vol 8, pp 213–229. Boston, Little, Brown, 1968

9. Diamond DJ: Intravitreal management of endophthamitis. In Shimizu K, Oosterhuis JA (eds): Acta XXIII Concilium Ophthalmologicum, Kyoto, 1978. Amsterdam, Excerpta Medica, 1979

10. Douvas NG: Anterior segment injuries and closed vitrectomy. In Freeman HM (ed): Ocular Trauma, pp 215–226. New York, Appleton-Century-Crofts, 1979

11. Duke-Elder S, MacFaul PA: System of Ophthalmology. Injuries. Part I: Mechanical Injuries, vol 14, pp 485–497; 512–541; 583–595. London, Henry Kimpton, 1972

12. Gaster RN, Duda EE: Localization of intraocular foreign bodies by computed tomography. Ophthalmic Surg 11:25–29, 1980

13. Graham RO, Peyman GA: Intravitreal injection of dexamethasone: Treatment of experimentally induced endophthalmitis. Arch Ophthalmol 92:149, 1974

14. Heimann K, Neubauer H, et al: Pars plana vitrectomy after intraocular foreign bodies. Mod Probl Ophthalmol 99:63, 1979

15. Hirose T, Schepens CL: Posterior segment reconstruction with open-sky vitrectomy in late complications of ocular trauma. In Freeman HM (ed): Ocular Trauma, pp 263–270. New York, Appleton-Century-Crofts, 1979

16. Hutton WL, Snyder WB, Vaiser A: Surgical removal of nonmagnetic foreign bodies. Am J Ophthalmol 80:838–843, 1975

17. Kollarits CR, DiChiro G, Christiansen J: Detection of orbital and intraocular foreign bodies by computerized tomography. Ophthalmic Surg 8 (1):45–53, 1977

18. Landers MB, Foulks GN, et al: Temporary keratoprosthesis for use during pars plana vitrectomy. Am J Ophthalmol: 615–619, 1981

19. Levy WJ: Intraocular foreign body. Br J Ophthalmol 42:610–616, 1958

20. Liu JH, Shiao CH, Huang SS: Localization of intraocular foreign body: A comparison of Comberg's technique, ultrasonogram and CT scan. Trans Soc Ophthalmol Sinicae 24:340–343, 1985

21. Liu JH: Vitreous surgery in the management of injuries due to intraocular foreign body. Trans Soc Ophthalmol Sinicae 21:74–84, 1982

22. Liu JH, Cheng CW: The lensectomy with anterior vitrectomy in the management of congenital and traumatic cataracts. Trans Asia-Pacific Acad Ophthalmol 9:334–337, 1983

23. Lobes LA, Grand MG, Reese J, et al: Computerized axial tomography in the detection of intraocular foreign bodies. Ophthalmology 33:26–29, 1981

24. Machemer R, Buettner H, Norton EWD: Vitrectomy: A pars plana approach. Trans Am Acad Ophthalmol Otolaryngol 75:813, 1971

25. Machemer R: A new concept for vitreous surgery. Two instrument techniques in pars plana vitrectomy. Arch Ophthalmol 92:407–412, 1974

26. Michels RG: Surgical management of nonmagnetic intraocular foreign bodies. Arch Ophthalmol 93:1003, 1975

27. Michels RG: Vitreous Surgery, pp 257–284. St Louis, CV Mosby Co, 1981

28. Neubauer H: Intraocular foreign bodies. Trans Ophthalmol Soc UK 95:496–502, 1975

29. Neubauer H: Management of nonmagnetic intraocular foreign bodies. In Freeman HM (ed): Ocular Trauma, pp 187–196. New York, Appleton-Century-Crofts, 1979

30. Oksala A: The echogram in the diagnosis of eye diseases. Klin Monatsbl Augenheilkd 137:72–87, 1960

31. Ossoinig K, Seher K: Ultrasonic diagnosis of intraocular foreign bodies. In Gitter K (ed): Ophthalmic Ultrasound, pp 311–320, St Louis, CV Mosby Co, 1969

32. Percival SPB: A decade of intraocular foreign bodies. Br J Ophthalmol 56: 454–461, 1972

33. Percival SPB: Late complications from posterior segment intraocular foreign bodies. Br J Ophthalmol 56:462–468, 1972

34. Peyman GA, Vastine DW, Crouch ER, et al: Clinical use of intravitreal antibiotics to treat bacterial endophthalmitis. Ophthalmology 78:862, 1974

35. Roper-Hall MJ: Review of 555 cases of intraocular foreign body with special reference to prognosis. Br J Ophthalmol 38:65–99, 1954

36. Runyan TE, Penner R: Comparison of localization of orbital foreign bodies by radiologic and ultrasonic methods. Arch Ophthalmol 81:512–517, 1969

37. Ryan ST, Allen AW: Pars plana vitrectomy in ocular trauma. Am J Ophthalmol 88:483, 1979

38. Schepens CL: Retinal Detachment and Allied

Diseases, vol 2, pp 687–692. Philadelphia, WB Saunders, 1983

39. Seymour EQ, Bane DB: A comparison of the accuracy of the Comberg and Sweet techniques of orbital foreign body localization. Radiology 96:75–76, 1970

40. Tate E, Cupples H: Detection of orbital foreign bodies with computed tomography: Current limits. AJR 137:493–495, 1981

41. Vastine DW, Peyman GA, Guth JB: Visual prognosis in bacterial endophthalmitis treated with intravitreal antibiotics. Ophthal Surg 10(3):76, 1979

26

Juvenile Rhegmatogenous Retinal Detachment in Taiwan

Wu-fu Tsai

While the incidence of rhegmatogenous retinal detachment in Taiwan is similar to that in Western countries, the disease appears to affect a younger population. The average age for rhegmatogenous retinal detachment is 39.02 years for men and 46.2 for women (average age of onset 41.68 years). In the West, rhegmatogenous retinal detachment is most frequently seen in the aged.[2,3,4,6] We studied the characteristic features of rhegmatogenous retinal detachment in Taiwanese patients under 20 years old.

FEATURES OF RHEGMATOGENOUS DETACHMENT IN THIS STUDY

Five million of the 18 million people in Taiwan are under 20 years old. An unusual characteristic of this population is the prevalence of myopia (40% from 6 to 12 years old, 55% from 13 to 15 years old, and 70% to 90% from 16 to 18 years old). An estimated 600 retinal detachment surgeries are performed annually in Taiwan.

From January 1979 through December 1982, I performed 861 retinal detachment operations on 820 patients, of whom 121 were under 20 years old. Of these patients, twenty had special pathogenetic factors affecting their retinal detachment that excluded them from this study. Two had retinoschisis, three had vitreous traction secondary to persistent hyperplastic primary vitreous, ten had ocular trauma, and four had surgical aphakia. Of the remaining 101 pa-

tients, eleven had bilateral retinal detachment. All patients were followed up for at least 6 months. The success of the surgery was determined at the latest visit, which ranged from 6 months to 4 years postoperatively.

The special features of juvenile rhegmatogenous retinal detachment in this study were as follows (Table 26–1 through 26–3):[1,7,9,10,12]

1. Of 101 patients, 88 (87.1%) were myopic. Myopia of less than 6 diopters was noted in 61 patients. The most common pathogenetic factor of the rhegmatogenous detachment in this group of patients was lattice degeneration associated with retinal hole (83 patients).
2. Macular involvement was common, and recovery of central vision was low. Of the treated patients, 91.1% had macular detachment, which might explain why reduced vision was the most common presenting symptom, with relatively poor recovery of central vision. Only 36 patients (35% to 64%) obtained best corrected vision of 20/50, the minimum required to read Chinese characters.
3. Proliferative vitreoretinopathy (PVR) seldom developed. Only 2.9% of the patients developed PVR. Although the reasons for the low rate of PVR are not clear, the atrophic retina and optic nerve in myopic eyes may be less conducive to PVR as proliferative diabetic retinopathy, which occurs less frequently in eyes with atrophic retina.

Table 26-1. Age Distribution of Patients With Juvenile Rhegmatogenous Retinal Detachment in Taiwan

Age Groups (yrs)	No. of Patients	Percentage
0–5	3	2.97
6–10	10	9.90
11–15	31	30.69
16–20	57	56.44

Table 26-3. Characteristics of Juvenile Retinal Detachment

Characteristics	No. of Patients	Percentage
Retinal detachment		
in lower quadrants	57	56.1
in temporal quadrants	22	21.7
Macular involvement	92	91.1
Development of proliferative vitreoretinopathy	3	2.9

4. Delay of surgical treatment. Only 25% of patients sought medical treatment within the first month of the onset of symptoms. Over half of the patients waited 1 to 6 months before seeking medical attention. Most patients had changed eyeglasses frequently for progressive myopia; it was easy for them to confuse the symptoms of progressive myopia with reduced vision secondary to retinal detachment. Frequency of surgical reattachment was high (95.4%). Since the retinal detachment most frequently occurred in the lower quadrants of the eye (Fig.26-1), and there was only a small risk of developing PVR, the rate of surgical reattachment remained high even though treatment was delayed.

THERAPEUTIC APPROACH

Special procedures have been adopted to treat retinal detachment in this age group of patients:

low scleral buckle, minimal diathermy, loose encircling band, complete subretinal fluid drainage, and vitrectomy, which is usually not necessary for this disease. Since most patients were young and myopic, we used diathermy instead of cryocoagulation to minimize the lengthening of the globe and the severity of myopia. Furthermore, as there was only a little vitreous traction, the scleral buckle was placed low, just to close the breaks. Also, a short postoperative course was achieved. Most of the patients were students and could not be absent from school longer than 2 weeks without jeopardizing a whole year of school work. To shorten this postoperative course, the subretinal fluid was drained completely during the operation.

Table 26-2. Presenting Symptoms of Juvenile Rhegmatogenous Retinal Detachments

Symptoms	No. of Patients	Percentage
Reduced central vision	41	40.6
Quadrantic visual defect	21	20.8
Distorted vision	16	15.84
Vitreous floaters	9	8.9
Light flash	7	6.9
Unknown	7	6.9

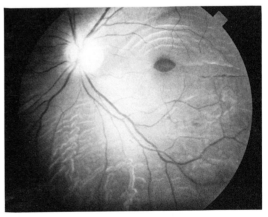

Figure 26-1. Retinal detachment involves lower quadrant and is associated with macular degeneration.

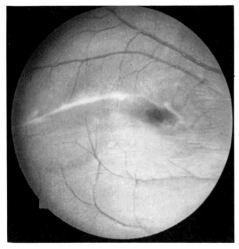

Figure 26-2. A subretinal strand extends across the macular area.

These procedures have been very effective, yielding a success rate of 95.1% of retinal reattachment. However, since most patients initially had a long-standing lower-quadrant retinal detachment with macular involvement, there was a tendency for them to develop subretinal strands across the macular area (Fig. 26-2). These patients did not have good vision even after the retina was reattached.

In 1978, Dr. Momose of Japan developed an operation he called *posterior scleral support.*[5] He used a strip of lyodura to support the macula external to the posterior sclera to inhibit the progression of chorioretinal degeneration and improve visual acuity by enhancing the vascular supply overlying the macular area. We combined Dr. Momose's technique with a scleral buckling procedure. Donor sclera was added to the sclera overlying the macular area and anchored by a piece of silicone band. Both ends of the silicone band were fixed under the encircling band of the buckle (Fig. 26-3).

We treated 12 patients with this combined procedure. The results have not yet been evaluted because induced vascularization from donor sclera was not to occur for 1 year after the operation. We believe, however, that since most patients are myopic, the prevention of retinal detachment through the treatment of lattice degeneration should be a public health priority.[8,11]

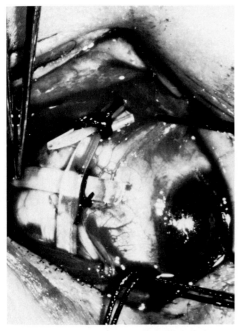

Figure 26-3. An encircling scleral buckle is placed with a posterior scleral support. The forceps indicate one end of the silicone band which holds the donor sclera over the macular area.

REFERENCES

1. Benson WE: Retinal Detachment, Diagnosis and Management. New York, Harper & Row, 1980
2. Cignell AH: Retinal Detachment Surgery. Berlin, Springer-Verlag, 1980
3. Folk JC, Burton TC: Bilateral phakic retinal detachment. Ophthalmology 89:815–821, 1980
4. Hilton GF, McLean EB, Norton EWD: Retinal Detachment, 3rd ed. Rochester, MN, American Academy of Ophthalmology, 1979
5. Michaelson IC: A National Cooperative Study in the Prevention of Retinal Detachment, Retina Congress, pp 661–667. New York, Appleton-Century-Crofts, 1972
6. Momose A: Posterior scleral support operation combined with extraction of lens in high myopia: Two-stage operation. Int XXIII Concilium Ophthalmologicum, pp 1232–1235. The Hague, Excerpta Medica, 1978
7. Schepens CL: Retinal Detachment and Allied Diseases. Philadelphia, WB Saunders, 1983
8. Scott JD: Congenital myopia and retinal detachment. Trans Opthalmol Soc UK 100:69–71, 1980

9. Sharf J, Zonis S: Juvenile retinal detachment. J Pediatr Ophthalmol 14:392–394, 1977

10. Verdaguer J: Juvenile retinal detachment. Pan American Association of Ophthalmology and American Journal of Ophthalmology Lectures. Am J Ophthalmol 93:145–156, 1982

11. Winslow RL, Tasman WS: Juvenile rhegmatogenous retinal detachment. Ophthalmology 85:607–618, 1985

12. Winslow RL, Tasman WS: Juvenile retinal detachment. Internal Ophthalmol Clin 16:96–105, 1976

27

Ultrasonography of Vitreoretinal Disease

Stanley Chang
D. Jackson Coleman

Ultrasonography is not only a fundamental diagnostic modality in the evaluation of vitreoretinal disease; it is a necessity when eyes have opaque media. Ultrasonography is the only means of localizing vitreoretinal disorders and obtaining accurate topographic characterizations of abnormal vitreoretinal relationships when the fundus cannot be visualized. The ultrasonographic findings provide the vitreoretinal surgeon with a basis for rational decisions regarding the necessity for, timing of, and prognosis of therapeutic intervention.

In the diagnosis and management of ocular tumors, acoustic tissue patterns are valuable in differentiating tumor types and malignant and benign neoplastic conditions. Although largely empirical, conventional methods of acoustic tissue characterization offer a high degree of accuracy. Computerized spectral analysis techniques, however, allow a more objective and quantitative assessment of acoustic tissue-reflectance properties that are determined by histologic structure. These analytic methods may also provide additional information on physiologic changes in the posterior ocular structures of both normal and diseased eyes.

TECHNIQUES AND INSTRUMENTATION

Current techniques of ocular ultrasonographic analysis employ pattern recognition of combined A- and B-scan images in real time. B-scan images represent cross-sectional displays of the topographic anatomy within the eye. The study of multiple two-dimensional B-scan images enables the examiner to define three-dimensional relationships among the vitreous membranes, retina, choroid, and sclera.

The A-scan pattern represents back-scattered echoes reflected from tissue interfaces along the path of the sound beam and provides information about structural features of the tissues. The acoustic reflectivity (echo amplitude) of an ocular tissue depends on the mismatch of acoustic impedance as the sound beam traverses tissue boundaries (reflection coefficient). As the sound beam passes through tissue, it may be absorbed and refracted, changes that can further alter the patterns observed. Isometric displays (D-scan) allow simultaneous presentation of A- and B-scan information. Electronically, the plane of the image can be rotated or tilted to enhance the viewing perspectives of reflectivity relationships in specific areas within the eye. This technique is especially useful in the analysis of vitreoretinal disorders.

Currently, two methods of ophthalmic examination are being used: the immersion method and the contact method. The examination techniques for each have been described previously.[2,5] The immersion technique offers the best B-scan resolution because the transducer is of high quality, its frequency can be altered, and the target organ can be placed within the focal zone of the transducer. The contact method offers convenience and ease of examination.

Table 27-1. Ultrasonographic Features of Vitreoretinal Disease

Location and extent of membranes	B-scan
Uniformity and thickness of membranes	B-scan
Membrane reflectivity	A-scan
Vitreous flow pattern	B-scan
Points of vitreoretinal contact	B-scan
Associated choroidal/scleral abnormalities	A- and B-scan
Foreign body localization	A- and B-scan

The examination process is dynamic, occurring in real time. The ultrasonographic features observed are listed in Table 27-1. The B-scan depicts the distribution and extent of membranous layers in the vitreous. The A-scan enables tissue differentiation according to acoustic reflectivity. The examiner observes the flow patterns of membranous structures within the vitreous during and following eye movement. Combined with information from A- and B-scan patterns, vitreous-flow patterns improve diagnostic accuracy.

Modern ophthalmic ultrasound equipment has incorporated digital signal processing technology. Images are stored in microprocessor memory and continuously displayed on the oscilloscope screen. Moreover, the gray scale is much better than analog instrumentation. At present, commercially available instrumentation offers six-bit or 64-level gray scale information. More sophisticated methods in the laboratory provide up to 256 levels of gray scale (eight-bit), which improve the quality of the image. Spectral-analysis techniques, which separate ultrasonic tissue signals into their constituent frequency components, are easily performed with digitized images. Algorithms for postacquisition signal processing and image enhancement may be applied. Image-processing techniques, such as logarithmic, linear, S-shaped amplifications and color-coded enhancement, are currently available. The advantages of each of these enhancement techniques for clinical diagnosis of various ocular disorders are currently under investigation.

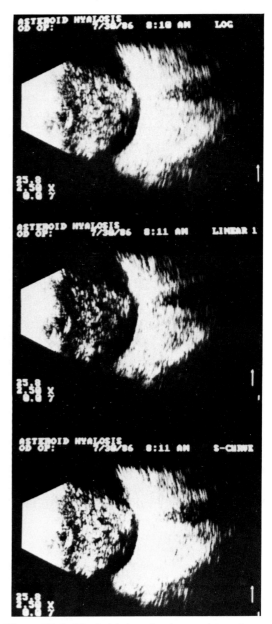

Figure 27-1. The brightly reflective particles of asteroid hyalosis are usually located only in cortical vitreous. The improved gray scale is shown with linear amplification *(middle)*, while S-scale amplification enhances low-amplitude echoes.

VITREOUS OPACITIES

Vitreous opacities that require examination by ultrasound usually result from hemorrhage, in-

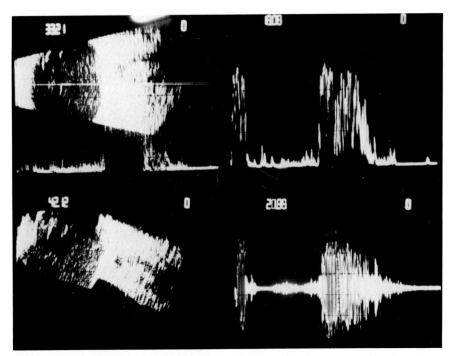

Figure 27-2. Recent diffuse vitreous hemorrhage emits low-reflective echoes on A-scan. Isometric viewing enhances the visual appreciation of the low-amplitude echoes contrasted with highly reflective sclera and orbital fat.

flammation, or trauma. Ultrasound, however, cannot differentiate hemorrhagic debris from inflammatory exudate. Metabolic causes or vitreous opacities also require ultrasonographic examination, such as asteroid hyalosis or amyloidosis.

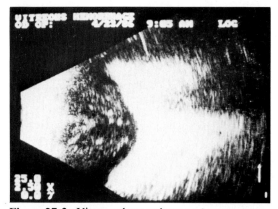

Figure 27-3. Vitreous hemorrhage and membranes are more acoustically reflective at seven months than initially.

Asteroid Hyalosis

Asteroid hyalosis (Fig. 27-1) appears as brightly reflective particulate echoes within the vitreous space. These calcium stearates are distributed in the cortical vitreous and are not seen in the subhyaloid space. The higher reflective echoes are emphasized by S-shaped amplification. The reflectivity on A-scan is usually moderate to high.

Vitreous Hemorrhage

Recent vitreous hemorrhage displays diffusely scattered echoes of low amplitude within the vitreous cavity (Fig. 27-2). Their amplitudes do not correlate with the density of the hemorrhage, because relatively few interfaces are present. As the hemorrhage matures, clumps of cellular aggregates and formed-vitreous membranes act as reflecting surfaces that increase the reflectivity of the hemorrhagic debris (Fig. 27-3). Approximately 7 to 10 days after a vitreous hemorrhage, the posterior hyaloid surface may separate from the retina. Hemorrhagic

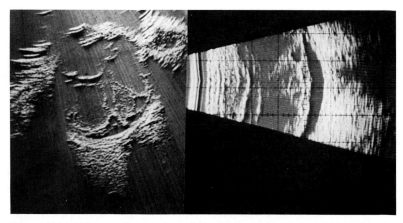

Figure 27-4. Vitreous hemorrhage following cataract surgery shows that layers of membranes with thickening have formed along the separated posterior hyaloid.

debris tends to cluster on the posterior hyaloid membrane and more prominently in the inferior vitreous cavity (Fig. 27-4). B-scan shows vitreous hemorrhage with posterior hyaloid separation as an irregularly thickened membrane of low to moderate reflectivity. The membranes are of irregular thickness with multiple layers (Fig. 27-5). A-scan usually shows the posterior hyaloid surface as being somewhat higher in reflectivity than hemorrhages in the cortical vitreous and often consists of multiple echoes. The echo amplitude of the posterior hyaloid, however, is usually not as high as those that form the sclera. As the patient moves the eye from side to side in the plane of the scan section, a completely separate posterior hyaloid surface appears, looking like a floating veil. The points where the hyaloid remains tethered to the retina are localized, often indicating a source of vitreous traction or the origin of vitreous hemorrhage, depending on the pathophysiologic processes involved (Fig. 27-6).

Diabetic Retinopathy

Abnormalities at the vitreoretinal interface in proliferative diabetic retinopathy are graphically demonstrated ultrasonographically. Fibrovascular proliferation develops around the optic disc and along the temporal vascular arcades. These fibrovascular membranes grow along the

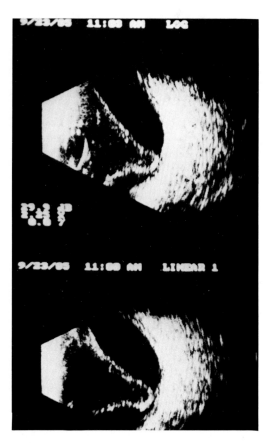

Figure 27-5. Vitreous hemorrhage with vitreous separation. The posterior hyaloid exhibits high mobility when the patient is asked to move the eye. Logarithmic amplification enhances low-amplitude echoes in the cortical vitreous.

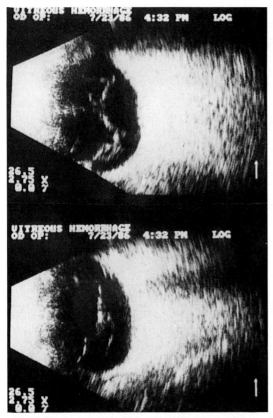

Figure 27-6. Vitreous hemorrhage in proliferative diabetic retinopathy. The points of vitreoretinal contact *(top)* indicate epicenters of fibroproliferation. The body of the vitreous hemorrhage is shown in the bottom figure.

posterior hyaloid surface or into the vitreous. Frequently, the posterior hyaloid incompletely separates, leaving vitreous attachments at areas of retinal neovascularization. The anteroposterior traction combined with tangential traction of the proliferative tissue may result in tractional retinal elevation.

The hyaloid surface may appear irregularly thickened on B-scan (Fig. 27-7) or may remain a thin sheet of moderately high reflectivity. When dense hemorrhage exists, locating the areas of greatest elevation of hyaloid separation can help the vitreous surgeon to identify regions where the hyaloid can be cut safely during initial stages of the operation. Preretinal or subhyaloid hemorrhages can be seen as low-amplitude echoes, usually under a membranous hyaloid surface (Fig. 27-8, 27-9). The slow-moving hemorrhage flows posteriorly as the patient reclines for the examination. In diabetic retinopathy, hemorrhagic echoes beneath a membrane are more likely to indicate that the membrane is of vitreous origin, since subretinal hemorrhage is observed less frequently in diabetic retinopathy.

Areas of localized tractional retinal detachment usually appear on B-scan as peaking of the retinal outline resulting from anteroposterior traction at the point of the hyaloid attachment (Fig. 27-10). The retina commonly assumes a concave appearance on either side of the point of vitreoretinal adhesion (Fig. 27-11). If the reti-

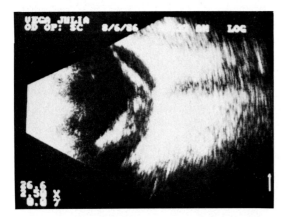

Figure 27-7. Diabetic vitreous hemorrhage exhibits thickened posterior hyaloid with remaining attachment at the optic disc. The membranes are irregular in thickness.

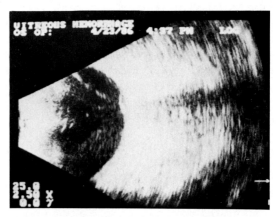

Figure 27-8. Preretinal hemorrhage reflects low-amplitude echoes in the subhyaloid space. A localized tractional retinal detachment is also present.

nal contour appears convex, a rhegmatogenous component should be suspected.

Broad areas of vitreoretinal adhesion can sometimes be identified, indicating that surgery may be more technically difficult (Fig. 27-12).

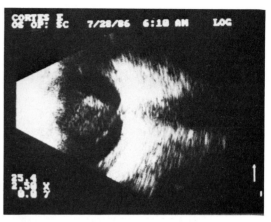

Figure 27-10. An opaque hyaloid membrane has anteroposterior traction, causing a peaked configuration of the localized retinal detachment.

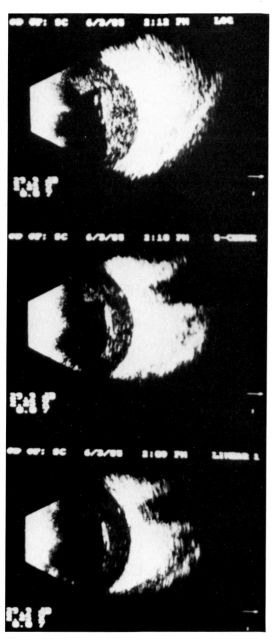

In assessing the topography of eyes with proliferative diabetic retinopathy before vitrectomy, it can be helpful to perform the examination with both serial horizontal and vertical sections. Involvement of the macula by tractional retinal detachment can be detected with accuracy. However, errors in diagnosis of macular involvement can occur because macular ectopia induced by fibroproliferation or shallow macular elevation cannot be detected acoustically.[14]

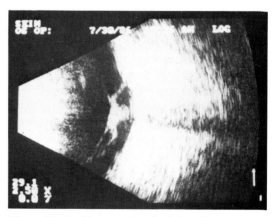

Figure 27-9. Preretinal hemorrhage produces echoes from blood in the subhyaloid space, which are enhanced by logarithmic amplification *(top)*.

Figure 27-11. Tractional retinal detachment demonstrates extensive fibrovascular proliferation with a concave retinal detachment resulting from traction.

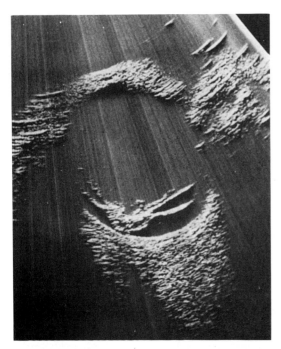

Figure 27-12. Broad areas of vitreoretinal proliferation in diabetic tractional retinal detachment may indicate increased technical difficulty in vitreous surgery.

RETINAL DETACHMENT

Retinal detachment appears by ultrasonography as a thin membrane of uniform thickness, usually extending from the optic disc to the ora serrata (Fig. 27-13, 27-14). A rhegmatogenous retinal detachment exhibits a convex contour. Because the retina is a strong acoustic reflector, on A-scan, the echo amplitude from the retinal surface is almost as high as that from the sclera. The extent of involvement with a subtotal retinal detachment can be determined in patients with miotic pupils or opaque media. A total retinal detachment would demonstrate retinal elevation in all quadrants. A partial retinal detachment can be mapped by localizing the two meridians of the borders where detached retina becomes attached. The configuration of the detachment may provide clues for locating the retinal breaks. Blumenkranz and Byrne found that in 87% of cases that the retinal break was located within 60 degrees of arc of the most superior margin of the retinal detachment indicated by ultrasound.[1] In 74%, the break occurred within 60 degrees of the highest elevation measured ultrasonographically.

A rhegmatogenous detachment cannot be differentiated from a serous retinal detachment because both can appear convex. A shifting of subretinal fluid may be observed as the position of the head is changed because the retina becomes more elevated as the denser subretinal fluid flows to more dependent areas. Retinal detachment has an undulating quality as the patient moves the eye. This movement is rapidly damped once eye movement ceases.

Long-standing retinal detachments develop epiretinal-membrane proliferation on all retinal

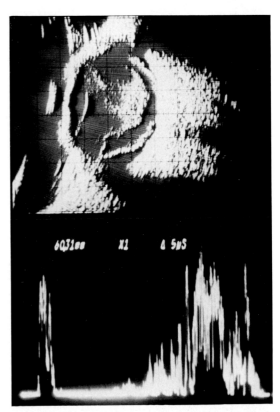

Figure 27-13. A retinal detachment and a dense vitreous hemorrhage from a retinal tear are present. The retina shows a continuous membrane of uniform thickness extending from the optic disc *(top)*. On A-scan the retinal echo is almost as high as that of the sclera *(bottom)*.

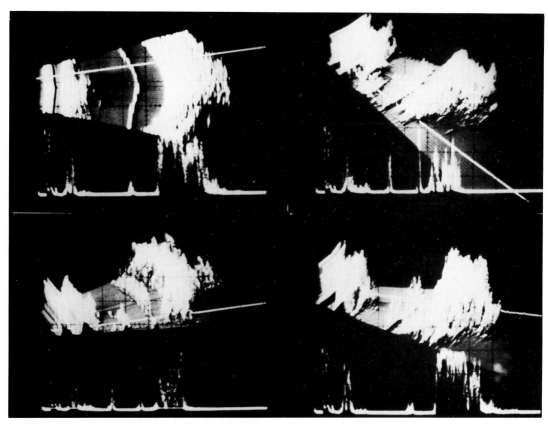

Figure 27-14. Isometric displays of retinal detachment enhance visualization of retinal detachment *(top left).* On isometric viewing, the retina appears as a highly reflective sheet of echoes with even height in the vitreous. The panes of viewing are changed electronically *(top right, bottom left,* and *bottom right).*

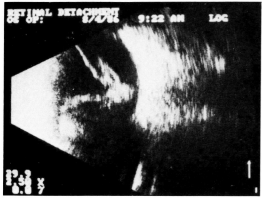

Figure 27-15. Retinal detachment demonstrates epiretinal proliferation with formation of fixed folds resulting in decreased retinal mobility.

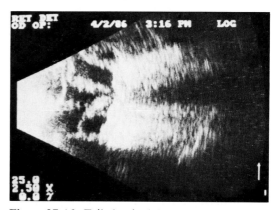

Figure 27-16. Failed retinal detachment surgery reveals shortening of the anteroposterior dimension of the retina. The choroid is diffusely thickened and the scleral buckle is seen peripherally.

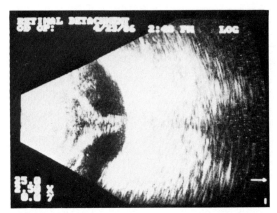

Figure 27-17. Retinal detachment, with advanced degrees of proliferative vitreoretinopathy, results in a triangular configuration from a closed funnel configuration.

surfaces, resulting in both circumferential traction around the vitreous base and anteroposterior shortening. Fixed folds within the retina and localized star-folds can be detected (Fig. 27-15). The shortening of retinal dimensions reduces retinal mobility with eye movement. In advanced degrees of proliferative vitreoretinopathy, the retinal detachment becomes less mobile on B-scan during eye motion (Fig. 27-16).

The anteriorly retracted posterior hyaloid surface shortens the retina in an anteroposterior direction, and the retina appears in a triangle or T configuration (Fig. 27-17). A giant retinal cyst may form with a chronic retinal detachment.

The images of special forms of retinal detachment vary with the pathophysiologic processes involved (Fig. 27-18, 27-19). A giant retinal tear shows disinserted peripheral retina.[11] Frequently, the tear folds over, and the posterior hyaloid surface retracts anteriorly. The torn edge of the retina often curls. In retrolental fibroplasia or sickle-cell retinopathy, peripheral fibrovascular proliferation results in contraction along the vitreous base. Because abnormal vitreoretinal relationships and areas of traction can be demonstrated ultrasonographically, their patterns may help determine the best surgical approach for these difficult cases.

OCULAR TRAUMA

Ultrasonographic evaluation is necessary following blunt or penetrating ocular injury that opacifies the media. Because ocular damage resulting from trauma varies in extent and sever-

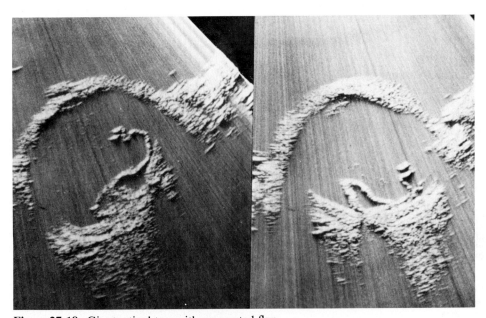

Figure 27-18. Giant retinal tear with an everted flap.

ity, ultrasonographic patterns cannot be categorized. Traumatic subluxation or dislocation of the lens into the vitreous shifts the lens position, producing a rounded lens contour as zonular tension relaxes (Fig. 27-20). In traumatic cata-

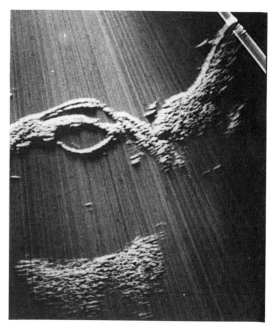

Figure 27-20. Traumatic subluxation of the lens appears as a shift in the location of the lens anteriorly, with a more rounded configuration resulting from zonular relaxation.

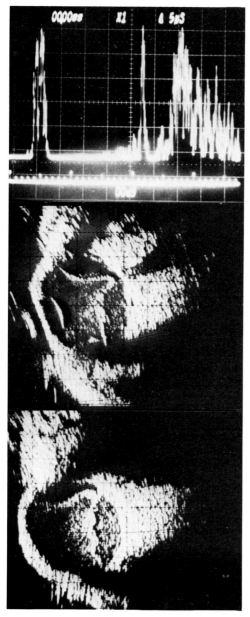

Figure 27-19. The total hemorrhagic retinal detachment with vitreous hemorrhage and extensive subretinal bleeding are from presumed ocular histoplasmosis.

ract, the integrity of the lens capsule can be determined (Fig. 27-21), which aids in the choice of surgical approach. An intact posterior capsule indicates cataract extraction by an anterior approach. If the posterior lens capsule is ruptured and mixed with vitreous, prompt intervention through the pars plana reduces the likelihood of cyclitic membrane formation.

With posterior penetrating injuries, a vitreous tract is commonly produced along the pathway of the injury. Ultrasonography demonstrates the extent of vitreous membranes and the presence of retinal detachment, influencing the timing of surgical intervention. When massive injury results in marked disorganization of the intraocular contents, it may be difficult to determine the status of the vitreoretinal structures. It may help to reduce the sensitivity of the amplifier, which allows echoes from more reflective structures, such as a retinal detachment or foreign body, to persist. Frequent follow-up examinations can also aid these situations. It is not always possible to detect a posterior scleral rupture ultrasonographically, because the adjacent

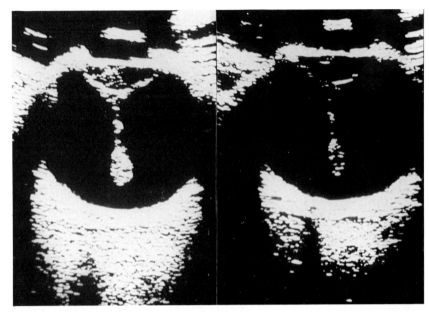

Figure 27-21. Traumatic rupture of the posterior lens capsule is visible in this eye with a swollen opaque lens *(left)*. Reduction of amplifier sensitivity *(right)* demonstrates capsular remnants.

orbital fat is highly reflective. A decision to explore the globe surgically for possible traumatic rupture should be based on clinical judgment rather than ultrasonographic findings.

Intraocular foreign bodies present characteristic ultrasonographic findings. An ultraocular foreign body has high acoustic reflectivity that persists on B-scan as sensitivity is reduced. The

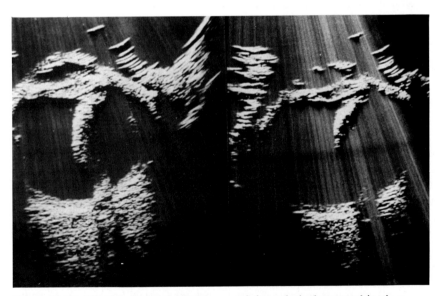

Figure 27-22. Metallic foreign body has passed through the lens, resulting in a cataract *(left)*. Reduction of amplifier gain demonstrates the strongly reflective nature of the foreign body *(right)*.

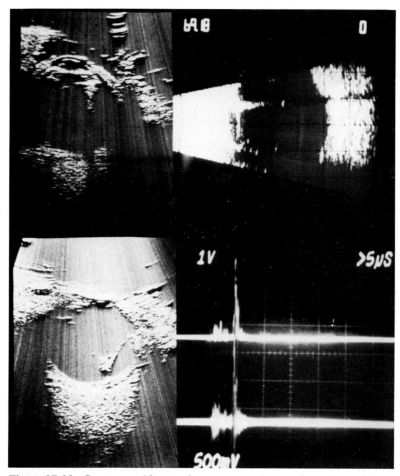

Figure 27-23. Contact and immersion scans are shown of a patient with a metallic foreign body located anteriorly. The acoustic shadowing resulting from sound absorption can be a helpful characteristic in localization *(top)*. Ultrasonography demonstrates related changes such as vitreous hemorrhage *(lower left)*.

strong sound absorption of the foreign body allows less energy to reach the posterior tissues; this is called *acoustic shadowing* (Fig. 27-22, 27-23). By decreasing the sensitivity of the amplifier, the acoustic shadowing can be enhanced. On A-scan, the echo amplitude from the foreign body often exceeds the scleral echo posteriorly. Round metallic foreign bodies, such as BB-gun pellets, produce reverberation artifacts as sound echoes internally between their two concave surfaces (Fig. 27-24). The isometric scan displays relatively high acoustic amplitudes from a foreign body well, which can aid localization

(Fig. 27-25). Occasionally, an air bubble may enter the wound with an intraocular foreign body, resulting in inaccurate localization. These air bubbles, however, rarely persist beyond 24 hours after injury.

We prefer to use computed tomography for ultrasonographic localization of intraocular foreign bodies. The tomographic scan should be performed with an overlapping section of 1.5 mm to maximize the detection of ocular or orbital foreign bodies. These scan techniques accurately detect foreign bodies around the globe; however, ultrasonographic techniques

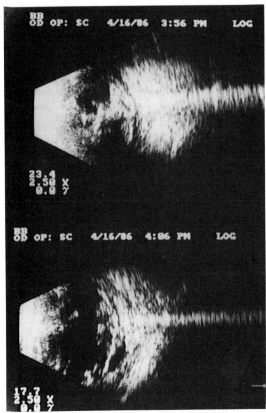

Figure 27-24. Intraocular BB pellet created vitreous tract. The reverberation artifacts aid in localizing the BB pellet, which is buried in the posterior ocular coats *(top)*. Reduction of amplifier gain improved localization *(bottom)*.

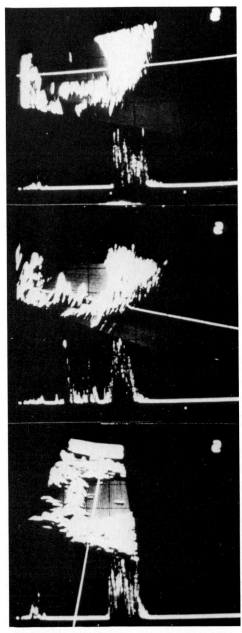

Figure 27-25. On isometric viewing, the highly reflective intraocular foreign body relative to adjacent ocular tissues is easily identified.

the vortex vein ampullae. Posteriorly, the contour of a large choroidal bulla forms an acute angle with the scleral surface. The presence of echoes in the subchoroidal space determines the nature of the fluid. Few or no low-reflective

are complementary, allowing an assessment of the intraocular topography resulting from the trauma. Vitreous hemorrhage or retinal detachment resulting from a penetrating injury are not visualized by computed tomography. An accurate evaluation of structural changes from the intraocular foreign body facilitates decisions concerning the surgical strategy.

CHOROIDAL DETACHMENT

Choroidal detachment on ultrasonography appears as a round, convex separation of choroidal and retinal layers from the sclera (Fig. 27-26). The choroidal separation is usually limited anteriorly by the ciliary body and posteriorly by echoes suggest serous detachment, while aggregates of higher reflectivity probably represent hemorrhagic clots in the suprachoroidal space (Fig. 27-27). Liquefaction of the hemorrhagic clots in the extensive hemorrhage can be observed as aftermovements in the suprachoroidal space as the patient moves the eye. On A-scan, the retina-choroid interface is thicker with retinal detachment alone. This interface usually demonstrates high acoustic reflectivity, approaching the scleral amplitude.

OCULAR TUMORS

Trends for the management of malignant melanomas of the choroid have changed markedly over recent years from enucleation to possibly sight-preserving techniques such as eye-wall resection, cobalt plaque therapy, and proton-beam irradiation. Ultrasonography has assumed an increasingly expanded role in the assessment and management of ocular tumors. Conventional ultrasonographic techniques to

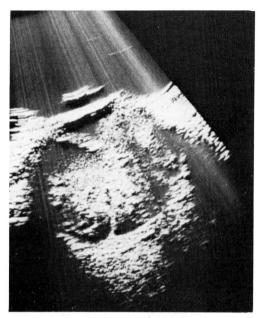

Figure 27-27. Choroidal hemorrhage produces solid echoes from the clotted blood located in the suprachoroidal space with appositional choroidal domes.

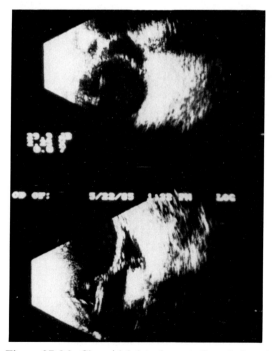

Figure 27-26. Choroidal detachment: the subchoroidal space contains few echoes indicative of probable serous fluid.

diagnose ocular tumors rely on pattern integration of A- and B-scan information. B-scan locates ocular tumors and defines their related structural abnormalities in the eye. A-scan tissue-pattern analysis allows differentiation of various ocular tumor types. These diagnostic techniques have been developed empirically over the years using the video A-scan signal, which is electronically processed to enhance visual identification of internal tissue characteristics. Diagnosis using amplitudes of reflected echoes as well as the general envelope pattern are helpful. Clinically, conventional techniques remain quite accurate and reliable in their ability to characterize ocular tumors. Unfortunately, these techniques are nevertheless empirical and rely heavily on the examiner's experience and familiarity with the instrument. For these reasons, it is believed that acoustic tissue characterization with power-spectrum techniques will provide truly standardized quantitative information.

The ultrasonographic differential diagnosis of ocular tumors is commonly separated into four categories: malignant melanoma of the choroid,

Table 27-2. Ultrasonographic Features of Choroidal Tumors

Tumor Type	*B-Scan Pattern*	*A-Scan Pattern (Linear Amplification)*
Choroidal melanoma	Solid, convex mass; collar-button pattern	Low-reflective, homogeneous internal texture, exponential envelope
Metastatic carcinoma	Flat, placoid, or convex, serous R.D. frequent	Medium-high internal reflectivity; irregular, sustained envelope
Choroidal hemangioma	Solid, convex mass or diffuse mass	Highly reflective throughout; regular, widely spaced internal texture
Subretinal hemorrhage	Solid, usually <3 mm, usually in macular region	Variable, fresh—low-reflective; disciform scar—high-reflective

metastatic carcinoma to the choroid, choroidal hemangioma, and subretinal hemorrhage. Table 27-2 lists the ultrasonographic features and diagnostic criteria of each category.

Malignant Melanoma

Malignant melanomas of the choroid usually assume one of two configurations on B-scan ul-

trasonography. The tumor is generally convex (Fig. 27-28, 27-29) or like a collar button when it has erupted through Bruch's membrane (Fig. 27-30). Frequently, large tumors have an associated retinal detachment or vitreous hemorrhage. Choroidal tumors exhibit low internal reflectivity, so there may be an area of acoustic "hollowing" or a "quiet zone" on B-scan. The replacement of choroidal tissue by an expand-

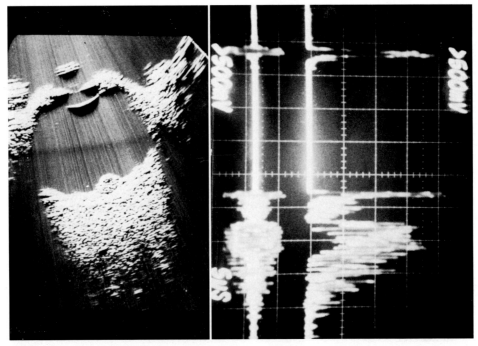

Figure 27-28. Choroidal melanoma appears as a small convex mass, demonstrating the choroidal excavation sign on B-scan *(left)*. A-scan is shown on the right.

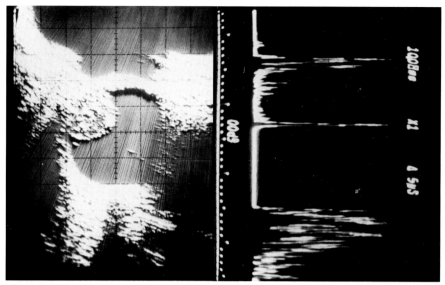

Figure 27-29. A large melanoma is detected near the ciliary body, with low internal reflectivity.

ing mass of low reflectivity accounts for the choroidal excavation appearance, described by Coleman and coworkers, which occurs in approximately 45% of cases.[3] Extrascleral extension can be detected only if it grossly infiltrates the scleral coats. Emissary vein extension of choroidal melanoma usually cannot be detected.

Within choroidal melanomas, A-scan pattern shows low-reflective internal echoes. With linear amplification, the envelope pattern of the echo signal appears to decay exponentially (Fig. 27-28). The internal acoustic texture of the echo amplitudes is relatively uniform and regular, corresponding to the relatively homogeneous histologic cytoarchitecture seen in melanomas.

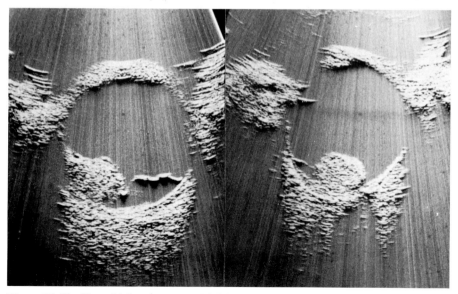

Figure 27-30. Choroidal melanoma exhibits collar-button appearance when the tumor erupts through Bruch's membrane. A retinal detachment is also present.

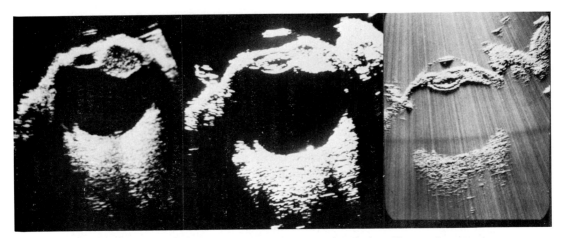

Figure 27-31. A ciliary-body melanoma was treated by proton irradiation. Six months later, advanced cataract developed while the tumor shrank. At 28 months, the tumor has further decreased in size.

Occasionally, the internal echoes are blurred (rapid spontaneous movements), attributed by Ossoning to vascular flow within the tumor. While it is often seen in melanomas, this sign is not specific for the tumor and can be observed in other rapidly growing masses.

Ultrasonographic biometry is the best technique for measuring the thickness of ocular tumors. Accurate thickness measurements are especially important because of the current trends to observe melanomas for longer periods and to treat them more conservatively (Fig. 27-31) than in the past. B-scan can localize the meridian of greatest tumor thickness. With the A-scan beam oriented perpendicular to the surface of the tumor and to the underlying sclera, the measurement is made electronically after tumor boundaries are identified. A focused beamed transducer should be at least 10 MHz. Our laboratory used a tissue velocity of 1600 meters per second. Recent measurements in human choroidal melanomas with the scanning laser acoustic microscope, however, indicate the actual velocity to be approximately 1665 meters per second.* With contact scans, notation of the meridian and orientation of the transducer should be made separately. The measurements of melanoma thickness will be reproducible if the scan planes and beam orientation are maintained consistently at each follow-up visit.

* Coleman, DJ: Personal communication

Metastatic Carcinoma

Metastatic carcinomas of the choroid often appear as tumors with a broad base and low height on B-scan (Fig. 27-32, 27-33), although they may also look like a solid convex mass. Frequently, an associated serous detachment of the retina overlies the area of the tumor. A-scan characteristics reveal moderate to high reflectivity, with irregular and heterogeneous echo amplitudes. The sustained echo envelope pattern on A-scan is typical of metastatic tumors; however, some variation in the echo pattern may be based on the histologic characteristics of the primary tumor. In the presence of a serous detachment and an irregular tumor surface, the leading edge of the tumor may be difficult to maximize with A-scan. Histologically, metastatic tumors infiltrate normal choroidal structures, creating areas of tissue heterogeneity that account for the A-scan pattern. We have observed quick spontaneous movements in rapidly growing metastatic tumors.

Choroidal Hemangioma

Choroidal hemangiomas may take on the B-scan appearance of a solid convex mass or they may diffusely involve the choroid (as in Sturge-Weber syndrome). As a convex mass, the tumor is usually located in the posterior pole, rarely more than 6.0 mm in height. When the B-scan

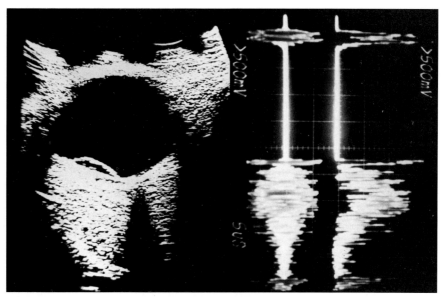

Figure 27-32. Metastatic carcinoma is placoid with overlying retinal detachment on B-scan. On A-scan, sustained echoes of moderately high amplitude are present internally.

appearance is that of a solid mass, the amplifier gain may have to be reduced to see the internal acoustic character of the tumor (Fig. 27-34). On A-scan, the internal reflectivity is high, with echoes reaching 95% to 100% of the scleral echo amplitude. The texture of the acoustic tissue is coarse, with broadly spaced echoes of high reflectivity, which is compatible with its histologic appearance of a tumor containing large vascular channels. The vascular walls are highly reflective structures that contrast with the blood, which has low reflectivity and excellent acoustic

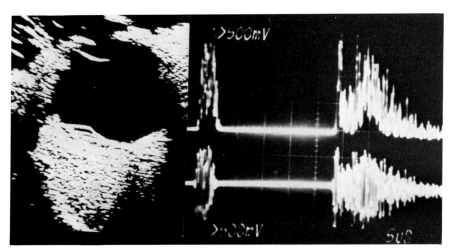

Figure 27-33. A metastatic carcinoma has a radio frequency signal on A-scan that appears to have an envelope with a sustained amplitude throughout the tumor *(right, lower trace)*. The B-scan is shown in the left figure.

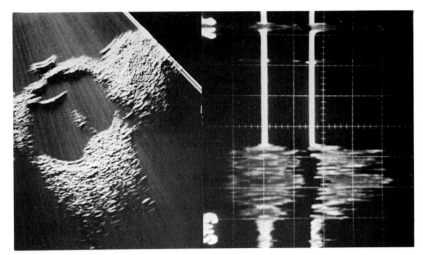

Figure 27-34. Choroidal hemangioma appears as a solid convex mass with overlying vitreous debris. The echo amplitudes are high throughout, with regular spacing.

transmission. Currently available instrumentation cannot depict the choroidal excavation sign in hemangiomas.

Subretinal Hemorrhage

Most frequently, subretinal hemorrhage occurs in age-related macular degeneration associated with a disciform scar. Although usually located in the macular region, eccentric hemorrhagic disciform scars may be clinically perplexing. The dark appearance of the subpigment epithelial hemorrhage resembles a malignant melanoma. Ultrasonographic differentiation of subretinal hemorrhage and melanoma may be difficult if the lesion is small. For accurate ultra-

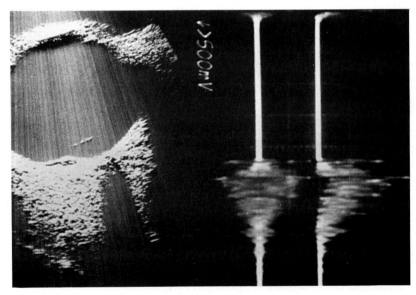

Figure 27-35. Recent subretinal hemorrhage is located in the macular region on B-scan. On A-scan, low-reflective echoes are seen without exponential decay, as observed in melanomas.

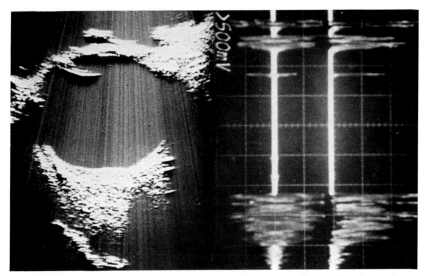

Figure 27-36. Subretinal hemorrhage. A disciform scar of age-related macular degeneration is usually less than 3.0 mm thick. A-scan may contain high-amplitude echoes.

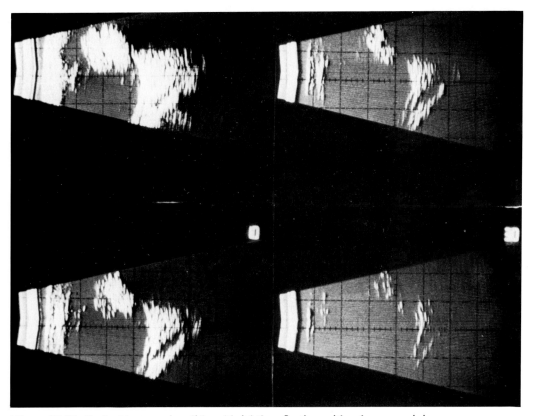

Figure 27-37. Retinoblastoma is solid and brightly reflective, with echoes remaining as sensitivity is reduced. The strong sound absorbency of the tumor results in acoustic shadowing.

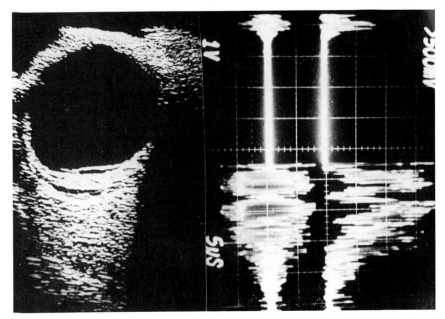

Figure 27-38. Scleritis is seen as a diffuse posterior inflammation of the sclera with overlying retinal detachment. The separation of Tenon's layer suggestive of edema is characteristic.

sonographic differentiation, a thickness of 2.5 to 3.0 mm is required. Most subretinal hemorrhages in macular degeneration are smaller. The ultrasonographic appearance of subretinal hemorrhage may vary depending on the stage at which it is examined. A recent hemorrhage on B-scan shows diffuse low-amplitude echoes under the retina (Fig. 27-35). On A-scan, the envelope pattern varies and is usually not the

exponential-decay type seen in choroidal melanomas. The internal echoes demonstrate low reflectivity with recent hemorrhage, but as the blood becomes organized and is replaced by cicatricial tissue, the internal reflectivity can increase, similar to the pattern seen in metastatic carcinoma (Fig. 27-36).

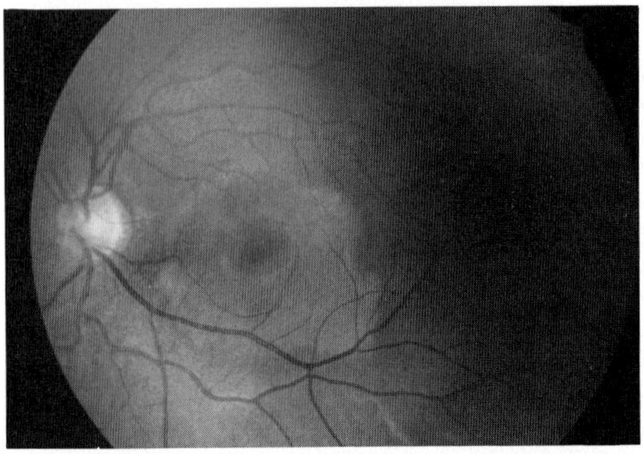

When differentiation is difficult, it may be necessary to perform serial examinations before a definitive diagnosis can be made. The growth of tumors may be observed, while subretinal hemorrhage involutes. When subretinal hemorrhage results from the growth of a choroidal tumor, monthly serial examinations can be extremely helpful in detecting an occult tumor.

Figure 27-39. The fundus appearance of the patient with a choroidal osteoma shown in Figure 27-40. The tumor is flat and light orange and has irregular borders. Visual acuity is 20/20.

Other Tumors

Retinoblastoma often appears on ultrasonography as a brightly reflective, irregularly shaped mass in the vitreous. The calcium-DNA precipitates both reflect and absorb sound, resulting in shadowing of the orbital fat. As amplifier sensitivity is reduced, these calcium complexes often persist at low gain (Fig. 27-37). Occasionally mistaken for a choroidal tumor is nodular or diffuse scleritis, in which diffuse or focal inflammatory thickening of the sclera occurs with an overlying retinal detachment. Ultrasonography can be extremely helpful in differentiating this condition from choroidal tumors. The inflammatory focus separates Tenon's layer posterior to the involved area, believed to represent edema (Fig. 27-38).

A characteristic ultrasonographic pattern is seen in choroidal osteomas. This osseous hamartoma of the choroid is often observed as a flat orange or creamy white mass adjacent to the optic disc or in the posterior pole (Fig. 27-39). The bony mass has high reflectivity and sound absorption, which blocks almost all sound energy from orbital penetration. A reduction of amplifier gain discloses a flat, persistently reflective structure (Fig. 27-40).

SPECTRAL ANALYSIS TECHNIQUES

The acoustic characterization of ocular tumors by spectral analysis is emerging as a useful technique with important clinical applications.[4,6,10] The video A-scan signal is electronically processed to enhance visual diagnosis of the tissue pattern. The amplified unprocessed reflected signal (radio frequency signal) contains additional information discarded electronically. By digitizing the radio-frequency signal and applying iterative computer processing techniques, acoustic tissue features of tumors can be characterized quantitatively.

In contrast to current methods based on empirical observation and clinical experience, new techniques classify tumors objectively on the basis of spectral reflectance criteria and use multivariate statistics to separate tumor types and subtypes. The power spectrum analysis uses frequency-dependent characteristics of tissue cytoarchitecture, similar to techniques for voice-print assessment. The tissue characteristics which are important in determining the power spectrum properties of a tissue are not completely understood; however, factors such as vascularity, scatter-size, fibrosis, necrosis, and melanin content may be important tissue features. A better understanding of tissue microarchitecture and theoretic principles related

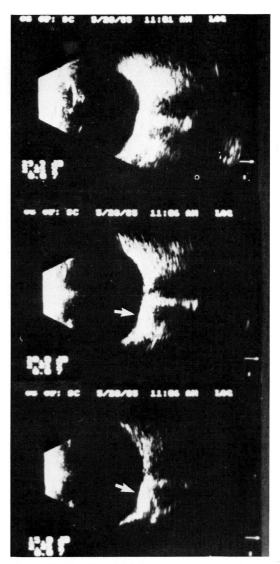

Figure 27-40. Choroidal osteoma occurs as a bony mass *(arrow)* that absorbs sound completely and is highly reflective *(top* and *center)*. Reduction of its sensitivity enhances visibility of the lesion because of its high reflectivity *(bottom)*.

to spectral patterns associated with tumors is currently under investigation.[8,13]

Ultrasonic signals are obtained from interfacing a digital computer with a conventional immersion diagnostic system.[12] A broad-band, focused transducer (10 MHz) is used, and the radio-frequency signals are digitized and acquired at a sampling rate of 100 MHz. B-scan

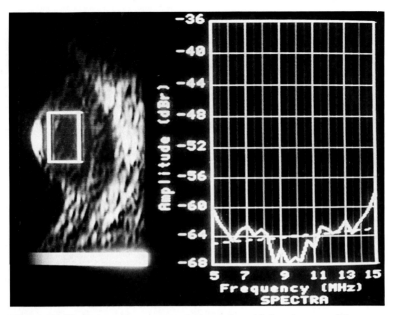

Figure 27-41. Power spectrum analysis of choroidal melanoma. The B-scan image *(left)* is displayed with 256 levels of gray scale from the A-scan radio frequency signals. The box is user-selected and represents the volume of tissue for spectral analysis.

images are displayed with 256 levels of gray scale from the original radio-frequency data. This image measures approximately 7.5 mm deep and 18 mm wide. For power spectrum analysis, a box of user-selected dimensions is placed over the region of interest. The power spectrum is calculated by averaging the squared magnitude of spectra from all scan lines in the region of interest and referenced to the system calibration spectrum, which is obtained by using the same data acquisition system to insonate a glass plate. This will minimize the effects of the measuring system on the tissue spectra.

The power spectrum analysis is based on Fourier transform techniques, which separate any signal into its constituent sine-wave frequencies. A family of sine-waves with different frequencies is derived which reproduce the original signal when summated. The power spectrum is plotted as the amplitude of the sine-wave components (decibels) as a function of frequency. Similar to voice-print analysis, these spectral patterns characterize an acoustic tissue "signature" for each ocular tumor type.

The calibrated power spectrum from a choroidal melanoma is shown in Figure 27-41. The dotted line represents the least squares fit to the power spectrum analysis. The plot consists of spectral amplitude against frequency (5 to 15 MHz, with a center frequency of 10 MHz). Characteristically, melanomas exhibit an expanding spectral amplitude with increasing frequency. The three spectral paramerters — spectral slope, spectral amplitude (measured from the zero-frequency intercept), and intercept residual (a measure of statistical variation in the intercept estimation), are used to separate tumor groupings. Individual spectral parameters vary from one tumor type to another, and multivariate analysis is used to separate the types. Linear discriminant analysis is a statistical technique that allows simultaneous evaluation of three variables to define canonical discriminant functions which maximize the separation of various tumor types. Our tumor data base of over 80 tumors is depicted in a three-dimensional spectral parameter space shown in Figure 27-42.

Boundaries enclose all data points for each type of tumor. Overlapping boundaries represent tumors of diagnostic uncertainty. Approximately 10% of tumors lie in these overlap re-

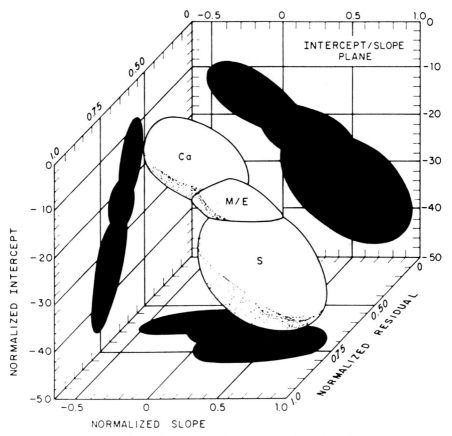

Figure 27-42. Three-dimensional spectral parameter plot. Three tissue types are separated from over 80 tumors in the data base (CA, metastatic carcinoma; S, spindle-cell melanomas; M/E, mixed epithelioid melanomas). (Feleppa EJ, Lizzi FL, Coleman DJ, et al: Diagnostic spectrum analysis in ophthalmology: A physical perspective. Ultrasound Med Bio 12:623–631, 1986; reprinted with permission)

gions, indicating that spectral parameters are highly separable for each tumor type. Tumor type S appears to be related histologically to Callender's classification of spindle B malignant melanoma. Tumor type M/E seems to correlate with Callender's mixed or epithelioid classification, and tumor type Ca is related to metastatic carcinoma. While this analysis is based on a retrospective evaluation, the library of pooled data defines an acoustic signature for each tumor type that can be used prospectively for diagnosis and characterization of unknown ocular tumors.

Acoustic staining techniques of B-scan images allow localization of areas within a tumor corresponding to spectral features of a specific tumor type (Fig. 27-43).[4] Spectral pa-rameters from all points within a tumor are compared to those representative of each tumor type, and areas of similarity are highlighted. Thus, when a stain specific for a melanoma is applied, most of the tumor is highlighted. When the melanoma stain is applied to metastatic carcinoma, little highlighting is observed.

The acoustic characteristics of uveal melanomas may also be useful in making a prognostication. Coleman and coworkers have shown that tumors acoustically classified as Type B (greater spindle cell population) exhibited greater regression of tumor thickness measurements following cobalt-plaque therapy than melanomas designated as Type E (mixed or epithelioid type).[7] In both groups, pretreatment and follow-up data from 6 to 12 months deter-

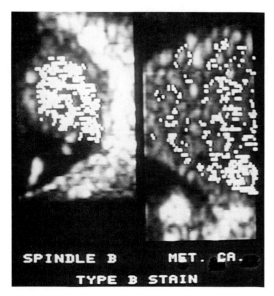

Figure 27-43. Acoustic staining is seen when representative spectral parameters for melanoma are applied to a melanoma and areas of the tumor are highlighted. When melanoma stain criteria are applied to metastatic carcinoma, little highlighting of the tumor results.

mined statistically significant decreases in the spectral slope, increased intercept, and increased residual following cobalt-plaque therapy. These factors may eventually help to decide the effectiveness of radiation treatment and the helpfulness in prognosticating the potential lethality of a given malignant melanoma.

REFERENCES

1. Blumenkranz MS, Byrne SF: Standardized echography (ultrasonography) for the detection and characterization of retinal detachment. Ophthalmology 89:821–831, 1982
2. Bronson NR, Fisher YL, Pickering NC, et al: Ophthalmic Contact B-scan Ultrasonography for the Clinician. Westport, Conn, Stratton Intercontinental, 1976
3. Coleman DJ, Abramson DH, Jack RL, et al: Ultrasonic diagnosis of tumors of the choroid. Arch Ophthalmol 91:344–354, 1974
4. Coleman DJ, Lizzi FL: Computerized ultrasonic tissue characterization of ocular tumors. Am J Ophthalmol 96:165–175, 1983
5. Coleman DJ, Lizzi FL, Jack RL: Ultrasonography of the Eye and Orbit. Philadelphia, Lea & Febiger, 1977
6. Coleman DJ, Lizzi FL, Silverman RH, et al: Acoustic biopsy as a means of characterization of intraocular tumors. In Henkind P (ed): ACTA: XXIV International Congress of Ophthalmology, pp 115–118. Philadelphia, JB Lippincott, 1982
7. Coleman DJ, Lizzi FL, Silverman RH, et al: Regression of uveal malignant melanomas following cobalt-60 plaque. Correlates between acoustic spectrum analysis and tumor regression. Retina 5:73–78, 1985
8. Coleman DJ, Lizzi FL, Silverman RH, et al: A model for acoustic characterization of intraocular tumors. Invest Ophthalmol Vis Sci 26:545–550, 1985
9. Dallow RL (ed): Ophthalmic Ultrasonography: Comparative Techniques, International Ophthalmology Clinics, Vol 19, No 4. Boston, Little, Brown, 1979
10. Feleppa EJ, Lizzi FL, Coleman DJ, et al: Diagnostic spectrum analysis in ophthalmology: A physical perspective. Ultrasound Med Biol 12:623–631, 1986
11. Jalkh AE, Jabbour N, Avila MP, et al: Ultrasonographic findings in eyes with giant retinal tears and opaque media. Retina 3:154–158, 1983
12. Lizzi FL, Coleman DJ, Feleppa E, et al: Digital processing and image modes for clinical ultrasound. Thijssen JM, Verbeek AM (eds): Proceedings of the 8th SIDUO Congress, pp 405–410. The Hague, Dr W Junk, 1981
13. Silverman RH, Coleman DJ, Lizzi FL, et al: Ultrasonic tissue characterization and histopathology in tumor xenografts following ultrasonically induced hyperthermia. Ultrasound Med Biol 12:639–645, 1986
14. Zakov AN, Berlin LA, Gutman FA: Ultrasonographic mapping of vitreoretinal abnormalities. Am J Ophthalmol 95:622–631, 1983

7

Tumors of the Retina and Choroid

28

Therapeutic Ultrasound in Ophthalmology

Stanley Chang
D. Jackson Coleman
Frederic L. Lizzi

High-intensity ultrasound energy can be focused to produce selective and controlled tissue damage that is beneficial in the treatment of ophthalmic diseases. While mechanisms for tissue injury are primarily thermal, ultrasound energy has unique properties that are not found in other treatment modalities. The effectiveness of this externally applied energy source depends on the acoustic absorption properties of the treated tissue. In contrast to the thermal lesions produced by laser energy, absorption of ultrasound is independent of the optical clarity of the propagating media and is relatively unaffected by the degree of pigmentation in the tissue undergoing treatment. Thus, ultrasound energy can be delivered despite the presence of corneal opacities, cataract, or vitreous hemorrhage. Tissue heating develops after application of ultrasound at high intensities, but the volume of affected tissue depends on the beam characteristics of the applied energy, the duration of the energy applied, the absorption properties of the tissue, and the location of the target organ in the sound field. Focused transducers allow concentration of large amounts of ultrasound energy to small areas in the eye while preserving the integrity of adjacent ocular tissues.

As early as 1938, the effects of ultrasound on the eye were reported by Zeiss.[1] Later, other investigators envisioned a therapeutic role for ultrasound in ophthalmology. Lavine and coworkers described the effects of plane and focused ultrasound waves on the eye.[2] They found lens opacities that occurred following application of focused ultrasound on the bovine lens in vitro. Early attempts to apply ultrasound therapy in ophthalmology were somewhat discouraging. Donn unsuccessfully tried to liquefy excised bovine vitreous using a 1 MHz tranducer at an energy level of 900 Watt (w)/cm² for 30 minutes.[3] Using a rabbit model, he observed vitreous liquefaction only after injection of an air bubble into the vitreous. After 24 hours, marked vitreous opacification was observed and histopathologic examination of the eyes revealed extensive damage to both lens and retina. Baum also insonified the rabbit eye at the level of 2.5 w to 3.0 w/cm² for 5 minutes and noted extensive and irreversible damage to anterior ocular structures, as well as eyelids and orbital tissue.[4] Later, Purnell and coworkers reported the production of focal chorioretinal adhesion using ultrasound.[5-7] They compared these lesions to laser therapy and applied their techniques to the treatment of experimental models of retinal detachment. They first suggested that focused ultrasound might be employed for treatment of retinal detachment, glaucoma, and ocular tumors. The major difficulties encountered with these uses were the variability in the

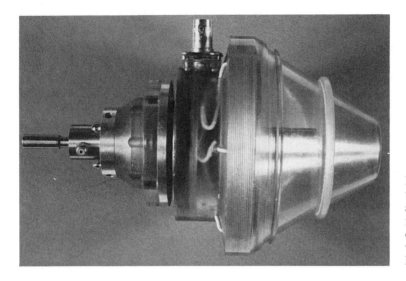

Figure 28-1. The therapeutic ultrasound transducer assembly measures approximately 8 cm in diameter. A coaxial diagnostic transducer with fiberoptic aiming light is located within the plastic cone.

amount of ultrasound energy entering the eye, which differed from exposure to exposure, and a high incidence of cataracts. Ocular lesions were also found outside the field of treatment, which probably resulted from the shape of the ultrasonic beam used.

In the 1970s, Coleman and Lizzi developed a focused therapeutic ultrasound system to evaluate the biologic effects of focused ultrasound on ocular tissues and to determine possible applications of this technique in experimental models of ocular disease.[8-12] Threshold levels for lens damage, chorioretinal lesions, and scleral damage were actively investigated.[8-13] In addition, experimental models of glaucoma, vitreous hemorrhage, traumatic cataract, retinal detachment, and intaocular tumors were used to evaluate the efficacy of this ultrasonic system for possible treatment of human diseases.[14-18] Currently, therapeutic ultrasound is undergoing clinical investigation in the treatment of advanced glaucoma and ocular tumors. This chapter summarizes the experimental and clinical results obtained in the treatment of glaucoma and choroidal tumors.

MATERIALS AND METHODS

Focused high-intensity ultrasound energy is best applied through a fluid medium. The therapeutic transducer is a concave ceramic crystal mea-suring approximately 8 cm in diameter (Fig. 28-1). Its basic resonant frequency is 1.46 MHz operated at the third harmonic, yielding a frequency of 4.6 MHz. The beam is focused at a distance of 90 mm from the center of the transducer and produces a focal zone that is 3 mm in length and 0.4 mm in diameter (−3-decibel beam width dimensions). A central aperture made in the center of the therapeutic transducer allows coaxial alignment of a diagnostic A-scan transducer and a fiberoptic aiming light. A plastic cone placed over the front of the transducer assembly reduces the streaming produced in the propagating medium, which occurs when the ultrasound energy is applied. During treatment, the aiming light is used visually to localize the area of treatment, and the diagnostic A-scan beam measures the distance of the transducer to the target tissue, using an electronic biometric interval counter. Once the correct distance has been measured, therapeutic energy is applied at predetermined exposure times. For hyperthermia treatment, a larger volume of low-temperature heating of tissue is desirable. During this treatment, the tumor is placed in the nonfocused portion of the ultrasound beam, in the near or far field, allowing a larger volume of tissue to be exposed. The diagnostic A-scan transducer is used to measure the distance of the focal zone from the anterior surface of the tumor. Spatial average intensities of up to 10,000 w/cm² can be obtained with the current system. The duration of each application of ultrasound energy ranges from 1 to 5 seconds for glaucoma treatment, to 60 minutes for hyperthermia treatment.

TREATMENT OF GLAUCOMA

Experimental Observations

Rosenberg and Purnell first reported the reduction of intraocular pressure in rabbits following focused ultrasound treatment of the ciliary body.[19] Using a transducer that functioned at 3 MHz or 7 MHz, they applied ultrasound energy to the sclera directly over the ciliary body and found a significant, although temporary, reduction in intraocular pressure. With their system, they noted difficulty delivering consistent levels of ultrasound energy to the sclera directly over the ciliary body, with variations from application to application. In addition, they noted extraciliary lesions in the posterior retina, which probably resulted from the shape of the beam used.

Coleman and coworkers observed scleral thinning in rabbit eyes following application of high intensities of ultrasound energy to produce chorioretinal lesions.[12] Subsequently, scleral lesions were made in the region of the pars plana of the rabbit eye, with marked thinning of the sclera in the area of treatment, and relatively minimal damage to the overlying conjunctiva. The ciliary body and ciliary epithelium also were partially affected. Immediately after the treatment, the conjunctiva becomes swollen, suggesting that the area of scleral injury might function as a filtration site. When fluorescein was injected into the vitreous, the dye was observed subconjunctivally only in the region of the bleb at 24 hours.[15] With continued observation, the conjunctiva gradually flattened over the ultrasound lesion, with persistent scleral thinning in the area of treatment, which could be demonstrated by transillumination.

An experimental model of glaucoma described by Sears and Sears was used in the rabbit eye to evaluate the potential application of ultrasound treatment in glaucoma.[20] Elevated intraocular pressure consistently developed after

0.25 ml (40 units of α-chymotrypsin) was injected into the posterior chamber of rabbit globes. The intraocular pressure was measured with a Schiotz tonometer at regular intervals. When elevated intraocular pressure was sustained for 2 weeks, insonification was performed. Two to four exposures were placed approximately 1 mm posterior to the limbus over the pars plana region. The immediate observations following ultrasound treatment revealed a grayish scleral lesion in the area of insonification, as well as elevation of the conjunctiva, suggesting either chemosis or filtration.[15] Spatial average intensities ranged from 600 w to 2000 w/cm^2. Within several minutes following insonification, there was an immediate reduction in the intraocular pressure in 12 of 14 treated globes (86%). In the treated globes, the intraocular pressure remained at or lower than the pressure level in the contralateral uninjected globe for 5 months. In two eyes, there was only a transient (2-week) reduction of intraocular pressure, compared to the normal contralateral eye. In two eyes, the pressure remained elevated following insonification, indicating treatment failure. These observations suggest that there is an immediate increase in outflow, probably resulting from the creation of a filtration bleb, in rabbit eyes following untrasound treatment. The late mechanisms for intraocular pressure reduction are probably related to ciliary body destruction and reduction of aqueous production.

Histologic evaluation of the sclera and ciliary body region following therapeutic insonification has been studied in both rabbit and pig eyes.[15,21] The latter animal was chosen because its scleral thickness more closely resembles that of the human eye. Immediately after insonification, there was a swelling of the scleral stroma as the thick 100- to 300-nm collagen fibrils were dissociated into thin filamentous components. The number of fibroblasts and production of new collagen increased over the next 2 weeks. At 3 months following insonification, the treated area showed marked thinning, which consisted of a small number of thick collagen fibrils that had survived insonification and numerous smaller collagen fibrils with a diameter of 30 to 40 nm filling the stromal space. There were also degenerative or vacuolar changes in the ciliary

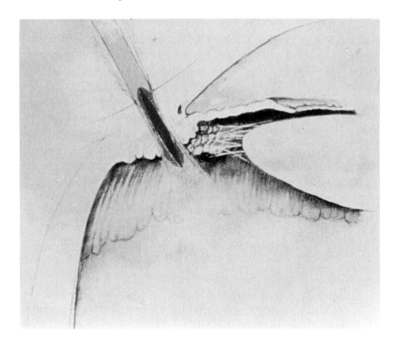

Figure 28-2. The ultrasound transducer is aimed perpendicularly to the sclera over the ciliary body. The focal zone is placed within the inner scleral surface.

epithelium noted in the region of insonification. The conjunctiva overlying the area of treatment was damaged but remained structurally intact.

A theoretical model was developed by Lizzi and coworkers to compute the spatiotemporal features of temperature rises induced in ocular tissue during exposure to high-intensity focal ultrasound.[22,23] By using the exposure parameters and the absorption coefficients of the tissue, the rate of heat generation and transfer can be computed to predict temperature rise within the sclera as functions of time and space. The elevation of temperature can then be used to compute a value called the *damage integral.* The damage integral predicts threshold values for scleral damage and lesion diameter. In rabbit experiments, this mathematical model predicted the diameter of scleral lesions to within 15% of experimentally observed values. Thus, this analysis allows accurate and effective estimation of heating effects in selected tissues and may be useful in planning treatment parameters in human clinical trials.

Clinical Evaluation

The use of focused ultrasound to treat refractory glaucoma in patients began in June 1982.[24,25]

The selection of patients progressed through several stages. Initially, patients who had elevated intraocular pressures and pain with no or minimal visual function were treated. Following successful pressure reduction in this group, a second group of patients with limited visual acuity and failed surgical attempts to lower intraocular pressure were treated. As experience continued to accumulate and results indicated minimal complications and significant pressure reduction using the technique, additional patients with mild reductions in visual acuity and failed surgical techniques were treated. Glaucoma types included congenital glaucoma, chronic open-angle glaucoma, and over 22 types of secondary glaucoma. In our laboratory, over 200 patients have been treated to date.

The treatment is usually administered on an ambulatory basis. Retrobulbar anesthesia, 2% lidocaine and 150 units of hyaluronidase, is administered to minimize patient discomfort and movement. A saline bath used in diagnostic immersion ultrasonography is draped around the eye. The ultasound transducer assembly is then lowered into the saline, and the beam is aimed perpendicularly 2 to 3 mm from the limbal margin. The focal zone is deeper than the inner scleral surface (Fig. 28-2). In this position, there

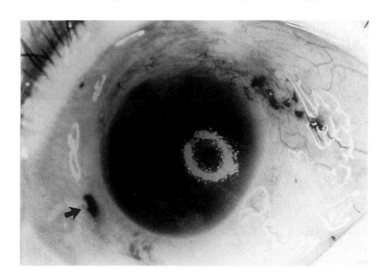

Figure 28-3. Following a clustered treatment, the scleral lesion appears as a focal area of grayish discoloration *(arrow)* in this aphakic patient.

is minimal chance of lens damage during treatment. For initial treatment, 6 to 10 exposures, each 5 seconds in duration, are applied. The exposure patterns on the sclera have varied. In some patients, clustered overlapping applications of ultrasound energy have been applied. In other patients, individual applications are equally spaced along the inferior, 180° over the ciliary body. These treatment patterns do not appear to affect the likelihood of successful treatment.[25]

Clinically, during the application of treatment a chemotic swelling of the conjunctiva develops, followed by a focal grayish discoloration of the underlying sclera measuring approximately 1 mm in diameter (Fig. 28-3). The chemosis allows the conjunctiva to be elevated, thus avoiding severe thermal change. In some patients who have undergone previous ocular surgery that resulted in conjunctival scarring, the balanced lesions also appeared to involve the conjunctiva. Within the first hour following treatment, an initial rise in intraocular pressure has occurred in 60% to 70% of patients. This rise in intraocular pressure usually can be controlled with additional carbonic anhydrase inhibitors or hyperosmotic agents. The pressure-lowering effect of ultrasound treatment is usually observed within 1 to 4 weeks following treatment and occurs in 70% to 85% of patients. Based on our experience in treatment of 170 eyes with refractory glaucoma, it appears reasonable to

allow 2 to 4 weeks after treatment for a satisfactory response to be seen before considering additional treatment. The long-term pressure-lowering response has been evaluated in 137 eyes using Kaplan – Meier survival analysis.[25] Treatment failure was defined as either the need for additional treatment with therapeutic ultrasound or alternative surgical treatment, or the elevation of intraocular pressures above pressure values of 18, 22, or 25 mm Hg. In general, medical treatment was continued following the ultrasound treatment. The clinical results are shown in Figure 28-4 and indicate an initial pressure reduction to 25 mm Hg or less in 80% of cases at 3 months, with a longer term success rate of 65% at 1 year. The 1-year success rates for 22 and 18 mm Hg thresholds were 56% and 50%, respectively. Patients with congenital glaucoma appeared to respond less than patients with open-angle glaucoma. Also, patients with angle closure secondary to uveitis or neovascularization appeared to have a somewhat lower success rate.

Complications of the treatment were of two major types: those related to inaccurate beam orientation and those related to an abnormal tissue response.[25]

Improper aiming or movement of the patient during treatment may result in corneal or lid burns. Retrobulbar anesthesia minimizes these complications. Following treatment, most patients develop a mild iritis, which usually heals

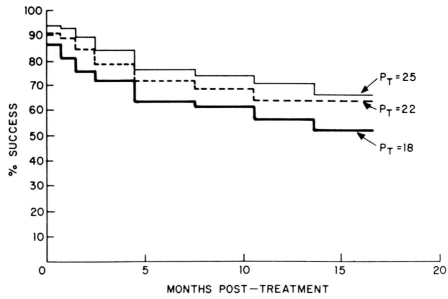

Figure 28-4. Clinical results in over 150 patients following treatment with therapeutic ultrasound for glaucoma using survival analysis indicate that in over 65% of patients intraocular pressure was below 25 mm Hg, and approximately 50% of patients had intraocular pressures below 18 mm Hg at 15 months.

spontaneously, without medication. A small number of patients have persistent flare after treatment. A focal area of scleral thinning in the region of ultrasound treatment was seen in 2.7% of adult patients and occurred more frequently in children (18.2%). In some cases, the uvea could be seen and a localized staphyloma was present, but no patient developed perforation of the globe. Choroidal effusions developed in 3 of 170 patients and were associated with a transient shallowing of the anterior chamber or hypotony. These effusions usually subsided spontaneously. One patient with glaucoma secondary to uveitis developed transient cystoid macular edema following ultrasound treatment.

Margo reported the light and electron microscopic findings in a human eye treated with therapeutic ultrasound and enucleated because of reduced vision and pain secondary to elevated intraocular pressure.[26] The histologic findings revealed areas of highly localized destruction of pigmented and nonpigmented ciliary epithelium with profound atrophy of the ciliary muscle and scleral thinning. Margo concluded that ultrasound damage was more pronounced than

that seen following cyclocyrotherapy. The histologic changes observed were localized to areas of treatment.

The mechanisms for lowering intraocular pressure following focused high-intensity ultrasound have been investigated by Yablonski.[27] In 15 phakic patients, total and true outflow facility was increased by 0.1 ml/min/mm Hg following treatment. Aqueous production decreased by approximately 50%. Pressure-independent outflow increased by 0.8 ml/min/mm Hg. Thus, there appears to be a threefold mechanism by which intraocular pressure is reduced. Focused high-intensity therapeutic ultrasound is an effective method for treating refractory glaucoma. Clinical evaluation of this procedure is being continued and compared to other available techniques.

TREATMENT OF OCULAR TUMORS

Experimental Model

Borda et al first reported the preliminary results of ultrasound treatment in an experimental model for ocular tumors.[28] Greene's melanoma was implanted into the anterior chamber of rabbit eyes, and ultrasound treatment of 1 w/cm[2] at 7 MHz was delivered to the eye for 10 minutes. After 3 days, treated tumors remained at or nearly the same size, while untreated tumors grew to fill the anterior chamber. In our laboratory, similar experiments were performed following implantation of Brown–Pearce carcinoma into the anterior chamber of rabbit eyes.[29] When growth of the tumor was visually evident, focal ablative treatment was given, using spatial average intensities up to 1000 w/cm[2]. Clinically, the tumors appeared to blanch because of the stagnant blood flow following treatment (Fig. 28-5). Histologically, focal areas of tumor cell death and necrosis in the field of treatment were found. Intravascular thrombosis within tumor vessels was also present.

Interest in studying the tumoricidal effects of hyperthermia in experimental ocular tumors is increasing.[17] The therapeutic ultrasound technique appears ideal for the induction of selective tissue heating. An experimental model of Greene's melanoma, modifying a technique described by Krohn and coworkers, was used.[30] The tumor was implanted into the subchoroidal space under a scleral flap and usually grew over 2 weeks to a size suitable for ultrasound treatment. The eye was treated by placing the tumor in the defocused portion of the ultrasound beam. Temperature was monitored throughout the procedure using thermocouples mounted in 29-gauge needles. The thermocouples were inserted into the tumor, overlying sclera, and normal regions around the eye. Treatment regimens used tumor temperatures ranging from 43°C to 67°C maintained for durations ranging from 75 seconds to 60 minutes. In 8 of 23 eyes treated with ultrasonic hyperthermia, there was complete regression of the tumor, which eventually appeared as a flat area of chorioretinal atrophy (Fig. 28-6). In seven eyes, there was initial regression of the tumor, but recurrence at the margin of the original mass was seen up to 6 weeks after treatment. In eight eyes, the tumor continued to grow, but at a slower rate than in control or sham treatment groups. Initial tumor regression was observed at temperatures of 45°C for 1 hour, while a complete regression

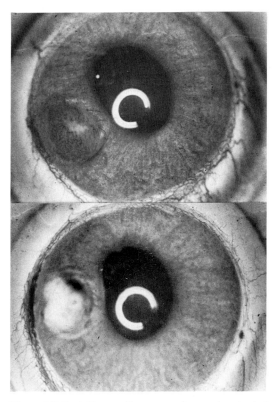

Figure 28-5. A Brown-Pearce carcinoma implanted on the iris of the rabbit eye (top) blanches immediately following focal treatment with therapeutic ultrasound (bottom). Frequently, small hemorrhages are also present on the tumor surface.

was most frequently observed at treatment temperatures of 49°C for 1 hour.

Riedel and coworkers, using the same techniques, reported similar findings using ultrasonically induced hyperthermia alone.[31] They also combined hyperthermia with proton-beam radiation, treating Greene's melanoma at 43°C for 1 hour followed by irradiation within 5 to 9 hours with ten to thirty gray. In ten of twelve tumors receiving the combined treatment modalities, complete tumor regression was confirmed both clinically and histologically. These studies suggested that hyperthermia could be used to enhance radiosensitivity of ocular tumors and to reduce the tumoricidal radiation dose required for the treatment of choroidal melanomas. Reduction of the levels of radiotherapy required for treatment of choroidal melanoma would lower the incidence of late adverse effects, such as radiation retinopathy.

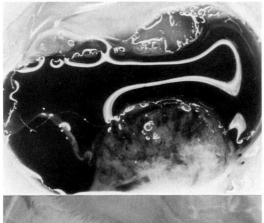

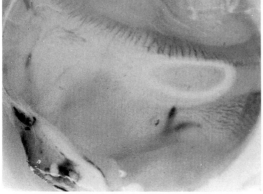

Figure 28-6. One month following implantation of Greene's melanoma untreated eyes developed growth of the tumor, overlying retinal detachment, and varying degrees of subretinal hemorrhage (top). Following ultrasonic hyperthermia, successfully treated tumors regressed completely, leaving a focal chorioretinal scar (bottom). The adjacent retina was normal on light microscopy.

Clinical Trials

Four patients with choroidal melanoma were treated with combined ultrasonic hyperthermia and radiation and were described by Coleman and coworkers.[32] Ultrasonically induced hyperthermia treatment was administered in either two or three 30-minute treatment sessions, heating the tumor to 43.5°C. Radiation therapy was administered between 3 and 6 hours following initial hyperthermia therapy. Radiation doses of approximately 3,900 rad were delivered to the apex of the tumor using a cobalt-60 episcleral plaque. In all patients, there was clinically observed arrest of growth or regression in the size of the tumor after at least 5 months of

follow-up. There was no evidence of cataract formation or retinal vasculopathy as a result of hyperthermia treatment. Ultrasound measurements of tumor height documented a serial decrease in tumor thickness in all patients.

The cellular mechanisms by which hyperthermia is effective in the treatment of tumors are uncertain. Malignant cells appear to be more thermally sensitive than normal cells, and the temperature must be carefully monitored so that normal tissues are not damaged. At a cellular level, there is denaturation of enzymes necessary for a DNA repair as well as direct inhibition of DNA, RNA, and protein syntheses.[33] Histologically, tumors show hypertrophy of the Golgi apparatus and an increase in acid phosphatase–positive lysosomes within 6 hours after hyperthermia treatment.[34] In addition, hyperthermia may cause stasis of blood flow within tumors and, consequently, tumor infarction and coagulative necrosis.

The resultant increase in aerobic glycolysis and lactic acid production may alter the local environment of *p*H within the tumor and further activate lysosomal enzymes. Synergy in treatment of ocular tumors may be achieved by combining radiotherapy with hyperthermia treatment, but it remains unclear which modality should be used first.

These preliminary experimental and clinical results suggest that ultrasonically induced hyperthermia with radiation therapy is effective in treatment of choroidal tumors. More extensive clinical evaluation is needed to evaluate these combined treatment modalities.

REFERENCES

1. Zeiss E: Uber Linsenveränderungen an herausgenommenen Rinderlinsen durch Ultraschalleinwirkung. Albrecht von Graefes Arch Clin Exp Ophthalmol 139:301–322, 1938
2. Lavine O, Langenstrass K, Bowyer C et al: Effect of ultrasonic waves on the refractive media of the eye. Arch Ophthalmol 47:204–219, 1952
3. Donn A: Ultrasonic wave liquefaction of vitreous humor in living rabbits. Arch Ophthalmol 53:204–219, 1955
4. Baum G: The effect of ultrasonic radiation upon the eye and ocular adnexae. Am J Ophthalmol 42:696–706, 1956

5. Purnell EW, Sokollu A, Holasek E: The production of focal chorioretinitis by ultrasound: A preliminary report. Am J Ophthalmol 58:953–957, 1964
6. Purnell EW, Sokollu A, Torchia R, Taner N: Focal chorioretinitis produced by ultrasound. Invest Ophthalmol Vis Sci 3:657–664, 1964
7. Torchia RT, Purnell EW, Sokollu A: Cataract production by ultrasound. Am J Ophthalmol 64:305–309, 1967
8. Coleman DJ, Lizzi FL, Burt WJ, Wen H: Properties observed in cataracts produced experimentally with ultrasound. Am J Ophthalmol 71:1284–1288, 1971
9. Coleman DJ, Lizzi FL, Weininger R, Burt W: Vitreous dispersion by ultrasound. Ann Ophthalmol 2:389–396, 1970
10. Lizzi FL, Packer AJ, Coleman DJ: Experimental cataract production by high-frequency ultrasound. Ann Ophthalmol 10:934–942, 1978
11. Lizzi FL, Coleman DJ, Driller J, Franzen LA: Experimental ultrasonically induced lesions in the retina, choroid, and sclera. Invest Ophthalmol Vis Sci 17:350–360, 1978
12. Coleman DJ, Lizzi FL, Jakobiec FA: Therapeutic ultrasound in the production of ocular lesions. Am J Ophthalmol 86:185–192, 1978
13. Lizzi FL, Coleman DJ, Driller J et al: Effects of pulsed ultrasound on ocular tissue. Ultrasound Med Biol 7:245–252, 1981
14. Coleman DJ, Lizzi FL, El-Mofty AA et al: Ultrasonically accelerated reabsorption of vitreous membranes. Am J Ophthalmol 89:409–499, 1980
15. Coleman DJ, Lizzi FL, Driller J et al: Therapeutic ultrasound in the treatment of glaucoma. Part I. Experimental model. Ophthalmology 92:339–345, 1985
16. Coleman DJ, Lizzi FL, Torpey JH et al: Treatment of experimental lens capsular tears with intense focused ultrasound. Br J Ophthalmol 69:645–649, 1985
17. Burgess SEP, Chang S, Svitra P et al: Effect of hyperthermia on experimental choroidal melanoma. Br J Ophthalmol 69:854–860, 1985
18. Rosecan LR, Iwamoto T, Rosado A et al: Therapeutic ultrasound in treatment of retinal detachment: Clinical observations and light and electron microscopy. Retina 5:115–122, 1985
19. Rosenberg RS, Purnell EW: Effects of ultrasonic radiation to the ciliary body. Am J Ophthalmol 63:403–409, 1967
20. Sears D, Sears M: Blood-aqueous barrier and alpha-chymotrypsin glaucoma in rabbits, Am J Ophthalmol 77:378–383, 1974
21. Burgess SEP, Coleman DJ, Iwamoto T et al: Histological studies of porcine eyes treated with high intensity focused ultrasound. Invest Ophthalmol Vis Sci (Suppl) 26:158, 1985
22. Lizzi FL, Coleman DJ, Driller J, Ostromogilsky M: Ultrasound. Med Biol 10:289–298, 1984
23. Lizzi FL, Coleman DJ, Driller J et al: Ultrasonic hyperthermia for ophthalmic therapy. IEEE Trans Sonic Ultrasonics SU-31:473–481, 1984
24. Coleman DJ, Lizzi FL, Driller J et al: Therapeutic ultrasound in the treatment of glaucoma. Part II. Clinical applications. Ophthalmology 92:347–353, 1985
25. Burgess SEP, Silverman RH, Coleman DJ et al: Treatment of glaucoma with high-intensity ultrasound. Ophthalmology 93:831–838, 1986
26. Margo CE: Therapeutic ultrasound: Light and electron microscopic findings in an eye treated for glaucoma. Arch Ophthalmol 104:735–738, 1986
27. Yablonski ME, Cook DJ, Coleman DJ: The effect of therapeutic ultrasound on aqueous humor dynamics. Invest Ophthalmol Vis Sci (Suppl) 26:158, 1985
28. Borda R, Proctor P, Kilpatrick D et al: Effects of ultrasound on ocular melanoma. Ultrasound Med 3b:2013, 1977
29. Coleman DJ, Lizzi FL, Chang S: Applications of therapeutic ultrasound in ophthalmology. Prog Med Ultrasound 2:263–270, 1981
30. Krohn DL, Brandt R, Morris DN: Subchoroidal transplantation of experimental malignant melanoma. Am J Ophthalmol 70:753–756, 1970
31. Riedel KG, Svitra PP, Seddon JM et al: Proton beam irradiation and hyperthermia: Effects on experimental choroidal melanoma. Arch Ophthalmol 103:1862–1869, 1984
32. Coleman DJ, Lizzi FL, Burgess SEP et al: Ultrasonic hyperthermia and radiation in the management of intraocular malignant melanoma. Am J Ophthalmol 101:635–642, 1986
33. Overgaard J, Skovgaard Poulsen H: Effect of hyperthermia and environmental acidity on the proteolytic activity of murine ascites tumor cells. J Natl Cancer Institute 58:1159–1161, 1977
34. Overgaard J: Histopathologic effects of hyperthermia. In Storm FK (ed): Hyperthermia in Cancer Therapy, pp. 163–185. Boston, GK Hall, 1983

29

Retinoblastoma: Diagnosis and Clinical Management

Charles Chia-Lee Lin

Retinoblastoma is the most common intraocular malignancy of childhood. The incidence has been estimated at 1 in 15,000 to 34,000 live births. Early diagnosis and prompt treatment are necessary, as intracranial and distal metastases may cause death. While enucleation of the diseased eye has been the treatment of choice to cure the tumor, more recently x- and cobalt-60 irradiation, laser photocoagulation, cryopexy, and chemotherapy have been used as alternate therapeutic modalities.

At a very early age, the heritable form of the disease presents as a bilateral retinoblastoma; sporadic tumors frequently occur unilaterally in late childhood. About 1% of the cases of retinoblastoma regress spontaneously to a benign form of retinoblastoma, termed *retinocytoma.* Advances in determining an oncogenetic hypothesis and developing methods for genetic counseling for retinoblastoma have been made by many investigators.

The pathologic features of retinoblastoma, which vary greatly, have fascinated ophthalmic pathologists. They range from undifferentiated retinoblastoma cells, rosettes, fleurettes, and photoreceptor differentiation to tumor necrosis, calcification, and DNA–like material precipitated along tumor vessels. This chapter deals with the clinical manifestations, pathologic features, therapeutic measures, genetic counseling, oncogenesis, and prognosis of retinoblastoma.

CLINICAL MANIFESTATIONS[4,21,35]

The highest incidence of retinoblastoma occurs in patients 2 or 3 years of age. However, Verhoeff has reported a case of retinoblastoma in a 48-year-old man that was verified microscopically. The tumor has no predilection for sex and may occur in either eye.[48] Most children with retinoblastoma exhibit no ocular abnormality at birth, but develop leukoma (Fig. 29-1) or strabismus (Fig. 29-2). Leukoma may be noted at age 12 months in bilateral cases and at 24 months in unilateral cases.

History
Differential diagnoses of retinoblastoma are listed in Table 29-1. In the history, maternal rubella, birth injury, prematurity, and oxygen inhalation should be investigated, in order to rule out ocular abnormalities such as congenital cataract, persistent hyperplastic primary vitreous (PHPV), retinopathy of prematurity, and retinal detachment. Contact by the child with puppies or the eating of raw fish or beef may suggest nematode endophthalmitis or a parasitic infection.

General Physical Examination
Systemic diseases, such as tuberous sclerosis, rubella embryopathy, tuberculosis, and syphilis may cause intraocular lesions that resemble retinoblastoma. Complete peripheral blood

Table 29-1. Differential Diagnosis of Ocular Diseases Simulating Retinoblastoma

I. Persistence and hyperplasia of embryonic ocular vasculature
   A. Persistent hyperplastic primary vitreous (PHPV)
   B. Posterior PHPV, epipapillary and peripapillary lesions, and congenital falciform fold
II. Retinal vascular anomalies with lipid exudation
   A. Coats' syndrome
   B. Leber's miliary aneurysms
   C. Von Hippel-Lindau angiomatosis
III. Toxic retinopathy — retinopathy of prematurity (retrolental fibroplasia)
IV. Inflammatory conditions
   A. Toxocariasis (nematode endophthalmitis)
   B. Uveitis, pars planitis
   C. Metastatic endophthalmitis
V. Conditions exhibiting abnormal retinal embryogenesis and/or retinal dysplasia as prominent features
   A. Norrie's disease
   B. Trisomy-13 syndrome
   C. Fundus colobomas
   D. Incontinentia pigmenti (Bloch-Sulzberger syndrome)
   E. Retinoschisis
VI. Trauma, organizing vitreous hemorrhage, massive retinal gliosis
VII. Neoplastic and proliferative lesions
   A. Neuroepithelial tumors of the ciliary body (medulloepithelioma)
   B. Miscellaneous proliferative lesions, hamartomas, and choristomas of the fundus

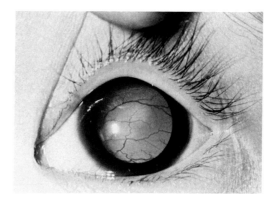

Figure 29-1. Leukokoria in a child with endophytic retinoblastoma.

tension will develop. In advanced cases, pseudohypopyon with retinoblastoma cells arises in the anterior chamber (Fig. 29-4). In endophytic tumors, white tumor cells appear in the vitreous or may be deposited anteriorly to form iris nodules. In exophytic tumors, the detached retina is displaced by the tumor mass and may be seen behind the lens. In more advanced cases, secondary glaucoma with rubeosis iridis develops.

Indirect or direct ophthalmoscopy often reveals a round or ovoid elevated, white tumor. Large tumors (3–10 mm) may appear as a chalky white mass (Fig. 29-5) supplied by dilated and tortuous vessels. The retina surrounding the tumor is sometimes detached, with clumping and proliferation of RPE. Multiple retinoblastoma nodules may occasionally appear throughout the retina. Scleral indentation should be used to verify the diagnosis of a tumorous mass at the peripheral retina.

Elevated tumors (>10 mm in diameter) fre-

studies, skull films, examinations of cerebrospinal fluid, and computed tomography (CT) may be necessary to arrive at an accurate diagnosis.

Ocular Examination

Patients with retinoblastoma may appear outwardly normal in the initial stages except for a white pupil, strabismus, or heterochromia. An opaque lens or a retrolental membrane may be considered in conjunction with other congenital abnormalities, such as PHPV, retrolental fibroplasia, or congenital rubella syndrome. If diagnosis or treatment is delayed marked proptosis (Fig. 29-3) with extraocular and intracranial ex-

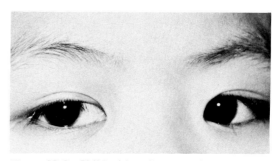

Figure 29-2. Child with unilateral retinoblastoma of the right eye has strabismus.

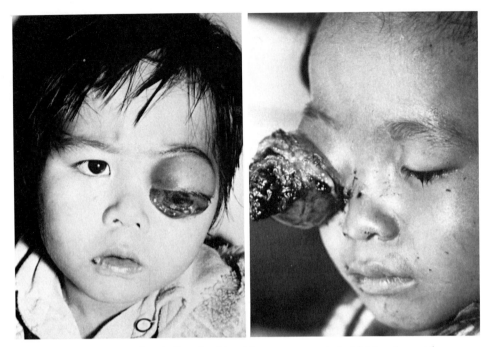

Figure 29-3. Proptosis of eyeball and orbit with severe necrosis in highly advanced retinoblastoma is due to delayed treatment in two small children.

quently contain multiple foci of calcified tumor necrosis. Ophthalmoscopically, three different tumor appearances represent tumor regression: type I, a white calcified mass resembling cottage cheese (Fig. 29-6); type II, a pink, translucent mass that looks like fish flesh (Fig. 29-7); and type III, a combination of types I and II.[1,6,7,33] These clinical features may also be seen after radiotherapy.

Fluorescein Angiography
Because tumor vessels frequently grow superficially on the retina, marked vascularity can be observed easily during the early phase on fluo-

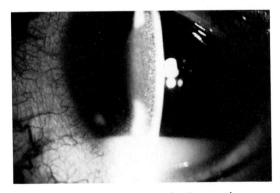

Figure 29-4. Pseudohypopyon in the anterior chamber is caused by advanced endophytic retinoblastoma.

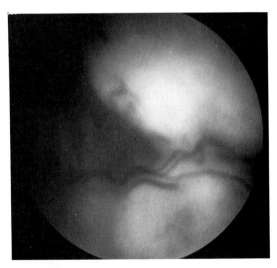

Figure 29-5. A chalky white retinal tumor is lined by dilated and tortuous tumor vessels. Note the surrounding retina is detached.

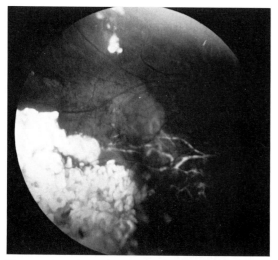

Figure 29-6. Cottage cheese–like regressed retinoblastoma is associated with calcification.

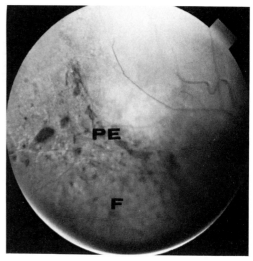

Figure 29-7. Fish-flesh (F) pattern of tumor regression in a 20-year-old woman whose other eye was enucleated for advanced retinoblastoma at the age of two. Note RPE degeneration and clumping (PE) surrounding the retina.

rescein angiograms (Fig. 29-8). Tumor staining may be seen in the later phases of the angiogram as hyperfluorescence. However, angiographic studies in small children may be difficult to perform.

Radiography

Calcification is a common feature of retinoblastoma and is often a hallmark in radiologic studies (Fig. 29-9). In a number of ocular diseases, such as nematode endophthalmitis, angiomatosis retinae, Coats' disease, or astrocytoma of retina, intraocular calcification may be considered in the differential diagnosis.

Ultrasonography

A- and B-scan ultrasonography is helpful in differentiating retinoblastoma from other leukocorias or pseudogliomas. The B-scan (Fig. 29-10) may show an acoustically solid mass with highly intense echoes and well-demarcated margins in the vitreous cavity. Foci of calcification within the tumor are noted as high reflections. When sensitivity is lowered, calcium echoes persist. The A-scan shows a very intense initial echo spike throughout the tumor extend-

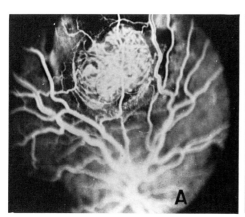

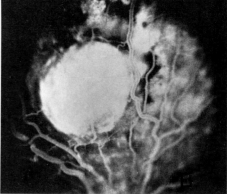

Figure 29-8. Fluorescein angiogram of retinoblastoma *(A)* early phase demonstrates prominent tumor vascularity; *(B)* late phase shows leakage of tumor vessels and tumor staining.

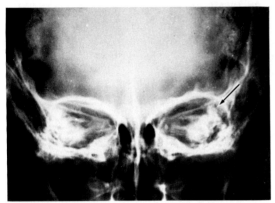

Figure 29-9. Radiograph shows calcification *(arrow)* as a shadow in the orbital tumorous mass.

ing from the anterior surface to the center of the elevated lesion. In diffuse or multifocal retino-blastomas, very intense internal reflections may be observed throughout the vitreous cavity, with marked attenuation of orbital echoes.

CT Scans

The CT scan (Fig. 29-11) is a most effective technique to diagnose retinoblastoma. Clinicians may observe intraocular tumors with many foci of calcification, and the scan may also detect the posterior extension of the tumor to the optic nerve, orbit, or brain. Furthermore, the CT scan can also assist in the detection of an independent brain tumor, such as a pinealoblastoma, or metastasis of the retinoblastoma to the brain.

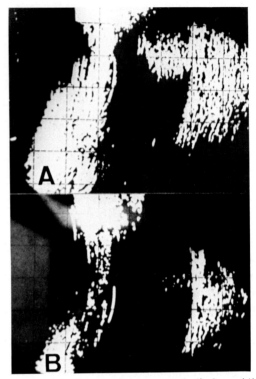

Figure 29-10. B-scan ultrasonograph discloses *(A)* highly reflective focal echoes representing a solid tumor within the eyeball *(B)*. When sensitivity is low, calcium echoes are persistent.

Aqueous Enzymes

The ratios of aqueous to plasma lactate dehydrogenase and phosphoglucose isomerase (PGI) are elevated in patients with retinoblas-

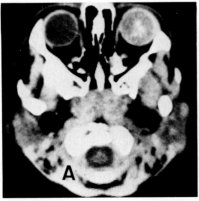
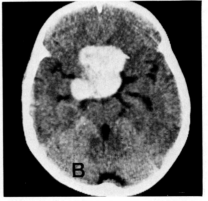

Figure 29-11. Computed tomograms of unilateral retinoblastoma with metastasis to the brain: *(A)* tumor seen as shadow in the right eye; *(B)* tumor revealed in the brain.

toma.[14,28,38] Anterior chamber paracentesis to obtain aqueous enzyme levels may help to determine the ratio, but is seldom necessary.

Cytologic Diagnosis

Aqueous and vitreous aspirate for cytologic smears may help differentiate the diagnosis of retinoblastoma from other intraocular lesions. A cytologic diagnosis is usually not necessary unless all other methods fail.

PATHOLOGIC FEATURES

Friable, chalky white tumor nodules (Fig. 29-12) may be seen on gross examination of an enucleated globe with retinoblastoma. Whitish to pearly pink areas may be present, depending on the vascularity of the tumor and cellular differentiation. Multifocal nodules may be observed within the globe. In the endophytic tumor, newly formed vessels run over the surface of the tumor and the calcium deposits appear cauliflower-like. In the exophytic, or diffuse form, extensive retinal detachment and thickening of the retina are seen. If retinoblastomas appear extensively necrotic and calcified, they may be undergoing spontaneous regression.[2,4,19]

Microscopically, retinoblastoma typically consists of small undifferentiated round or po-

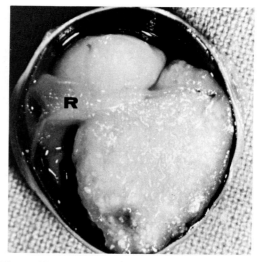

Figure 29-12. Gross inspection discloses a chalky white exophytic retinoblastoma with numerous foci of calcification. Note the overlying retina (R) is detached and pushed toward the center of the vitreous cavity.

lygonal cells (Fig. 29-13*A*), with hyperchromatic nuclei and scanty cytoplasm. These cells are usually gathered in nests around a central blood vessel to form pseudorosettes (Fig. 29-14). Foci of dense basophilic tumor necrosis and calcium plaques are scattered in the tumor, and mitotic figures are common. Some retinoblastomas exhibit more advanced differentiated areas, marked by the presence of Flexner-Wintersteiner rosettes and fleurettes.[44-47] The

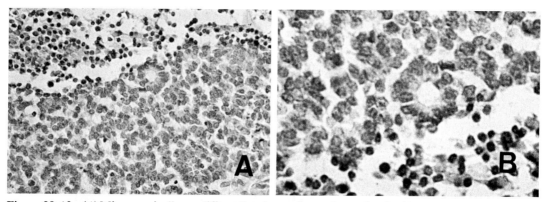

Figure 29-13. *(A)* Microscopically, undifferentiated round or polygonal retinoblastoma cells with hyperchromatic nuclei and minimal cytoplasm arise from the retinal cells. *(B)* Some of the tumor cells are arranged as Flexner-Wintersteiner rosettes representing a well-differentiated retinoblastoma. Note the central cavity is lined by thin external limiting membrane. (H & E; original magnifications, *A* × 200; *B* × 400)

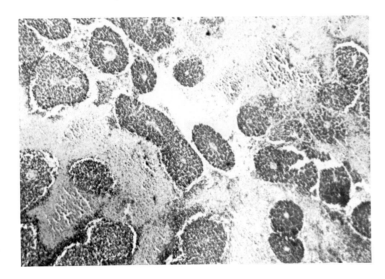

Figure 29-14. Pseudorosettes are a gathering of tumor nests around central tumor vessels. (H & E; original magnification ×75)

cells in Flexner-Wintersteiner rosettes (Fig. 29-13*B*) are arranged around a central lumen lined by a thin membrane simulating the external limiting membrane of the retina and containing mucopolysaccharides in the lumen. Tumor cells may form Homer-Wright rosettes in which the cell processes of a ring of tumor cells intertwine without forming a lumen (Fig. 29-15). Fleurettes (Fig. 29-16) are highly differentiated tumor cells, grouped like a bundle of flowers, which develop photoreceptor elements. Some retinoblastomas arise from neuronal elements of the retina. Highly differentiated retinoblastomas have a better prognosis than less-

differentiated ones, but there are other influential factors, such as tumor infiltration into portions of the optic nerve, including the resection line (Fig. 29-17); tumor invasion of the choroid; and intracranial extension.[31] With extensive invasion, the prognosis may be poor even though the tumor is differentiated. However, the presence of an independent brain tumor (pinealoblastoma) should be carefully ruled out, as it may have had a common embryologic origin, as Zimmerman has proposed ("trilateral retinoblastoma").[51,52]

In some areas within the tumor, irregular, globular basophilic deposits, which are histolog-

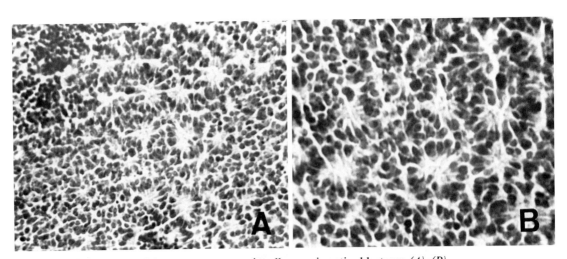

Figure 29-15. Homer-Wright rosettes are occasionally seen in retinoblastoma *(A)*. *(B)* Some features are shown under high magnification (H & E; original magnification, *A* × 200; *B* × 400)

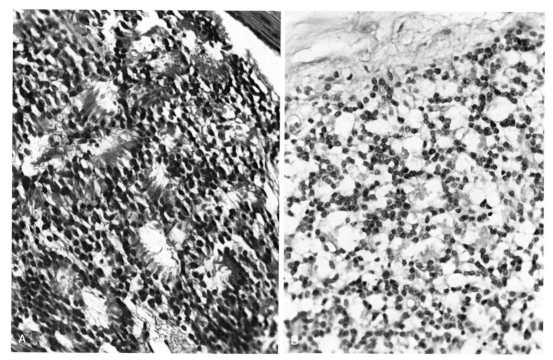

Figure 29-16. *(A)* Well-differentiated fleurettes in retinoblastoma. The tumor cells cluster together to produce well-aligned photoreceptor elements. *(B)* Moderately differentiated fleurettes in retinoblastoma. (H & E; original magnifications, $A \times 300$; $B \times 265$)

ically Feulgen positive, are seen around the tumor vessel wall or at the edge of the focal tumor necrosis.[26] Staining may diminish if there is pretreatment with purified deoxyribonuclease. However, Feulgen staining of globular deposits is abolished by pronase-deoxyribonu-

clease pretreatment of the sections, suggesting that these deposits may consist of DNA protein complex.

To study the pathogenesis of tumor regression and calcification in retinoblastoma, an electron microscopic study was performed.[24] In

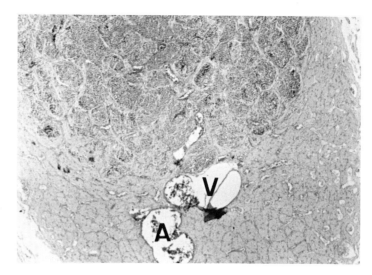

Figure 29-17. Half of the axon bundle of the optic nerve is occupied by poorly differentiated retinoblastoma cells (H & E; original magnification ×150). A, central retinal artery; V, central retinal vein.

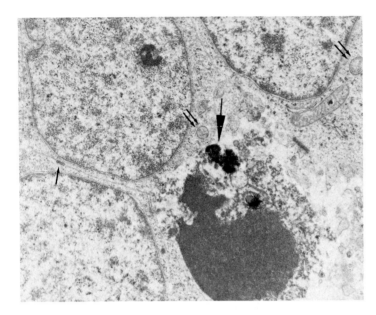

Figure 29-18. Viable retinoblastoma cells have an intact plasmalemma. Macula adherente–type cell junctions *(small arrow)* and normal-looking mitochondria *(double arrows)* are noted. In contrast, degenerative tumor cells show focal disruption of plasmalemma with clumping of nuclear chromatin, dense cytoplasmic granules, and calcium deposits *(large arrow)*. (Original magnification ×8000) (Lin CCL, Tso MOM: An electron microscopic study of calcification of retinoblastoma. Am J Ophthalmol 96:765–774, 1983; with permission from the American Journal of Ophthalmology)

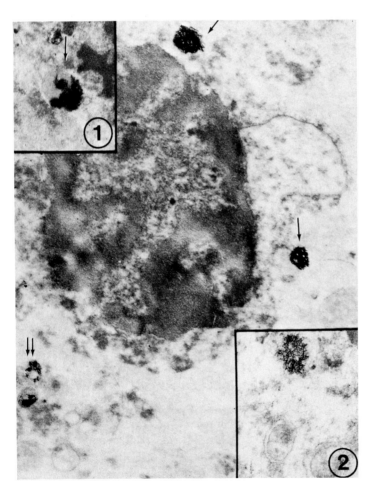

Figure 29-19. Tumor cells with partially ruptured plasmalemma exhibit calcium deposits in calcified mitochondria *(single arrows)*. Some of the mitochondria retain the membrane architecture *(double arrows)*. (Inset 2) Crystalline calcium deposits are seen in mitochondria under high magnification. (Original magnifications, large photo ×10,000; inset 2 ×25,000) (Lin CCL, Tso MOM: An electron microscopic study of calcification of retinoblastoma. Am J Ophthalmol 96:765–774, 1983; with permission from the American Journal of Ophthalmology)

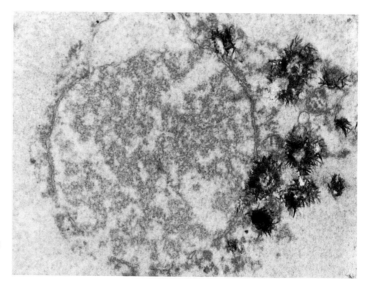

Figure 29-20. Crystalline calcium deposits occur in mitochondria of tumor cells and form calcium microbodies. (Original magnification × 11,000) (Lin CCL, Tso MOM: An electron microscopic study of calcification of retinoblastoma. Am J Ophthalmol 96:765–774, 1983; with permission from the American Journal of Ophthalmology)

the area of tumor necrosis, the tumor cell showed disruption of the plasmalemma (Fig. 29-18). Extracellular needle-like calcium deposits were observed within the mitochondria of tumor cells (Fig. 29-19). With progressive tumor necrosis and liquefaction, calcium microbodies (Fig. 29-20) characterized by a central calcified core and surrounded by an electron-translucent zone and coarse needle-like calcium deposits on the tumor surface were seen (Fig. 29-21). It is suggested that the pathologic process of calcification and spontaneous regression may depend on the process of plasmalemma disruption and cell necrosis.

CLINICAL MANAGEMENT

Preferred treatment depends on the size and extension of the tumor, unilateral involvement or bilateral, and the patient's systemic status.[7,8,11,12,17,30,36,37]

Enucleation

Enucleation is indicated for (1) all unilateral cases in which the tumor is large and no useful vision is preserved; (2) bilateral cases in which the extensively affected eye may be enucleated and the less-involved eye may be managed by radiation therapy or other methods; (3) involve-

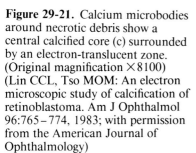

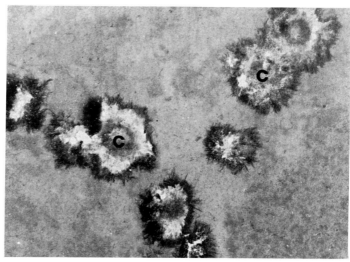

Figure 29-21. Calcium microbodies around necrotic debris show a central calcified core (c) surrounded by an electron-translucent zone. (Original magnification × 8100) (Lin CCL, Tso MOM: An electron microscopic study of calcification of retinoblastoma. Am J Ophthalmol 96:765–774, 1983; with permission from the American Journal of Ophthalmology)

ment of both eyes by advanced tumors and no hope of retaining any vision.

A "gentle" or "nontouch" technique is recommended for enucleation to prevent dissemination of loosely cohesive malignant tumor cells. A long segment of the optic nerve should be excised to include tumor extensions that may be involved. Detailed pathologic examination of the enucleated globe is necessary to determine whether tumor cells have extended beyond the lamina cribrosa of the optic nerve. Postoperative radiation therapy is needed if extraocular extension is present.

External Radiation Therapy

It is reported that mortality is comparable whether patients undergo external radiation therapy or enucleation. Radiation therapy is generally indicated in the following situations:

1. To save the second involved eye after the eye with the more advanced tumor has been enucleated.
2. For bilateral tumors when some useful vision remains or when the tumor is less than one half the size of the globe.
3. If there are small tumors but another treatment such as photocoagulation or cryotherapy cannot be applied.
4. If residual orbital tumor or tumor extension beyond the optic nerve is present following enucleation.

With the patient under general anesthesia, a linear accelerator utilizing gamma rays via an anterior or temporal portal approach may be used. A total of 3500 to 4000 rads may be delivered within a 3-week period at the rate of three sessions per week.

Radiation cataract and retinopathy are late complications of radiation therapy. Dry eye, sunken orbit with atrophy of the temporal fossa, and optic atrophy are occasionally seen. If radiation doses do not exceed 3500 rads, the incidence of postradiation tumors, such as orbital sarcoma, is quite low.

Episcleral Plaque Radiation

Radiation may be administered via a scleral platinum envelope containing a cobalt-60 (^{60}Co) plaque. This modality has the advantage of limiting the irradiated area of the eye. Indica-

tions for treatment are: the tumor is between 6 and 15 mm in diameter; or the tumor is at least 3 mm from the optic disc or fovea; or there are residual tumors that have not been completely controlled with external radiation, photocoagulation, or cryotherapy.

After the tumor location is marked by indirect ophthalmoscopy and scleral depression, a gamma-ray (^{60}Co) or beta-ray (^{90}Sr, ^{90}Y, ^{106}Ru) plaque may be sutured onto the sclera. The radiation dosage is calculated according to the size and thickness of the tumor. After 3000 to 4000 rads are delivered to the apex of the tumor, the plaque may be surgically removed. Complications of episcleral plaque radiation include cataract, radiation retinopathy, and induced sarcomas, but the incidence is usually quite low.

Radiation therapy of most retinoblastomas yields satisfactory results. A few days after treatment, edema, exudate, and hemorrhage may appear on the surface of the tumor. Tumor volume decreases progressively. The outline of the tumor becomes irregular, assuming a cottage cheese–like appearance. Whitish calcification spots on the surface of the tumor increase in number, imparting a look of white coral. Normal retinal tissue around the tumor mass is pigmented. Complete tumor regression may take many months, and calcification may be gradually absorbed in the ensuing years. If the tumor recurs, a new course of irradiation may be indicated, with a cumulative dose of 6000 to 8000 rads.

Photocoagulation

Photocoagulation therapy may be indicated for small tumors without involvement of the optic disc, fovea, or pars plana and for tumors without vitreous seeding.[12,20] One or two rows of xenon-arc or laser photocoagulation may be applied around the tumor. The power should be high enough to cause a deep whitening of the surrounding retina and closure of the feeder vessels. Repeated treatment will be necessary if a single dose is not sufficient to obliterate the retinal vessels. Possible complications of this treatment are retinal hemorrhage or tractional retinal detachment.

Cryotherapy

Cryotherapy may be applied to a small peripheral retinoblastoma near the ora serrata or to residual or recurrent tumors in the peripheral fundus following incomplete irradiation with external beam therapy.[32,42] The triple freeze-thaw technique at 10- to 15- second intervals is usually adequate to shrink the tumor to a flat, well-defined pigmented scar.

Chemotherapy

When a patient with retinoblastoma shows evidence of systemic metastasis, chemotherapy may be administered. Cyclophosphamide, 30 mg/kg, and vincristine, 0.05 mg/kg, may be given intravenously every 3 weeks for as long as 1 year.

The general guidelines for therapy are summarized as follows:

1. Isolated or multiple tumors, up to four discs in diameter and 3 diopters of elevation in a peripheral location, should receive cryopexy, with or without photocoagulation. Such tumors located at the equator or posterior pole, except for those on the optic disc and macula, should be administered photocoagulation.
2. Isolated or multiple tumors, from four to ten discs in diameter or more than 3 diopters of elevation, should be given cobalt application at a dosage of 3500 to 4000 rads, with or without photocoagulation.
3. Isolated tumors, more than ten discs in diameter, or those located on the optic disc or in the macular area, should receive external radiation of 3500 to 4000 rads.
4. Multiple tumors, over ten discs in diameter, should be given external beam radiation of 3500 to 4000 rads, with or without complementary photocoagulation.
5. Massive tumors involving more than half of the retina should undergo enucleation with maximum excision of the optic nerve.

CLINICAL FOLLOW-UP EXAMINATION

Patients should be observed at regular intervals following treatment. General anesthesia may be used if a child is uncooperative. The orbital socket is inspected and palpated for residual or recurrent tumor. The fellow eye must also be examined. Indirect binocular ophthalmoscopy after pupillary dilation should be carried out with scleral indentation for peripheral tumors. Lesions should be photographed or diagramed after each examination.

If the tumor involves the optic nerve, clinical examination should be performed every 4 to 6 months until the child reaches 5 years of age, and every 6 to 12 months thereafter. Other studies such as a bone marrow biopsy, lumbar puncture, hepatic test, or a CT scan may be needed.

GENETIC COUNSELING

The genetic risk may vary according to the clinical situation, as follows:[13,15,49,50]

1. For healthy parents with one child, the risk of having another child with retinoblastoma is 1% to 4%. If more than one family member is affected, the risk increases to 40%.
2. The risk for descendants of a retinoblastoma survivor is 40% if there are other members in the family affected, suggesting a hereditary disease. The risk of transmitting the disease is 8% to 10% in unilateral cases and 40% in bilateral cases.

Children suffering from bilateral retinoblastoma have an increased probability of developing a second, nonocular tumor.[3,15,34] The incidence is 10% to 30% depending on the life expectancy of the patient, and the mortality is 85% in this group. This second tumor is frequently an osteogenic sarcoma, although other neoplasms have been reported.

ONCOGENESIS OF RETINOBLASTOMA[5,10,17,19,27,41]

Some retinoblastoma patients have been noted to develop various congenital anomalies associated with a deletion of specific bands of chromosome 13q14. The simplest hypothesis is that, in genetically predisposed retinoblastoma, a submicroscopically mutated gene is inherited, and that this gene is located interstitially in the long arm of chromosome 13. Although constitutional chromosomal deletion including 13q14 has been found in all retinoblastoma patients whose esterase D activity is 50% of normal, one female patient was noted to have 50% esterase D activity in all normal cells on examination but no deletion of 13q14.

Knudson used simple clinical observations to show the relationship of age and diagnosis.[22,23] Nonhereditary unilateral cases were diagnosed at a slightly older age, and when similarly plotted, they showed a more complex curve, indicating that two or more events were required for malignancy in the absence of the hereditary tendency. Bilateral cases were diagnosed earlier than unilateral cases, presumably because less time is required for one mutational event than for two.

The first mutation (M1) may be inherited as an autosomal-recessive trait or may occur postzygotically in somatic cells that form the retina. Any retinal cell harboring M1, whether through inheritance or via somatic mutation may acquire a mutation (M2) at the other allele. This doubly mutated cell can then form a malignancy due to complete loss of this genetic function.

The retinoblastoma gene is considered a model for a class of recessive human cancer genes that have a suppressor function. The loss or inactivation of both alleles of this gene appears to be a primary mechanism in the development of retinoblastoma. Such a mechanism is in direct contrast to that of the dominant human cancer genes which are actually activated by mutation. These genes require mutation at only one allele in order to be activated and lead to tumor formation. Dominant cancer genes cause tumors by providing an altered genetic function instead of experiencing loss of function as is the case with retinoblastoma. Genetic rearrangements can be identified by the use of restriction fragment length polymorphism (RFLP).

PROGNOSIS

Clinical prognosis may be based on tumor size and location. The following five groups indicate the prognosis for the amount of future vision and life outcome:

Group 1, very favorable:
- Single tumor smaller than 4 discs in diameter, at or behind the equator.
- Multiple tumors, none greater than 4 discs in diameter, at or behind the equator.

Group 2, favorable:
- Single tumor, 4 to 10 discs in diameter, on or behind the equator.
- Multiple tumors, 4 to 10 discs in diameter, on or behind the equator.

Group 3, uncertain:
- All lesions anterior to the equator.
- Single tumors larger than 10 discs in diameter situated behind the equator.

Group 4, unfavorable:
- Multiple tumors, some larger than 10 discs in diameter.
- All lesions extending anterior to the ora serrata.

Group 5, very unfavorable:
- Massive tumors involving more than half of the retina.
- Seeding into the vitreous.

CONCLUSION

Retinoblastoma is the most common potentially fatal, malignant ocular tumor of childhood. Prognosis depends on early diagnosis. A complete ophthalmologic examination of children suspected of having retinoblastoma and all children with family history of retinoblastoma is helpful. Prompt treatment according to the clinical, radiologic, and histopathologic features of the disease and regular follow-up examinations to rule out residual, recurrent, or distal metastasis are necessary.

REFERENCES

1. Abramson DH: Retinoma, retinocytoma, and retinoblastoma gene. Arch Ophthalmol 101: 517–1518, 1983
2. Abramson DH, Ellsworth RM, Zimmerman LE: Nonocular cancer in retinoblastoma survivors. Trans Am Acad Ophthalmol Otolaryngol 81:454–456, 1976

3. Abramson, DH, Ronner HJ, Ellsworth RM: Second tumors in nonirradiated bilateral retinoblastoma. Am J Ophthalmol 87:624–627, 1979

4. Balmer A, Gaillourd C: Retinoblastoma: Diagnosis and treatment. In Straub W (ed): Turning Points in Cataract Formation Syndrome and Retinoblastoma, pp 36–100. New York, S Karger, 1983

5. Benedict WF, Banerjee A, Spina CA, et al: Patient with 13 chromosome deletion: Evidence that the retinoblastoma gene is a recessive cancer gene. Science 219:973–975, 1983

6. Benson WE, Cameron JD, Furgiuele FP, et al: Presumed spontaneously regressed retinoblastoma. Ann Ophthalmol 10:897–899, 1978

7. Binder P: Unusual manifestations of retinoblastoma. Am J Ophthalmol 77:674–679, 1974

8. Cassady JR, Sagerman RH, Tretter P, et al: Radiation therapy in retinoblastoma. Radiology 93:405–409, 1969

9. Margo C, Hidayat A, Kopelman J, et al: Retinocytoma, a benign variant of retinoblastoma. Arch Ophthalmol 101:1519–1531, 1983

10. Dryja TP, Carence W, White R, et al: Homozygosity of chromosome 13 in retinoblastoma. N Engl J Med 310:550–553, 1984

11. Ellsworth RM: Treatment of retinoblastoma. Am J Ophthalmol 66:49–51, 1968

12. Ellsworth RM: The practical management of retinoblastoma. Trans Am Ophthalmol Soc 67:462–534, 1969

13. Falls HF: Inheritance of retinoblastoma. JAMA 133:171–174, 1947

14. Felberg NT, McFall R, Shields JA: Aqueous humor enzyme patterns in retinoblastoma. Invest Ophthalmol 16:1039–1046, 1977

15. Francois J, Matton MT, DeBie S, et al: Genesis and genetics of retinoblastoma. Ophthalmologica 170:405–425, 1975

16. Gallie BL, Ellsworth RM, Abramson DH, et al: Retinoma: Spontaneous regression of retinoblastoma or benign manifestation of the mutation? Br J Cancer 45:513–521, 1982

17. Gallie BL, Phillips RA: Retinoblastoma: A model of oncogenesis. Ophthalmology 91:666–672, 1984

18. Gallie BL, Phillips RA, Ellsworth RM, et al: Significance of retinoblastoma and phthisis bulbi for retinoblastoma. Ophthalmology 89:1393–1399, 1982

19. Godbout R, Dryja TP, Squire J, et al: Somatic inactivation of genes on chromosome 13 is a common event in retinoblastoma. Nature 304:451–453, 1983

20. Hopping W, Meyer-Schwickerath G: Light coagulation treatment in retinoblastoma. In Boniuk M (ed): Ocular and Adnexal Tumors: New and Controversial Aspects, pp. 192–200. St Louis, CV Mosby, 1964.

21. Kabak J, Romano PE: Aqueous humor lactic dehydrogenase isoenzymes in retinoblastoma. Br J Ophthalmol 59:268–269, 1975

22. Knudson AG Jr: Mutation and cancer: A statistical study of retinoblastoma. Proc Natl Acad Sci USA 68:820–823, 1971

23. Knudson AG, Meadows AT, Nichols WW, et al: Chromosome deletion and retinoblastoma. N Engl J Med 295:1120–1123, 1976

24. Lin CL, Tso MOM: An electron microscopic study of calcification of retinoblastoma. Am J Ophthalmol 96:765–774, 1983

25. Margo C, Hidayat A, Kopelman J, et al: Retinocytoma, a benign variant of retinoblastoma. Am J Ophthalmol 80:263–265, 1975

26. Mullaney J: Retinoblastomas with DNA precipitation. Arch Ophthalmol 82:454–456, 1969

27. Murphee AL, Benedict WF: Retinoblastoma: Clues to human oncogenesis. Science 223:1028–1033, 1984

28. Piro PA, Abramson DH, Ellsworth RM, et al: Aqueous humor lactate dehydrogenase in retinoblastoma patients. Arch Ophthalmol 96:1823–1825, 1978

29. Redler LD, Ellsworth RM: Prognostic importance of choroidal invasion in retinoblastoma. Arch Ophthalmol 90:294–296, 1973

30. Reese AB, Ellsworth RM: The evaluation and current concept of retinoblastoma therapy. Trans Am Acad Ophthalmol Otolaryngol 67:164–172, 1963

31. Rootman J, Ellsworth RM, Hofbauer J, et al: Orbital extension of retinoblastoma: A clinicopathological study. Can J Opthalmol 13:72–80, 1978

32. Rubin ML: Cryopexy treatment for retinoblastoma. Am J Ophthalmol 66:870–871, 1968

33. Rubin ML, Kaufman HE: Spontaneously regressed probable retinoblastoma. AJR 105:529–535, 1969

34. Sagerman RH, Cassady JR, Tretter P, et al: Radiation induced neoplasia following external beam therapy for children with retinoblastoma. Arch Ophthalmol 81:442–445, 1969

35. Shields JA: Current methods in the diagnosis of retinoblastoma. Contemp Ophthalmol 1(3):1–4, 1980

36. Shields JA: Current methods in the management of retinoblastoma. Contemp Ophthalmol 1(4):1–5, 1980

37. Shields JA: Diagnosis and Management of Intraocular Tumors, pp 437–533. St Louis, CV Mosby, 1983

38. Shields JA, Leonard BC, Michelson JB, et al: B-scan ultrasonography in the diagnosis of atypical retinoblastomas. Can J Ophthalmol 11:42–51, 1976

39. Shields JA, Lerner HA, Felberg NT: Aqueous cytology and enzymes in nematode endophthalmitis. Am J Ophthalmol 84:319–322, 1977

40. Sparkes RS, Murphree AL, Lingua RW, et al:

Gene for hereditary retinoblastoma assigned to human chromosome 13 by linkage to ES-D. Science 219:971–973, 1983

41. Sparkes RS, Sparkes MC, Wilson MG, et al: Regional assignment of genes for human esterase D and retinoblastoma to chromosome band 13q14. Science 208:1042–1044, 1980

42. Thompson RW, Small RC, Stein JJ: Treatment of retinoblastoma. AJR 114:16–23, 1972

43. Tolentino FI, Tablante RT: Cryotherapy of retinoblastoma. Arch Ophthalmol 87:52–55, 1972

44. Tso MOM, Fine BS, Zimmerman LE: The Flexner-Wintersteiner rosettes in retinoblastoma. Arch Pathol 88:665–671, 1969

45. Tso MOM, Fine BS, Zimmerman LE: The nature of retinoblastoma. II: Photoreceptor differentiation: An electron microscopic study. Am J Ophthalmol 69:350–359, 1970

46. Tso MOM, Fine BS, Zimmerman LE, Vogel MH: Photoreceptor elements in retinoblastoma: A preliminary report. Arch Ophthalmol 82:57–59, 1969

47. Tso MOM, Zimmerman LE, Fine BS: The nature of retinoblastoma. I: Photoreceptor differentiation: A clinical and histopathologic study. Am J Ophthalmol 69:339–349, 1970

48. Verhoeff FH: Retinoblastoma: Report of a case in a male age forty-eight. Arch Ophthalmol 2:643–650, 1929

49. Vogel F: Genetics of retinoblastoma. Hum Genet 52:1–54, 1979

50. Warburg M: Retinoblastoma. In Goldberg MF (ed): Genetic and Metabolic Eye Disease, pp 447–460. Boston, Little, Brown, 1974

51. Zimmerman LE: Trilateral retinoblastoma. In Blodi FC (ed): Contemporary Issues in Ophthalmology. vol II: Retinoblastoma. pp 185–210. New York, Churchill Livingstone, 1985

52. Zimmerman LE, Burns RP, Wankum G, et al: Trilateral retinoblastoma: Ectopic intracranial retinoblastoma associated with bilateral retinoblastoma. J Pediatr Ophthalmol Strab 19:310–315, 1982

Index